Sixth Edition

Spirituality in Nursing

STANDING ON HOLY GROUND

MARY ELIZABETH O'BRIEN, PhD, RN, MSW, MTS, FAAN

Professor Emeritus
School of Nursing
The Catholic University of America
Washington, DC

JONES & BARTLETT
LEARNING

World Headquarters
Jones & Bartlett Learning
5 Wall Street
Burlington, MA 01803
978-443-5000
info@jblearning.com
www.jblearning.com

Jones & Bartlett Learning books and products are available through most bookstores and online booksellers. To contact Jones & Bartlett Learning directly, call 800-832-0034, fax 978-443-8000, or visit our website, www.jblearning.com.

Substantial discounts on bulk quantities of Jones & Bartlett Learning publications are available to corporations, professional associations, and other qualified organizations. For details and specific discount information, contact the special sales department at Jones & Bartlett Learning via the above contact information or send an email to specialsales@jblearning.com.

Production Credits
VP, Executive Publisher: David D. Cella
Executive Editor: Amanda Martin
Associate Acquisitions Editor: Rebecca Stephenson
Editorial Assistant: Christina Freitas
Vendor Manager: Sara Kelly
Senior Marketing Manager: Jennifer Scherzay
Product Fulfillment Manager: Wendy Kilborn
Composition and Project Management: S4Carlisle Publishing
  Services

Cover Design: Kristin E. Parker
Rights & Media Specialist: Wes DeShano
Media Development Editor: Troy Liston
Cover Image: © Cyril Leclerc/EyeEm/Getty
Chapter opener image: © Herzlinde Vancura/Dreamstime.com
Printing and Binding: Edwards Brothers Malloy
Cover Printing: Edwards Brothers Malloy

Library of Congress Cataloging-in-Publication Data

Names: O'Brien, Mary Elizabeth, author.
Title: Spirituality in nursing : standing on holy ground / Mary Elizabeth
  O'Brien.
Description: Sixth edition. | Burlington, Massachusetts : Jones & Bartlett
  Learning, [2018] | Includes bibliographical references and index.
Identifiers: LCCN 2016047291 | ISBN 9781284121001
Subjects: | MESH: Spirituality | Nurse-Patient Relations | Religion and
  Medicine | Christianity | Nursing Care—ethics | Philosophy, Nursing
Classification: LCC RT85.2 | NLM WY 87 | DDC 610.7301—dc23 LC record available at https://lccn.loc.gov/2016047291

6048

Printed in the United States of America
21 20 19 18 17   10 9 8 7 6 5 4 3 2

Dedication

*This book is dedicated to the many patients,
family members, and caregivers, including
nurses, physicians, chaplains, firefighters,
and police officers, who so generously shared
their beliefs and experiences in the hope of
clarifying the importance of spirituality in
nursing. Some have crossed over to a new
life; others continue to live courageously,
finding meaning and hope in the experience
of illness or in ministering to those who
are ill. Their words, quoted extensively in
the following pages, are their legacy. I am
privileged to be the storyteller.*

God called to Moses out of the bush: "Remove the sandals from your feet, for the place on which you are standing is holy ground."

Exodus 3:4–5

The nurse's smile warmly embraces the cancer patient arriving for a chemotherapy treatment.
   This is holy ground.

The nurse watches solicitously over the pre-op child who tearfully whispers, "I'm scared."
   This is holy ground.

The nurse gently diffuses the anxieties of the ventilator-dependent patient in the ICU.
   This is holy ground.

The nurse tenderly takes the hand of the frail elder struggling to accept life in the nursing home.
   This is holy ground.

   The nurse
      reverently touches and is touched by
         the patient's heart,
            the dwelling place of the living God.

   This is spirituality in nursing,
      this is the ground of the practice of nursing,
         this is holy ground!

Contents

Preface

In this third millennium, our society is looking more and more to its spiritual traditions and philosophies for understanding, guidance, and comfort. This is witnessed by the fact that the concept of spirituality, encompassing numerous definitions, is being widely explored in such media as books, newsmagazines, websites, and television documentaries. The nursing community, also, has experienced a resurgence of interest in spirituality, especially in relation to the spiritual needs of those who are ill.

The purpose of this text is to explore the relationship between spirituality and the practice of nursing from a number of perspectives, including nursing assessment of patients' spiritual needs, the nurse's role in the provision of spiritual care, the spiritual nature of the nurse–patient relationship, the spiritual history of the nursing profession, and the contemporary interest in spirituality within the nursing profession. The work is undergirded by the author's research in spirituality and nursing over the past three decades. The text's subtitle and theme, *Standing on Holy Ground*, which describes the nurse's posture in providing spiritual care, was derived from nursing studies of the spiritual needs of chronically and acutely ill adults and children experiencing the sequelae of such conditions as cancer (including leukemia and lymphoma), cardiovascular disease, diabetes, depression, arthritis, Alzheimer's disease, chronic renal failure, and human immunodeficiency virus (HIV) infection and acquired immunodeficiency syndrome (AIDS). The research included both formal and informal interviewing and observing of patients at home as well as in hospital and long-term care settings. The spiritual needs of fragile patient populations—the poor, the elderly, and ventilator-dependent patients in the intensive care unit—were also explored. Data on the spiritual needs and concerns of patients' family members were obtained through interaction with significant others.

In order to expand the database of patient spiritual needs appropriate to nursing intervention, qualitative interviews were conducted with a cadre of contemporary nurses from a variety of clinical backgrounds, including medical–surgical nursing, perioperative nursing, critical care nursing, emergency nursing, community health nursing, psychiatric–mental health nursing, pediatric nursing, gerontological nursing, and parish nursing; the group included nurse clinicians, nurse educators, nurse administrators, and nurse researchers. In addition to providing data on patient spiritual needs, numerous reports of spiritual care provided by practicing nurses were documented. The data derived from patient, family, and nurse interviews are supplemented by materials excerpted from the author's journal maintained both during the research and while serving as a chaplain intern in a research-oriented medical center. Pseudonyms are used in all instances where naming of study respondents is warranted.

The text presents study findings and implications for care in chapters on nurse–patient interaction, the nurse's role in spiritual care, the spiritual needs of acute and chronically ill persons, the spiritual needs of ill children and the families of those who are ill, the spiritual needs of the frail older adult, spiritual needs in mass casualty disasters, the spirituality of parish nursing, spiritual needs at the end of life, spiritual needs in death and bereavement, the spirituality of servant leadership in nursing, the importance of prayer in nursing, and the spirituality of nurses' caring behaviors.

In this sixth edition of *Spirituality in Nursing: Standing on Holy Ground*, a new chapter has been added. Chapter 18 presents a lived experience of the spirituality of caring employing the ministry of Catherine of Siena, patroness of nursing, as exemplar. In this chapter, Catherine's tender compassion for the ill and infirm is documented through numerous case study examples of her care for the poor and the marginalized, especially those suffering from such diseases as leprosy and the plague. The relevance of Catherine's nursing ministry for contemporary caregivers is explained.

Chapter 1, "Spirituality In Nursing," includes a new discussion of "Nursing as a Vocation: The Call to Serve," and in Chapter 2, "The Spiritual History of Nursing," both Old and New Testament Biblical roots of nursing are now explored, as well as the role of Jesus, as healer; also described are additional nursing role models in terms of both individuals and nursing communities. These include Florence Nightingale, Catherine of Siena, Patroness of Nursing, Veronica of Jerusalem, the Alexian Brothers Nursing Community, and Mary Breckinridge and the Frontier Nursing Service, among others. The chapter is grounded in the nursing and theological literature, documenting the historical role of the nurse in the provision of spiritual care.

Chapter 3, "Nursing Assessment of Spiritual Needs," contains a Spiritual Assessment Scale with established validity and reliability, which can be used by nurses in both practice and research. Also included is identification of nursing diagnoses related to alterations in spiritual integrity. Chapter 3 also contains a subsection discussing the impact of contemporary Health Insurance Portability and Accountability Act (HIPAA) regulations on patients' spiritual and pastoral needs.

In Chapter 4 there is a discussion of the construction of spirituality in nursing theory as well as commentary on the contemporary relevance of nursing theory in practice, research, and education and, in Chapter 6 myriad new literature citations document the value of the nurse's role in spiritual care as well as placing emphasis on this role in undergraduate nursing education. Chapter 8 provides new information on the spiritual needs of the mentally challenged person. Chapter 10 incorporates information describing the long-term care setting of the continuing care retirement community (CCRC), as well as the spiritual needs of CCRC residents. In Chapter 13, "Parish/Faith Community Nursing" a discussion of the recent title change (for some practitioners) from "parish nursing" to "faith community nursing" is explained. Chapter 13 contains information on the latest edition (2012, second edition) of the *Scope and Standards of Faith Community Nursing*, published by the American Nurses Association (ANA) in collaboration with the Health Ministries Association (HMA). Also included are criteria for certification in "Faith Community Nursing" as identified by the ANA and HMA (2014).

Chapter 14 contains descriptions of recent research on the spiritual needs of post-9/11 survivors and witnesses. A new section on spirituality and international terrorism has been added focusing on three recent events: the Boston Marathon Bombings, the Paris Terrorist Attacks, and the Brussels Multisite Explosions. Chapter 15 includes current nursing research on the concept of servant leadership in nursing and health care. Chapter 16 explores the concept of prayer in nursing. Prayer is described as the catalyst for contemplative nursing; among the topics included are a history of prayer in nursing, finding time for prayer in nursing, and the ethics of praying with patients. Chapter 17 presents a newly developed "Sacred Covenant Model of Caring for Nursing Practice"; the spirituality of caring is explored both broadly and in terms of theory development for nursing practice.

New material and references have been added in all chapters in order to update the concepts in terms of current thinking on spirituality in nursing. Each chapter opens with a quote from a contemporary practicing nurse expressing his or her perceptions and/or experiences related to the spirituality of the nursing profession and the chapter topic.

It is understood that a text dealing with spiritual issues must, to a large degree, be influenced by the personal spiritual and religious élan of the writer. Thus, it is important to acknowledge that the author's Christian philosophy of life inspired, guided, and supported the writing of *Spirituality in Nursing*. Although an effort has been made to include examples of patient spiritual needs, supported by both data and literature, relative to other religious affiliations, the overall orientation of the work is derived primarily from the Judeo-Christian tradition. It is believed, nonetheless, that nurse readers whose spirituality is guided by another religious ethic will find meaning and inspiration in the poignant nursing examples of spiritual care and compassion as well as in the case examples of patients' spiritual needs.

Acknowledgments

The author's loving thanks is extended to the many patients and caregivers, both professional and family, who graciously and generously shared their thoughts and experiences, included in the text, in the hope of helping others who may one day tread a similar path.

Much appreciation must also be expressed to the editorial and production staff of Jones & Bartlett Learning, who have continued to support the work of preparing the revised and updated editions of *Spirituality in Nursing: Standing on Holy Ground.*

And, finally, my deepest and most abiding gratitude is to God, the source of my strength and the center of my life; to the Father who provides me with the courage and energy to write, to His Divine Son, Jesus Christ, whose care for the ill and infirm provides the model for ministry to the sick and to the Holy Spirit, without whose inspiration and guidance these pages would never have been completed.

Text Credits

The Scripture quotations contained herein are from *The New Revised Standard Version Bible: Catholic Edition*, copyright © 1993 and 1989 by the Division of Christian Education of the National Council of the Churches of Christ in the U.S.A. Used by permission. All rights reserved.

Chapter 2 contains material from pages 32, 33–34, 52–54; and nursing quotes at the beginning of all chapters are taken from pages 102–103, 143, 148, 159, 162–163, 201, 205, 224–225, 237, 242, 253, 263, 278, 299, 302–303, and 308 of *Servant Leadership in Nursing: Spirituality and Practice in Contemporary Health Care*. Burlington, MA: Jones & Bartlett Learning, 2011. Used with permission of the publisher.

Chapter 3, pages 66–67; Chapter 6, page 128; and Chapter 7, page 155, quotes from M. E. O'Brien (1982), The need for spiritual integrity. In H. Yura and M. Walsh (Eds.), *Human needs and the nursing process*, vol. 2. Norwalk, CT: Appleton-Century-Crofts. Used with permission of the editors.

One section of Chapter 3, "Nursing Assessment of Spiritual Needs," describing the patient spiritual assessment and care mandated by The Joint Commission, has been reprinted from *A Nurse's Handbook of Spiritual Care: Standing on Holy Ground*, p. 15, Jones & Bartlett Learning, 2004, used with permission of the publisher.

Major sections of Chapter 4, "A Middle-Range Theory of Spiritual Well-Being in Illness," have been taken from Chapter 5, "Conceptual Models of Parish Nursing Practice: A Middle-Range Theory of Spiritual Well-Being in Illness," in *Parish Nursing: Healthcare Ministry Within the Church*, Jones & Bartlett Learning, 2003, used with permission of the publisher.

Major sections of Chapter 15, "The Spirituality of Servant Leadership in Nursing," have been taken from Chapters 1, 4, 5, and 8 in *Servant Leadership in Nursing: Spirituality and Practice in Contemporary Health Care*. Jones & Bartlett Learning, 2011. Used with permission of the publisher.

Major sections of Chapter 16, "Prayer in Nursing," were taken from portions of Chapters 1, 3, 4, and 5 in *Prayer in Nursing: The Spirituality of Compassionate Caregiving*, Jones & Bartlett Learning, 2003, as well as one passage in Chapter 17, "The Spirituality of Caring," taken from pp. 83–84, in *Prayer in Nursing: The Spirituality of Compassionate Caregiving*. Used with permission of the publisher.

Major sections of Chapter 18, "A Lived Experience of Caring in Nursing Practice: The Ministry of Catherine of Siena" have been taken from pages 162–188 in *Catherine of Siena: A Sacred Covenant of Caring for the Sick*, New Priory Press, 2015. Used with permission of the publisher.

▶ Other Jones & Bartlett Learning titles By Mary Elizabeth O'Brien

A Nurse's Handbook of Spiritual Care: Standing on Holy Ground

Parish Nursing: Healthcare Ministry within the Church

Prayer in Nursing: The Spirituality of Compassionate Caregiving

A Sacred Covenant: The Spiritual Ministry of Nursing

Servant Leadership in Nursing: Spirituality and Practice in Contemporary
  Health Care

CHAPTER 1

Spirituality in Nursing: Standing on Holy Ground

God called to Moses out of the bush: "Moses, Moses!" And he said, "Here I am." "Come no closer," God said. "Remove the sandals from your feet, for the place on which you are standing is holy ground."

Exodus 3:4–5

> Nursing is really about being intuitive and spiritual. . . . When you see nursing as a calling, you go to this higher level which is the vocation level, which has a spiritual dimension to the profession. . . . I think that whenever there is another human being involved, you see yourself as in a vocation, you really understand . . . "I can make it better. That is the ministry way of looking at nursing; that is the spiritual way of looking at it.

Anne, Supervisor of a Critical Care Unit

Perhaps no scriptural theme so well models the spiritual posture of nursing practice as the Old Testament depiction of Moses and the burning bush. In the biblical narrative, God reminded Moses that, when he stood before his Lord, the ground beneath his feet was holy. When the nurse clinician, nurse educator, nurse administrator, or nurse researcher stands before a patient, a student, a staff member, or a study participant, God is also present, and the ground on which the nurse is standing is holy. For it is here, in the act of serving a brother or sister in need, that the nurse truly encounters God. God is present in the nurse's practice of caring just as surely as He was present in the blessed meeting with Moses so many centuries ago. In an editorial in the *Journal of Christian Nursing*, Judy Shelly (2003) reminded us that "the holy ground we as nurses are called to enter may be . . . difficult . . . we face pain, suffering, fear, communication barriers, cultural and ethnic prejudice, injustice, impossible working conditions and constant obstacles" (p. 3). However, Shelly added, although we may at times "feel inadequate and defeated . . . God is with us. He offers us his peace" (p. 3). This, I believe, is the gift and the grace of our nursing vocation of "standing on holy ground." This is the blessing; the precious knowledge that, however great or small our nursing task may be, God is with us and will give us His peace.

This introductory chapter addresses the nurse's spiritual posture, "standing on holy ground," while also offering a historical perspective on the spiritual ministry of nursing. The overall relationship between spirituality and nursing practice is explored; the concepts of spirituality—as distinguished from religiosity or religious practice—and nursing are defined with a view to understanding their meaning for the contemporary nurse. Nursing practice is examined in relation to the nurse's spiritual stance in caring for patients, the nurse's participation in the provision of holistic care, and the nurse's role as healer. Finally, a practice model, labeled a "Nursing Theology of Caring," is described.

The empirical data on the spiritual concerns and needs of the ill in the present chapter, as well as those in the following chapters, are derived from nursing research with persons suffering from a multiplicity of illness conditions in a variety of settings. The author conducted both formal and informal interviewing and observation with these patients, their family members, and their nurse caregivers. The interview and observational data are supplemented by materials excerpted from journals maintained during the conduct of the research and also during a hospital chaplaincy experience.

▶ The Spiritual Ministry of Nursing: A Historical Perspective

In a small but classic volume, *The Nurse: Handmaid of the Divine Physician*, written in the early 1940s, Franciscan Sister Mary Berenice Beck articulated what a great number of nurses of her era, especially those of the Judeo-Christian tradition, understood as the spirituality of their practice. Historically, nursing was viewed in large part as a vocation of service, incorporating a clearly accepted element of ministry to those for whom the nurse cared. A nurse's mission was considered to be driven by altruism and empathy for the sick, especially the sick poor. The practicing nurse of the early and middle 20th century did not expect much in terms of worldly rewards for her efforts. She envisioned her caregiving as commissioned and supported by God; to Him alone were the thanks and the glory to be given. This vision of nursing as a spiritual ministry is reflected in Sr. Mary Berenice's nurse's prayer:

> I am Thine Own, great Healer, help Thou me to serve Thy sick in humble charity;
>
> I ask not thanks nor praise, but only light to care for them in every way aright.
>
> My charges, sick and well, they all are Thine. (Beck, 1945, p. xvii)

Other nursing authors of the time also supported the concept of nursing as a calling, with a decidedly spiritual element undergirding its practice. As nurse historian Minnie Goodnow (1916) asserted, "Nursing is not merely an occupation, temporary and superficial in scope; it is a great vocation" (p. 17). She added, "It [nursing] is so well known to be difficult that it is seldom undertaken by a woman who has not, in the depths of her consciousness, an earnest purpose to serve humanity" (p. 17). And, in the introduction to an early fundamentals of nursing textbook, *The Art, Science and Spirit of Nursing* (1954), author Alice Price observed, "Nursing is possessed of a spiritual quality, in that its primary aim is to serve humanity, not only by giving curative care to the bodies of the sick and injured, but by serving the needs of the mind and spirit as well" (p. 3). For the Christian nurse, the frequently quoted scriptural text supporting practice was that of Matthew 25:35–40, "For I was . . . sick and you took care of me. . . . I tell you, just as you did it to one of the least of these . . . you did for me."

A condition that kept the original spiritual ministry of nursing alive in this country was the fact that many early to mid-20th century nurses received their education in nursing schools affiliated with one of the predominant religious denominations. Prior to the development of contemporary undergraduate and graduate programs in nursing, the three-year diploma schools that were the norm were generally not associated with academic institutions. Rather they were sponsored by individual hospitals, many of which were religiously affiliated. These schools tended to be small and insular in character, taking on the spiritual élan of the hospital with which they were connected. This was evident in the rituals of passage such as "capping" and graduation that were often conducted in places of worship with the blessing of a cleric included as part of the ceremony.

In the latter half of the 20th century, however, although some U.S. nursing schools did retain a strong spiritual milieu as a characteristic feature, many of the newer university and college-affiliated programs began to focus on the professional character of nursing. Nursing publications and conferences described the characteristics of a profession, and much debate centered around how nursing incorporated specified professional criteria, particularly the criterion of autonomy of practice. These discussions were appropriate, as advanced health-care technology and burgeoning knowledge generated by the behavioral sciences resulted in the practicing nurse requiring and receiving ever more sophisticated education related to patient care. For a time, at least, the proverbial pendulum appeared to swing toward the science, rather than the art, of nursing. This represented a concerted effort to bring nursing practice up to standard alongside medical practice and that of other caregiving professions.

During the 1970s and 1980s, however, despite the fact that curricula in baccalaureate and newly emerging master's and doctoral programs in nursing were becoming increasingly more complex in terms of the biologic and behavioral sciences, many were beginning to acknowledge the need for holistic health care. With the advent of the concept of holism, came a reawakening of the importance of the ill person's spiritual nature and a heightened concern for spiritual needs. In identifying a model for holistic nursing, nurse clinician and researcher Cathie Guzzetta (1988) described holistic concepts as incorporating "a sensitive balance between art and science, analytic and intuitive skills, and the ability and knowledge to choose from a wide variety of treatment modalities to promote balance and interconnectedness of body, mind and spirit" (p. 117). Thus, in the holistic nursing model, patients' spiritual nature and needs are brought into equal focus with their cognitive and physiologic needs.

Nursing literature, both professional and lay, now began to address the spiritual component of the human person. Books and articles abounded relating to such topics as prayer, spiritual counseling, "near-death" experiences, interactions with angels, and volunteer activities undertaken for spiritual motives. Many individuals in our society were seeking to find transcendent meaning in their lives. It was not surprising, then, that nurses, now more solidly entrenched in their professional identities, should follow suit. As theorist Barbara Barnum (1994) pointed out, whereas nursing's focus in the past was on the "biopsychosocial" model of care, more recently nurse scholars have demonstrated a renewed interest in the spiritual dimension of caregiving (p. 114). Barnum's assertion was reflected in an increase in the nursing literature in conceptual and research-based articles related to the association between spirituality and health/illness. One example was the work of Jean Watson (1995) who observed, "At its most basic level nursing is a human-caring, relational profession. It exists by virtue of an ethical-moral ideal, and commitment to provide care for others" (p. 67). Watson's comment reflected a newer understanding of the spiritual ministry of nursing practice.

▶ Spirituality and Nursing Practice

In order to provide some basis for beginning a discussion of spirituality and contemporary nursing practice, there must be a common understanding of the concepts of spirituality and nursing. Spirituality, as a personal concept, is generally understood in terms of an individual's attitudes and beliefs related to transcendence (God) or to the nonmaterial forces of life and of nature. Religious practice or religiosity, however, relates to a person's beliefs and behaviors associated with a specific religious tradition or denomination. Nurses need to have a clear understanding of this distinction or they may neglect spiritual needs in focusing only on a patient's religious practice (Emblen, 1992, p. 41).

The latter point is strongly supported by nurse practitioner Patricia Alpert (2010) in the article "Spirituality Goes beyond Religiosity: A Much Needed Practice in Nursing." In the article Alpert asserts, as noted previously, that "religion and spirituality are not synonymous" and points out that religiosity may only be "a partial expression of one's spirituality" and that "in health care, spiritual care may be viewed as religious care" (p. 140). Alpert defines *spiritual care* as "any act that nourishes the soul or spirit" (p. 141) and describes spiritual care as "fundamental to nursing practice" (p. 141).

Reinert and Koenig (2013) propose "defining spirituality in the context of religious involvement when conducting research, while using a broader definition of spirituality when providing spiritual care" (p. 2622). As noted by scholar Barbara Pesut (2013), spirituality, as well as religion "will likely continue to play an enduring role in providing fundamental meaning for nursing work" (p. 5).

Spirituality

Spirituality, as related to holistic nursing, has been described by Dossey (1989) as "a broad concept that encompasses values, meaning, and purpose; one turns inward to the human traits of honesty, love, caring, wisdom, imagination, and compassion; existence of a quality of a higher authority, guiding spirit or transcendence that is mystical; a flowing, dynamic balance that allows and creates healing of body-mind-spirit; and may or may not involve organized religion" (p. 24). Pamela Reed (1992) presented a paradigm with which to explore spirituality in nursing by defining *spirituality* as "an expression of the developmental capacity for self-transcendence" (p. 350). Nurse anthropologist Madeleine Leininger (1997, p. 104) identified spirituality as a relationship with a supreme being that directs one's beliefs and practices.

Spirituality viewed as a human need has been described as "that dimension of a person that is concerned with ultimate ends and values. . . . Spirituality is that which inspires in one the desire to transcend the realm of the material"

(O'Brien, 1982, p. 88). For many individuals, especially those adhering to the Western religious traditions of Judaism, Christianity, and Islam, the concept of transcendence incorporates belief in God. This is reflected explicitly in the conceptualization of spirituality articulated by nurse Ruth Stoll (1989) who asserted, "Through my spirituality I give and receive love; I respond to and appreciate God, other people, a sunset, a symphony and spring" (p. 6). Prayers as indicating a meaning in life have been identified as indications of spirituality (Meraviglia, 1999); spirituality may thrive, however, outside the sphere of organized religion (Kendrick & Robinson, 2000).

Three characteristics of spirituality posited by Margaret Burkhardt (1989) include "unfolding mystery," related to one's attempt to understand the meaning and purpose of life; "harmonious interconnectedness," or an individual's relationship to other persons and/or to God; and "inner strength," which relates to one's personal spiritual resources and "sense of the sacred" (p. 72). Spirituality was proposed as a "cornerstone" of holistic nursing by Nagai-Jacobson and Burkhardt (1989) who suggested that questions appropriate to exploring a patient's spirituality might include how the individual understands God and what things give meaning and joy to life (p. 23). Each nurse needs to understand his or her own spirituality, keeping in mind that this personal belief system may differ significantly from that of a patient and family.

The nursing literature offers no one clear definition of *spirituality*. As pointed out by Verna Benner Carson in the *Journal of Christian Nursing* (1993), "Definitions of spirituality represent a variety of worldviews and the opinions of people from divergent walks of life" (p. 25). Common to most descriptions of spirituality, as reflected in the early and later nursing literature, are the elements of love; compassion; caring; transcendence; relationship with God; and the connection of body, mind, and spirit.

Nurse educator Janice Clarke presents a critical view of nursing's definition of *spirituality* by suggesting that theology may provide needed insight into the concept. Clarke (2009) concludes that the broad explanations of spirituality existing in some of the nursing literature has led to "definitions which have the tendency to result in a type of spiritual care which is indistinguishable for psychosocial care, hard to explain to patients and difficult to put into practice" (p. 1666).

In an article on the "range and diversity of definitions" of spirituality within the nursing literature, however, Swinton and Pattison (2010) argue that "It is in fact the vagueness of the concept that is its strength and value" (p. 226). These authors feel that a "thin" definition of spirituality will increase the usefulness of the concept in practical situations (p. 232). Other authors agree that the concept of spirituality in nursing is appropriately "open to interpretation" (Noble & Jones, 2010, p. 565); that "the concept (of spirituality in nursing) and its application have been the subject of much debate" (Pike, 2011, p. 743); and that "spirituality in nursing is a subject that is not easily defined, interpreted or understood" (Ellis & Narayanasamy, 2009, p. 886).

This diversity in the definitions of spirituality in nursing literature, accepted by Swinton and Pattison, is also supported by Bruce, Shields, and Molzahn in the paper "Language and the (Im)possibilities of Articulating Spirituality" (2011). The authors assert that incompleteness or differences in definitions of spirituality are "perhaps necessary and to be welcomed" (p. 44). They conclude that "lack of agreement [of definitions of *spirituality*] may suggest a way to protect profound human experiences" from being too cavalierly dismissed and/or the differences in definition may simply reflect "the impossibility of solidifying in language what is too fluid and experiential" (p. 50).

Ultimately the meaning of spirtualty in nursing practice will be guided by the spirituality and spiritual attitudes of those providing care; attitudes and behaviors such as presence and patient centeredness (Ramezani, Ahmadi, Mohammadi, & Kazemnejad, 2014, p. 11); kindness, compassion, and tenderness (Meehan, 2012, p. 990); and empathy and humility (Narayanasamy, 2015, p. 246).

Nursing

Writing in the early 1950s, Alice Price (1954), offered a definition of *nursing* that incorporated not only the concept of the patient's spiritual nature, but the altruistic vocation of the nurse as well. She described nursing as neither pure science nor true art, but as a combination of both. "Nursing, as a profession, will embrace more than an art and a science; it will be a blending of three factors: of art and science, and the spirit of unselfish devotion to a cause primarily concerned with helping those who are physically, mentally or spiritually ill" (p. 2). Price ultimately defined *nursing* as "a service to the individual which helps him to regain, or to keep, a normal state of body and mind; when it cannot accomplish this, it helps him gain relief from physical pain, mental anxiety or spiritual discomfort" (p. 3). Although Price was writing some 25 to 30 years prior to the widespread acceptance of the term *holistic nursing*, her vision of the professional nurse's role clearly included attention to the needs of a patient's spirit, as well as to the needs of the body and the mind.

In their book *Introduction to Nursing*, written 40 years after publication of Price's 1954 text, coauthors Lindberg, Hunter, and Kruszewski (1994) argued that, because of the continual growth and development of the profession, no single definition of nursing can be accepted (p. 7). The authors presented excerpts of nursing definitions articulated by a cadre of theorists from Florence Nightingale in 1859 to Martha Rogers in 1970 but, ultimately, suggested that each practicing nurse develop a definition of his or her own. Lindberg and colleagues did, however, express the hope that, whatever one's definition, it will contain an emphasis on caring or nurturing as a motivating factor for choosing nursing (p. 7).

Following the suggestions of Price in 1954 and Lindberg, Hunter, and Kruszewski in 1994, a potential working definition of nursing follows:

> Nursing is a sacred ministry of health care or health promotion provided to persons both sick and well, who require caregiving, support, or education to assist them in achieving, regaining, or maintaining a state of wholeness, including wellness of body, mind, and spirit. The nurse also serves those in need of comfort and care to strengthen them in coping with the trajectory of a chronic or terminal illness, or with experiencing the dying process.

The spiritual dimensions of the definition relate to two concepts: first, the sacred ministry of caring on the part of the nurse; and second, the ultimate goal of the patient's achievement of a state of wholeness, including the wellness of body, mind, and spirit. These concepts are next explored in terms of the nurse's spiritual posture, the patient's spiritual wholeness, and the nurse–patient spiritual interaction.

Later nursing authors also focused on the importance of spirituality in nursing. Some examples included a discussion of spirituality as a key concept in the nursing models of Betty Neuman, Margaret Newman, Rosemary Parse, and Jean Watson (Young & Koopsen, 2011, p. 7); a critique of nursing's definitions of spirituality (Clarke, 2009); an analysis of the current debate about spirituality in nursing

(Gray, 2009); identification of philosophical approaches to the study of spirituality in nursing (Tinley & Kinney, 2007); and literature reviews on spirituality and nursing and health outcomes (Como, 2007; Pesut, 2008).

▶ The Nurse's Spiritual Posture: Standing on Holy Ground

Spiritual writer Sister Macrina Wiederkehr (1991) advised, "If you should ever hear God speaking to you from a burning bush, and it happens more often than most of us realize, take off your shoes for the ground on which you stand is holy" (p. 2). How appropriate, it seems, to envision practicing nurses, who must come together with their patients in caring and compassion, as standing on holy ground. God frequently speaks to us from a "burning bush," in the fretful whimper of a feverish child, in the anxious questions of a preoperative surgical patient, and in the frail moans of a fragile elder. If we "take off our shoes," we will be able to realize that the place where we stand is holy ground; we will respond to our patients as we would wish to respond to God in the burning bush.

But what does it really mean to "take off one's shoes"? Sister Macrina asserted that it means stripping away "whatever prevents us from experiencing the holy" (1991, p. 3). She added that God speaks to us in many "burning bushes of today" and that "the message is still one of holy ground"; it is a message that is often missed "because of [our] unnecessary shoes" (p. 3). In the contemporary conduct of nursing practice, nursing education, nursing administration, and nursing research, some of us may admit to having a number of unnecessary pairs of shoes littering our professional closets. First, there are running shoes, which many of us wear as we rush pell-mell from task to task in order to manage the day. As we fly about, feet barely touching the ground, it is easy to forget, in the busyness, that where we are standing is a holy place. Another often relied on pair of shoes are sturdy walking brogues, which provide protection against unwanted intrusions. Unfortunately, their insulated soles, which keep us safe and secure, may also prevent our feet from feeling the holy ground on which we walk. And then there are old, favorite loafers, well-worn and cozy. When we are wearing these shoes, we can so rest in their comfort that we need not be troubled by any disturbing bumps in the holy ground. We nurses probably have, I am sure, many more unnecessary pairs of shoes that prevent our feet from experiencing holy ground. But recollections of times past when, literally or figuratively, we have been able to take off our shoes, even if only briefly, well validate the Old Testament message.

▶ Holistic Nursing: The Body, Mind, and Spirit Connection

At times we hear an individual described as being truly healthy. The assumption underlying such a remark may relate not so much to the physical health or well-being of the person as to the fact that he or she is perceived as solidly grounded spiritually. One can be possessed of a healthy attitude toward life, even if suffering from a terminal illness. In order to achieve such a spiritual grounding in the face of physical or psychological deficit, the individual must be closely attuned to the body, mind, and spirit connection; one must understand and accept the value of the spiritual dimension in the overall paradigm of holistic health.

As our society advanced scientifically during the past half century, it became increasingly more difficult for some in the health-care community to give credence to the importance of the spiritual nature of the human person, especially in relation to health/illness issues. Ultimately, however, caregivers began recognizing that sensitivity to a patient's spiritual needs was critical if they were to provide truly "holistic" health care. Nurse and minister Ann Robinson (1995) believed that nurses must "embrace the spirituality of the human community" in order to support their patients' holistic health behaviors (p. 3).

Authors Dossey and Keegan (1989) defined the concept of holism, which undergirds holistic health and holistic nursing care, including the body, mind, and spirit connection, as "the view that an integrated whole has a reality independent of and greater than the sum of its parts" (p. 4). They described holism as consisting of a philosophy of positive, interactionally based attitudes and behaviors that can exist not only in one who is well but also in one who is seriously or terminally ill (p. 5). Nurses practicing care supportive of such holism need to envision the spiritual needs of a patient as deserving of attention equal to that provided in response to physical and psychosocial concerns.

Overall, holistic nursing is supported by and alternately supports the intimate connection of body, mind, and spirit. Nursing of the whole person requires attention to the individuality and uniqueness of each dimension, as well as to the interrelatedness of the three. In *The Wholeness Handbook*, Emeth and Greenhut (1991) described the body, mind, and spirit elements: The body is the physical substance of a person that can be perceived in empirical reality; the mind is that dimension of an individual that conceptualizes; and the spirit is the life principle that is shared with all humanity and with God. "It is the dimension of personhood that drives us to create, love, question, contemplate and transcend" (pp. 27–28). Those practicing holistic nursing today truly "appreciate the need to integrate the body, mind and spirit within the delivery of health care" (Boswell, Cannon, & Miller, 2013, p. 329).

For the nurse seeking to provide holistic health care, then, the spiritual dimension and needs of the person must be carefully assessed and considered in all therapeutic planning. Spiritual care cannot be separated from physical, social, and psychological care (Lo & Brown, 1999; O'Connor, 2001). Often it is uniquely the nurse, standing either literally or figuratively at the bedside, who has the opportunity and the entreé to interact with patients on that spiritual level where they strive to create, love, question, contemplate, and transcend. Here, truly, the nurse is standing on holy ground.

▶ The Nurse as Healer

The nurse, standing as he or she does on the holy ground of caring for the sick, is well situated to be the instrument of God's healing. In the sacred interaction between nurse and patient, the spiritual healing dimension of holistic health care is exemplified and refined. The nurse stands as God's surrogate and as a vehicle for His words and His touch of compassionate care.

Healing has been described variously as facilitating openness to the "communication of the Holy Spirit, whose message is always wholeness" (Johnson, 1992, p. 21); "the process or act of curing or restoring to health or wholeness, the body, the mind and the spirit" (Haggard, 1983, p. 235); and "to make whole" (Burke, 1993, p. 37). The concept of the nurse as healer incorporates the characteristics of all three definitions; that is, the nurse healer must listen to the voice of God; desire to restore health either of body or of spirit; and attempt to assist the patient in achieving wholeness and integrity of body, mind, and spirit. For the nurse of the Judeo-Christian tradition, spiritually oriented scriptural models of healing abound in both the Old and the New Testaments.

Yahweh's healing power is reflected in Old Testament Scripture in such narratives as Elijah's healing of the widow's son (1 Kings 17:17–23) and Elisha's cleansing of Naaman's leprosy (2 Kings 5:1–14). In the New Testament account of the ministry of Jesus, 41 healings are identified (Kelsey, 1988, p. 43). Jesus healed by word and by touch, sometimes even using physical materials such as mud and saliva. Always, Jesus' healings were accompanied by love and compassion for the ill persons or their families, as in the case of Jairus' young daughter, who her parents thought to be dead. Jesus comforted Jairus with the words, "The child is not dead but sleeping" (Mark 5:39). And then, "He took her by the hand and said to her, 'Talitha cum,' which means 'Little girl, get up!' And immediately the girl got up and began to walk about" (Mark 5:41).

In her doctoral dissertation entitled "Biblical Roots of Healing in Nursing," Maria Homberg (1980) posited that an established biblical tradition reflecting the healing power of such concepts as respect for human dignity and positive interpersonal relationships has parallels in contemporary nursing (p. 2). Homberg suggested that the biblical history of healing can be used by nurse educators to support the importance of these concepts. Dossey (1988) identified the characteristics of a nurse healer as having an awareness that "being present" to the patient is as essential as technical skills, respecting and loving all clients regardless of background or personal characteristics, listening actively, being nonjudgmental, and viewing time with clients as times of sharing and serving (p. 42). These characteristics reflect the spiritual nature of healing described in the Old and the New Testament Scriptures. Finally, nurse educator Brenda Lohri-Posey (2005) says that to become a "compassionate healer" a nurse must "recognize the ability to be a healer" and understand that "healing occasions are unique for each patient" and that "the healing occasion" may change a nurse's "beliefs about pain and suffering" (p. 37).

The Nurse as Wounded Healer

When a nurse is described as a healer, one tends to focus on his or her ability to relieve suffering. The label "healer" evokes the concept of a strong and gifted individual whose ministry is directed by care and compassion; this is an appropriate image. What may be forgotten in such a description is the fact that sometimes the gift of healing has emerged from, and indeed has been honed by, the healer's own experiences of suffering and pain. In exploring the nurse's healing role as an "anonymous minister," a gerontologic nurse practitioner, Sharon, describes using her own pain in counseling patients: "I may not talk about my pain . . . [but] I understand where they're coming from if they're hurting." Sharon, who imagined this experience as being "united in suffering" with those she cared for, reflected Henri Nouwen's (1979) classic conceptualization of the wounded healer. Nouwen described the wounded healer as one who must look after personal wounds while at the same time having the ability to heal others. The wounded healer concept is derived from a Talmudic identification of the awaited Messiah:

> He is sitting among the poor covered with wounds. The others unbind all their wounds at the same time and bind them up again, but he unbinds one at a time and binds it up again, saying to himself: "Perhaps I shall be needed; if so, I must always be ready so as not to delay for a moment." (Tractate Sandhedren, as cited in Nouwen, 1979, p. 82)

The nurse, as any person who undertakes ministry, brings into the interaction personal and unique wounds. Rather than hindering the therapeutic process, the caregiver's wounds, when not unbound all at once, can become a source of strength, understanding, and empathy when addressing the suffering of others. The nurse as a wounded healer caring for a wounded patient can relate his or her own painful experiences to those of the ill person, thus providing a common ground of experience on which to base the initiation of spiritual care.

Two discussions that validate the meaning and importance of the "wounded healer" concept in nursing and health care are those presented by Niven on the meaning of the wounded healer concept for nurses (2008) and teaching the concept of the wounded healer Graves (2008).

▶ A Nursing Theology of Caring

In the previous pages the nurse is described as having the opportunity to heal and to facilitate wholeness, and in the process, to be in the posture of standing on holy ground. But what is it that initiates and supports such nursing practice? What theological or spiritual understanding and beliefs guide the nursing activities of contemporary practitioners? Perhaps these questions can best be answered in the exploration of a nursing theology of caring. The theology of caring encompasses the concepts of being, listening, and touching and was derived from the author's clinical practice with a variety of acutely and chronically ill patients. The nursing theology of caring is supported by the Christian parable of the Good Samaritan:

> A man was going down from Jerusalem to Jericho, and fell into the hands of robbers who stripped him, beat him and went away leaving him half dead. . . . But a Samaritan, while traveling . . . saw him and was moved to pity. He went to him and bandaged his wounds, having poured oil and wine on them. Then he put him on his own animal, brought him to an Inn, and took care of him. (Luke 10:30, 33–34)

The Gospel relates Jesus' parable of the Good Samaritan, told in response to a question posed by a scholar of the law who asked, "Teacher," he said, "what must I do to inherit eternal life?" (Luke 10:25). Jesus said to him, "What is written in the Law?" In response to Jesus' question, the scholar replied, "You shall love the Lord your God with all your heart . . . and your neighbor as yourself" (Luke 10:27). To justify himself, however, the scholar added, "And who is my neighbor?" (Luke 10:29). Jesus related the parable of the Good Samaritan in reply. At the conclusion of the parable, Jesus asked the scholar, of all those who had seen the beaten man, which one was truly a neighbor. The scholar replied, "The one who showed him mercy." Jesus said to him, "Go and do likewise" (Luke 10:36–37).

In a commentary on the parable of the Good Samaritan, Kodell (1989) noted that Jesus' story was intended to challenge a prevailing but discriminating attitude in the society of the time—the fact that a Samaritan, a member of an ethnic group despised by some, could behave so lovingly. The parable, Kodell pointed out, exemplified the love commandment: while the lawyer suggests that not all persons are his neighbors, Jesus' reply indicates that one must consider everyone a neighbor regardless of nationality or religious heritage and affiliation (p. 62). This Gospel narrative provides nurses with a model of unequivocal concern and nondiscrimination in providing care to those in need; it reflects the conceptual framework to support a nursing theology of caring.

Prior to discussing a theology of caring, on which nursing practice may be based, the key concepts of theology and caring will be explored briefly.

Theology

The term *theology* comes originally from the Greek words *theos* meaning "God," and *logos* or "science." The contemporary meaning of theology is "an intellectual discipline, i.e., an ordered body of knowledge about God" (Hill, 1990, p. 1011). The study of theology is often described according to Anselm of Canterbury's conceptualization as "faith seeking understanding." In this context, faith is viewed as "a stance of the whole person towards God, characterized by radical trust, hope, love and commitment" (Fehr, 1990, p. 1027). Each nurse's personal understanding of theology will be informed by myriad factors: religious or denominational heritage, formal and informal religious education, religious and spiritual experience, and current faith practices.

Caring

James Nelson (1976), in his exploration *Rediscovering the Person in Medical Care*, reported that "Underneath . . . important assumptions about the unity of the person and the individual's and community's participation in the healing process lies a fundamental truth: the importance of caring" (p. 62). Nelson added that in health-care facilities (clinics, hospitals, nursing homes) staff have a primary interest in "curing" certain disease and illness conditions. Ministers and nurses must, however, remember the importance of their vocational call to care (p. 62). Nelson defined caring as "an active attitude which genuinely conveys to the other person that he or she does really matter. . . . It is grounded in the sense of uniqueness and worth which, by the grace of God, the other has" (p. 63).

One of the earliest nursing theorists of caring is Madeleine Leininger (1978), who defined the concept as referring to "direct (or indirect) nurturant and skillful activities, processes and decisions related to assisting people in such a manner that reflects behavior attributes which are empathetic, supportive, compassionate, protective, succorant, educational and otherwise dependent upon the needs, problems, values and goals of the individual or group being assisted" (p. 489). In her later writings, Leininger described caring as the central focus or dimension of nursing practice (Leininger, 1980, 1988, 1991). Nurse authors Eriksson (1992); Montgomery (1992); and Benner, Tanner, and Chesla (1996) also identified caring as a central concept of nursing, as did Simone Roach (1992), who postulated five attributes of the concept: "compassion, competence, confidence, conscience, and commitment" (p. 1). In their practice, nurses have always embraced the concept of caring as integral to the essence of the profession (Picard, 1995; Pinch, 1996). And ultimately, through the manifestation of caring nursing practice, nurses engender the kind of trust and confidence in their patients that leads to the promotion of good health (Bishop & Scudder, 1996, p. 41).

Finally, seven characteristics of caring were identified in a study of 200 nurses' stories describing patient care; these were "caring, compassion, spirituality, community outreach, providing comfort, crisis intervention, and going the extra distance" (Hudacek, 2008, p. 124).

The following section, "Dimensions of Caring," encompasses the characteristics of caring as identified in the theological and health-care literature and the goal of a healing outcome as understood in the clinical practice of nursing. Patient examples are drawn from the author's journal chronicling a chaplaincy experience at a research medical center.

▶ Dimensions of Caring

For the nurse practicing spiritual caring, three key activities may serve as vehicles for the carrying out of the theological mandate to serve the sick: being with patients in their experiences of pain, suffering, or other problems or needs; listening to patients verbally express anxieties or emotions, such as fear, anger, loneliness, depression, or sorrow, which may be hindering the achievement of wellness; and touching patients either physically, emotionally, or spiritually to assure them of their connectedness with others in the family of God.

In and of themselves the acts of being with, listening to, or touching a patient may not constitute spiritual care. These behaviors, however, grounded in a nurse's spiritual philosophy of life such as that articulated in the parable of the Good Samaritan, take on the element of ministry; they constitute the nurse's theology of caring.

Being

Being with a sick person without judgment creates space for meaning to emerge and for the holy to be revealed.

—**E. Emeth and J. Greenhut**, 1991, p. 65

The concept of "being" indicates the idea of a nurse's presence or of simply being with a patient or family member during a time of need. Often, after the therapeutic procedures have been completed, the medications have been given, and the formal nursing interventions have been carried out, ill persons and/or family members long for a nurse to just be with them for a few minutes; to be a caring presence, not listening for they may be too fatigued to talk; not touching for they may be in too much pain for physical contact. But just to be there, to be present during their time of loneliness and suffering.

The association between spirituality and nursing presence was highlighted in an article describing a unique clinical experience for nursing students during which the students worked with the poor and homeless, taking on an advocacy posture for their clients. The students affirmed that the clinical practicum provided "an experience of self-discovery and maturation in understanding spirituality and nursing presence in nursing practice" (Rankin & DeLashmutt, 2010, p. 282).

In fact, a nurse's presence is viewed as such a well-accepted nursing activity that two nurse theorists have developed a "mid-range theory of nursing presence" (McMahon & Christopher, 2011). In the theory, professional nursing presence is described as "dependent upon the combination of five variables: individual nurse characteristics, individual client characteristics, shared characteristics within the nurse-client dyad, and environment conducive to relational work, and the nurse's intentional decisions within the practice domain" (p. 71). This theory, the authors believe, contributes to an understanding of the "relational aspects of nursing practice within the contemporary healthcare environment" (p. 71).

A description from the author's journal of an experience with a young cancer patient reflects the importance of being present with a patient in need.

> This morning a young man, Michael, who was facing mutilating surgery in hope of slowing the progress of advanced rhabdomyosarcoma, asked to talk to me; he said, "I need you to help me understand why this is happening. I need you to help me deal with it." I sought consultation both in prayer and from my own spiritual mentor before the meeting. I entered Michael's room, however, with much trepidation; how could I possibly help him "understand why" God seemed to be allowing his illness. As it turned out, Michael was the one who helped me. As soon as I sat down, he said, "There are some things I've been thinking about that I need to tell you," and the conversation continued with Michael sharing much about his own faith and his attempt to understand God's will in his life. As I prepared to leave, Michael got up, hugged me, and said, "Our talk has helped a lot"; we prayed together for the coming surgery. Simply being with Michael as he struggled with the diagnosis of cancer in light of his own spirituality constituted the caring. I did not have, nor did I need, any right words; I only needed to be a caring presence in Michael's life.

Emeth and Greenhut (1991), in their discussion of understanding illness, described the importance of being with patients and families, especially when, as with Michael, they need to ask questions for which there are no answers. "We cannot answer the question, 'Where is God in this experience?' for anyone else; rather, we must be willing to be with others in their experience as they live with the questions and wait for their personal answers to emerge. This 'being with' is at the heart of health care" (p. 65).

Listening

Many people are looking for an ear that will listen … He who no longer listens to his brother will soon no longer be listening to God either … One who cannot listen long and patiently will presently be talking beside the point and never really speaking to others, albeit he be not conscious of it.

—**Dietrich Bonhoeffer**, 1959, p. 11

The concept of listening is an integral part of being with a person, as was learned from the interaction with Michael. However, as his illness progressed, there were also times when being with Michael in silence was a significant dimension of caring. In some situations, however, active listening, with responsive and sensitive feedback to the person speaking, is important in providing spiritual care.

Ministering to Philip, a young man diagnosed with anaplastic astrocytoma, revealed the importance of such listening. Philip, because of his neurologic condition, had difficulty explaining his thoughts, especially in regard to spiritual matters, yet he very much wanted to talk. Philip described himself as a born-again Christian, a fact of which he was very proud.

> On my first visit Philip showed me a well-worn Bible in which he had written comments on favorite Scripture passages. As our meetings continued, I began to realize that if I opened the Bible and focused on a particular passage, Philip's speech was helped by looking at the words. I tried to listen carefully, to follow and comprehend Philip's thoughts on the Scripture and its meaning in his life. Our sharing was validated one day when Philip reached out and took my hand and said, "I'm glad you're here; I really like our talking about God together."

In a discussion of spirituality and the nursing process, Verna Carson (1989) recognized the importance of such listening. "The ability to listen is both an art and a learned skill. It requires that the nurse completely attend to the client with open ears, eyes and mind" (p. 165). And, in a poignant case study entitled "A Lesson Learned by Listening," palliative care nurse Katie Jantzi affirmed the importance of listening to a dying patient, reminding us that patients are our "best teachers" (2005, p. 41).

Touching

And there was a leper who came to Him, and knelt before Him saying: "Lord, if you choose you can make me clean." He stretched out His hand and touched him saying: "I choose. Be made clean." Immediately his leprosy was cleansed.

—**Matthew** 8:2–3

The Christian Gospel message teaches us compellingly that touch was important to Jesus; it was frequently used in healing and caring interactions with His followers. Loving, empathetic, compassionate touch is perhaps the most vital dimension of a nursing theology of caring. At times the touch may be physical: the laying on of hands, taking of one's hand, holding, or gently stroking a forehead. At other times a nurse's touch may be verbal: a kind and caring greeting or a word of comfort and support. Physical touch has been described in the nursing literature as encompassing five dimensions of caring: physical comfort, emotional comfort, mind–body comfort, social interaction, and spiritual sharing (Chang, 2001).

Perhaps one of the most rewarding experiences with the use of caring touch occurred during an interaction with Erin, a nine-year-old newly diagnosed with acute lymphocytic leukemia.

> Erin was about to begin chemotherapy and was terrified at the thought of having IVs started; the staff asked if I would try to help calm her during the initiation of treatment. One of the pediatric oncology nurses pulled up a stool for me next to Erin so that I could hold and comfort her during the needle insertion. After the procedure was finished and I was preparing to leave, Erin trudged across the room dragging her IV pole, wrapped her arms around me, and said, "Thank you for helping me to get through that!"

It is not surprising that Carson (1989) identified touch, associated with being with a patient, as critical to the provision of spiritual caring. She suggested that the nurse's "presence and ability to touch another both physically and spiritually" is perhaps his or her most important gift (p. 164). And, in describing the power of "compassionate touch," Minister Victor Parachin asserts, "Whenever we reach out with love and compassion to touch another life, our contact makes the burden a little lighter and the pain more bearable. . . . By reaching out and touching someone through deed or word, we provide the extra push that person needs to carry on, rather than give up" (2003, p. 9). "The human touch," Parachin concludes, "can make the difference between life and death" (p. 9).

Ultimately the activities of being, listening, and touching, as exemplified in Jesus' parable of the Good Samaritan and in a nursing theology of caring, will be employed in a variety of ways as needed in the clinical setting. This is what constitutes the creativity of nursing practice; this is what constitutes the art of the profession of nursing.

▶ Nursing as a Vocation: Called to Serve

Nursing, as a profession, has developed significantly during the past half century. The vocation or spiritual calling to care for the sick, addressed earlier in the chapter, somewhat diminished during nursing's heightened concern with professionalism, is experiencing a reawakening among contemporary nurses. This may be related to the interest in spiritual and religious issues manifested in the larger society. Taking a historical perspective, Nightingale scholar JoAnn Wiederquist pointed out that Florence Nightingale did, from the inception of the nursing profession, consider nursing a spiritual vocation. Wiederquist cited founder of nursing Nightingale's assertion, "A new art and science (nursing) has been created since and within the last 40 years and with it a new profession, so they say; we say *calling*" (Nightingale, as cited in Wiederquist, 1995, p. 6).

A number of nursing articles have addressed the topic of nursing as a "vocation" or "calling" to serve the sick. A variety of nurse authors have sought to explain why 21st-century professional nursing may be also appropriately described as an altruistic or spiritual vocation of service. In the book *The Nurse Apprentice 1860–1977,* British nurse educator Ann Bradshaw supports the concept of nursing as a vocation (2002). While admitting the importance of current nursing education, Bradshaw laments the fact that some professional nurses have lost their initial sense of vocation or calling (2002). In a 2010 article on the understanding of the nursing "vocation," Bradshaw observed that "whether the historical ideal of vocation remains important, negatively or positively, to the attitudes, values and motivations of the clinical nurse and the quality of patient care, is a relevant and significant issue" (p. 3465).

Theologian Mikael Lundmark provided an analysis of nursing as a vocation, commenting on the work of both Bradshaw and Eriksson; their writings, he concluded, both explicitly and implicitly advocated "a vocational understanding of nursing" (2007, p. 778). And, in exploring the concept of professional nursing from an ethical perspective, Karolyn White observed that "nursing is best understood as a vocational occupation" (2002, p. 279). White's argument was based on Blum's model of vocations, which identifies a vocation as a calling in which workers identify with "traditions, norms and meanings" (p. 279).

Finally, anecdotal nursing journal articles abound describing a nurse's personal identification with nursing as a vocation of service, including "Answering God's Call"

(Schmidt, 1997); "Hearing the Call to Nursing" (Jeffries, 1998); "Childhood Interest in Nursing Has Become Lifelong Vocation" (King, 2003); "Responding to God's Call" (McKoy, 2004); and "God's Call" (Folta, 2005).

Nursing, as both a vocation and a profession, encompasses a unique commitment to provide both care and compassion for those one serves. The subject of spirituality in nursing practice includes concern not only with the personal spiritual and religious needs of the patient and nurse, but with the spiritual dimension of the nurse–patient interaction as well.

▶ References

Alpert, P. T. (2010). Spirituality goes beyond religiosity: A much needed practice in nursing. *Home Health Care Management & Practice, 22*(2), 140–143.

Barnum, B. S. (1994). *Nursing theory: Analysis, application, evaluation.* Philadelphia, PA: J. B. Lippincott.

Beck, M. B. (1945). *The nurse: Handmaid of the divine physician.* Philadelphia, PA: J. B. Lippincott.

Benner, P., Tanner, C. A., & Chesla, C. A. (1996). *Expertise in nursing practice: Caring, clinical judgment and ethics.* New York, NY: Springer.

Bishop, A. H., & Scudder, J. R. (1996). *Nursing ethics: Therapeutic caring presence.* Sudbury, MA: Jones & Bartlett Learning.

Bonhoeffer, D. (1959). *Life together.* New York, NY: Harper & Brothers.

Boswell, C., Cannon, S. B., & Miller, J. (2013). Students' perceptions of holistic nursing care. *Nursing Education Perspectives, 34*(5), 329–333.

Bradshaw, A. (2002). *The nurse apprentice 1860–1977.* Aldershot, UK: Ashgate.

Bradshaw, A. (2010). An historical perspective on the treatment of vocation in the Briggs Report (1972). *Journal of Clinical Nursing, 19*(23–24), 3459–3467.

Burke, B. H. (1993, September). Wellness in the healing ministry. *Health Progress, 74*(7), 33–39.

Burkhardt, M. A. (1989). Spirituality: An analysis of the concept. *Holistic Nursing Practice, 3*(3), 69–77.

Bruce, A., Shields, L., & Molzahn, A. (2011). Language and the (im)possibilities of articulating spirituality. *Journal of Holistic Nursing, 29*(1), 44–52.

Carson, V. B. (1993, Winter). Spirituality: Generic or Christian. *Journal of Christian Nursing, 10*(1), 24–27.

Carson, V. B. (Ed.). (1989). Spirituality and the nursing process. In *Spiritual dimensions of nursing practice* (pp. 150–179). Philadelphia, PA: W. B. Saunders.

Chang, S. O. (2001). The conceptual structure of physical touch in caring. *Journal of Advanced Nursing, 33*(6), 820–827.

Clarke, J. (2009). A critical view of how nursing has defined spirituality. *Journal of Clinical Nursing, 18*(1), 1666–1673.

Como, J. M. (2007). Spiritual practice: A literature review related to spiritual health and health outcomes. *Holistic Nursing Practice, 21*(5), 224–236.

Dossey, B. M. (1988). Nurse as healer: Toward an inward journey. In B. M. Dossey, L. Keegan, C. E. Guzzetta, & L. G. Kolkmeier (Eds.), *Holistic nursing: A handbook for practice* (pp. 39–54). Rockville, MD: Aspen.

Dossey, B. M. (1989). The transpersonal self and states of consciousness. In B. M. Dossey, L. Keegan, L. G. Kolkmeier, & C. E. Guzzetta (Eds.), *Holistic health promotion: A guide for practice* (pp. 23–35). Rockville, MD: Aspen.

Dossey, B. M., & Keegan, L. (1989). Holism and the circle of human potential. In B. M. Dossey, L. Keegan, L. G. Kolkmeier, & C. E. Guzzetta (Eds.), *Holistic health promotion: A guide for practice* (pp. 3–21). Rockville, MD: Aspen.

Ellis, H. K., & Narayanasamy, A. (2009). An investigation into the role of spirituality in nursing. *British Journal of Nursing, 18*(14), 886–890.

Emblen, J. D. (1992). Religion and spirituality defined according to current use in nursing literature. *Journal of Professional Nursing, 8*(1), 41–47.

Emeth, E. V., & Greenhut, J. H. (1991). *The wholeness handbook: Care of body, mind and spirit for optimal health.* New York, NY: Continuum.

Eriksson, K. (1992). Nursing: The caring practice, "Being There." In D. A. Gaut (Ed.), *The presence of caring in nursing* (pp. 201–210). New York, NY: National League for Nursing Press.

Fehr, W. L. (1990). The history of theology. In J. A. Komonchak, M. Collins, & D. A. Lane (Eds.), *The new dictionary of theology* (pp. 1027–1035). Collegeville, MN: The Liturgical Press.

Folta, R. (2005). God's call. *Christian Nurse International, 11*(1), 7.

Goodnow, M. (1916). *Outlines of nursing history.* Philadelphia, PA: W. B. Saunders.

Graves, L. (2008). Teaching the wounded healer. *Medical Teacher, 30,* 217–219.

Gray, J. (2009). Debate on spirituality needed. *Nursing Standard, 23*(23), 10.

Guzzetta, C. E. (1988). Nursing process and standards of care. In B. M. Dossey, L. Keegan, C. E. Guzzetta, & L. G. Kolkmeier (Eds.), *Holistic nursing: A handbook for practice* (pp. 101–126). Rockville, MD: Aspen.

Haggard, P. (1983, fall). Healing and health care of the whole person. *Journal of Religion and Health, 22*(3), 234–240.

Hill, W. J. (1990). Theology. In J. A. Komonchak, M. Collins, & D. A. Lane (Eds.), *The new dictionary of theology* (pp. 1011–1027). Collegeville, MN: The Liturgical Press.

Homberg, M. (1980). *Biblical roots of healing in nursing* (Unpublished doctoral dissertation). Teacher's College, Columbia University, New York, NY.

Hudacek, S. S. (2008). Dimensions of caring: A qualitative analysis of nurses' stories. *Journal of Nursing Education, 47*(3), 124–129.

Jantzi, K. (2005). A lesson learned by listening. *Journal of Christian Nursing, 22*(1), 41.

Jeffries, E. (1998). Hearing the call to nursing. *Nursing, 3*(2), 71–72.

Johnson, R. P. (1992). *Body, mind, spirit: Tapping the healing power within you.* Liguori, MO: Liguori.

Kelsey, M. T. (1988). *Psychology, medicine and Christian healing.* San Francisco, CA: Harper & Row.

Kendrick, K. D., & Robinson, S. (2000). Spirituality: Its relevance and purpose for clinical nursing in a new millennium. *Journal of Clinical Nursing, 9*(5), 701–705.

King, J. (2003, January). Childhood interest in nursing has become lifelong vocation. *The Catholic Herald, 16,* 6.

Kodell, J. (1989). *The gospel according to Luke.* Collegeville, MN: The Liturgical Press.

Leininger, M. M. (1978). *Trans-cultural nursing: Concepts, theories and practice.* New York, NY: John Wiley & Sons.

Leininger, M. M. (1980). Caring: A central focus of nursing and health care services. *Nursing and Health Care, 1*(3), 135–143.

Leininger, M. M. (1988). *Care: The essence of nursing and health.* Detroit, MI: Wayne State University Press.

Leininger, M. M. (1991). Foreword. In D. A. Gaut & M. M. Leininger (Eds.), *Caring: The compassionate healer.* New York, NY: National League for Nursing Press.

Leininger, M. M. (1997). Transcultural spirituality: A comparative care and health focus. In M. S. Roach (Ed.), *Caring from the heart: The convergence of caring and spirituality* (pp. 99–118). New York, NY: Paulist Press.

Lindberg, J. B., Hunter, M. L., & Kruszewski, A. Z. (1994). *Introduction to nursing: Concepts, issues, and opportunities.* Philadelphia, PA: J. B. Lippincott.

Lo, R., & Brown, R. (1999). Holistic care and spirituality: Potential for increasing spiritual dimensions of nursing. *Australian Journal of Holistic Nursing, 6*(2), 4–9.

Lohri-Posey, B. (2005). Becoming a compassionate healer. *Journal of Christian Nursing, 22*(4), 34–37.

Lundmark, M. (2007). Vocation in theology-based nursing theories. *Nursing Ethics, 14*(6), 767–780.

McKoy, Y. D. (2004). Responding to God's call. *Journal of Christian Nursing, 21*(2), 35–37.

McMahon, M., & Christopher, K. (2011). Toward a mid-range theory of nursing presence. *Nursing Forum, 46*(2), 71–82.

Meehan, T. C. (2012). Spirituality and spiritual care from a careful nursing perspective. *Journal of Nursing Management, 20*(8), 990–1001.

Meraviglia, M. G. (1999). Critical analysis of spirituality and its empirical indicators: Prayers and meaning in life. *Journal of Holistic Nursing, 17*(1), 18–33.

Montgomery, C. L. (1992). The spiritual connection: Nurses' perceptions of the experience of caring. In D. A. Gaut (Ed.), *The presence of caring in nursing* (pp. 39–52). New York, NY: National League for Nursing Press.

Nagai-Jacobson, M. G., & Burkhardt, M. A. (1989). Spirituality: Cornerstone of holistic nursing practice. *Holistic Nursing Practice, 3*(3), 18–26.

Narayanasamy, A. (2015). Reflexive account of unintended outcomes from spiritual care qualitative research. *Journal of Research in Nursing, 20*(3), 234–248.

Nelson, J. B. (1976). *Rediscovering the person in medical care.* Minneapolis, MN: Augsburg.

Niven, E. (2008). The wounded healer: What has the concept to offer nursing? *Nursing Ethics, 15*(3), 287–288.

Noble, A., & Jones, C. (2010). Getting it right: Oncology nurses understanding of spirituality. *International Journal of Palliative Care Nursing, 16*(11), 565–569.

Nouwen, H. J. (1979). *The wounded healer.* Garden City, NY: Image Books.

O'Brien, M. E. (1982). The need for spiritual integrity. In H. Yura & M. Walsh (Eds.), *Human needs and the nursing process* (Vol. 2, pp. 82–115). Norwalk, CT: Appleton-Century-Crofts.

O'Connor, C. I. (2001). Characteristics of spirituality, assessment and prayer in holistic nursing. *Nursing Clinics of North America, 36*(1), 33–46.

Parachin, V. M. (2003). The power of compassionate touch. *Journal of Christian Nursing, 20*(2), 8–9.

Pesut, B. (2008). A conversation on diverse perspectives of spirituality in nursing literature. *Nursing Philosophy, 9*, 98–109.

Pesut, B. (2013). Nursings' need for the idea of spirituality. *Nursing Inquiry, 20*(1), 5–10.

Picard, C. (1995). Images of caring in nursing and dance. *Journal of Holistic Nursing, 13*(4), 323–331.

Pike, J. (2011). Spirituality in nursing: A systematic review of the literature from 2006–2010. *British Journal of Nursing, 20*(12), 743–749.

Pinch, W. J. (1996). Is caring a moral trap? *Nursing Outlook, 44*(2), 84–88.

Price, A. L. (1954). *The art, science and spirit of nursing.* Philadelphia, PA: W. B. Saunders.

Ramezani, M., Ahmadi, F., Mohammadi, E., & Kazemnejad, A. (2014). Spiritual care in nursing: A concept analysis. *International Nursing Review, 61*(2), 211–219.

Rankin, E., & DeLashmutt, M. (2010). Finding spirituality in nursing presence: The student's challenge. *Journal of Holistic Nursing, 24*(4), 282–288.

Reed, P. G. (1992). An emerging paradigm for the investigation of spirituality in nursing. *Research in Nursing and Health, 15*, 349–357.

Reinert, K. G., & Koenig, H. G. (2013). Re-examining definitions of spirituality in nursing research. *Journal of Advanced Nursing, 69*(12), 2622–2634.

Roach, S. (1992). *The human act of caring.* Ottawa, Canada: Canadian Hospital Association.

Robinson, A. (1995). Spirituality and risk: Toward an understanding. *Holistic Nursing Practice, 8*(2), 1–7.

Schmidt, K. (1997). Answering God's call. *Journal of Christian Nursing, 14*(1), 11.

Shelly, J. A. (2003). Walking on holy ground. *Journal of Christian Nursing, 20*(3), 3.

Stoll, R. I. (1989). The essence of spirituality. In V. B. Carson (Ed.), *Spiritual dimensions of nursing practice* (pp. 4–23). Philadelphia, PA: W. B. Saunders.

Swinton, J., & Pattison, S. (2010). Moving beyond clarity: Towards a thin, vague and useful understanding of spirituality in nursing care. *Nursing Philosophy, 11*, 226–237.

Tinley, S. T., & Kinney, A. Y. (2007). Three philosophical approaches to the study of spirituality. *Advances in Nursing Science, 30*(1), 71–80.

Watson, J. (1995, July). Nursing's caring-healing paradigm as exemplar for alternative medicine. *Alternative Therapies, 1*(30), 64–69.

White, K. (2002). Nursing as vocation. *Nursing Ethics, 9*(3), 279–290.

Wiederkehr, Sr. M. (1991). *Seasons of your heart.* New York, NY: HarperCollins.

Wiederquist, J. (1995). Called to serve. *Christian Nurse International, 11*(1), 4–6.

Young, C., & Koopsen, C. (2011). *Spirituality, health and healing: An integrative approach* (2nd ed.). Sudbury, MA: Jones & Bartlett Learning.

CHAPTER 2

A Spiritual History of Nursing

Nursing is an art, and if it is to be made an art, it requires as exclusive a devotion, as hard a preparation, as any painter's or sculptor's work. For what is having to do with dead canvas or cold marble compared with having to do with the living body, the temple of God's spirit.

Florence Nightingale, 1867, as cited in Baly, 1991, p. 68

I've always viewed nursing as a calling. I read nursing articles and nursing books. I like to read about history (of nursing) and lives of other nurses like Florence Nightingale who have made contributions to nursing or medical fields to keep me in touch with the meaning of nursing as a caring vocation. I don't think that will change. . . . I think nursing should always be a calling. It should be a profession where you care for people but you don't only consider their medical needs, but also their spiritual and emotional needs.

Cathy, Charge Nurse on a Medical–Surgical Unit

Recently there has been a resurgence of nursing publications directed toward the spiritual concerns of those who are ill. To better understand practicing nurses' contemporary interest in spirituality and the spiritual vocation of nursing, it is important to walk briefly in the world of our ancient and medieval past, as well as to examine the post-Reformation period, to explore the powerful and compelling spiritual history of nursing up to the modern era.

It is said that we stand on the shoulders of those who have gone before us; in the stories of the pre-Christian and early Christian caregivers are found many strong shoulders on which to stand. They are exemplary models whose ministries of love and care for the sick speak eloquently to us as nurses today. The spirit and spirituality of these pioneer nurses provide a foundation and a vision that informs, strengthens, and supports contemporary caregiving as nursing moves into the 21st century. Nurse historian Sonya Grypma (2012) reminds us that "historical amnesia is dangerous" (p. 12); such amnesia related to the spiritual history of nursing could prevent us from reflecting on the beautiful models of caring and compassion that have informed our profession from its earliest days. British nursing scholar and historian Ann Bradshaw (2013) noted that nurse educators have, for the past century, asserted the importance of "the religious ideal of developing virtue" as being "fundamental to being a good nurse" (p. 90). Nursing history "matters" (Chatterton, 2012, p. 612) especially in such subfields as public health nursing (Hogan, 2015) and trauma care (Ayers, 2014).

In this chapter, selected caregivers to the sick, whose activities prefigure the role and posture of the modern nurse, are described. The spiritual attitudes and behaviors of these individuals and communities are presented chronologically, beginning with the pre-Christian era, and continuing through the early and later Christian period, up to the present day. The common thread unifying the persons and communities discussed is their concern with the spiritual as well as the physical and psychosocial needs of those who are ill or infirm; these caregivers viewed nursing the sick as a religious vocation supported by the individual's personal spiritual belief system. The present chapter is based on the extant nursing and theological literature that documents the historical role of the nurse in providing spiritual care.

▶ Nursing in the Pre-Christian Era

Whatsoever they receive for their wages . . . they do not keep as their own, but bring into the common treasury for the use of all, nor do they neglect the sick who are unable to contribute their share.

—Philo, writing of the "Essenes," as cited in Robinson, 1946, p. 6

Prior to discussing the Christian influence on care of the sick, health care in the pre-Christian era should be examined briefly. Medicine and nursing in ancient civilizations provided the foundations on which many of the health-care practices of Christian nurses rested. These ancient cultures also influenced the concept of Christian charity in relation to caring for those who are ill (Bullough & Bullough, 1987). Archeological study of the pre-Christian cultures has revealed two related yet distinct types of nurses. One group consisted of skilled women who "nursed for hire"; more commonly identified, however, were "nurses" whose positions were those of slaves in wealthy households (Dolan, Fitzpatrick, & Herrmann, 1983, p. 81). These nurses practiced their art according to the established medical models of their respective societies.

Nursing might be explored in a number of early cultures. In Babylonia, the "Code of Hammurabi" suggested that nursing care was provided for patients between physician visits (Walsh, 1929, p. x). Early Buddhist discoveries in China of the curative value of many plants led to nursing therapeutics employing herbology (Sellew & Nuesse, 1946, p. 6). Hindu medical practice in India included a role for the male nurse (Grippando, 1986, p. 3). In Ireland, ancient druidic priests and priestesses advised on care and healing in illness (Dolan et al., 1983, p. 40). The four key societies, however, whose spiritual and cultural contributions are most frequently cited as supporting the art and the science of modern medicine and nursing are those of Egypt, Greece, Rome, and Israel.

Egypt

Egyptian medicine contained a strong element of religious magic in its origins; however, the practice of embalming taught the Egyptians human anatomy, from which they were able to derive surgical procedures (Deloughery, 1977, p. 7). Egyptian history boasts the first physician, Imhotep, as well as the first medical textbook, Ebers Papyrus (Frank, 1953, p. 9).

The Egyptians were concerned about public health problems such as famine and malnutrition. While offering prayers and sacrifices to religious deities, they also took preventive measures such as storing grain against future need. Researchers have determined that a school for the education of Egyptian physicians existed as early as 1100 B.C., and as a result a number of practical therapeutic remedies for care of the sick were developed. Nurse historians Dietz and Lehozky (1967) concluded, thus, that "undoubtedly some form of instinctive nursing care must have existed at this time" (p. 10).

Greece

History documents the fact that "nursing in the Greco-Roman era was largely the responsibility of members of the patient's own family or that of slaves employed to provide specific skills. The spiritual rationale for providing nursing care was duty to and love for a relative" (Swaffield, 1988, pp. 28–30). The consummate ancient Greek physician, of course, was Hippocrates (460–370 B.C.), who instructed caregivers to "use their eyes and ears, and to reason from facts rather than from gratuitous assumptions" (Deloughery, 1977, p. 8). Hippocrates cautioned those who tended the sick to be solicitous to their patients' spiritual well-being and "to do no harm" (Frank, 1953, p. 17).

Although Hippocrates did not identify nursing as a profession, many of his prescribed therapies fall within the realm of nursing practice. Some examples include the teachings that "fluid diet only should be given in fevers"; "cold sponging [should be used] for high temperatures"; and "hot gargles [should be taken] for acute tonsillitis" (Dietz & Lehozky, 1967, p. 16).

Researchers have explored the characteristics and role of the "nurse" in Greek life by studying the literature, art, and culture of Grecian society. From a study of the early Greek world, Gorman (1917) determined that the nurse "though usually a slave, was sometimes manumitted; that a preference was frequently shown at Athens for the foreign-bred nurse; and, that, on occasion, free women resorted to nursing as a means of gaining a livelihood" (p. 15). The nurse's role was considered a noble one among the Greeks of the era, and, Gorman pointed out, "instances of love and devotedness of nurses are not wanting in the [Greek] literature" (p. 30).

It is also noted that Greek religious mythology introduced the concept of women's involvement in the healing arts, in the tale of Aesculapius, the god of healing: "One of his five children, Hygeia, became the Goddess of Health and another, Panacea (from whom comes our word for 'cure all'), the Restorer of Health" (Deloughery, 1977, p. 9).

Rome

Rome did not offer great advances in medical and nursing practice prior to Christianity but depended greatly on the knowledge of the Greek physicians. Prior to the advent of Greek medicine, care of the sick in Roman households was guided primarily by the use of natural or folk remedies. For example, in the writings of the early Roman scholar, Cato the Elder, is found "advice for the treatment and care of gout, colic, indigestion, constipation, and pain in the side" (Bullough & Bullough, 1969, p. 24). Religion was influential in nursing the sick; Roman gods were offered libations in petition for favors related to health and illness needs. Following the conquest of Corinth many Roman youth began to study in Athens and personally achieved the skills of Greek healing (Pavey, 1952, p. 78). Together with this professional education, however, appreciation and respect for the favor of the gods continued as an important adjunct to therapeutic procedures. Prayer to a god, or to several gods, was considered a critical adjuvant therapy in nursing a sick Roman.

Israel

The Hebrew people of Israel identified in their Mosaic Law much concern for the provision of nursing care for the ill and infirm. There were religious proscriptions concerning general health and hygiene: "Rules of diet and cleanliness, and hours of work and rest" (Sellew & Nuesse, 1946, p. 35). Sellew and Nuesse observed that "Since these rules were enforced by the group and not left to the will of the individual, they were, in effect, rules of public health" (p. 34). Robinson (1946) asserted that the people of Israel actually "laid the foundations of public health nursing on enduring principles, [as they] naturally regarded visiting the sick ('bikkur holim') as a religious duty incumbent upon all" (p. 4). The Israelites articulated specific rules regarding the nursing of those with contagious diseases, and were particularly noted for their care of children and of the elderly. Another religious tradition of the Hebrew people related to nursing of the sick encompassed the concepts of "hospitality" and "charity" for anyone in need. This resulted in a system of "houses for strangers," supported by each citizen tithing a 10th of his or her possessions toward charitable work (Pavey, 1952, p. 29).

Finally, the Hebrew Scriptures contain references to the "nurse"; one who "appears at times as a combination servant, companion and helpmate" (Bullough & Bullough, 1969, p. 14). An example from Genesis 24, verse 59, describes Rebekah's going forth to meet Isaac, her future husband, accompanied by her nurse, Deborah: ". . . they allowed Rebekah and her nurse to leave, along with Abraham's servant and his men." Grippando (1986) asserted that "Deborah was the first nurse to be recorded in history" (p. 3).

▶ Biblical Roots of Nursing

The Bible, recognized by Christian nurses as a guide to their lives and their nursing practice, contains scriptures identified as being those of both the Old and the New Testaments.

Old Testament

There are many concepts in the Old Testament that provide models for the nurse–patient relationship, such as God's covenant with the people of Israel (Isaiah 49:15–16). The history of God's faithfulness to his people, even when they displeased him, provides a powerful example of the faithfulness required of a nurse–patient covenant of caring and support. Other particularly helpful Old Testament scriptures for nursing are those of the Psalms. The Psalms, 150 Hebrew songs, contain a variety of messages that may provide care, support, strength, courage, and an understanding of God's love and mercy both for nurses and their patients in times of stress or suffering.

The Old Testament scriptures include the following books: *The Pentateuch* (Genesis, Exodus, Leviticus, Numbers, and Deuteronomy), which relate the story of creation to the death of Moses; *The Historical Books* (Joshua, Judges, Ruth, Samuel 1 and 2, Kings 1 and 2, Chronicles 1 and 2, Ezra, Nehemiah, and Esther [and Tobit, Judith, and Maccabees 1 and 2 in the Roman editions]) containing Israel's history; *The Wisdom and Poetic Books* (Job, Psalms, Proverbs, Ecclesiastes, and Song of Songs [and Wisdom and Sirach in the Roman editions]), which describe the Lord's love and concern for His people; and *The Prophetic Books* (Isaiah, Jeremiah, Lamentations, Ezekiel, Daniel, Hosea, Joel, Amos, Obadiah, Jonah, Micah, Nahum, Habakkuk, Zephaniah, Haggai, Zechariah, and Malachi [and Baruch in the Roman editions]), which relate God's care for and expectations of the people of Israel.

New Testament

Many Christian nurses believe that their vocational call to serve is derived directly from Jesus' message in the New Testament: "And whoever gives even a cup of cold water to one of these little ones in the name of a disciple—truly I tell you none of these will lose their reward" (Matthew 10:42). Jesus also explained that in caring for the least members of his family we were caring for Him: "For I was hungry and you gave me food, I was thirsty and you gave me something to drink, I was a stranger and you welcomed me, I was naked and you gave me clothing, I was sick and you took care of me, I was in prison and you visited me" (Matthew 25:35).

The New Testament scriptures consist of the four *Gospels* (Matthew, Mark, Luke, and John), which contain the life and teachings of Jesus; the *Acts of the Apostles* describing the early Church after Jesus' death; the *Letters of St. Paul* (Romans, Corinthians 1 and 2, Galatians, Ephesians, Philippians, Colossians, Thessalonians 1 and 2, Timothy 1 and 2, Titus, Philemon, and Hebrews), which were instructions written by Paul, an early disciple of Jesus; the *Letters of James, Letters of Peter, Letters of John,* and *Letters of Jude*, which provided guidance and support for the early Christians; and the *Book of Revelation*, which focuses on the end times employing symbolic language in its instruction.

▶ Christianity and Care of the Sick

Then Jesus went about all the cities and villages, teaching in their synagogues, and proclaiming the good news of the Kingdom, and curing every disease and sickness.

—Matthew 9:35

Jesus as Healer

In the New Testament Gospels, described earlier as relating the life and teachings of Jesus, much of Jesus' activity is identified as a ministry of healing. In fact, physician John Wilkinson estimates that the healing narratives consist of over one-third of the entire gospel message; he asserts that "all four gospel writers regard the healing activity of Jesus as an important part of his ministry" (1998, p. 65). The book entitled *The Nurse with an Alabaster Jar: A Biblical Approach to Nursing* (O'Brien, 2006) suggests that there was such a variety of Jesus' healing narratives reported in the gospels that they might actually be categorized according to nursing specialty areas (p. 30). A table categorizing Jesus' healings includes such headings and examples as: Acute Illness—Peter's Mother-in-Law (Matthew 8:14–15); Chronic Illness—A Paralytic (lowered through the roof; Matthew 9:1–8); Infectious Disease—The Cleansing of a Leper (Matthew 8:1–4); Women's Health—The Woman with the Twelve-Year Hemorrhage (Matthew 9:20–22); Orthopedic Conditions—The Bent-over Woman (Matthew 21:14); Ophthalmology—The Blind Beggar (Matthew 20:29–34); Critical Care—Jairus' Daughter (Matthew 9:18–19); Pediatrics—Boy with a Demon (Matthew 17:14); Gerontology—The Man Ill for 38 Years (John 5:1–9); Mental Health—The Gerasene/Gaderene Demoniac (Matthew 8:28–34); and Community Health—Healing Among the Crowds (Matthew 8:16–17) (pp. 30–31).

In these and other healings, Jesus modeled how nurses should care for those who were ill or injured; he touched the sick, visited their homes, allowed them to touch him, and showed compassion whenever asked for mercy by one who was in need of his caring support.

Thus, it is not surprising to learn that in the early Christian Church, nursing of the sick or injured was accorded a place of honor and respect, associated as it was with one of the primary messages of Jesus: to love one's neighbor. Scripture described so many instances of Christ's healing the sick; His teaching regarding the need for each individual's care for brothers and sisters is also reflected especially in the parable of the Good Samaritan (Luke 10:30–36).

Nurse historian Josephine Dolan (1973) pointed out that the way in which Jesus interacted with the sick provides our example. "Instead of 'saying the word' and healing the sick, Christ gave individual attention to the needs of all by touching, anointing, and taking the hand" (p. 47). She concluded, "The least gesture of human kindness" was important to Jesus, and even "a cup of cold water given in His name did not pass unrewarded" (p. 47). Christ, in His own ministry of healing and teaching, prepared the way for his early followers to serve, with care and tenderness, the needs of their ill brothers and sisters. Central among the early Christians involved in nursing the sick were those persons identified as having a diaconal role in the young church.

In Christianity, Sister Charles Marie Frank asserts, "nursing as an organized service to society had its inception and development" (1953, p. 60). This thought is echoed by M. Patricia Donahue in the comment: "Christ's teachings of love and brotherhood transformed not only society at large but also the development of nursing. 'Organized nursing' was a direct response to these teachings and epitomized the concept of pure altruism initiated by the early Christians" (1996, p. 74).

It is asserted that "there is little evidence that any organized group of women nurses existed before the Christian era; ideals such as 'service,' 'charity,' and 'self-sacrifice,' derived from Christian teaching, now supported groups of workers whose main function was to care for the sick and the needy" (Deloughery, 1977, p. 5).

Early Christian Nurses

Veronica of Jerusalem

One of the first recorded acts of nursing heroism and courage was, I believe, reflected in the actions of the holy woman Veronica of Jerusalem who, according to legend, was present during Christ's painful journey to Calvary and who cleansed His bleeding face with her veil. As described by Franciscan Matthew Miller, "Veronica, a woman, risking the physical punishment of the guards, bravely broke through their ranks and with tender, womanly sympathy wiped the bleeding countenance of the Master" (1954, p. 19).

I have always thought of Veronica as a "nurse." I believe that only one deeply imbued with the calling to provide care for the sick and suffering would have had the courage and the compassion to step out of an anonymous crowd, risking the wrath of spear-wielding Roman soldiers, to comfort her injured Rabbi.

In looking at the older nursing literature, one finds Veronica frequently cited as a model for nurses. Some examples include a 1939 editorial in *The Trained Nurse and Hospital Review* in which Veronica is extolled as a nursing example (Heyward, p. 346); a 1953 article encouraging nurses to care for patients even as Veronica cared for her Lord ("The Nurse's Mass," p. 54); and two 1954 articles, both of which describe Veronica as the nurse's role model (Hawley, p. 17; Miller, p. 20). A 1958 article, describing the nurse as a "modern Veronica," suggests that nurses should show their patients the "compassion which Veronica showed to Christ on the Via Dolorosa" (Meyer, p. 47); and several articles in the 1960s demonstrated similar themes. One author pointed out that on the journey to Calvary "no one offered Jesus physical comfort except Veronica . . . Could it be that she was experienced in giving care to those who suffered?" (Ridgway, 1960, p. 67). Another paper asserted that Veronica was the model for "our public health nurses" (George, 1964, p. 57).

In her 1978 nursing history, Josephine Dolan asserted that nursing practice was indeed fostered by the examples of early caregivers such as Veronica who wiped the face of Jesus and who "will be recorded for all time for (her) example in comforting the afflicted" (p. 49). Finally, British spiritual writer Caryll Houselander pointed out that it is Veronica's compassion that inspires the "Veronicas of today." Nurses were identified as contemporary "Veronicas" by Houselander: "Nurses who comfort the dying in hospitals . . . who go into the homes of the sick and the poor to serve" (1955, p. 69).

Whether the legend of the holy woman Veronica is accurate in all of its details or not, the image of a caring, compassionate woman, brave enough to step out of a group of curious onlookers to comfort her wounded spiritual leader, whom some considered a criminal, is a magnificent guide for nurses, especially those engaged in caring for the marginalized.

Deacons and Deaconesses

I give you a new commandment, that you love one another . . . by this everyone will know that you are my disciples.

—John 13:34–35

Among the first "titled" followers of Jesus for whom care of the sick and infirm was an identified task were the deacons and deaconesses, the term *deacon* being derived from the Greek verb *diakonen* meaning "to serve." These men and women were obliged, by their positions, to visit and nurse the sick (Frank, 1953).

And whoever gives even a cup of cold water to one of these little ones in the name of a disciple, truly, I tell you, none of these will lose their reward.

—Matthew 10:42

Following the exhortation of Jesus to give "a cup of cold water" in His name, these early disciples of Christianity opened their homes, as well as their hearts, to those in need of physical and emotional care. "The Deacons and Deaconesses were especially zealous in seeking out cases of need, and not only nursed the sick by a system of visiting, but brought them into their own homes to be cared for" (Nutting & Dock, 1935, Vol. 1, p. 118). These settings, precursors to the modern hospital, were called diakonias, associating, again, the diaconate with the work of nursing. The diakonias were, in the very early days of the Church, called "Christrooms," suggesting a direct association with Jesus' teaching, "I was a stranger and you took me in" (Dolan, 1973, p. 56). A well-known deacon, Lawrence, was asked to bring the treasures of the Church before a Roman prefect, prior to his trial for being a Christian. He brought to the prefect a group of the "halt, the blind, and the very ill who were unable to care for themselves, and presented them . . . as the treasures of the Church" (Walsh, 1929, p. 2). For his trouble, Lawrence was roasted on a gridiron in martyrdom.

An early Christian woman, Phoebe, described as a friend of St. Paul, is identified as a deaconess in the New Testament. "I commend to you our sister Phoebe, a deacon of the Church . . . for she has been a benefactor of many" (Romans 16:1–2). Phoebe, who lived around 55 A.D., was known as a woman of great dignity and social status; she is said to have spent many hours nursing the poor in their homes (Grippando, 1986, p. 4).

These deacons and deaconesses and their later counterparts, the Roman matrons, were the earliest forerunners of professional nursing in the Christian Church.

Roman Matrons

A number of Roman matrons who had converted to Christianity served the early Church around the third and fourth centuries. These women were able to use their power and wealth to support the charitable work of nursing the sick. The matrons founded hospitals and convents, living ascetic lives dedicated to the care of the ill and infirm. Three of the most famous Roman matrons were Saints Helena, Paula, and Marcella.

St. Helena, or Flavia Helena, was empress of Rome and mother of Constantine the Great. After embracing Christianity, she devoted her life to care of the sick poor. She is identified as having started the first "gerokomion" or home for the aged infirm in the Roman Empire (Dolan, 1973).

St. Paula, a learned woman of her time, founded the first hospice for pilgrims in Bethlehem (Frank, 1953). Paula also built hospices for the sick along the roads to the city; she both managed the institutions and personally nursed the tired and the sick for almost 20 years. St. Jerome wrote of her, "She was oft by them that were sick, and she laid their pillows aright; and . . . she rubbed their feet and boiled water to wash them. And it seemed to her that the less she did to the sick in service, so much the less service she did to God" (Jameson, 1855, as cited in Nutting & Dock, 1935, Vol. 1, p. 141).

St. Marcella, who has been described as the leader of the Roman matrons (Pavey, 1952, p. 102), was known as a scholar and a deeply spiritual woman. She founded a community of religious women whose primary concern was care of the sick poor. Marcella instructed her followers in the care of the sick, while also devoting herself personally to charitable works and prayer.

Although individual deacons, deaconesses, and Roman matrons cared for many of the sick, especially the sick poor, during the early Christian era, it was with the advent and rise of monasticism that the work of nursing began to become institutionalized.

Early Monastic Nurses

The care of the sick is to be placed above and before every other duty, as if indeed Christ were being directly served by waiting on them.

—Rule of St. Benedict, 529 A.D.

The monasticism of the fourth, fifth, and sixth centuries was born out of a desire of many Christian men and women to lead lives of sanctity, withdrawing from the world to be guided by the vows of poverty, chastity, and obedience. At first the monks' daily work consisted primarily of prayer and manual labor. This began to change with the advent of such communities as that of St. Benedict of Nursia, whose rule was written in 529 A.D. Although early monasteries, such as those of Benedict, were centers of learning, eventually "nursing of the sick became a chief function and duty of community life" (Donahue, 1985, p. 127). In this era, twin communities of men and women also developed. Three of the most famous abbesses who ruled these groups were St. Radegunde at Poitiers (559 A.D.); St. Hilda of Whitby (664 A.D.); and St. Brigid (487 A.D.), who was the first woman to rule an abbey in Ireland (Donahue, 1985, pp. 129–130).

St. Radegunde, daughter of a Thuringian king, initially took poor patients into her own palace to nurse them. She later founded Holy Cross Monastery, with a community of more than 200 nuns (Goodnow, 1916). Radegunde also established a hospice where she herself cared for the patients; she is reputed to have cared lovingly and tenderly especially for those afflicted with leprosy. Radegunde's work is said to have encouraged many other women to make a life commitment to caring for the sick.

St. Hilda, a cultured and scholarly woman, directed her monastic community in the care of the sick; she nursed the sick poor, including lepers, herself. Hilda also supported a group of associate members of the monastery, called oblates, who assisted in the nursing of those who came under her care (Seymer, 1949).

St. Brigid, who became one of the most famous abbesses in Ireland, was the daughter of an Ulster chieftain and also a disciple of St. Patrick. Brigid founded the great monastery of Kildare, where the ill were received with charity and compassion. Dolan (1973) related that "In Fifth Century Ireland, when leprosy was an incurable scourge ... they [lepers] came in droves to Kildare to be bathed and treated by Brigid" (p. 60). Brigid became known as the "Patroness of Healing."

Although the monastic communities initiated a more formalized nursing care program for the physically ill and infirm, a greatly neglected and significantly stigmatized population in need of support were those suffering from mental illness or other cognitive impairments.

Mental Illness in the Middle Ages
Dymphna of Belgium

The people of Gheel have learned from childhood to live with the patients; their reception and care have been passed on from generation to generation.

—"Foster Family Care in Gheel," 1991, p. 15

Dymphna, the seventh-century Irish saint, identified to this day as the patroness of the mentally ill, devoted her life to care of the sick poor in the manner of the early monastic nurses ("Foster Family Care," 1991; Matheussen, Morren, & Seyers, 1975).

According to legend, Dymphna traveled to Gheel, Belgium, to assist the Irish missionaries. Once there, she focused her compassion and care especially on persons with impaired mental health. Dymphna was martyred at a young age, but after her death the Belgian women of Gheel believed that she could still intercede for the needs of the ill. Thus, a church and small clinic were erected in Dymphna's honor in the town. Many pilgrims traveled there hoping for a cure and, as the clinic could not house all of these visitors, local Gheel families began offering hospitality to mentally challenged pilgrims (Dolan et al., 1983, pp. 59–60). The practice has continued for centuries, and the Flemish community of Gheel, with its own psychiatric hospital under the supervision of the Belgian government, has been considered a model for home health care of the mentally ill ("Foster Family Care," 1991).

The system remains functional today. This was reflected in two 21st century articles on the Gheel system of deinstitutionalization published in scholarly journals. In 2003, the *Community Mental Health Journal* published a paper entitled "The Legend and Lessons of Gheel, Belgium: A 1500-Year-Old Legend, a 21st Century Model," which explains how the Gheel foster family care system for mental patients provides a model case study that can help other communities "identify significant factors that contribute to successful community mental health programs" (Goldstein & Godemont, 2003, p. 441). And in a 2007 article on deinstitutionalization for the mentally ill, the author points out that "the oldest example of community care for mental patients, the historic colony for mental patients in Gheel, Belgium" contains important lessons for contemporary mental health care (Tuntiya, 2007, p. 469).

During the early Middle Ages, the concept of free-standing institutions or hospitals to care for both the mentally and physically ill was beginning to emerge in Christian nursing history. These early facilities were staffed primarily by men and women inspired by religious motives to care for their less fortunate brothers and sisters.

Medieval Hospital Nursing

Augustinian nuns began their attendance at the Hôtel Dieu; for twelve hundred years immured within these walls; alive yet not of this world; aloof from the human race, with the breath of God upon their faces. To and fro they walked the wards, back and forth throughout the days and years and centuries.

—Robinson, 1946, p. 50

Two of the most famous medieval Christian hospitals built outside monastic walls were the Hôtel-Dieu of Lyon (542 A.D.) and the Hôtel-Dieu of Paris (650 A.D.). The title Hôtel-Dieu, or "House of God," was often chosen as the name for a French hospital of the era (Grippando, 1986, p. 10). In the beginning, these "hospitals" served as almshouses and orphanages, as well as facilities for care of the sick. Goodnow (1916) reported that the early nurses in these facilities were "religious women who devoted their lives to charity" (p. 29).

The Hôtel-Dieu of Lyon eventually added to its cadre of women nurses a group of men called "brothers" who also assisted with the care of the sick. The hospital was designed to care for pilgrims, orphans, the poor, and the sick. It was one of the first hospitals to separate those with contagious illnesses from those with more ordinary ills (Nutting & Dock, Vol. 1, 1935).

The Hôtel-Dieu of Paris began as a hostel providing care for a small number of the sick poor. After a brief period, the group of women who had ultimately been constituted as a religious community known as the Augustinian Sisters took over the hospital (Dietz & Lehozky, 1967, p. 25). The Sisters lived under a very strict rule; following profession of religious vows their entire world became the hospital where they both lived and worked with no thought of ever returning home even to visit. The Sisters gave excellent care to the patients; for each the work was her life. As Nutting and Dock (1935) observed, "Their home is the 'Hôtel-Dieu.' From the day of their profession they live and die there" (Vol. 1, p. 296).

Although these early hospitals served the civilian populations until about the 10th century, it was recognized with the undertaking of the Crusades that casualties generated by the wars would overwhelm existing nursing facilities. It was anticipated that following the conflicts large numbers of wounded crusaders would return home weakened and battle scarred, many in need of extensive nursing care. Thus an entirely new cadre of nurses was created whose mission was centered on the care of wounded crusaders; these nursing communities were called the military nursing orders.

Military Nursing Orders

To the Knights Hospitallers of St. John of Jerusalem:

With regard to the hospital which thou hast founded in the city of Jerusalem . . . that House of God . . . shall be placed under the protection of the Apostolic See.

—Bull of Pope Pascal II, February 15, 1113

Out of the 11th-, 12th-, and 13th-century Crusades to the Holy Land came the military nursing orders, orders of men who were committed by their religious ministry to the care of those wounded in battle. The three major groups were the Knights Hospitallers of St. John of Jerusalem, the Teutonic Knights, and the Knights of St. Lazarus. The three general classes of members in the orders were knights, priests, and serving brothers (Kalisch & Kalisch, 1995). The knights participated in the Crusades and helped to care for the injured, the priests served the religious needs in camps and hospitals, and the serving brothers were responsible for general care of the sick (Pavey, 1952, pp. 163–164). All members of the orders, however, professed religious commitment of their lives as exemplified in the Rule of the Order of St. John of Jerusalem, as written by its first grand master, Raymond du Puy:

> Firstly, I ordain that all the brethren engaging in the service of the sick shall keep with God's help the three promises that they have made to God, . . . poverty, chastity, obedience . . . and to live without any property of their own, because God will require of them at the last judgement the fulfillment of these three promises. (Austin, 1957, p. 73)

The largest of the orders, the Knights Hospitallers of St. John of Jerusalem, is thought to have been created around 1050 A.D. to staff the two Jerusalem hospitals organized to care for those wounded in the Crusades: one for men, dedicated to St. John; the other for women, dedicated to St. Mary Magdalene (Seymer, 1949). Historians assert that the order was originated under the guidance of Peter Gerard, a deeply religious man. An associated order for women was also created to nurse the sick, under Agnes of Rome (Jensen, Spaulding, & Cady, 1959). The knights of St. John were characterized by a specific dress: a black robe with white linen cross.

A second community, the German order of Knights Hospitallers or Teutonic Knights, was founded in 1191 A.D. at the time of the Third Crusade. These knights, who followed the rule of the Knights of St. John, taking the usual vows of poverty, chastity, and obedience, also took a vow of care of the sick (Donahue, 1985, p. 155). The Teutonic Knights were in charge of many German hospitals and later became a separate organization under the Rule of St. Augustine (Jensen et al., 1959).

The Knights of St. Lazarus were organized primarily to care for the lepers in Jerusalem; they also admitted lepers to their order. There were two categories of knights: warriors and hospitallers. The latter group had a special commitment to care for those with leprosy. The community's first grand master was himself a leper (Seymer, 1949). It might be suggested here that the military nursing orders of the 11th, 12th, and 13th centuries—which were founded specifically to care for the Crusaders, the soldiers of the day, fallen or injured in battle—were indeed the forebears of contemporary military nurses in this country and throughout the world. Members of the early military nursing orders, as military nurses today, took an oath of obedience and promised a willingness to risk their lives in order to care for those wounded in war (see O'Brien, 2003, "Navy Nurse: A Call to Lay Down My Life").

During the period of the Crusades and afterward, while the military nursing orders cared for those wounded in war, medieval monastics continued to provide nursing care for civilians. Some of these monastic nurses were highly respected and honored for their care and compassion, as well as for their healing powers.

Medieval Religious Community Nursing
Catherine of Siena: Patroness of Nursing

Then in her sacred saving hands
She took the sorrows of the lands,
With maiden palms she lifted up
The sick times blood-embittered cup,
And in her virgin garment furled
The faint limbs of a wounded world,
Clothed with calm love and clear desire
She went forth in her soul's attire,
A missive fire.

—Algernon Swinburne, 1911, p. 162

Historian of nursing James Walsh (1929) poignantly described Catherine of Siena's commitment to the sick poor:

> According to . . . legend, her devotion to the ailing poor was so pleasing to the Master, who had gone about healing the ailing, that she had a number of visits from celestial personages. Above all the Christ Child was so much interested in this young woman, who, when scarcely more than a child, had

insisted on devoting herself to His ailing poor, that He put a ring on her finger as an indication of the fact that she was to be His heavenly spouse. (Walsh, 1929, pp. 121–122)

Catherine of Siena (1347–1380), known to contemporary health-care providers as the "Patroness of Nursing," entered the Tertiaries of St. Dominic while still in her teens. As a Tertiary or "Mantellate," a "Dominican laywoman, Catherine tended terminally ill patients at La Scala Hospital. Many legends of Catherine's generous work evolved around her hospital activities" (Vinje, 1990, p. 21). Biographer Sigrid Undset wrote of her: "Catherine would sometimes spend the night at La Scala Hospital . . . to take over the watch in the small hours, the cold and comfortless hours before dawn when the patient's life is at its lowest ebb and the nurses are worn out and without courage" (1954/2009, p. 71). Undset observed that it was reported that Catherine "gladly took on herself the charge of hopeless cases and the most difficult and ungrateful patients" and that "the good Sisters of La Scala were more than willing to let her take them over as soon as they learned of her indefatigable patience and her unquenchable good humor and serenity" (p. 71).

Catherine died young, at the age of 33, yet during her life she became renowned as a teacher, nurse, and mystic (Sellew & Nuesse, 1946, pp. 129–130). Catherine worked extensively with the ill, especially lepers, and when Siena was overwhelmed with the Black Plague epidemic in 1372, she is said to have "walked night and day in the wards, only resting for a few hours now and then in an adjacent house" (Nutting & Dock, 1935, Vol. I, p. 230).

During the time of the plague it is also reported that Catherine "organized groups of young men as stretcher bearers to transport the stricken from all over the city to the wards of the hospital, which she supervised" (Donahue, 1996, p. 136). Throughout the epidemic historians note that "Catherine could be seen going about the streets of Siena at night. With a lighted lantern she would look for forsaken victims so that she might comfort them" (Dolan et al., p. 72). In a sense, one might view Catherine of Siena as the first "lady with the lamp."

An anecdote is told about an indigent woman of Siena suffering from leprosy who was so diseased that no caregiver, even in the hospital, had the courage to assist her. "When Catherine heard of this . . . she hastened to the hospital, visited the leper, kissed her, and offered not only to supply all her necessities, but also to become her servant during the remainder of her life" (Raymond of Capua, 1853, pp. 93–94). In summarizing St. Catherine's extraordinary commitment to the sick, Blessed Raymond of Capua (1853) wrote, "Catherine was wonderfully compassionate to the wants of the poor, but her heart was even more sensitive to the sufferings of the sick (cited in Austin, 1957, p. 94).

In his classic biography of Catherine of Siena, Raymond of Capua, who was her spiritual director, also wrote that "for those who were ill [Catherine's] pity was unbounded. As a result of this pity, she performed unprecedented labors" (1934/2011, p. 111). In addition to the anecdote told here, Raymond described another case, this one of a woman critically ill with advanced cancer of the breast. Because of the unpleasantness of the disease no one would care for the woman. When Catherine learned of this "she realized that heaven had reserved this unfortunate woman especially for herself, and she immediately went off to see her, comforting her with a kind and cheerful countenance and joyfully offering her services for as long as the illness lasted" (p. 121).

Catherine of Siena truly earned the title "patroness of nursing" for her early commitment to those most in need of nursing care and compassion several centuries before the formal establishment of the profession. She is a teacher and role model for 21st-century nurses facing different, yet nevertheless challenging, patient and family needs.

The Alexian Brothers

It is somewhat difficult to know where to situate the Alexian Brothers' community chronologically in nursing history. This is because the community has a long and magnificent history of caring for the sick from, some sources suggest, the mid-13th century. The Brothers' more formal ministry of nursing the sick, however, seems to have been highlighted during the terrible era of the "Black Plague" that swept Europe during the middle of the 14th century (Dietz & Lehozky, 1967, p. 112; Dolan, 1978, p. 76; Whittock & Leonard, 2003, p. 243). In a comprehensive description of the community, Christopher Kauffman noted: "The plague marks a turning point in the history of the Alexian Brothers" (1976, p. 53). In the previous century the community consisted of a loosely organized group of dedicated laymen caring for the sick poor in a variety of venues. These individuals chose a life of poverty and apostolic service based on the teachings of Christ and the example of the early church. Kauffman reported that while "there is an abundance of documents to verify the pre-plague existence of the "Poor Brothers," the plague seems to have acted as a catalyst in bringing this thoroughly amorphous lay ministry movement into some primitive form of organization" (p. 54).

The nursing literature suggests that after the end of the plague epidemic, the Poor Brothers or "Cellites," as they were sometimes called (Seymer, 1949, p. 46), sought to formally become a religious community, and "in 1431 they became an organized body of religious nurses and adopted the Augustinian Rule, taking vows of poverty, chastity, and obedience (Pavey, 1952, p. 187). With recognition by the Pope in 1472, "the Society adopted St. Alexius Santelli as their patron saint" (Gibba, 1949, p. 29). Alexius is described as a holy man of God who chose to become a humble beggar in order to devote himself to prayer, penance, and care of the sick and the poor.

The history of the Brothers in the United States may be marked by the establishment of the Alexian Brothers' Hospital in Chicago, in 1866, which, Wall observed, confirms "their long tradition of caring for the poor and the destitute" (2009a, p. 159). Early 20th-century American ministries were initiated in such institutions as The Alexian Brothers Hospital School of Nursing, described as "the largest all-male nursing school in the United States" (Dolan, 1978, p. 76); Memorial Hospital and Clinic at Boystown, Nebraska; and The Alexian Brothers Nursing School in St. Louis (Sellew & Nuesse, 1946, p. 287). Notable among the Alexian Brothers' commitments to justice and equal care for all was the community's 1953 decision to desegregate the wards of their Chicago Hospital. This was done, the Brothers asserted, to "better fulfill the objectives of their hospital: 'care for the sick, regardless of color, race, creed or financial status' " (Wall, 2009b, p. 88).

A contemporary model of the Alexian Brothers' continued response to societal needs of the era is Alexian Village of Tennessee (AVT), a "Life Care Community," which provides a home for over 600 of the country's elders needing a place to live and receive care as they age. The Brothers first began to minister to frail elderly men in the mid-20th century. Over time the Village expanded its ministry to admit women as well as men. The 21st-century AVT has developed into a modern, nonprofit life care community housing elders seeking independent living, assisted care, and/or skilled nursing care.

▶ Post-Reformation Nursing: The Catholic and Protestant Nursing Orders

Nurse historian Patricia Donahue (1985) reported that in the 16th century alone "more than 100 female [religious] orders were founded specifically to do nursing" (p. 216). The growth of nursing communities continued, though more slowly, during the 17th, 18th, and 19th centuries, with a few new groups being founded in the early to mid-20th century. Some orders have survived and attained a notable history and tradition in the care of the ill and infirm; others were short-lived with little historical information available about them. For the present exploration, examples of Catholic and Protestant communities with significant historical involvement with nursing and health-care activities are discussed. These groups are the Daughters of Charity of St. Vincent de Paul, the Kaiserswerth Deaconesses, the Nightingale nursing community, and Mary Breckinridge and the Frontier Nursing Service. Although not all are formally constituted as religious orders, groups such as Florence Nightingale and her nursing community, who served in the Crimean War, undertook their work out of spiritual motivation. Briefly described is one other women's religious community that continues to maintain a significant commitment to nursing as a contemporary ministry, the Servants for Relief of Incurable Cancer, also referred to as the Dominican Sisters of Hawthorne, New York.

Daughters of Charity of St. Vincent de Paul

One of the largest and best known of the early religious communities of women are the Daughters of Charity founded in Paris, France, in 1633 by St. Vincent de Paul, in conjunction with St. Louise de Marillac. Some years after ordination to the priesthood, Vincent became concerned about the lack of care for the poor and needy, especially the sick poor, in 17th-century France. His personal spirituality was centered on seeing Christ in the person of the poor; he was much attracted to the Lukan Gospel of Jesus, especially such passages as Luke 4:18. "The Spirit of the Lord . . . has sent me to bring glad tidings to the poor, to proclaim liberty to captives, recovery of sight to the blind. . . ." (Maloney, 1992, p. 14).

In 1617, Vincent began gathering together a band of laity to visit and care for the sick and the poor, naming them the Confraternity of Charity. As some of the women, later named the Ladies of Charity, encountered the overwhelming needs of the sick, both in hospitals where they observed the exhaustion of the overworked Augustinian nuns and in the homes of the poor, they recognized a great need for more nursing Sisters. One of the women, Louise de Marillac, a wealthy widow, was directed by Vincent to become the first leader of the small community. "She would give the Dames de Charité instructions. She accompanied them on their rounds helping them, advising them, assisting them in their duties and making suggestions about other ways of giving care to patients" (Dolan, 1973, p. 100).

The Daughters of Charity were formally established as a religious community dedicated to serving the "poorest of the poor" in 1633. The first Sisters "nursed the sick poor in their homes" as well as caring for patients in the famous Hôtel-Dieu in Paris (Daughters of Charity National Health Services, 1994, p. 1). Many of the early Daughters were young Frenchwomen raised in rural areas. "They wore the French peasant costume, a heavy coarse dress of blue woolen cloth with a full skirt and tight fitting waist, a blue apron of washable material, and a large white linen headdress . . . [T]hey were not nuns but 'pious women of the world' prepared to nurse on the battlefields in time of war or to be sent to care for the sick in any disaster" (Sellew & Nuesse, 1946, pp. 198–199).

Dock and Stewart (1920) noted that St. Vincent de Paul would not let the Daughters pronounce permanent vows; they took vows for one year only, as they do today. The vows can, however, be renewed indefinitely on an annual basis. Vincent's advice to his Sisters "if they were to be useful as nurses, was uncompromising in the extreme: 'My daughters,' he said, 'You are not religious in the technical sense, and if there should be found some marplot among you to say, it is better to be a nun, Ah! Then, my daughters, your company will be ready for extreme unction. Fear this, my daughters, and while you live permit no such change; never consent to it. Nuns must needs have a cloister, but the Daughters of Charity must needs go everywhere" (p. 102). Vincent directed also that the Daughters were to have neither convent nor cell; his emphasis in this regard has been preserved in a well-known quote from the community's rule:

> Your convent will be the house of the sick; your cell, a hired room; your chapel, the parish church; your cloister, the streets of the city, or the wards of the hospital. (Daughters of Charity, 1993)

Stepsis and Liptak (1989) observed that, given the Church's history, in the era of mandating cloistered community life for all women religious "the successful efforts of Saint Vincent de Paul and Saint Louise de Marillac to create and maintain a noncloistered congregation of women in France, during the seventeenth century and beyond . . . were monumental" (p. 18). They added, "Vincent's attempt at bridging the gap between cloistered and active religious community became the American model" (p. 19). A historical overview of Vincent's vision for health care identifies the "essential attributes" as including such characteristics as "spiritually rooted," "holistic," "integrated," "flexible," and "creative" (Sullivan, 1997, p. 49).

Today the Daughters of Charity comprise one of the largest international Catholic religious communities of women in existence, with over 20,000 Daughters worldwide. Daughters of Charity are involved in a variety of ministries with health care, education, and social ministry being the major categories of service.

In the United States, the Daughters of Charity National Health Services (DCNHS) was, in the 20th century, one of the most extensive health-care systems in the world, with Sisters serving primarily in the arenas of administration, nursing, and pastoral care. In addition to ministering in hospitals and nursing homes, the Daughters served the sick poor in settings such as "free clinics in poor neighborhoods in the cities, in rural areas, with migrant workers in the deep south, and in drug treatment centers" (Daughters of Charity, 1995, p. 1).

Kaiserswerth Deaconesses

The Kaiserswerth Deaconesses, an important Protestant community of women with a primary ministry of nursing the sick, was founded by a young Lutheran minister,

Theodor Fliedner, around 1836 in Kaiserswerth, Germany (Kalisch & Kalisch, 1995). Pastor Fliedner, who was concerned about the overall social and health-care needs of his poor parishioners, enlisted his wife, Frederika Munster, to gather a group of women who would visit and nurse the sick poor in their homes. The Fliedners attempted to attract a group of young women of good character; in this era, prior to Florence Nightingale, nurses were generally considered to be prostitutes, alcoholics, and generally unseemly women.

Frank (1953) described the education of the Kaiserswerth Deaconesses. "Their course of training lasted three years, their uniform was simple, and they were taught domestic duties associated with caring for the sick" (p. 95). Nutting and Dock (1935, Vol. 2) quoted Pastor Fliedner's own description of the essentials of the Deaconess vocation. "In organization the work is a free religious association, not dependent on state or church authorities. It takes its stand on the mother nature of the church founded by Christ" (p. 33). The four key branches of the Deaconesses' work were described as "Nursing; relief of the poor; care of children; and work among unfortunate women" (Nutting & Dock, 1935, Vol. 2, pp. 33–34).

In commenting on the Deaconesses' religious commitment, Woolsey (1950) observed, "The Deaconess Vows are taken for five years . . . however, women are expected to declare that they intend to adopt the office of Deaconess for life. Those trained as nurses are more apt . . . to regard [the] vows and retain their connection with the order . . . and the settled resolution, no doubt, is one of the elements that contributes to make them good nurses" (pp. 30–31).

The Kaiserswerth Deaconesses began their work in the United States in 1849 when four deaconesses were sent to Pennsylvania. "They were to assume responsibility for the Pittsburgh Infirmary [Passavant Hospital]. This was the first Protestant Church hospital in the United States" (Dolan, 1973, p. 123). The Pittsburgh infirmary was founded by Lutheran minister William Passavant, a founder of the Lutheran deaconess movement in this country. The American Lutheran Deaconess Foundation continued to grow in the years following Passavant's initiation, spreading to such places as Philadelphia, New York, and Baltimore (Olson, 1992, see "Lutheran Deaconesses in America," pp. 243–339).

The role of the Lutheran deaconess is to "serve God's people through spiritual care and works of mercy" (Concordia University, 1994). Central to diaconal ministry are the concepts of "agape love and love of neighbor" as well as a sense of "mercifulness and community" (Zetterlund, 1997, p. 11). Deaconess roles are encompassed in such professions as nursing, social work, parish ministry, chaplaincy, counseling, and missionary work. A deaconess may serve within a Lutheran Church congregation, she may be employed by a caregiving institution such as a hospital or nursing home, or she may accept a domestic or foreign missionary assignment.

Three Lutheran deaconess communities that provide diaconal education in the United States are the Evangelical Lutheran Deaconess Association community motherhouse at Gladwyne, Pennsylvania; the Center for Diaconal Ministry of the Lutheran Deaconess Association at Valparaiso University, Valparaiso, Indiana; and the Deaconess Program at Concordia University, River Forest, Illinois. Deaconess education programs may vary but generally include the study of theology and ministry as well as liberal arts and courses to prepare the future deaconess for a professional role. A yearlong deacon internship is usually included in the program of study. Following diaconal education, a woman may be consecrated in the role of deaconess within the Lutheran Church.

Nightingale Nurses: Mission to the Crimea

The Nightingale Pledge

I solemnly pledge myself before God and in the presence of this assembly:

To pass my life in purity and to practice my profession faithfully.

I will abstain from whatever is deleterious and mischievous, and will not take or knowingly administer any harmful drug.

I will do all in my power to elevate the standard of my profession, and

will hold in confidence all personal matters committed to my keeping, and all

family affairs coming to my knowledge in the practice of my profession.

With loyalty will I endeavor to aid the physician in his work, and devote

myself to the welfare of those committed to my care.

—as cited in Kalisch & Kalisch, 1995, p. 117

Although, as noted earlier, Florence Nightingale's community (1820–1910) is not considered a religious "order," it was, however, the first Christian community of nurses sent by the English government in 1854 to care for the wounded soldiers during the Crimean War. Nightingale trained under Pastor Fliedner at his Deaconess School in Kaiserswerth, as well as under the Daughters of Charity of St. Vincent de Paul in France. In exploring the historical roots of spirituality in nursing, Patricia Maher observed that prior to the 19th century "there was little beside spiritual care with which to heal. Within an overtly religious society, spiritual care was seen as a formidable and credible endeavor and people were suspicious of medical care for good reason" (2006, p. 419). Florence Nightingale, Maher asserts, "was one of the first nurses to bring spirituality and science together to improve the care of the sick" (p. 419).

Nurse historian Deloughery (1977) offered a glimpse of Nightingale's personal spirituality in reporting that in 1847, "after a busy 'social summer,' . . . she went into retreat for ten days in the convent of the Trinita dei Monti, where she absorbed much of the spirit of the Church and where her religious belief greatly matured" (p. 52). Deloughery added that Nightingale, a member of the Church of England, "remained deeply religious throughout her life" (p. 52). Central to Florence Nightingale's spirituality was her belief in the greatness of God, as the "Spirit of Truth" (Widerquist, 1992, p. 49). Nightingale felt spiritually called to model the greatness and generosity of God in service to the sick; her first experience of this vocational call occurred immediately before her 17th birthday (Selanders, 1993, p. 8). At the age of 24, Florence wrote to her friend and mentor, Dr. Samuel Howe, to ask "if there would be anything unsuitable or unbecoming to a young Englishwoman, if she should devote herself to works of charity in hospitals and elsewhere as the Catholic Sisters do?" Howe replied, "Go forward if you have a 'vocation' for that way of life . . . and God be with you" (Dolan, 1973, p. 167). Florence Nightingale sought to instill her sense of "spiritual vocation" into the team of "Nightingale Nurses" who accompanied her on the Crimean Mission. An excerpt from a work of one of the world's greatest poets is illustrative of the spiritual heritage Nightingale left to the nurses who would follow in her footsteps.

Santa Filomena
Thus thought I as by night I read
of the great army of the dead,
The trenches cold and damp,
The starved and frozen camp.
The wounded from the battle plain,
In dreary hospitals of pain,
The cheerless corridors,
The cold and stony floors.
Lo, in that house of misery,
A lady with a lamp I see
pass through the glimmering gloom
and flit from room to room.
And slow, as in a dream of bliss,
the speechless sufferer turns to kiss
her shadow as it falls,
upon the darkening walls.

—Henry Wadsworth Longfellow, 1857, p. 23

The latter stanza of Longfellow's poem was based on factual reports from wounded soldiers in the Scutari hospital. The young Englishmen described in letters the peace they felt in simply seeing the "Lady with the Lamp"; her shadow falling across one's cot, it was said, brought comfort and relief.*

Professional nursing literature reflects a renewed interest in the spirituality of Florence Nightingale, one example being the 1995 article by Janet Macrae entitled "Nightingale's Spiritual Philosophy and Its Significance for Modern Nursing." In the piece, Macrae reported, "For Nightingale, spirituality is intrinsic to human nature and is our deepest and most potent resource for healing" (p. 8). Macrae also noted Florence Nightingale's attraction to mysticism, particularly the writings of Francis of Assisi and John of the Cross. She cited an excerpt from the preface to Nightingale's own unpublished book on mysticism. "Where shall I find God; In myself. That is the true mystical doctrine. But then I myself must be in a state for Him to come and dwell in me. This is the whole aim of the mystical life" (as cited in Macrae, 1995, p. 10). Ultimately, Macrae argued, Nightingale's spiritual philosophy, which views "spirituality as intrinsic to human nature and compatible with science," may provide important

---

*Longfellow's poem, although entitled "Santa Filomena," has long been considered to have been written for Florence Nightingale; thus her identification throughout history as "the lady with the lamp." Benet (1948) offered an explanation: "Longfellow called Florence Nightingale 'Saint Filomena,' not only because 'Filomena' resembles the Latin word for 'nightingale,' but also because the Saint, in Sabatelli's picture, is represented as hovering over a group of the sick and maimed, healed by her intervention" (p. 970).

direction for the current and future development of nursing theory and practice (p. 8). Similar to nurse theorist Janet Macrae, historian Barbara Dossey also considers Florence Nightingale a mystic, as reflected in her article: "Florence Nightingale: A 19th Century Mystic" (2010). In the paper, Dossey discusses Nightingale's life and nursing ministry in the context of mysticism and compares Florence's attitudes and behaviors to that of three recognized women mystics: Catherine of Siena, Catherine of Genoa, and Teresa of Avila. Dossey concluded that perhaps the reason so many have been "captivated" by Florence Nightingale's life is that "we sense in her the wisdom that is demonstrated by the great mystics throughout history" (p. 26). Nightingale, Dossey pointed out, "shows us that it is possible to honor our spiritual vision and integrate it with the highest standards of nursing practice" (p. 27).

Ultimately, Nightingale felt that "the nurse was to acquire and apply knowledge about God's laws of health and thus move humankind closer to perfection" (Dolamo, 2010, p. 22). Florence Nightingale's spiritual legacy is also advanced for current practitioners of nursing by Ann Bradshaw (1996) who asserted that holistic nursing must include attention to the spiritual needs and concerns of both patient and family as envisioned by Nightingale (p. 42).

Nurse educator Deva-Marie Beck observed that "as a global thinker, Nightingale would have loved the 21st century. She noted cultural, social and economic concerns, particularly in relation to health and to the discipline of nursing. She urged nurses to progress in their practice and to think outside their official domains" (2010, p. 291). Beck asserted, "As we remember and further study the extraordinary panorama that is our Nightingale legacy, we are creating and shaping our relevant, emerging 21st century nursing practice" (p. 291). "Nurses can," Beck added, "like Nightingale, become global visionaries for the health of humanity. As we stand at the crossroads, her light can help us see" (p. 292).

The Frontier Nursing Service: Mary Breckinridge

Surely one of the most important and beloved nursing leaders of the early 20th century was Mary Breckinridge (1881–1965), founder of the Frontier Nursing Service in Hayden, Kentucky, in 1928. After graduating from a basic nursing education program, Mary married and had two children, both of whom died early in life; following these tragedies Mary Breckinridge decided to dedicate her life to the care of children.

At the close of World War I, Mary traveled to France with an American nursing committee seeking to assist those devastated by the occupation. During her stay she became acquainted with a number of British trained nurse midwives and after some consideration, Mary Breckinridge decided to introduce nurse-midwifery to rural areas of America where there was no medical care available for poor mothers and babies. In order to accomplish this goal, Mary moved to London and trained to become a certified English midwife.

At the end of her training, Mary returned to Leslie County, Kentucky, a poverty-stricken rural area of the state where at the time "medical care was virtually nonexistent, with no hospitals and only one licensed physician to serve the entire area" (Raines & Wilson, 1996, p. 124). It was here in 1925 that Mary created the "Kentucky Committee for Mothers and Babies . . . three years later its name would be changed to the 'Frontier Nursing Service'" (McKown, 1966, p. 175).

Mary Breckinridge and her first frontier nurses traveled on horseback to the mountain hollows as there was no other way to reach the mothers and babies in need. Mary and her early frontier nurses visited "hundreds of cabins, delivering babies, providing prenatal care as well as other types of preventive care such as typhoid vaccines, and instructing families in methods to improve the sanitary conditions of their homes" (Raines & Wilson, 1996, p. 125).

Ultimately Miss Breckinridge built her center for frontier nursing in an area near Hayden, Kentucky, and established the first graduate nursing school of midwifery in the country. She had also started a small clinic where seriously ill patients could be cared for; several years later this was replaced by the Hayden Hospital and Health Center. In the hospital Mary commissioned the construction of Saint Christopher's Chapel, containing a stained glass window displaying an image of St. Christopher carrying the Christ child across a stream; the stream, Mary observed was "like ours" (Breckinridge, 1981, p. 362). Mary explained: "If the Frontier Nursing Service had a patron saint, it could be none other than Saint Christopher, on whose help we counted when we carried children on the pommels of our saddles through treacherous fords" (p. 362).

Today Mary Breckinridge's legacy of leadership in frontier nursing lives on in the hearts and spirits of the many nurses who have embraced, and continue to embrace, her vision. While horses have now been replaced by jeeps, and the Hayden Hospital by the more modern Mary Breckinridge Hospital, 21st-century frontier nurses continue to serve disenfranchised families in the rural mountains of Kentucky.

Servants for Relief of Incurable Cancer: Dominican Sisters of Hawthorne

Around the year 1895, the American Roman Catholic Nursing community, the Servants for Relief of Incurable Cancer, now referred to as the Dominican Sisters of Hawthorne, was founded in New York by Rose Hawthorne Lathrop (1851–1926). According to the accounts of her life, Rose Hawthorne had both a good friend and an employee who were afflicted by cancer, resulting in painful and prolonged deaths. Following these experiences, Rose determined to study nursing and to commit her life to caring for the victims of cancer who, in her era, were stigmatized outcasts. After a brief period of training, she and another friend, Alice Huber, opened a free house for those with incurable cancer in New York City (Joseph, 1965).

Robinson (1946) reported that "without distinction of race, or creed, or color or sex, there was only one passport to St. Rose's Free Home: poverty with Cancer" (p. 279). Gradually others came to join the two founders of St. Rose's Home, and Rose Hawthorne Lathrop became Mother Alphonsa, superior of a new community to care for those with incurable cancer. As Robinson (1946) observed, "Mother and the Sisters loved [the patients]; they were outcasts of society because of their terrible affliction, but they were honored guests in the home" (p. 280).

An important point about the work of the community, which also reflects the character of Mother Alphonsa, was made by historian Walsh (1929). "Until her death Mother Alphonsa made it a rule to assume her share of the duty of taking personal care of the patients" (p. 272); she also directed her Sisters to always take a "personal share" in the work of caring for the sick.

In a newsletter, the community of the Servants for Relief of Incurable Cancer (Hawthorne Dominicans) asserted again that "the congregation has one apostolate: to nurse incurable cancer patients, providing them with a free home" where they can end their days (Dominican Sisters, 1994, p. 1). The Dominican Sisters of Hawthorne currently administer three free homes in three different states in the United States.

Since the community's founding by Rose Hawthorne Lathrop, the Sisters have cared for more than 135,000 men, women, and children suffering from cancer. The community's early mission statement asserts, "Middle-class or poor, black or white, Christian or Jew, each finds a home with us where they can spend their precious final days in dignity. We see in each the image of Christ. We minister to each with the same tender care we give our beloved Savior" (Dominican Sisters, 1994, p. 1). To this day the Dominican Sisters of Hawthorne maintain loving and caring homes for patients with incurable cancer who are unable to pay for care; the contemporary skilled-care Dominican homes are located in Hawthorne, New York; Atlanta, Georgia; and Philadelphia, Pennsylvania.

As American society moves into this time of potential health-care reform, the magnificent examples of caring and commitment of pre-Christian and Christian forebears, presented in this chapter, can serve to strengthen the contemporary nurse's sensitivity to the needs of those who are ill, especially the poor and disadvantaged. In such an atmosphere of care for brothers and sisters in need, the spiritual history of the profession will take on new and treasured meaning for those who strive to live a nursing commitment of compassion and love.

▶ References

Austin, A. L. (1957). *History of nursing sourcebook*. New York, NY: C. P. Putnam's Sons.

Ayers, K. (2014). How did Florence Nightingale survive being a trauma coordinator? *Journal of Trauma Nursing, 9*(4), 89–92.

Baly, M. (Ed.). (1991). *As Miss Nightingale said . . . Florence Nightingale through her sayings—A Victorian perspective*. London, UK: Scutari Press.

Beck, D. (2010). Remembering Florence Nightingale's panorama: 21st century nursing at a critical crossroads. *Journal of Holistic Nursing, 28*(4), 291–301.

Benet, W. R. (Ed.). (1948). *The reader's encyclopedia*. New York, NY: Thomas Y. Crowell.

Bradshaw, A. (1996). The legacy of Nightingale. *Nursing Times, 92*(6), 42–43.

Bradshaw, A. (2013). Godamer's two horizons: Listening to the voices in nursing history. *Nursing Inquiry, 20*(1), 82–92.

Breckinridge, M. (1981, published posthumously). *Wide neighborhoods: A story of the Frontier Nursing Service*. Lexington, KY: The University of Kentucky Press.

Bullough, V. L., & Bullough, B. (1969). *The emergence of modern nursing* (2nd ed.). New York, NY: Macmillan.

Bullough, V. L., & Bullough, B. (1987). Our roots: What we should know about nursing's Christian pioneers. *Journal of Christian Nursing, 4*(1), 10–14.

Chatterton, C. (2012). Mental health nursing: An overview of its development. *Journal of Healthcare Assistants, 6*(12), 612–617.

Concordia University. (1994). Just what is a deaconess? *Deaconess Beacon: A Student Publication of the Deaconess Program, 8*(2), 3–4. Retrieved from http://tcmnet.com/ncc/lcms/deaconess/html

Daughters of Charity. (1993). *Daughters of Charity Vocation Program* (Video). Emmitsburg, MD: Author.

Daughters of Charity. (1995). *Reflection of the apostolic works of the province*. Emmitsburg, MD: Author.

Daughters of Charity National Health Services. (1994, September). *Audit Services Newsletter*, 4. Washington, DC: Author.

Deloughery, G. L. (1977). *History and trends of professional nursing.* St. Louis, MO: C. V. Mosby.

Dietz, L. D., & Lehozky, A. R. (1967). *History and modern nursing* (2nd ed.). Philadelphia, PA: F. A. Davis.

Dock, L. L., & Stewart, I. M. (1920). *A short history of nursing.* New York, NY: G. P. Putnam's Sons.

Dolamo, B. (2010). Can one's religion make a nurse a better practitioner? A reflection on Florence Nightingale. *Nursing Update, 34*(4), 22–24.

Dolan, J. A. (1973). *Nursing in society: A historical perspective.* Philadelphia, PA: W. B. Saunders.

Dolan, J. A. (1978). *Nursing in society: A historical perspective* (2nd ed.). Philadelphia, PA: W. B. Saunders.

Dolan, J. A., Fitzpatrick, H. L., & Herrmann, E. K. (1983). *Nursing in society: A historical perspective.* Philadelphia, PA: W. B. Saunders.

Dominican Sisters of Hawthorne. (1994, Fall). *Hawthorne happenings, 1.* Hawthorne, NY: Author.

Donahue, M. P. (1985). *Nursing: The finest art, an illustrated history.* St. Louis, MO: C. V. Mosby.

Donahue, M. P. (1996). *Nursing: The finest art, an illustrated history* (2nd ed.). St. Louis, MO: C. V. Mosby.

Dossey, B. M. (2010). Florence Nightingale: A 19th century mystic. *Journal of Holistic Nursing, 28*(1), 10–35.

Foster Family Care in Gheel. (1991). *Flanders: The Magazine of the Flemish Community, 9,* 15–17.

Frank, C. M. (1953). *Foundations of nursing.* Philadelphia, PA: W. B. Saunders.

George, M. (1964). A way of the cross for nurses. *The Catholic Nurse, 12*(3), 56–58.

Gibba, M. S. (1949). The Alexian Brothers. *RN, 12*(10), 29–30.

Goldstein, J. L., & Godemont, M. L. (2003). The legend and lessons of Gheel, Belgium: A 1500-year-old legend, a 21st century model. *Community Mental Health Journal, 39*(5), 441–447.

Goodnow, M. (1916). *Outlines of nursing history.* Philadelphia, PA: W. B. Saunders.

Gorman, M. R. (1917). *The nurse in Greek life* (Unpublished doctoral dissertation). The Catholic Sisters College of The Catholic University of America, Washington, DC.

Grippando, G. (1986). *Nursing perspectives and issues* (3rd ed.). Albany, NY: Delmar.

Grypma, S. (2012). Historically informed nursing. *Journal of Christian Nursing, 29*(1), 12.

Hawley, W. L. (1954). The lay apostolate in nursing. *The Catholic Nurse, 2*(3), 17–20.

Heyward, M. E. (1939). The Golden Jubilee at The Catholic University School of Nursing.

Hogan, D. (2015). Public health nursing: A rich history. *The Florida Nurse, 9*(10), 10.

Houselander, C. (1955). *The way of the cross.* New York, NY: Sheed & Ward.

Jensen, D. M., Spaulding, J. F., & Cady, E. L. (1959). *History and trends of professional nursing.* St. Louis, MO: C. V. Mosby.

Joseph, Sr. M. (1965). *Out of many hearts: Mother M. Alphonsa Lathrop and her work.* Hawthorne, NY: The Servants for Relief of Incurable Cancer.

Kalisch, P. A., & Kalisch, B. J. (1995). *The advance of American nursing.* Philadelphia, PA: J. B. Lippincott.

Kauffman, C. J. (1976). *Tamers of death: The history of the Alexian Brothers from 1300 to 1789.* New York, NY: The Seaburg Press.

Longfellow, H. W. (1857, November). Santa Filomena. *Atlantic Monthly, 1,* 22–23.

Macrae, J. (1995). Nightingale's spiritual philosophy and its significance for modern nursing. *Image, 27*(1), 8–10.

Maher, P. (2006). Reclaiming spirituality in nursing. In L. Andrist, P. Nicholas, & K. Wolf (Eds.), *A history of nursing ideas* (pp. 417–420). Sudbury, MA: Jones & Bartlett Learning.

Maloney, R. P. (1992). *The way of Vincent de Paul: A contemporary spirituality in the service of the poor.* New Rochelle, NY: New City Press.

Matheussen, H., Morren, P., & Seyers, J. (1975, January). *The state psychiatric hospital: A center for family care in Gheel.* Gheel, Belgium (paper obtained from the Belgian Embassy, Washington, DC).

McKown, R. (1966). *Heroic nurses*. New York, NY: G.P. Putnam's Sons.

Meyer, A. G. (1958). The Catholic nurse: A modern Veronica. *The Catholic Nurse, 7*(1), 45–47.

Miller, M. (1954). Modern Veronicas. *The Catholic Nurse, 2*(3), 20–22.

The nurse's Mass. (1953). *The Catholic Nurse, 2*(2), 53–54.

Nutting, M. A., & Dock, L. L. (1935). *A history of nursing* (Vols. 1–2). New York, NY: G.P. Putnam's Sons.

O'Brien, M. E. (2003). Navy nurse: A call to lay down my life. *Journal of Christian Nursing, 20*(4), 32–33.

O'Brien, M. E. (2006). *The nurse with an alabaster jar: A biblical approach to nursing*. Madison, WI: NCF Press.

Olson, J. E. (1992). *One ministry many roles: Deacons and deaconesses through the centuries*. St. Louis, MO: Concordia.

Pavey, A. E. (1952). *The story of the growth of nursing*. Philadelphia, PA: J. B. Lippincott.

Raines, K. H., & Wilson, A. (1996). Frontier Nursing Service: A historical perspective on nurse-managed care. *Journal of Community Health Nursing, 13*(2), 123–127.

Raymond of Capua. (1853). *Life of St. Catherine of Siena* (Ladies of the Sacred Heart, Trans.). New York, NY: P. J. Kenedy & Sons.

Raymond of Capua. (2011). *The life of St. Catherine of Siena: The classic on her life and accomplishments as recorded by her spiritual director*. Charlotte, NC: TAN Books. (Original work published 1934)

Ridgway, E. (1960). Veronica. *The Catholic Nurse, 12*(3), 67.

Robinson, V. (1946). *White caps: The story of nursing*. Philadelphia, PA: J. B. Lippincott.

Sellew, G., & Nuesse, C. J. (1946). *A history of nursing*. St. Louis, MO: C. V. Mosby.

Seymer, L. R. (1949). *A general history of nursing*. New York, NY: Macmillan.

Stepsis, M., & Liptak, D. A. (1989). *Pioneer healers: The history of women religious in American health care*. New York, NY: Crossroad.

Sullivan, L. (1997). *Vincentian mission in health care*. Emmitsburg, MD: Daughters of Charity National Health System.

Swaffield, L. (1988, September 14). Religious roots. *Nursing Times, 84*(37), 28–30.

Swinburne, A. (1911). *The poems of Algernon Charles Swinburne*. London, UK: Chatto and Windus.

Tuntiya, N. (2007). Free-air treatment for mental patients: The deinstitutionalization debate of the nineteenth century. *Sociological Perspectives, 50*(3), 469–488.

Undset, S. (2009). *Catherine of Siena*. San Francisco, CA: Ignatius Press. (Original work published 1954)

Vinje, P. (1990). *Praying with Catherine of Siena*. Winona, MN: Saint Mary's Press.

Wall, B. M. (2009a). Religion and gender in a men's hospital and school of nursing, 1866–1969. *Nursing Research, 58*(3), 158–165.

Wall, B. M. (2009b). Catholic nursing Sisters and Brothers and racial justice in mid-20th century America. *Advances in Nursing Science, 32*(2), 81–93.

Walsh, J. J. (1929). *The history of nursing*. New York, NY: P. J. Kenedy & Sons.

Whittock, M., & Leonard, L. (2003). Stepping outside the stereotype: A pilot study of the motivations and experiences of males in the nursing profession. *Journal of Nursing Management, 11*(1), 242–249.

Widerquist, J. G. (1992). The spirituality of Florence Nightingale. *Nursing Research, 41*(1), 49–55.

Wilkinson, J. (1998). *The Bible and healing: A medical and theological commentary*. Grand Rapids, MI: Eerdman's.

Woolsey, A. H. (1950). *A century of nursing*. New York, NY: G.P. Putnam's Sons.

Zetterlund, J. (1997). Kaiserswerth revisited: Putting the care back into health care. *Journal of Christian Nursing, 14*(2), 10–13.

CHAPTER 3

Nursing Assessment of Spiritual Needs

The healer has to keep striving for ... the space ... in which healer and patient can reach out to each other as travelers sharing the same broken human condition.

Henri J. M. Nouwen, *Reaching Out*, 1986, p. 93

When you view nursing as a vocation, it helps you to assess the patient as a whole. You know, to really think about what their needs are physically, mentally, and spiritually. You see the whole person and are able to help them better by doing that; by assessing everything that's going on.

Terri, Team Leader on a Pediatric Unit

The first step in planning spiritual care for one who is ill is conducting a needs assessment; this may be done formally in the context of nursing research, or informally through interaction with the patient and family. The ill individual's level of spiritual development and religious tradition and practice are important variables to be explored. In this chapter, tools to assess spiritual and religious beliefs and needs are presented; these tools were developed through nursing research with persons living with a variety of illness conditions. Nursing diagnoses related to alterations in spirituality, derived from patient assessment, are examined, and selected nursing studies in which patients' spiritual and religious beliefs and needs were identified are described.

▶ Nursing Assessment

During the past few decades, nursing assessment of hospitalized patients' problems and needs has become increasingly more sophisticated. Assessment tools vary depending on the care setting, for example, intensive care versus a general care unit; nevertheless, today's nursing assessment instruments are much more detailed than the medical model–oriented database forms of the past. Recently nurses' comfort level in conducting assessment of patients' spiritual needs has also received significant attention (Taylor, 2013, p. 178). Although it is admitted that some nurses may feel uncomfortable or unprepared to discuss spiritual or religious topics with patients (Ameling & Povilonis, 2001; Brush & Daly, 2000), a systematic approach to assessing spiritual well-being (SWB) is recommended (Govier, 2000). In addition to assessing physiologic parameters, caregivers also assess psychological and sociological factors that may impact patients' illness conditions. A significant weakness, however, among many contemporary nursing assessment tools is the lack of evaluation of a patient's spiritual needs. Frequently, the spiritual assessment is reflected in a single question asking the religious affiliation of the individual. The assumption is that the patient's spiritual care can then be turned over to a hospital chaplain assigned to minister to persons of that religious tradition.

Although the important role of the hospital chaplain is in no way devalued, the nurse, if he or she is to provide holistic care, should have first-hand knowledge of the spiritual practices and needs of a patient. If no detailed spiritual assessment is carried out, such information, even if revealed during a chaplain's visit, might never be communicated to the nursing staff. A patient may, however, reveal a spiritual problem or concern in some depth to the primary nurse during an assessment at the bedside. In health-care facilities with well-functioning departments of spiritual ministry, excellent communication often takes place between pastoral caregivers and nursing staff. This is the ideal. In such situations, chaplains attend nursing care conferences and share in holistic health planning for patients. If the nursing staff has performed a spiritual assessment, this information, combined with the chaplain's insight and advice, can serve to round out the spiritual dimension of the holistic health-care plan.

In the contemporary era of home health care, assessment of a patient's spiritual beliefs and needs is also critical to developing a holistic home nursing care plan. Frequently the home care patient experiencing or recuperating from illness is isolated from sources of spiritual support such as attendance at worship services and interaction with other members of a church or faith group. In such a case, the home health-care nurse may be able to assist the patient in verbalizing his or her spiritual or religious needs; the nurse can then offer creative strategies for meeting those needs. The nurse may also provide a bridge between the patient and family and their church, recommending counseling from an ordained pastoral caregiver if this seems warranted.

Nursing authors continue to discuss the importance of assessing patients' spiritual needs (Young & Koopsen, 2011, pp. 149–152), as well as the value of continuing to develop spiritual assessment tools (Power, 2006). The need for spiritual assessment is identified specifically for such populations as intensive care unit (ICU) and coronary care unit (CCU) patients (Timmins & Kelly, 2008) and families of those who are ill (Tanyi, 2006). Assessment of the spiritual needs of terminally ill patients is a current concern for palliative care nurses (Smyth & Allen, 2011).

In light of current understanding of the need to evaluate patients' spiritual concerns, a number of recently developed spiritual assessment tools, appropriate for nurses' use with patient populations, are currently being proposed and tested. Some of these include: the "Hope Tool" (Blaber, Jones, & Willis, 2015); the "Spiritual Health Scale" (Hsiao, Chiang, Lee, & Han, 2013); the "FACIT-SP Spiritual Well-Being Scale" (Haugen, 2014); and the "Two Stage Spiritual Assessment in Health Care Settings" instrument (Hodge, 2015).

▶ The Joint Commission Mandate on Assessment of Spiritual Needs

During the past several decades, The Joint Commission (formerly the Joint Commission for Accreditation of Healthcare Organizations) has recognized the importance of spiritual and religious beliefs and traditions for persons who are ill or disabled. This concern is reflected in The Joint Commission's standards relating to spiritual assessment and spiritual care both for those who are hospitalized (Standard R1.1.3.5) and those living in nursing homes (Standard PE1.1.5.1) (The Joint Commission, 2003). The Joint Commission's standards "reflect the need to recognize and meet the spiritual needs of patients" (Sanders, 2002, p. 107).

The Joint Commission has "acknowledged that patients' psychosocial, spiritual and cultural values affect how they respond to care and has addressed spirituality and emotional well-being as aspects of patient care" (Clark, Drain, & Malone, 2003, p. 659). Standards refer to both spiritual services and pastoral care for health-care patients (p. 659). Care of patients' spiritual needs is now considered central to care provided in health-care organizations, which The Joint Commission recommends "(1) acknowledge patients' rights to spiritual care and (2) provide for these needs through pastoral care and a diversity of services that may be offered by certified, ordained or lay individuals" (La Pierre, 2003, p. 219).

The Joint Commission website suggests that assessment of patients' spiritual needs should be carried out not only to determine religious denomination, but also to identify spiritual and religious beliefs and practices, especially as related to coping with illness or disability. Some questions to be included in a spiritual assessment include: "Who or what provides the patient with strength and hope?"; "Does the patient use prayer in (his/her) life?"; "What type of spiritual/religious support does the patient desire?"; "What does dying mean to the patient?"; "Is there a role of church/synagogue in the patient's life?"; and "How does faith help the patient cope with illness?" (The Joint Commission, 2008).

The importance of the identified Joint Commission standard for the patient's spiritual assessment continues to be supported in contemporary health care–related chapters and articles (Hodge, 2006; Young & Koopsen, 2011). It is now understood that nurses must be involved in patients' spiritual care in the United States as "the Joint Commission (formerly JCAHO) requires spiritual assessment as part of health care" (Pesut, Fowler, Reimer-Kirkham, Taylor, & Sawatzky, 2009, p. 342).

▶ HIPAA Regulations and Spiritual Assessment

As noted, The Joint Commission, which accredits health-care organizations, has essentially mandated that nurses pay attention to patients' spiritual needs. Staff nurses, as members of the health-care team, have access to records for the patients under their care, and thus it seems that the confidentiality dimension (privacy standards) of the Health Insurance Portability and Accountability Act (HIPAA) should not be a concern. The HIPAA regulations may, however, impact patients' spiritual needs/care indirectly by limiting access to patients' personal clergy person or pastoral care provider.

In an article published in the newsletter of the Lutheran Services in America (2004), one pastor complained that since the advent of HIPAA his access to general information about hospitalized parishioners has been limited. He observed that before HIPAA he was "able to provide better pastoral care when [he] could see the entire patient list" (p. 1).

The situation appears to be somewhat different for the minister who is a hospital chaplain. In a series of three articles in consecutive issues of the *Association of Professional Chaplains (APC) News*, the authors raised the topic of HIPAA's impact on hospital chaplains and their clinical pastoral education (CPE) students (White, 2003; White & Pierce, 2002a, 2002b). The conclusion seemed to be that patient records would be available and accessible to these pastoral care providers as they were, in fact, clinically trained members of the health-care team with responsibility for patients' spiritual care. A distinction in title was suggested by the president and CEO of the National Association of Catholic Chaplains (NACC) as follows: "The chaplain is a health care professional; the clergyperson is a religious leader; the chaplain tends to the spiritual needs of all the patients; the clergyperson tends to the religious needs of his or her congregants" (Driscoll, 2003, p. 4). Thus, it seems that a pastoral care provider's role description might significantly impact his or her access to patient records as controlled by HIPAA regulations.

Spiritual Development

Central to assessing a patient's spirituality is a basic knowledge of the spiritual development of the human person. A number of theories attempt to track spiritual development; significant among these is James Fowler's (1981) paradigm set forth in his book *Stages of Faith Development*. Fowler's theory, encompassing seven stages of faith development, emerged from data generated from research with persons across the life span from 3.5 to 84 years of age.

Fowler (1981) described faith as "not always religious in its content or context" (p. 4). He explained that faith has to do with one's finding coherence in life, with seeing oneself in relation to others "against a background of shared meaning and purpose" (p. 4). Faith is viewed as deeper and more personal than organized religion, as relating to one's transcendent values and relationship with a higher power, or God. Although Fowler admitted that more research needs to be done, his work demonstrated a preliminary pattern of relationships between the stages of faith development and chronological age. Fowler's seven faith stages and their approximate corresponding age categories are as follows:

1. Undifferentiated Faith is a "prestage" (infancy) in which the seeds of trust, courage, hope, and love are joined to combat such issues as possible "inconsistency and abandonment in the infant's environment" (p. 121). This faith stage has particular relevance for the maternal–infant nurse concerned with issues of parental–infant bonding.
2. Intuitive–Projective Faith (3–6 years) is an imitative "fantasy-filled" period in which a young child is strongly influenced by "examples, moods, actions and stories of the visible faith of primarily related adults" (p. 133). Pediatric nurses, especially those working with chronically or terminally ill children, will find guidance for dealing with the child's spiritual and emotional needs from Fowler's conceptualization of this stage.

3. Mythic–Literal Faith (7–12 years) is described as the time when the child begins to internalize "stories, beliefs and observances that symbolize belonging to his or her own faith community" (p. 149). In working with slightly older pediatric patients, the concept of mythic–literal faith can help the nurse to support the child's participation in rites, rituals, and/ or worship services of his or her tradition, which may provide support and comfort in illness.

4. Synthetic–Conventional Faith (13–20 years) describes the adolescent's experiences outside the family unit: at school, at work, with peers, and from the media and religion. Faith provides a "basis for identity and outlook" (p. 172). Fowler's definition of this faith stage provides an understanding of how the ill adolescent may relate to both internal (family) and external (peer) support and interaction during a crisis situation.

5. Individuative–Reflective Faith (21–30 years) identifies a period during which the young adult begins to claim a faith identity no longer defined by "the composite of one's roles or meanings to others" (p. 182). This is a time of personal creativity and individualism that has important implications for the nurse, including patient autonomy in planning care for the ill young adult patient.

6. Conjunctive Faith (31–40 years) is a time of opening to the voices of one's "deeper self" and the development of one's social conscience (p. 198). Nurses caring for patients in this faith stage must be sensitive to the adult's more mature spirituality, especially in relation to finding meaning in his or her illness.

7. Universalizing Faith (40 years and above) is described by Fowler as a culmination of the work of all of the previous faith stages, a time of relating to the "imperatives of absolute love and justice" toward all humankind (p. 200). Nurses need to be aware that patients may vary significantly in terms of degree of accomplishing the imperatives of this final stage. Assessing approximately where the mature adult patient is, related to such faith, will help in understanding both the patient's response to an illness condition and his or her need for external support in coping with the crisis.

Although a nurse may not be able to identify every patient's stage of faith development chronologically, Fowler's theory with its approximate age-associated categorization does present some guidelines to assist in broadly estimating a patient's level of spiritual development.

▶ Nursing Assessment of Spiritual Needs

The Spiritual Assessment Scale

In their fundamentals of nursing text, Taylor, Lillis, and LeMone (1993) asserted that assessment of a patient's spirituality should be considered part of any "comprehensive nursing history" because, they reasoned, "a person's spirituality and religious beliefs have the potential to influence every aspect of being" (p. 1173). Although an initial spiritual assessment or history can provide baseline information regarding a patient's spirituality, it is important to remember that spiritual needs may change, or new spiritual concerns may arise during an illness experience. And, because a patient may find it difficult to discuss spiritual problems, the nurse is advised to look for signs of possible spiritual distress such as "sudden changes in spiritual practices [rejection, neglect, fanatical devotion]; mood changes [frequent crying, depression, apathy, anger]; sudden interest in spiritual matters [reading religious books or watching religious programs on television, visits to clergy]; and disturbed sleep" (p. 1174).

Nurse researchers Sessanna, Finnell, Undershill, Chang, and Peng (2011) assert that "Assessing spiritual needs and preferences is an essential and critical aspect of holistic and multidisciplinary patient care practice" (p. 1692). The authors admit, however, that "conceptual and operational definitions of spirituality vary greatly among nursing and health related literature" (p. 1692). They found that the concept of "religiosity" was often included in the ostensible measuring of "spirituality."

One set of questions describing a patient's spirituality that may be included as part of a nursing history are those contained in the spiritual history guide developed by Ruth Stoll (1979). The guide is divided into four subsections or "areas of concern": "The person's concept of God or deity; the person's source of strength and hope; the significance of religious practices and rituals to the person; and the person's perceived relationship between his spiritual beliefs and his state of health" (p. 1574). Some standardized spiritual assessment tools created by nurses include the Spiritual Perspective Scale, which measures adult spiritual views (Reed, 1991); Kerrigan and Harkulich's (1993) Spiritual Assessment Tool, developed to identify the spiritual needs of nursing home residents; the JAREL Spiritual Well-Being Scale, a tool to assess the spiritual attitudes of older adults (Hungelmann, Kenkel-Rossi, Klassen, & Stollenwerk, 1996); Puchalski's (2000) "Spiritual History," which includes four domains: "Faith, Importance, Community, and Address" (p. 129); the multidimensional "Spiritual Needs Survey," which includes seven major constructs: "belonging, meaning, hope, the sacred, morality, beauty, and acceptance of dying" (Galek, Flannelly, Vane, & Galek, 2005, p. 62); the spiritual assessment model, including focus on one's "spiritual belief system, personal spirituality, integration/involvement in a spiritual community, ritualized practices and restrictions, implications for care and terminal events planned (advanced directives)" (Dameron, 2005, p. 16); the "Serenity Scale," which measures spirituality and well-being and has three subscales that explore "acceptance, inner haven and trust" (Kreitzer, Gross, Waleekhachonloet, Reilly-Spong, & Byrd, 2009); and the "Spiritual Care Inventory," which measures nurses' attitudes toward and behaviors in providing patients' spiritual care (Burkhart, Schmidt, & Hogan, 2011).

The author's standardized instrument to assess adult, cognitively aware individuals' spiritual beliefs and practices, entitled the "Spiritual Assessment Guide," was initially developed and published in 1982 (O'Brien, 1982a, pp. 99–102). The 53-item tool contained six subscales: General Spiritual Beliefs, Personal Spiritual Beliefs, Identification with Institutionalized Religion, Spiritual/Religious Support Systems, Spiritual/Religious Rituals, and Spiritual Deficit/Distress. Items contained in the instrument were derived from content analysis of qualitative data generated in interviews with 126 chronically ill hemodialysis patients. The patients had been asked to discuss their spiritual beliefs, practices, concerns, and needs in relation to living with a long-term life-threatening illness. It was admitted at the time of construction that this early version of the tool, which contains a mix of both closed- and open-ended questions, was more detailed than appropriate for nursing use in short-term care but could prove valuable in nursing research on the spiritual beliefs and behaviors of the chronically ill patient.

During the past two decades, the Spiritual Assessment Guide has been revised several times and selected items were used in research with such populations as nursing home residents (O'Brien, 1989), persons living with human immunodeficiency virus (HIV) and acquired immunodeficiency syndrome (AIDS) (O'Brien, 1992, 1995; O'Brien & Pheifer, 1993), and the homebound elderly (Brennan, 1994).

The Spiritual Assessment Guide has recently been significantly revised again and retitled the Spiritual Assessment Scale (SAS). The standardized instrument, which measures the construct of SWB, now contains 21 items organized into three subscales: Personal Faith (PF), 7 items; Religious Practice (RP), 7 items; and Spiritual Contentment (SC), 7 items. In its newly abbreviated form, the SAS, which takes approximately 3 to 4 minutes to complete, can be used by practicing nurses in the health-care setting, as well as being employed as a research instrument. The tool, as revised, will provide nursing staff and nurse researchers with a broad overview of a patient's personal faith beliefs, the type of spiritual support he or she receives from religious practices, and the type and degree of spiritual contentment/distress the patient is currently experiencing. The 21-item scale is organized with Likert-type scale response categories (SA—Strongly Agree, A—Agree, U—Uncertain, D—Disagree, SD—Strongly Disagree) following each item to facilitate administration; the appropriate categories may be checked by the patient or read aloud and marked by the nurse if a patient is unable to write.*

Validity and Reliability of the SAS

The construct measured by the SAS, SWB, includes the dimensions of both spirituality and religiousness, or "religiosity," operationally defined in terms of three discrete concepts: Personal Faith, Religious Practice, and Spiritual Contentment.

Spiritual Well-Being

The term *spiritual well-being* is described historically as having emerged following a 1971 White House Conference on Aging. Sociologist of religion David Moberg (1979) identified SWB as relating to the "wellness or health of the totality of the inner resources of people, the ultimate concerns around which all other values are focused, the central philosophy of life that guides conduct, and the meaning-giving center of human life which influences all individual and social behavior" (p. 2). The concept of hope is central to a number of definitions of SWB. In a discussion of holistic nursing care, SWB is described as "an integrating aspect of human wholeness, characterized by meaning and hope" (Clark, Cross, Deane, & Lowry, 1991, p. 68). Lindberg, Hunter, and Kruszewski (1994) included "the need to feel hopeful about one's destiny" (p. 110) in a litany of patient needs related to SWB; and Droege (1991), in discussing the "faith factor" in healing, suggested that when an individual does not experience SWB, serious "spiritual maladies" may occur, such as "depression, loneliness, existential anxiety and meaninglessness" (p. 13).

---

*The Spiritual Assessment Scale does assume belief in a Supreme Being, or God.

Most notions of SWB also contain some reference to philosophy of life and transcendence. Blaikie and Kelson (1979) described SWB as "that type of existential well being which incorporates some reference to the supernatural, the sacred or the transcendental" (p. 137); and Barker (1979) observed that SWB is "to be in communication, in communion with that which goes beyond oneself in order to be whole in oneself" (p. 154). For the Christian, SWB is identified as "a right relationship of the person to God, and, following that, a right relationship to neighbor and self" (Christy & Lyon, 1979, p. 98).

Spirituality is generally identified as being related to issues of transcendence and ultimate life goals. Nurse theorist Barbara Dossey (1989) explained spirituality as encompassing "values, meanings, and purpose" in life; it includes belief in the existence of a "higher authority"; and it may or may not involve "organized religion" (p. 24). O'Brien (1989), in reporting on research with the chronically ill, suggested that spirituality is a broad concept relating to transcendence [God]; to the "non-material forces or elements within man [or woman]; spirituality is that which inspires in one the desire to transcend the realm of the material" (p. 88).

Religiousness, or "religiosity," as it is sometimes identified in the sociological literature, refers to religious affiliation and/or practice. Kaufman (1979) described religiousness as "the degree to which religious beliefs, attitudes and behaviors permeate the life of an individual" (p. 237). In their classic work, Stark and Glock (1968) identified five primary elements of religiousness: belief, religious practice (ritual, devotional), religious experience, religious knowledge, and consequence of religious practice on day-to-day living.

The "spirituality" dimension of SWB is measured in terms of the concepts of Personal Faith and Spiritual Contentment; the "religiousness" element of the construct is reflected in the concept of Religious Practice.

▶ Personal Faith

Personal faith, as a component concept of the SWB construct, has been described as "a personal relationship with God on whose strength and sureness one can literally stake one's life" (Fatula, 1993, p. 379). Personal faith is a reflection of an individual's transcendent values and philosophy of life.

Religious Practice

Religious practice is primarily operationalized in terms of religious rituals such as attendance at formal group worship services, private prayer and meditation, reading of spiritual books and articles, and/or the carrying out of such activities as volunteer work or almsgiving.

Spiritual Contentment

Spiritual contentment, the opposite of spiritual distress, is likened to spiritual peace (Johnson, 1992), a concept whose correlates include "living in the now of God's love," "accepting the ultimate strength of God," knowledge that all are "children of God," knowing that "God is in control," and "finding peace in God's love and forgiveness" (pp. 12–13). When an individual reports minimal to no notable spiritual distress, he or she may be considered to be in a state of "spiritual contentment."

Construct Validity of the SAS

In research with young adults, Moberg (1979) identified eight correlates or characteristics of SWB: Peace with God (PG), Inner Peace (IP), Faith in Christ (God) (FG), Good Morals (GM), Faith in People (FP), Helping Others (HO), Good Health (GH), and Being Successful (BS) (p. 8). Moberg reported that study participants placed greatest importance on the concepts Peace with God, Inner Peace, and Faith in Christ. The majority of respondents believed that Good Health and Being Successful were not critical elements to SWB. Those persons, however, who did not seem to possess SWB were reported as being "more likely to interpret these [health and success] as essential or most likely to be present" with overall SWB (p. 9).

The SAS, developed to assess SWB, was constructed to broadly reflect Moberg's eight correlates. In some cases a liberal interpretation of the characteristic was accepted; for example, Faith in Christ is understood also as Faith in God, to include the tradition of the non-Christian believer; Good Health, which Moberg described as physical, may also include good mental health, for the person whose body is suffering the ravages of illness; and Being Successful may relate to an individual's positive feeling about self related to the strength of his or her spiritual beliefs.

The SAS items relate to Moberg's conceptualization of SWB as follows: Peace with God—item 2; Inner Peace—items 13, 14; Faith in God/Christ—items 1, 3, 5, 6; Good Morals—items 8, 9; Faith in People—items 7 (also GH), 11, 12; Helping Others—item 10; Good Health—item 7 (also FP); Being Successful—item 4.[*]

Construct validity of the SAS is also derived, in part, from the association of individual items with James Fowler's (1981) conceptualization of the stages of faith development (p. 113), proceeding from the prestage, infancy (Undifferentiated Faith), to the late adult stage (Universalizing Faith):Prestage (trust, courage, hope, and love): items 3, 6

Stage 1 (child learns examples of faith from related adults): items 11, 12

Stage 2 (internalization of stories of one's own faith community): items 1, 4

Stages 3 and 4 (religious faith as a basis for identity and world outlook): items 2, 5

Stage 5 (conjunctive faith): items 7, 13, 14

Stage 6 (universalizing faith; one recognizes imperatives of love and justice toward all humankind): items 8, 9, 10[*]

---

[*]SAS items 15–21 assessing spiritual contentment/spiritual distress explore negative or lack of negative experiences associated with Moberg's correlates of Inner Peace and Faith in God.

[*]SAS items 15–21 assessing spiritual contentment/spiritual distress explore negative or lack of negative experiences associated with Fowler's stages of faith development; focus is placed especially on internalization of trust and hope (stage 1) and the development of one's personal reflective faith (stage 5).

Content Validity of the SAS

Content validity of the SAS was established through submission of the revised items to a panel of experts in the area of spirituality and health/illness. Following the expert judges' review, certain tool items were modified and/or reworded.

Reliability of the SAS

Reliability of the newly revised 21-item SAS was determined through administration to a sample population of 179 chronically ill persons who agreed to respond to the tool items for the purpose of statistical analysis.

The sample group, employed for the purpose of establishing instrument reliability, consisted of 36 men and 143 women. One hundred thirty-eight members of the group (76 percent) were Roman Catholic; 34 were Protestant; 3 were Jewish; and 4 identified no specific religious belief system. Sixty-three persons attended church services weekly; 26 individuals attended daily church services; and 6 persons reported never going to church or synagogue. The mean age of the sample group was 49 years, with ages ranging from 19 to 89. Seventy-seven persons were single; 79 individuals were married. The participants were well educated, with 70.3 percent reporting some level of college education; the range was from 16.2 percent with 2 years of college or AA degrees to 5 percent who had achieved an MD or PhD.

Selected occupations of the sample group members included physician, nurse, teacher, social worker, secretary, pastoral minister, nursing aide, counselor, engineer, chaplain, and speech pathologist. Some examples of the chronic illnesses reported by the study population, as categorized by body system, included gastrointestinal—ulcer, gastroesophageal reflux disease (GERD), colitis, esophageal cancer, colorectal cancer; genitourinary—end-stage renal disease (ESRD), nephritis, polycystic kidneys; cardiovascular—hypertension, rheumatic heart disease, prolapsed mitral valve, pernicious anemia; respiratory—chronic obstructive pulmonary disease (COPD), asthma, lung cancer, emphysema; neurologic—brain cancer, epilepsy; musculoskeletal—osteoarthritis, osteoporosis, arthritis, multiple sclerosis; gynecological—uterine cancer, breast cancer, ovarian tumors, herpes; psychiatric—chronic depression, bipolar disease, transient amnesia, bulimia/anorexia.

Statistical reliability was calculated for a sample of 171 cases (11 cases were deleted because of missing data). Items 15–21, comprising a subscale measuring the degree of spiritual distress, were recorded in the opposite direction to reflect the concept of Spiritual Contentment.

Cronbach's alpha coefficients for the overall SAS and the subscales Personal Faith (PF), Religious Practice (RP), and Spiritual Contentment (SC) demonstrated statistically significant reliability for the instrument, both in regard to the overall tool and its subscales as examined individually:

SPIRITUAL ASSESSMENT SCALE (SAS)—21 ITEMS
   Alpha coefficient = 0.92
Personal Faith (PF)—7 items
   Alpha coefficient = 0.89
Religious Practice (RP)—7 items
   Alpha coefficient = 0.89
Spiritual Contentment (SC)—7 items
   Alpha coefficient = 0.76

Mean total scale and subscale scores reflected a sample population with a strongly positive sense of SWB. The overall mean SAS score was 91.7, out of a possible total scale score of 105. The subscales reflected a similar pattern with a PF subscale mean of 32.2 (possible total subscale score of 35); and RP and SC subscale means of 29.7 and 29.6, respectively (possible total scores of 35 for each subscale).

Spiritual Assessment Scale

Instructions: Please check the response category that best identifies your personal belief about the item (response categories: SA—Strongly Agree; A—Agree; U—Uncertain; D—Disagree; SD—Strongly Disagree).

A. Personal Faith
1. There is a Supreme Being, or God, who created humankind and who cares for all creatures.
    SA _____ A _____ U _____ D _____ SD _____
2. I am at peace with God.
    SA _____ A _____ U _____ D _____ SD _____
3. I feel confident that God is watching over me.
    SA _____ A _____ U _____ D _____ SD _____
4. I receive strength and comfort from my spiritual beliefs.
    SA _____ A _____ U _____ D _____ SD _____
5. I believe that God is interested in all the activities of my life.
    SA _____ A _____ U _____ D _____ SD _____
6. I trust that God will take care of the future.
    SA _____ A _____ U _____ D _____ SD _____
7. My spiritual beliefs support a positive image of myself and of others, as members of God's family.
    SA _____ A _____ U _____ D _____ SD _____

B. Religious Practice
8. Belonging to a church or faith group is an important part of my life.
    SA _____ A _____ U _____ D _____ SD _____
9. I am strengthened by participation in religious worship services.
    SA _____ A _____ U _____ D _____ SD _____
10. I find satisfaction in religiously motivated activities other than attending worship services, for example, volunteer work or being kind to others.
    SA _____ A _____ U _____ D _____ SD _____
11. I am supported by relationships with friends or family members who share my religious beliefs.
    SA _____ A _____ U _____ D _____ SD _____
12. I receive comfort and support from a spiritual companion, for example, a pastoral caregiver or friend.
    SA _____ A _____ U _____ D _____ SD _____
13. My relationship with God is strengthened by personal prayer.
    SA _____ A _____ U _____ D _____ SD _____
14. I am helped to communicate with God by reading or thinking about religious or spiritual things.
    SA _____ A _____ U _____ D _____ SD _____

C. Spiritual Contentment
15. I experience pain associated with my spiritual beliefs.
SA _____ A _____ U _____ D _____ SD _____
16. I feel "far away" from God.
SA _____ A _____ U _____ D _____ SD _____
17. I am afraid that God might not take care of my needs.
SA _____ A _____ U _____ D _____ SD _____
18. I have done some things for which I fear God may not forgive me.
SA _____ A _____ U _____ D _____ SD _____
19. I get angry at God for allowing "bad things" to happen to me, or to people I care about.
SA _____ A _____ U _____ D _____ SD _____
20. I feel that I have lost God's love.
SA _____ A _____ U _____ D _____ SD _____
21. I believe that there is no hope of obtaining God's love.
SA _____ A _____ U _____ D _____ SD _____

▸ Nursing Diagnoses: Alterations in Spiritual Integrity

Nursing diagnoses are currently used in selected health-care facilities to label those patient conditions whose treatment falls within the purview of the nurse. From early in the nursing diagnosis movement, spiritual issues have been addressed with such diagnoses as "alterations in faith" (Gebbie, 1976; Gebbie & Lavin, 1975) and "nursing diagnoses related to spiritual distress" (Campbell, 1978). This concern for the identification of patients' spiritual needs and deficits has continued among contemporary theorists of nursing diagnosis. The nursing diagnosis "high risk for spiritual distress related to confrontation with the unknown" was described by Holloway (1993). Two other diagnoses related to faith beliefs, "potential for spiritual well-being" and "spiritual distress," were identified in 1994 by the North American Nursing Diagnosis Association (Brennan, 1994, p. 852). The potential for SWB is associated with "the process of an individual's developing an unfolding of mystery through harmonious interconnections that spring from inner strength"; "spiritual distress is a disruption of the life principle that pervades a person's entire being and that integrates and transcends one's biological and physiological nature" (Brennan, 1994, p. 852). A recently advanced nursing diagnosis for human response in the domain of spirituality is that of "enhanced spirituality" (Cavendish et al., 2000).

As contemporary nurses become more involved with diagnosis and intervention in the spiritual arena, some basic knowledge of the beliefs and behaviors associated with the major religious cultures is essential (Engebretson, 1996). This information will allow nurses to accurately identify and address significant spiritual needs and problems exhibited or reported by their patients.

Seven nursing diagnoses related to "alterations in spiritual integrity," which were identified from the author's research (O'Brien, 1982a) on spirituality and life-threatening illness, include:

"Spiritual Pain, as evidenced by expressions of discomfort or suffering relative to one's relationship with God; verbalization of feelings of having a void or lack of

spiritual fulfillment, and/or a lack of peace in terms of one's relatior
ator" (O'Brien, 1982a, p. 106). A terminally ill patient, experienci
pain," may verbalize a fear that he or she has not lived "according
concern is exacerbated as the possibility of imminent death appre

"Spiritual Alienation, as evidenced by expressions of loneliness, or the teeuug
that God seems very far away and remote from one's everyday life; verbalization that
one has to depend upon oneself in times of trial or need; and/or a negative attitude
toward receiving any comfort or help from God" (O'Brien, 1982a, p. 106). Often, a
chronically ill person expresses frustration in terms of closeness to God during sickness; the comment may be heard: "Where is God when I need Him most?"

"Spiritual Anxiety, as evidenced by an expression of fear of God's wrath and
punishment; fear that God might not take care of one, either immediately or in the
future; and/or worry that God is displeased with one's behavior" (O'Brien, 1982a,
p. 106). Some cultural groups entertain a concept, although not held by all members
of the culture, that illness may be a "punishment" from God for real or imagined
faults or failures.

"Spiritual Guilt, as evidenced by expressions suggesting that one has failed to do
the things which he or she should have done in life, and/or done things which were
not pleasing to God; articulation of concerns about the 'kind' of life one has lived"
(O'Brien, 1982a, p. 106). Certain individuals, especially those schooled in more fun-
damentalist religious traditions, experience "guilt" related to their perceived failure to
follow God's will, as they understand it. This "guilt" frequently is exacerbated during
times of physical or psychological illness.

"Spiritual Anger, as evidenced by expressions of frustration, anguish or outrage
at God for having allowed illness or other trials; comments about the 'unfairness' of
God; and/or negative remarks about institutionalized religion and its ministers or
spiritual caregivers" (O'Brien, 1982a, p. 107). Family members of those who are ill
may express anger at God for allowing a loved one to suffer.

"Spiritual Loss, as evidenced by expression of feelings of having temporarily lost or
terminated the love of God; fear that one's relationship with God has been threatened;
and/or a feeling of emptiness with regard to spiritual things" (O'Brien, 1982a, p. 107).
A sense of "spiritual loss" may frequently be associated with psychological depression;
for an individual who feels useless and powerless, there may also be a resultant feeling
of alienation from anything or any person perceived as good, such as God.

"Spiritual Despair, as evidenced by expressions suggesting that there is no hope
of ever having a relationship with God, or of pleasing Him; and/or a feeling that
God no longer can or does care for one" (O'Brien, 1982a, p. 107). Although spiritual despair is generally rare among believers, such a diagnosis may be associated
with serious psychiatric disorders. If such thoughts or feeling are expressed by a
patient, the nurse needs to be alerted, also, to the potential for suicidal ideation or
possible behavior.

▶ Spirituality and Nursing Research

Although clinical nursing research efforts in the area of spirituality and nursing practice
have not been extensive, some nurse investigators have addressed the spiritual needs of
particular patient groups. Examples include Soeken and Carson (1987), "Responding
to the Spiritual Needs of the Chronically Ill"; Clifford and Gruca (1987), "Facilitating

̣piritual Care in the Rehabilitation Setting"; Reed (1991), "Preferences for Spiritually Related Nursing Interventions Among Terminally Ill and Nonterminally Ill Hospitalized Adults and Well Adults"; Toth (1992), "Faith in Recovery: Spiritual Support After an Acute M.I."; Highfield (1992), "Spiritual Health of Oncology Patients"; Mickley, Soeken, and Belcher (1992), "Spiritual Well-Being, Religiousness, and Hope Among Women with Breast Cancer"; Harris et al. (1995), "The Role of Religion in Heart-Transplant Recipients' Long-Term Health and Well-Being"; Smith (1995), "Power and Spirituality in Polio Survivors: A Study Based on Roger's Science"; Twibell, Wieseke, Marine, and Schoger (1996), "Spiritual and Coping Needs of Critically Ill Patients: Validation of Nursing Diagnoses"; and Post-White et al. (1996), "Hope, Spirituality, Sense of Coherence, and Quality of Life in Patients with Cancer."

Nursing studies, especially those in the arena of chronic illness, have frequently included the concepts of spirituality, religion, and/or religiosity (religious practice) as key variables in a larger matrix. Some examples include the author's research with chronic renal failure (CRF) patients, migrant farmworkers, nursing home residents, and persons living with HIV infection and AIDS. Brief examples of the studies are described here; more detailed qualitative data elicited in the research can illustrate instances of spiritual need and spiritual care.

Study Title: Religious Faith and Adaptation to Maintenance Hemodialysis

The purpose of this study was to examine the relationship between religious faith and adaptation to chronic renal failure and its treatment regimen of maintenance hemodialysis. The religious faith question represented one variable in a multivariate study of adaptation to renal disease and dialysis. The study subjects consisted of 126 adult hemodialysis patients who were interviewed first to obtain baseline data and again in a three-year follow-up, when 63 of the original sample were identified (O'Brien, 1982c, p. 75).

Study Title: Spirituality and Health Beliefs and Practices of Migrant Farmworkers

The research consisted of an exploratory descriptive qualitative study of the overall health attitudes and behaviors of a sample group of Mexican American migrant farmworkers. Central to the study was an examination of the spirituality and religious beliefs of the population, as related to health/illness beliefs and practices. The methods of data collection were observation and focused interview. During the three-month data collection phase of the study, the investigator attended many of the group's religious services and rituals, including weekly Spanish Masses, evening Mass in migrant camps, Baptisms, First Communion services, a Mass of departure as the migrants moved from one work setting to another, and a "coming of age" religious service for a teenage girl. The author visited several Mexican American religious shrines and interviewed three practitioners of folk religion/medicine. Focused interviews were also conducted with 125 adult migrant workers in three Midwestern states (O'Brien, 1982b, p. 13).

Study Title: Spiritual Beliefs and Behaviors of the Institutionalized Elderly

The purpose of this exploratory case study, conducted over a two-year period, was to examine and describe the overall institutional nursing home setting, as well as the patterns of attitude and behavior exhibited by the residents, family members, medical and nursing caregivers, and ancillary staff. A key variable of interest was spirituality, or the spiritual perceptions, attitudes, behaviors, and needs of the residents. The nursing home studied was a 230-bed residential facility that provided three levels of care: skilled, semiskilled, and domiciliary. The author collected data by means of direct and participant observation, as well as through focused interviews with staff, family members, and 71 alert and cognitively aware residents (62 women and 9 men). Variables of particular interest related to the spiritual/religious attitudes, experiences, and practices of the residents. Selected data on religion and spirituality are presented as excerpted from verbatim interview transcripts (O'Brien, 1989, p. 47).

Study Title: Religious Faith and Living with HIV Infection

Personal faith beliefs, as well as the support of an individual's church group or religious denomination, were examined in a study of coping response in HIV infection. The overall aim of the longitudinal project was to establish a database of physical, psychosocial, and spiritual needs associated with HIV infection, from which appropriate caregiving strategies could be derived. The study population consisted initially of 133 men and 3 women, all of whom were categorized within the CDC IV classification: "Constitutional Disease, Secondary Infections, Secondary Cancers, or Other Conditions Related to HIV Infection." A number had diagnoses of AIDS. A subgroup of 41 men with HIV/AIDS was followed over a five-year period, as long-term survivors of the infection. Data were collected by both quantitative (interview schedule) and qualitative (tape-recorded focused interview) measures. Data on the relationship of religion and spirituality revealed the importance of personal faith beliefs and church affiliation in coping with HIV (O'Brien, 1992, 1995).

Although not all nurses may or must feel comfortable in providing spiritual care, the assessment of a patient's spiritual needs is a professional responsibility. Contemporary holistic health care mandates attention to the problems and concerns of the spirit as well as to those of the body and mind. In carrying out an assessment of the patient's SWB, a nurse may glean information important to supporting the medical and nursing therapies planned for the ill person. Following a spiritual assessment, appropriate spiritual or religious interventions may be provided either by the nurse or through referral to a designated pastoral caregiver.

▶ References

Ameling, A., & Povilonis, M. (2001). Spirituality, meaning, mental health and nursing. *Journal of Psychosocial Nursing & Mental Health Services, 39*(4), 15–20.

Barker, E. (1979). Whose service is perfect freedom. In D. O. Moberg (Ed.), *Spiritual well-being: Sociological perspectives* (pp. 153–171). Washington, DC: University Press of America.

Blaber, M., Jones, J., & Willis, D. (2015). Spiritual care: Which is the best assessment tool? *Journal of Palliative Nursing, 21*(9), 430–438.

Blaikie, N. W., & Kelson, G. P. (1979). Locating self and giving meaning to existence. In D. O. Moberg (Ed.), *Spiritual well-being: Sociological perspectives* (pp. 133–151). Washington, DC: University Press of America.

Brennan, M. R. (1994). *Spirituality in the homebound elderly* (Unpublished doctoral dissertation). The Catholic University of America. Ann Arbor, MI.

Brush, B. L., & Daly, P. R. (2000). Assessing spirituality in primary care practice: Is there time? *Clinical Excellence for Nurse Practitioners, 4*(2), 67–71.

Burkhart, L., Schmidt, L., & Hogan, N. (2011). Development and psychometric testing of the spiritual care inventory. *Journal of Advanced Nursing, 67*(11), 2463–2472.

Campbell, C. (1978). *Nursing diagnosis and intervention in nursing practice*. New York, NY: Wiley.

Cavendish, R., Luise, B. K., Horne, K., Bauer, M., Medefindt, J., Gallo, M. A., . . . Kutza, T. (2000). Opportunities for enhanced spirituality relevant to well adults. *Nursing Diagnosis, 11*(4), 151–163.

Christy, R. D., & Lyon, D. (1979). Sociological perspectives on personhood. In D. O. Moberg (Ed.), *Spiritual well-being: Sociological perspectives* (pp. 91–98). Washington, DC: University Press of America.

Clark, C. C., Cross, J. R., Deane, D. M., & Lowry, L. W. (1991). Spirituality: Integral to quality care. *Holistic Nursing Process, 3*(1), 67–76.

Clark, P., Drain, M., & Malone, M. (2003). Addressing patients' emotional and spiritual needs. *Joint Commission Journal on Quality and Safety, 29*(12), 659–670.

Clifford, M., & Gruca, J. (1987). Facilitating spiritual care in the rehabilitation setting. *Rehabilitation Nursing, 12*(6), 331–333.

Dameron, C. (2005). Spiritual assessment made easy . . . with acronyms. *Journal of Christian Nursing, 22*(1), 14–16.

Dossey, B. M. (1989). The transpersonal self and states of consciousness. In B. M. Dossey, L. Keegan, L. G. Kolkmeier, & C. E. Guzzetta (Eds.), *Holistic health promotion* (pp. 23–35). Rockville, MD: Aspen.

Driscoll, J. (2003). HIPAA: Calling the question. *Vision, 13*(5), 4–5.

Droege, T. (1991). *The faith factor in healing*. Philadelphia, PA: Trinity Press International.

Engebretson, J. (1996). Considerations in diagnosing in the spiritual domain. *Nursing Diagnosis, 7*(3), 100–107.

Fatula, M. A. (1993). Faith. In M. Downey (Ed.), *The new dictionary of Catholic spirituality* (pp. 379–390). Collegeville, MN: The Liturgical Press.

Fowler, J. W. (1981). *Stages of faith development*. New York, NY: HarperCollins.

Galek, K., Flannelly, K., Vane, A., & Galek, R. (2005). Assessing a patient's spiritual needs: A comprehensive instrument. *Holistic Nursing Practice, 19*(2), 62–69.

Gebbie, K. M. (1976). *Summary of the second national conference, classification of nursing diagnoses*. St. Louis, MO: C. V. Mosby.

Gebbie, K. M., & Lavin, M. A. (1975). *Classification of nursing diagnoses, proceeds of the first national conference*. St. Louis, MO: C. V. Mosby.

Govier, I. (2000). Spiritual care in nursing: A systematic approach. *Nursing Standard, 14*(17), 32–36.

Harris, R. C., Dew, M. A., Lee, A., Amaya, M., Bushes, L., Rettz, D., & Coleman, G. (1995). The role of religion in heart-transplant recipients' long-term health and well-being. *Journal of Religion and Health, 34*(1), 17–32.

Haugan, G. (2014). The FACIT-SP spiritual well-being scale: An investigation of the dimensionality, reliability and construct validity in a cognitively intact nursing home population. *Scandinavian Journal of Caring, 29*(1), 152–164.

Highfield, M. (1992). Spiritual health of oncology patients. *Cancer Nursing, 15*(1), 1–8.

Hodge, D. R. (2015). Administering a two-stage assessment in healthcare settings: A necessary component of ethical and effective care. *Journal of Nursing Management, 23*(1), 37–38.

Hodge, D. R. (2006). A template for spiritual assessment: A review of the JCAHO requirements and guidelines for implementation. *Social Work, 51*(4), 317–326.

Holloway, N. M. (1993). *Medical surgical care planning* (2nd ed.). Springhouse, PA: Springhouse Corporation.

Hsaio, Y., Chiang, Y., Lee, H., & Han, C. (2013). Psychometric testing of the properties of the Spiritual Health Care Scale Short Form. *Journal of Clinical Nursing, 22*(21/22), 2981–2990.

Hungelmann, J., Kenkel-Rossi, E., Klassen, L., & Stollenwerk, R. (1996). Focus on spiritual well-being: Harmonious interconnectedness of mind-body-spirit—Use of the JAREL spiritual well-being scale. *Geriatric Nursing, 17*(6), 262–266.

Johnson, R. P. (1992). *Body, mind, spirit: Trapping the healing power within you.* Liguori, MO: Liguori.

Joint Commission. (2003). *Comprehensive accreditation annual for hospitals: The official handbook.* Oakbrook Terrace, IL: The Joint Commission.

Joint Commission. (2008). *Standards FAQ details: Spiritual assessment.* Retrieved from http://www.jointcommission.org/standards_information/jcfaqdetails.aspx?StandardsFaqId=290&ProgramId=1

Kaufman, J. H. (1979). Social correlates of spiritual maturity among North American Mennonites. In D. O. Moberg (Ed.), *Spiritual well-being: Sociological perspectives* (pp. 237–254). Washington, DC: University of America Press.

Kerrigan, R., & Harkulich, J. T. (1993). A spiritual tool. *Health Progress, 74*(5), 46–49.

Kreitzer, M. J., Gross, C., Waleekhachonloet, O., Reilly-Spong, M., & Byrd, M. (2009). The brief serenity scale: A psychometric analysis of a measure of spirituality and well-being. *Journal of Holistic Nursing, 27*(1), 7–16.

LaPierre, L. (2003). JCAHO safeguards spiritual care. *Holistic Nursing Practice, 17*(4), 219.

Lindberg, J. B., Hunter, M. L., & Kruszewski, A. Z. (1994). *Introduction to nursing: Concepts, issues and opportunities.* Philadelphia, PA: J. B. Lippincott.

Lutheran Services in America. (2004, July). Intersections of HIPPA and pastoral care. *Q & A, Lutheran Services in America Newsletter,* 1.

Mickley, J., Soeken, K., & Belcher, A. (1992). Spiritual well-being, religiousness and hope among women with breast cancer. *Image, 24*(4), 267–272.

Moberg, D. O. (Ed.). (1979). The development of social indicators of spiritual well-being and quality of life. In *Spiritual well-being: Sociological perspectives* (pp. 1–13). Washington, DC: University of America Press.

North American Nursing Diagnosis Association (NANDA). (1994). *NANDA, nursing diagnoses: Definitions and classification, 1995–1996.* Philadelphia, PA: Author.

Nouwen, H. J. M. (1986). *Reaching out.* New York, NY: Doubleday.

O'Brien, M. E. (1982a). The need for spiritual integrity. In H. Yura & M. Walsh (Eds.), *Human needs and the nursing process* (Vol. 2, pp. 82–115). Norwalk, CT: Appleton-Century-Crofts.

O'Brien, M. E. (1982b, April). Pragmatic survivalism: Behavior patterns affecting low level wellness among minority group members. *Advances in Nursing Science, 4*(3), 13–26.

O'Brien, M. E. (1982c). Religious faith and adjustment to long-term hemodialysis. *Journal of Religion and Health, 21*(1), 68–80.

O'Brien, M. E. (1989). *Anatomy of a nursing home: A new view of resident life.* Owings Mills, MD: National Health Publishing.

O'Brien, M. E. (1992). *Living with HIV: Experiment in courage.* Westport, CT: Auburn House.

O'Brien, M. E. (1995). *The AIDS challenge: Breaking through the boundaries.* Westport, CT: Auburn House.

O'Brien, M. E., & Pheifer, W. G. (1993). Nursing care of persons infected with HIV. In M. Maas, K. Buckwalter, & M. Titler (Eds.), *Nursing clinics of North America, 23*(2), 303–315.

Pesut, B., Fowler, M., Reimer-Kirkham, S., Taylor, E., & Sawatzky, R. (2009). Particularizing spirituality in points of tension: Enriching the discourse. *Nursing Inquiry, 16*(4), 337–346.

Post-White, J., Ceronsky, C., Kreitzer, M. J., Nickelson, K., Drew, D., Mackey, K. W., . . . & Gutknecht, S. (1996). Hope, spirituality, sense of coherence, and quality of life in patients with cancer. *Oncology Nursing Forum, 23*(10), 1571–1579.

Power, J. (2006). Spiritual assessment: Developing an assessment tool. *Nursing Older People, 18*(2), 16–18.

Puchalski, C. (2000). Taking a spiritual history allows clinicians to understand patients more fully. *Journal of Palliative Medicine, 3*(1), 129–137.

Reed, P. G. (1991). Preferences for spiritually related nursing interventions among terminally ill and nonterminally ill hospitalized adults and well adults. *Applied Nursing Research, 4*(3), 122–128.

Sanders, C. (2002). Challenges for spiritual care-giving in the millennium. *Contemporary Nurse, 12*(2), 107.

Sessanna, L., Finnell, D., Underhill, M., Chang, Y., & Peng, H. (2011). Measures assessing spirituality as more than religiosity: A methodological review of nursing and health-related literature. *Journal of Advanced Nursing, 67*(8), 1677–1694.

Smith, D. W. (1995). Power and spirituality in polio survivors: A study based on Roger's science. *Nursing Science Quarterly, 8*(3), 133–139.

Smyth, T., & Allen, S. (2011). Nurses' experiences assessing the spirituality of terminally ill patients in acute clinical practice. *International Journal of Palliative Care Nursing, 17*(7), 337–343.

Soeken, K., & Carson, V. B. (1987). Responding to the spiritual needs of the chronically ill. *Nursing Clinics of North America, 22*(3), 603–611.

Stark, R., & Glock, C. (1968). *American piety: The nature of religious commitment.* Berkeley, CA: University of California Press.

Stoll, R. I. (1979). Guidelines for spiritual assessment. *American Journal of Nursing, 79*(9), 1574–1577.

Tanyi, R. A. (2006). Spirituality and family nursing: Spiritual assessment and interventions for families. *Journal of Advanced Nursing, 53*(3), 287–294.

Taylor, E. J. (2013). New Zealand hospice nurses' self-rated comfort in conducting spiritual assessment. *International Journal of Palliative Nursing, 19*(4), 178–185.

Taylor, C., Lillis, C., & LeMone, P. (1993). *Fundamentals of nursing: The art and science of nursing care* (2nd ed.). Philadelphia, PA: J. B. Lippincott.

Timmins, R., & Kelly, J. (2008). Spiritual assessment in intensive and cardiac care nursing. *Nursing in Critical Care, 13*(3), 124–131.

Toth, J. C. (1992). Faith in recovery: Spiritual support after an acute M.I. *Journal of Christian Nursing, 9*(4), 28–31.

Twibell, R. S., Wieseke, A. W., Marine, M., & Schoger, J. (1996). Spiritual and coping needs of critically ill patients: Validation of nursing diagnoses. *Dimensions of Critical Care Nursing, 15*(5), 245–253.

White, L. (2003). Pastoral care providers are members of the health care team in accordance with the regulations of the Department of Health and Human Services. *APC News, 6*(1), 1–2.

White, L., & Pierce, R. (2002a). HIPPA regulations raise questions for chaplains. *APC (Association of Professional Chaplains) News, 5*(1), 1–2.

White, L., & Pierce, R. (2002b). HIPPA regulations impact on visitation by clergy, lay ministers and faith group representatives. *APC News, 5*(3), 1–2.

Young, C., & Koopsen, C. (2011). *Spirituality, health and healing: An integrative approach.* Sudbury, MA: Jones & Bartlett Learning.

CHAPTER 4

A Middle-Range Theory of Spiritual Well-Being in Illness

For everything there is a season, and a time for every matter under heaven: a time to be born and a time to die; a time to plant and a time to pluck up what is planted.

Ecclesiastes 3:1

I believe that spirituality is a very healing thing, not only for the patient but also for nurses. It is a reflection of who you are as a person. . . . You have to have some kind of belief in yourself and in a higher being in a meaningful, purposeful way to give of yourself. . . . You've got to have the spiritual aspect in your nursing to survive.

Jessica, Supervisor of a Medical-Surgical Outpatient Clinic

Nursing theorists, as the author of the Book of Ecclesiastes would say, recognize that in their world of caring for the sick there is indeed "a time to be born and a time to die"; a time for planting and a time to harvest what has been planted. They know that in their patients' lives there is "a time for every matter under heaven." Thus, the early "grand theorists" of nursing developed conceptual schemas that attempted to address, in some way, all of a patient's possible "seasons" of life.

More recently, however, nurse metatheorists, also sensitive to the varied and unique seasons of patients' lives, have encouraged the development of theories of the middle range. That is, those theories that address specific health- and illness-related phenomena of concern to practicing nurses.

To respond to the call for such theories, a middle-range theory of spiritual well-being (SWB) in illness was developed based on the author's many years of clinical nursing research with persons experiencing chronic and life-threatening illnesses.[*]

---

[*]Major sections of this chapter have been taken from Chapter 5, "Conceptual Models of Parish Nursing Practice: A Middle-Range Theory of Spiritual Well-Being in Illness" in Mary Elizabeth O'Brien, *Parish Nursing: Healthcare Ministry within the Church*, 2003, Jones & Bartlett Publishers. Used with permission of the publisher.

63

▶ A Brief History of Theory Development in Nursing

During the decades of the 1970s and 1980s, especially, both academicians and practicing nurses began to incorporate theories of nursing into their research and practice. The majority of these early nursing models fell into the category of "grand theories" of nursing, or those conceptual frameworks that attempted to present a way of describing and understanding the overall discipline of professional nursing practice. Each model contained some exploration of the concepts: person, health, nursing, and environment. There were a number of nursing theory conferences organized to analyze and discuss the logical adequacy and practicality of these theories for use in research and practice. The meetings often included presentations by key nursing theorists of the day, such as Dorothea Orem, Callista Roy, Martha Rogers, and Betty Neuman. Some of the most frequently cited conceptual frameworks were Orem's self-care model for nursing, the Roy adaptation model, the Neuman systems model, and Rogers's model of unitary person. Despite focus on the work of the theorists of the late 20th century, as contemporaries of that era, most nurse metatheorists, however, acknowledged and still acknowledge Florence Nightingale as the first nursing theorist; this accolade is based on Nightingale's exploration and understanding of the need for a framework for nursing practice as described in her 1859 book *Notes on Nursing*.

While some nurse researchers have attempted to use grand theories of nursing to undergird their studies, the breadth of these models makes such efforts difficult. Usually, the grand theory is dissected by an investigator, a portion of the model being employed to provide the framework for research. While the grand theories of nursing provide valuable parameters to delineate and explain the practice of professional nursing, metatheorists have called for and continue to advocate the development of middle-range nursing theories, or those theories that strive to explain more discrete phenomena of interest to practicing nurses.

Distinct from the grand theories of nursing, which attempt to incorporate myriad concepts representing a broad range of phenomena within the discipline, a number of middle-range theories have begun to emerge in the professional literature. Some of these include frameworks dealing with such issues as pain control, chronic sorrow, end of life, uncertainty of the illness experience, and skill acquisition. The concept of "middle-range theory" was introduced in the sociological literature by Robert Merton (1957, p. 9); midrange theories were viewed as bodies of knowledge that would encompass a more limited number of variables than grand theories and could be empirically tested. Middle-range nursing theories cluster "around a concept of interest" (Chinn & Kramer, 1995, p. 40), such as those identified previously. They are also described as "theories that focus on specific nursing phenomena that reflect clinical practice" (Meleis, 1997, p. 18); "not covering the full range of phenomena that are of concern within the discipline" (Chinn & Jacobs, 1987, p. 205); sharing "some of the conceptual economy of grand theories but also [providing] the specificity needed for usefulness in research and practice" (Walker & Avant, 1995, p. 11); and "made up of a limited number of concepts and propositions that are written at a relatively concrete . . . level" (Fawcett, 1992, p. 5). As middle-range theories address a specific phenomenon, their goal is thus to "describe, explain or predict phenomena" (Fawcett, 1992, p. 5). In sum, middle-range theories fall somewhere between the more abstract or grand theories/conceptual models and circumscribed practice theories.

Despite this history documenting the value of nursing theory over the past several decades, the title of a recent editorial by distinguished nurse theorist Rosemarie Rizzo Parse (2016) posed the question "Where have all the nursing theories gone?". Parse's concern was raised particularly by a 2015 *Nursing Outlook* issue devoted to nursing science, which, she noted, was "devoid of any mention of what is commonly known as nursing theory" (p. 101). The journal, Parse contended, ignored the work of "a century of nurse theorists and scholars who strove to design theories that make up the body of nursing knowledge" (p. 101). These theories, Parse noted, "must be acknowledged if nursing is to have a unique body of knowledge differing from that of the biological and behavioral sciences" (p. 101).

Theorist Patricia Donohue-Porter (2014) also argues that "when nursing theory is not fully valued by the profession, not only knowledge is lost but also the language that helps nurses to lead" (p. 330). To encourage the "future development of the theoretical bases of the nursing discipline . . . diverse ways of theory evaluation" need to be identified (Im, 2015, p. 2268). New nursing theories continue to be called for (Morgan & Georges, 2015) and nursing curricula need to continue to include the teaching of nursing theory in order to provide nurses with "the theoretical foundation to inform research, practice and education" (Yancey, 2015, p. 274).

Construction of Spirituality in Nursing Theory

While there has been only minimal focus on spirituality in early nursing theories, both grand theories and theories of the middle range, more recently metatheorists in nursing and health care have begun to address the concept. Some examples include a discussion of the "construction of spirituality" in nursing theory (Henery, 2003, p. 550); development of a model for advancing spiritual care in nursing and health care (McSherry, 2006); and presentation of an evolving framework for exploring the concept of spirituality in nursing (Miner-Williams, 2006).

One of the first steps in the development of theory is that of concept analysis. Several 21st-century nursing articles reflecting the process of concept analysis in the area of spirituality are: "Spiritual Crisis: A Concept Analysis" (Agrimson & Taft, 2008), which employs the Walker and Avant method to explore the impact of spiritual crisis on meaning of life (p. 454); "Spirituality: Concept Analysis and Model Development" (Buck, 2006), employing Chinn and Kramer's method of conceptual development; "Spirituality in Nursing and Health-Related Literature" (Sessanna, Finnell, & Jezewski, 2007), using Walker and Avant's framework to identify the attributes of spirituality as a concept; and "Faith: A Concept Analysis" (Dyess, 2011). The latter paper explores the concept of faith "within the lens of Margaret Newman's Health as Expanding Consciousness" model (p. 2723).

The "construction of spirituality," noted previously, is examined in contemporary nursing theory using the method of discourse analysis (Henery, 2003), and the meaning of the concept of spirituality for practicing nurses is explored through literature review (Miner-Williams, 2006). Miner-Williams attempts to clarify spirituality in the evolving framework by using definitions in the literature and through identifying component concepts: "connectedness, meaning, transcendence, values and beliefs, energy and emotion" (p. 811). Miner-Williams also presents six practical guidelines to assist nurses in the provision of spiritual care in a clinical setting.

Three other more recently developed models for spirituality in nursing include: "An Experiential Theory of Spiritual Care in Nursing Practice" (Burkhart & Hogan, 2008); "Spirituality and Psychological Well-Being: Testing a

Theory of Family Interdependence Among Family Caregivers and Their Elders," which looked at the relationship between the spirituality of the caregiver and the spirituality of the care receiver (Kim, Reed, Hayward, Kang, & Koenig, 2011); and "T.R.U.S.T.: An Affirming Model for Inclusive Spiritual Care" (Barss, 2012).

Finally, nurse theorists Mary White, Rosalind Peters, and Stephanie Schim (2011) have undertaken to expand the existing Dorothea Orem's Self-Care Deficit Theory by including and describing the concepts of spirituality and spiritual self-care into the framework. These authors consider the "integration of the concepts of spirituality and spiritual self-care with Orem's self-care deficit nursing theory as a critical step in theory development" (p. 48). A model of self-care deficit theory, including the construct of spiritual self-care, is presented; spiritual self-care is described as being "based on an individual's mind/spirit/body connection, upbringing, moral and religious background and life experiences that originate from faith, feelings and emotions" (p. 53).

The importance of the continued interest in nursing theory development in the area of spirituality is supported by Barbara Pesut, a nurse philosopher who points out the current universal interest in things spiritual described as the "sacralization" of society. Pesut (2009) notes that this is also evidenced in "nursing discourse where it is common to find claims about the nature of persons as inherently spiritual, about what a spiritually healthy person looks like and about the environment as spiritually energetic and interconnected" (p. 15).

▶ A Middle-Range Theory of Spiritual Well-Being in Illness

A middle-range theory of SWB in illness can be useful in orienting the practice of any nurse carrying out holistic health care, which includes attention to the needs of body, mind, and spirit. Such a theoretical orientation is especially important for nurses caring for those experiencing long-term chronic illness, life-threatening and terminal illness, as well as any illness or injury that affects an individual's personal and/or professional life goals. In such cases, patients frequently struggle mightily to find some reason that can help them find meaning in the illness or disability. Regardless of religious affiliation or its lack, individuals coping with life-altering conditions generally strive to make some sense of the state in which they find themselves. Or, this seeming impossible, most patients try to achieve a sense of acceptance, and even peace, in the midst of their suffering.

A middle-range theory of SWB in illness can help both nurse practitioners and nurse researchers working with seriously ill persons to assess and evaluate their patients' spiritual needs and, if warranted, to institute appropriate spiritual care interventions.

▶ Development of the Theory of Spiritual Well-Being in Illness

The nursing literature suggests that "middle-range theories generally emerge from combining research and practice, and building on the work of others" (McEwen, 2002, p. 207).

The latter point is validated by nurse theorists who assert that middle-range theories may be derived or deduced from grand theories or conceptual frameworks (Ruland & Moore, 1998, p. 170) or from established clinical guidelines (Good, 1998, p. 120). The midrange nursing theory of SWB in illness was derived from earlier conceptualizations in the area of SWB and also from the nursing model conceived by Joyce Travelbee, in which a central focus of the framework is the concept of finding meaning in an illness experience.

The core component of the nursing theory of SWB in illness is the concept of finding spiritual meaning in the experience of illness. While Travelbee (1971) introduced the importance of spiritual concerns—"the spiritual values a person holds will determine to a great extent his [sic] perception of illness" (p. 16)—she never explicitly described the concept of "spiritual well-being" in her model. Rather, Travelbee developed an interactional framework based on "human-to-human," nurse–patient relationships, viewing the nurse's role as assisting "the ill patient to experience hope as a means of coping with illness and suffering" (Chinn & Kramer, 1995, p. 176); illness was envisioned as a "spiritual, emotional and physical" experience that might be defined both "subjectively and objectively" (Chinn & Jacobs, 1987, p. 188).

For Travelbee, one's definitions of illness and suffering depended very much on "the symbolic meaning attached to these concepts by the individual" (Thibodeau, 1983, p. 90); she further postulated that "a person's attitude toward suffering ultimately determines how effectively he [sic] copes with illness" (Meleis, 1997, p. 361). Finally, Travelbee (1971) taught that "the professional nurse practitioner must be prepared to assist individuals and families not just to cope with illness and suffering but to find meaning in these experiences" (p. 13). "This is the difficult task of professional nursing," she admitted, but "it must not be evaded" (p. 13).

Joyce Travelbee, a psychiatric nurse practitioner and educator, died at age 47 just as she was beginning doctoral study; thus, we do not know how she might have expanded her beginning conceptual model for nursing practice. Travelbee has been described as a deeply spiritual woman, whose human-to-human vision of nursing practice was importantly influenced by her early educational experience at Charity Hospital in New Orleans, by the work of the great psychotherapist Viktor Frankl, and by the writings of nurse theorist Ida Orlando. Although Joyce Travelbee did not live to further explain and validate her interaction model, her groundbreaking work on the concept of a sick person finding meaning in the experiences of illness and suffering provides a solid and scholarly basis for the development of a midrange-level theory exploring and describing the spiritual meaning of illness and suffering: a nursing theory of SWB in illness.

As noted, the middle-range theory of SWB in illness was also inductively derived and concretized through a number of nursing studies exploring the importance of SWB in coping with chronic illness and disability. Overwhelmingly positive associations, both quantitatively and qualitatively, were found between SWB and quality of life. That is, those persons who reported a higher degree of personal faith, spiritual contentment, and religious practice were much more positive about and satisfied with other aspects of their lives and had greater hope for the future, despite sometimes painful and debilitating illnesses. Several case examples of the positive association between SWB and quality of life reported by Parish Nursing Study participants (discussed in more detail later in the book) were those of a 62-year-old Methodist parishioner who was suffering from leukemia; an 82-year-old Lutheran parishioner with a multiplicity of disease conditions, including osteoporosis, congestive heart failure, and diabetes; and a 75-year-old Roman Catholic parishioner who was disabled with rheumatoid arthritis, among other diagnoses. In completing the Spiritual Assessment Scale (Chapter 3), which measures SWB, all three scored very positively on the items measuring faith, religious practice, and spiritual contentment or lack of spiritual distress. Similarly, all three study participants were most positive in their responses related to quality of life: hope for the future, for example, being positive about life, being able to get through difficulties, and feeling loved; and life satisfaction, for example, agreeing that they are "just as happy as when younger" (O'Brien, 2001). In looking back, they agreed they were "fairly well satisfied" with their lives.

Philosophy and Key Concepts

Every theory must have a philosophical basis undergirding the concepts and relationships articulated in the framework. The middle-range theory of SWB in illness is grounded in the belief that the human person, as well as being possessed of a physical and psychosocial nature, is also a spiritual being capable of transcending and/or accepting such experiences as pain and suffering in the light of his or her higher nature. Over and over, clinical nurses have witnessed ill or disabled patients rise above constraining physical or psychosocial deficits to live extraordinarily positive and productive lives. This ability to accept, and in some cases even embrace, illness and suffering is primarily a function of the patients' personal spiritual resources. It is for the purpose of identifying, supporting, and strengthening the influence of these spiritual resources, in relation to sickness or disability, that the nursing theory of SWB in illness has been developed.

The key concept of the middle-range theory of SWB in illness is, of course, that of SWB itself. In the conceptual model (**FIGURE 4-1**), an ill individual is presented as having the ability to find spiritual meaning in the experience of illness, which can ultimately lead to an outcome of SWB for the sick person. The capacity to find spiritual meaning in an occasion of illness or suffering is influenced by a number of factors. First and foremost, an individual's perception of the spiritual meaning of an illness experience is influenced by personal spiritual and religious attitudes and behaviors. These attitudes and behaviors include variables related to personal faith: belief in God, peace in spiritual and religious beliefs, confidence in God's power, strength received from personal faith beliefs, and trust in God's providence; spiritual contentment: satisfaction with faith, feeling of closeness to God, lack of fear, reconciliation, security in God's love, and faithfulness; and religious practice: support of a faith community, affirmation in worship, encouragement of spiritual companions, consolation from prayer, and communication with God through religious practices.

The impact of these spiritual and religious attitudes and behaviors on one's finding spiritual meaning in illness may also be mediated by such potentially intervening variables as severity of illness: degree of functional impairment; social support: support of family, friends, and/or caregivers; and current stressful life events: emotional, sociocultural, and/or financial.

The first step in developing a middle-range theory is to conduct an analysis of the core concepts in the model. Nurse metatheorists Walker and Avant (1995) identify a series of "steps" to be included in a "concept analysis," which include (among others) determining the "aims of the analysis," identifying "uses of the concept," and "defin[ing] empirical referents" (p. 39). The aim of exploring the concept of SWB is

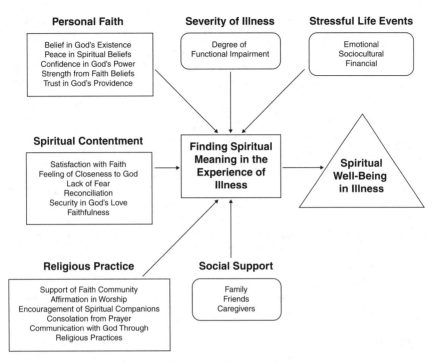

FIGURE 4-1   A conceptual model of spiritual well-being in illness.

to identify and describe its meaning in terms of contemporary usage, especially in relation to experiences of illness and suffering. The usage and empirical referents of the concept have been examined from the extant literature as well as nursing practice and nursing research. The concept of SWB was explored in both the nursing and sociological literature in the process of developing the earlier referenced Spiritual Assessment Scale (SAS).

Based on prior nursing practice and nursing research, I envision the concept of SWB as consisting of two dimensions: that of spirituality or one's personal relationship with God or the Transcendent; and religiosity or religiousness, reflecting an individual's practice of his or her faith beliefs (this dimension of SWB may or may not involve participation in an organized religious tradition). Thus, empirical referents of SWB are conceptualized in terms of personal faith and spiritual contentment (spirituality) and religious practice (religiosity or religiousness).

Theory Synthesis

Theory synthesis is defined as "a strategy aimed at constructing theory, an interrelated system of ideas, from empirical evidence" (Walker & Avant, 1995, p. 155). In theory synthesis "a theorist pulls together available information about a phenomenon. Concepts and statements are organized into a network or whole, a synthesized theory" (Walker & Avant, 1995, p. 155). In the preceding discussion, a diagrammatic model of the theory of SWB in illness is presented (Figure 4-1) to identify the relationships between key concepts and potentially mediating variables relevant to the framework. A sick or disabled individual's ability to find spiritual meaning in an experience of illness or suffering is perceived as being influenced by his or her spiritual and religious attitudes, beliefs, and practices, including those reflecting the concepts of personal faith, spiritual contentment, and religious practice.

An ill person's personal faith—not only whether or not he or she believes in the existence of God, but also his or her trust in the power and the goodness of God's care, sense of peacefulness about these beliefs, and courage and strength derived from them—is critical to whether the individual will be able to identify and/or accept an illness experience as having a spiritual dimension. If one believes in God, yet does not truly trust in or feel at peace in accepting His loving providence, an illness experience may be considered an unwarranted and unfair burden at best, or a punishment for some perceived past indiscretion at worst. In terms of the concept of spiritual contentment, an ill person may indeed believe in God's existence, His power, His care for all of humankind, and yet not personally feel close to the Lord; his or her faith may be based on a relationship that incorporates fear of God's judgment rather than security in His love. In such a situation, again, it may be very difficult for the individual to perceive an experience of illness or suffering as anything more than a possible retaliation or punishment for past sins.

While religious practice, in the formal sense of attending church services, may not be necessary for one to find a spiritual meaning in illness or disability, coping with illness can be greatly facilitated if a sick person has the support of such devotions as prayer or spiritual reading. The encouragement of a faith community with whom one may occasionally share worship or whose members pray for sick parishioners during communal worship services and/or the guidance of a pastor or spiritual companion can also be very comforting spiritual supports in times of illness and suffering.

A practicing nurse can provide important nursing intervention in helping an ill patient who may be struggling with a number of spiritual issues. Very often, as will be seen in the many empirical examples presented throughout this text, nurses facilitate either the enhancement of, or in some cases the return to, religious practices that may have waned or even been abandoned by a patient during the onset of an illness experience.

Also, as demonstrated in the diagrammatic model presented in Figure 4-1, there are a number of potentially confounding variables that may interfere with a sick person's ability to achieve a sense of SWB in his or her illness. A nurse may have the opportunity to intervene in relation to a number of these factors hindering the ability to find meaning in the illness experience. For example, a nurse may be able to serve as a referral agent assisting sick persons in finding some relief for a functional impairment. For instance, if an ill individual is hard of hearing, the nurse may recommend audiology testing if this has not been done and/or may assist the individual in obtaining a hearing aid if necessary.

A nurse may also serve as a "bridge" facilitating communication with family and friends if these relationships have become strained due to illness or disability. Finally, through the various roles of educator, referral agent, counselor, and patient advocate, the nurse may have the opportunity to guide, advise, teach, or support an ill patient in regard to a variety of emotional, sociocultural, and even financial concerns that may interfere with the individual achieving a sense of SWB in the illness experience.

Hypotheses Derived from the Theory

Based on the middle-range theory of SWB in illness, as described, several hypotheses might be derived related to the association between spiritual well-being and quality of life for those dealing with illness and/or disability. First, it can be proposed that there will be a significant relationship between the degree of a sick person's personal faith and his or her perceived quality of life in an illness experience. Second, there will be a significant relationship between the activity of a sick person's religious practice and his or her perceived quality of life in an illness experience. Third, there will be a significant relationship between the degree of a sick person's feeling of spiritual contentment and his or her perceived quality of life in an illness experience. An overall hypothesis might be stated as follows: there will be a significant relationship between SWB (personal faith, spiritual contentment, and religious practice) and quality of life among sick persons experiencing illness or disability, controlling for the variables of severity of illness, social support, and stressful life events.

Empirical Testing

Testing of these relationships has already begun. Empirical findings support both the subhypotheses and the overall hypothesis, correlating SWB (as a total concept and in its subcomponents: personal faith, spiritual contentment, and religious practice) with quality of life. The research was conducted among chronically ill adults at the end of life experiencing myriad illness conditions; study participants belonged to a variety of religious traditions and faith communities. It is anticipated that future nursing studies might be carried out with other patient populations experiencing both similar and different illness conditions and disabilities. Such research would greatly assist in validating the importance of the nursing role of spiritual caregiving; positive findings would strengthen and potentially expand the spiritual care role of the nurse while also supporting the health-care dimension of the nursing ministry.

It is suggested that, as in the studies presented in this text, nursing research to test the middle-range theory of SWB in illness employ methodological triangulation; that is, the collecting of both quantitative and qualitative data to explore the relationship of SWB to coping with illness and disability. While the quantitative data would provide a strong statistical basis for the relationship, the qualitative data elicited in focused conversational interviews with ill persons could provide the detailed narrative examples from which guidelines for the nurse's role of integrator of faith and health could be further expanded and clarified.

▶ References

Agrimson, L. B., & Taft, L. B. (2008). Spiritual crisis: A concept analysis. *Journal of Advanced Nursing,* 65(2), 454–461.

Barss, K. (2012). T.R.U.S.T.: An affirming model for inclusive spiritual care. *Journal of Holistic Nursing, 30*(1), 24–34.

Buck, H. (2006). Spirituality: Concept analysis and model development. *Holistic Nursing Practice, 20*(6), 288–292.

Burkhart, L., & Hogan, N. (2008). An experiential theory of spiritual care in nursing practice. *Qualitative Health Research, 18*(7), 928–938.

Chinn, P. L., & Jacobs, M. K. (1987). *Theory and nursing: A systematic approach* (2nd ed.). St. Louis, MO: C. V. Mosby.

Chinn, P. L., & Kramer, M. K. (1995). *Theory and nursing: A systematic approach* (4th ed.). St. Louis, MO: C. V. Mosby.

Donohue-Porter, P. (2014). The creative élan of nursing theory: Indispensable to leadership. *Nursing Science Quarterly, 27*(4), 330–335.

Dyess, S. M. (2011). Faith: A concept analysis. *Journal of Advanced Nursing, 67*(12), 2723–2731.

Fawcett, J. (1992). *The relationship of theory and research* (3rd ed.). Philadelphia, PA: F. A. Davis.

Good, M. (1998). A middle-range theory of acute pain management: Use in research. *Nursing Outlook, 46*(3), 120–124.

Henery, N. (2003). Constructions of spirituality in contemporary nursing theory. *Journal of Advanced Nursing, 42*(6), 550–557.

Im, E. O. (2015). The current status of theory evaluation in nursing. *Journal of Advanced Nursing, 71*(10), 2268–2278.

Kim, S., Reed, P., Hayward, R., Kang, Y., & Koenig, H. (2011). Spirituality and psychological well-being: Testing a theory of family interdependence among family caregivers and their elders. *Research in Nursing & Health, 34*(2), 103–115.

McEwen, M. (2002). Middle-range nursing theories. In M. McEwen & E. M. Wills (Eds.), *Theoretical basis for nursing* (pp. 202–225). Philadelphia, PA: Lippincott, Williams, & Wilkins.

McSherry, W. (2006). The principal components model: A model for advancing spirituality and spiritual care within nursing and health care practice. *Journal of Clinical Nursing, 15*, 905–917.

Meleis, A. I. (1997). *Theoretical nursing: Development and progress* (3rd ed.). Philadelphia, PA: Lippincott.

Merton, R. K. (1957). *Social theory and social structure*. Glencoe, IL: Free Press.

Miner-Williams, D. (2006). Putting a puzzle together: Making spirituality meaningful for nursing using an evolving theoretical framework. *Journal of Clinical Nursing, 15*, 811–821.

Morgan, S. N., & Georges, J. M. (2015). Refocusing a nursing lens distorted by perfection: The call for a mid-range theory. *Journal of Theory Construction & Testing, 19*(1), 26–32.

O'Brien, M. E. (2001). *Spiritual well-being in chronic illness* (Unpublished study report). Catholic University of America, Washington, DC.

O'Brien, M. E. (2003). *Parish nursing: Healthcare ministry within the church*. Sudbury, MA: Jones & Bartlett Learning.

Parse, R. R. (2016). Where have all the nursing theories gone? *Nursing Science Quarterly, 29*(2), 101–102.

Pesut, B. (2009). Ontologies of nursing in an age of spiritual pluralism: Closed or open worldview. *Nursing Philosophy, 11*, 15–23.

Ruland, C. M., & Moore, S. M. (1998). Theory construction based on standards of care: A proposed theory of the peaceful end of life. *Nursing Outlook, 46*(4), 169–175.

Sessanna, L., Finnell, D., & Jezewski, M. (2007). Spirituality in nursing and health-related literature. *Journal of Holistic Health, 25*(4), 252–262.

Thibodeau, J. A. (1983). *Nursing models: Analysis and evaluation*. Monterey, CA: Wadsworth Health Sciences Division.

Travelbee, J. (1971). *Interpersonal aspects of nursing*. Philadelphia, PA: F. A. Davis.

Walker, L. O., & Avant, K. C. (1995). *Strategies for theory construction in nursing* (3rd ed.). Norwalk, CT: Appleton & Lange.

White, M., Peters, R., & Schim, S. (2011). Spirituality and spiritual self-care: Expanding self-care deficit theory. *Nursing Science Quarterly, 24*, 48–56.

Yancey, N. R. (2015). Why teach nursing theory? *Nursing Science Quarterly, 28*(4), 274–278.

CHAPTER 5

The Nurse–Patient Relationship: A Caring Ministry

"Therefore, since it is by God's mercy that we are engaged in the ministry, we do not lose heart."

2 Corinthians 4:1

"When I do nursing, when I care for someone who is sick, I have a real feeling that I'm ministering to that person; that I am doing ministry. That goes back to the idea that the gospel tells us, as Christians, to care for the sick and that when we care for them we care for the Lord. Nursing is definitely a ministry".

Megan, Nurse Practitioner in Community Health

▶ The Nurse–Patient Relationship

For centuries, the nurse–patient relationship has been unique and individualized. Both patient and nurse bring into the partnership a multiplicity of personal life variables, including such factors as demographics (age, gender, marital status, ethnicity, religion, and socioeconomic status), family history, illness experience, and spiritual orientation. All of the characteristics associated with these variables may affect how the nurse–patient relationship is played out during the course of an interaction. Recent literature has also begun to explore, in more specificity, the topic of professional boundaries related to the nurse–patient relationship (Griffith, 2013), focusing especially on such issues as: the nurse's power and the patient's vulnerability (Benbow, 2013, p. 30); trust in nurse–patient relationships (Dinc & Gastmans, 2013); person-centered practice (Devenny & Duffy, 2014); communication (Reblin, Otis-Green, Ellington, & Clayton, 2014); and spirituality and the nurse's penchant for innate compassion (Wright &

Neuberger, 2012). Any or all of these variables, as well as sociodemographic characteristics, may impact the nurse–patient relationship.

The research data in this chapter poignantly describe the ministerial dimension of the nurse–patient relationship as identified by a cadre of practicing nurses. The nurses' own words are employed to label concepts in a paradigm of interaction that reveals the nurse as an anonymous minister. In this ministerial role, the nurse enters into a sacred covenant of caring for the sick.

▶ Spirituality and the Nurse

In discussing nurses' spiritual needs, Philip Burnard (1988) posed a number of questions that may help a nursing practitioner explore his or her own spirituality in relation to caregiving. These questions focus on such topics as understanding the term *spiritual*, religious education, the importance of spirituality to the nurse, feelings about spiritual beliefs different from one's own, the potential for changing personal spiritual beliefs, feelings regarding talking about spiritual beliefs with other nurses, and the perception of how one's own spiritual beliefs affect patient care (p. 36). For seasoned nurses, these questions may have been well explored in the course of their own faith development; for the newer clinician, exploring spiritual beliefs can be a valuable and growth-producing faith experience. Ultimately, responses to Burnard's questions may have an important impact on the nurse–patient ministerial relationship. Writing on the subject of a nurse's spirituality in 1912, distinguished nurse educator Isabel Hampton Robb (1912) asserted that indeed "the nurse's work is a ministry; it should represent a consecrated service, performed in the spirit of Christ, who made Himself of no account but went about doing good. The woman who fails to bring this spirit into her nursing misses the pearl of greatest value that is to be found in it" (p. 38). Nursing's spiritual dimension has been described as including the fact that attention to the "spirit should be regarded as an important part of spiritual care" (Myers, 2009, p. 22); that there should be "a systematic provision of spiritual care to patients" (Dunn, 2008, p. 4); that the concept of spiritual care should be included in nursing fundamentals textbooks (Pesut, 2008); and that nurses have a duty to facilitate the meeting of patients' spiritual and/or religious needs (Ledger, 2005).

In a 2010 literature review exploring the integration of spirituality into nursing practice, Tiew and Creedy identified five themes that impact spiritual care: these include "a lack of shared understanding of spirituality, lack of emphasis on spirituality in nursing education, attitudes, organizational and cultural factors, and individuality" (p. 15). Among these authors' recommendations following the review was the notion that "more research is required to develop a better understanding of how nurses perceive spirituality and the types of difficulties or barriers they face integrating spirituality into practice" (p. 19). A paper in *Nursing Ethics* addresses one of the themes identified by Tiew and Creedy, that of a lack of emphasis on spirituality education. Annette Becker (2009) asserts that "despite the evidence in college students indicating a hunger for spiritual insight and spirituality's application in health care, there continues to be a guardedness within the academy toward the inclusion of curricula that address spirituality" (p. 697). Becker offers a model for teaching spirituality and health that contains four guidelines: "approach teaching spirituality as any other 'difficult topic'";

"develop . . . a pragmatic course including learning activities that engage depth of learning"; "create and sustain a secure environment of learning"; and "be a trustworthy citizen of the college community" (p. 703).

In line with Becker's concept of creating activities that promote learning, one nurse author suggests that "creative modalities offer nurses a new perspective on how to care for patients" in an article entitled "Creativity and Spirituality in Nursing: Implementing Art in Healing" (Lane, 2005, p. 122). Dr. Mary Lane focuses on the accomplishment of healing using such arts as music, painting, and sculpture (p. 122). Other authors who link the concepts of spirituality with healing include: Glen McCabe (2008), who suggests the integration of body, mind, and spirit with traditional healing practices in psychotherapy; Dr. Jane Hart, of the Center for Spirituality and Healing at the University of Minnesota, which offers programs based on an integrative healing model (2010, p. 50); and Pipe, Hansen, Hentz, and Hartsell, who describe a program of spirituality and healing using "Watson's Theory of Human Caring (as) the framework guiding the project" (2010, p. 47).

Tyler and Raynor (2006) remind nurses that "there has been consistent use of spiritual practices to address health concerns by individuals for thousands of years" (p. 63); they note further that "incorporating spiritual care into practice is an integral dimension of holistic care that is the crux of nursing practice in the 21st century" (p. 63). Research employing focus groups, including patients, nurses, and hospital chaplains, showed that spirituality "played various roles in patients' lives during their illness" (van Leeuwen, Tiesinga, Jochemsen, & Post, 2007, p. 482), and myriad investigations have revealed that "spirituality is a fundamental quality that contributes to health and wellness" (Shores, 2010, p. 8).

Although the author's interviews with practicing nurses described in the following pages did address the nurses' own spiritual needs, only a modest amount of data was elicited on the topic. Nurses who participated in the study were clearly more interested in talking about the spiritual concerns and needs of their patients, how they had attempted to meet these, and how they might better practice spiritual care in the future. Nursing has historically been a discipline of service to others; the concern with one's personal well-being, spiritual or otherwise, was secondary to meeting the needs of the ill. The study nurses who did speak about their own spirituality, however, described the importance of such religious activities as prayer and Scripture reading in providing support for their practice.

Ellie, a pediatric oncology nurse practitioner who had worked with terminally ill children for more than 15 years, explained the significance of her personal spirituality:

> In this job, in this work I do with little ones, some of them are so, so sick. It hurts a lot to watch them get sicker and sicker; they are so brave, some of them. And the parents! It can get to you. Some days you just want to run away and say "no more!" I can't keep doing this job. You want to forget that babies are dying. . . . I truly do believe it's my faith in God, in the Lord Jesus, that holds me up. I try to pray every morning while I'm getting myself together for work. And when I can steal a few minutes I read some Scripture or something like Henri Nouwen; I love his books. And my church, they're a big, big support. I guess I could say that it is the spiritual that keeps me in oncology nursing.

▶ The Nurse: The Anonymous Minister

In addition to the nurse's personal spirituality, a number of other factors are relevant to the spiritual dimension of nurse–patient interactions, including the nurse's comfort level in discussing spiritual issues with patients, the degree of spiritual support provided in the care setting (i.e., support for both patients' and caregivers' spiritual needs), and the emphasis or lack of emphasis on providing spiritual care to patients in the course of professional nursing education. "Ministry denotes service and servanthood," asserts nurse educator Do-rhen Angking (2012). Although "the notion of nursing as a service has been de-emphasized, mainly due to the vigorous efforts to raise nursing to the realms of science as a profession," Angking points out that "for many nurses, especially Christian nurses, nursing is indeed the ministry they are called to by Christ" (p. 59). In order to explore, empirically, these questions and issues regarding spirituality and the covenantal nurse–patient relationship, the author conducted focused interviews with 66 contemporary nurses employed in two East Coast metropolitan areas, soliciting individual experiences, attitudes, and behaviors regarding the relationship between spirituality and nursing practice. The nursing cadre was purposely chosen to include a broad range of experience and education. The 6 men and 60 women comprising the population of nurses reported the following religious affiliations: 39 Roman Catholics; 25 Protestants (4 Baptists, 3 born-again Christians, 2 Methodists, 2 Episcopalians, 2 Presbyterians, 1 Lutheran, 1 "Christian," and 10 persons who described themselves broadly as "Protestant"); 1 Jewish nurse; and 1 nurse who reported having no religious affiliation.

Two members of the group were licensed practical nurses, five were diploma registered nurses, and one had an associate in arts nursing degree. Eleven individuals had baccalaureate degrees in nursing, 25 had master's in nursing degrees, 14 had doctorates in nursing science, and 8 were registered nurses with doctorates in the biologic or behavioral sciences.

The largest subgroup of 38 nurses identified a history of 16 to 25 years of nursing experience; 19 had been nurses for 26 to 40 years; and only 9 had practiced nursing for less than 15 years. Thirty-three percent of the group described their specialty area as medical–surgical nursing. Seven nurses worked in the area of psychiatric-mental health, and seven worked in pediatrics. Five critical care nurses and five cardiovascular nurses were included in the group; there was one oncology nurse, as well as three hospice and five gerontologic nurses. Three nurses worked in the area of maternal–child health, and two each represented the areas of community health, emergency room, and operating room nursing. Three of the study nurses worked with the mentally retarded/developmentally disabled, and three worked in home health-care nursing; one of the latter group of nurses was primarily involved with the health care of homeless persons.

Sixteen of the study nurses were employed at military health-care facilities; 10 were faculty members in schools of nursing. Ten nurses were employed by medical centers, 7 by research institutions, 12 by private religiously affiliated hospitals, 3 by hospice facilities, 7 by city-run health-care facilities, and 1 nurse worked for an HMO. More than half of the group were identified as working in the area of nursing practice; 10 were nurse educators, 10 were nurse administrators, and 4 were employed as nurse researchers.

Interviews with the nursing group explored experiences and attitudes associated with nursing and spirituality, focusing on such topics as nurse–patient interactions related to patients' spiritual needs and/or spiritual care, the nurse's personal spirituality and/or spiritual needs, spiritual support provided in the health-care setting, and the inclusion or lack of inclusion of spiritual concepts in the nurse's educational program. Discussions were tape-recorded to preserve the nurses' attitudes, perceptions, and experiences in their own words. Confidentiality was assured to the nurses participating in the interviews; wherever naming is warranted, pseudonyms are used.

Tape-recorded interviews were transcribed and content analyzed to identify dominant themes related to nursing and spirituality. A multiplicity of concepts emerged associated with such broad areas as nurses' attitudes toward spirituality and spiritual care, the identification of patients' spiritual needs, nursing behaviors regarding the spiritual care of patients, and nurses' perceptions of their roles in ministering to patients' spiritual needs. All dominant themes and related concepts are derived from the practicing nurses' own words.[*]

Study Findings

Ultimately, an overall construct describing the association between spirituality and the nurse–patient relationship emerged from analysis of the interview data and was labeled "The Nurse: The Anonymous Minister."

This construct, which identifies the nurse's frequently unrecognized role in spiritual ministry, consists of three dominant themes: A Sacred Calling, Nonverbalized Theology, and Nursing Liturgy. Each theme incorporates six key concepts reflective of the category's content and orientation (see **TABLE 5.1**).

A Sacred Calling

The first concept of the empirically derived construct, The Nurse: The Anonymous Minister, is reflected in a dominant theme derived from the nurses' interviews and labeled A Sacred Calling. This theme relates to a perceived professional nursing role in ministering to the spiritual needs of patients. A majority of the nurse practitioners, educators, administrators, and researchers interviewed described nursing as being a vocation or calling, reflecting a spiritual element incorporated within their profession.

---

*The nurses who participated in the Nursing and Spirituality interviews were identified through informal sampling. The author requested key nurses, in the various types of health-care facilities described, to approach members of their staff who might be willing to meet and discuss the topic of spirituality. No criteria regarding the nurses' religious affiliations were specified. As demonstrated in the demographic profile, 64 of the overall group of 66 nurses who agreed to participate in the project identified themselves as Christian. Thus, many of the themes and concepts relating to spirituality and the nurse–patient relationship presented in this chapter are undergirded by Christian theology and spirituality. It is expected, however, that the reader affiliated with another religious tradition will be able to appreciate the universal themes of love, caring, compassion, and ministry to those in need.

TABLE 5.1 The Nurse: The Anonymous Minister		
A Sacred Calling	Nonverbalized Theology	Nursing Liturgy
A Send of Mission	United in Suffering	Healing Rituals
Messenger of Good Faith	Proddings of the Holy Spirit	Experiencing the Divine
The Almost Sacred	The Day the Lord has Made	Touching the Core
Touching the Hand of God	Crying for More	Being Present
Sensing the Vibrations	Needing Ventilation	Midwifing the Dying
A Healing Ministry	Praying a Lot	Privileged Moments

Peg, a master's-prepared psychiatric–mental health nurse with eight years of experience in the field, observed:

> When I was 16 I felt a "calling" to be a nurse; it's like a Sacred Calling. Over time you develop a devotion. I can't imagine doing anything else.

And Catherine, a doctorally prepared medical–surgical practitioner with 25 years of experience, perceived nursing as a calling from early on in her education:

> I went to school because I felt called to be a nurse. I see nursing as a spiritual vocation. It's much more than work; I find it a way of serving.

The term *vocation*, which is derived from the Latin word *vocare*, "to call," has been identified as a key theme "in both Hebrew and Christian scriptures" (O'Connell, 1993). "[V]ocation is central to understanding the relationship between Divine initiative and human response" (O'Connell, 1993, p. 1009). The concept of vocation is broadly understood as defining an individual's felt call to a particular ministry or work. In theological terminology the word *vocation* generally refers to "a Divine call to undertake a particular activity or embrace a particular 'stage of life' on behalf of God or the community" (Holland, 1990, p. 1087).

One of the younger study discussants, Amy, a 24-year-old baccalaureate-prepared nurse with one year of experience in the pediatric intensive care unit, asserted that although it had been a real "challenge" to master the health-care technology used in the care of critically ill children, it was the spiritual dimension of nursing that appealed to her: "When the day comes that I don't minister spiritually to that child or the family, then I need to get out. This is why I felt called to go into nursing; I don't just want to be a technician."

Supportive of envisioning nursing as a vocation, also, is the recent resurgence of interest among nurse researchers and educators in the relationship of moral belief to the practice of nursing. Ray (1994) observed that nurse theorist Jean Watson "illuminated caring as the moral ideal in nursing where protection, preservation, and enhancement of human dignity are the mandates for the nurse" (p. 106).

The theme of vocation, or a Sacred Calling, may be further explained in terms of six key concepts derived from the data elicited in the Nursing and Spirituality discussions. These include A Sense of Mission, Messengers of Good Faith, The Almost Sacred, Touching the Hand of God, Sensing the Vibrations, and A Healing Ministry.

A Sense of Mission

A number of nurses described their perceptions of and experiences with spiritual care in terms of a call to mission or ministry. For Christians, all are called to ministry as pointed out in the New Testament:

> Then the king will say to those at his right hand, "Come you that are blessed by my Father, inherit the kingdom prepared for you from the foundation of the world; for I was hungry and you gave me food, I was thirsty and you gave me something to drink, I was a stranger and you welcomed me, I was naked and you gave me clothing, I was sick and you took care of me, I was in prison and you visited me . . . I tell you, just as you did it to one of the least of these . . . you did it to me. (Matthew 25:34–36; 40)

Although several terms are used to indicate the concept of ministry in the New Testament, interestingly, one used at least 20 times is the word *therapeu*, which means "to care for," "attend," "serve," "treat," especially by a physician, hence, "to heal" (Rademacher, 1991, pp. 39–40). Rademacher pointed out as well that "since the Jews, unlike some of the Greeks, did not divide the person into body and soul, we must assume the word describes a holistic healing of the total person" (p. 40). Most practicing nurses used the terms *ministry* and *mission* interchangeably; they also linked the concept of holistic nursing assessment and nursing care with a sense of ministering to the "whole" person, which they perceived as including the patient's spiritual needs.

Sarah, a baccalaureate-prepared nurse with 12 years of experience in hospice care and pediatric oncology, explained that, although she did need to work for financial reasons, she would not have chosen nursing if it were not for the ministry aspect, "I feel a real 'sense of mission' in nursing. It's a spiritual ministry. If I didn't feel that, I wouldn't be here." She added:

> I really depend on God to direct me. Every morning I try to spend some time in prayer and reading Bible verses to give myself strength. I try, when I have time off, to be alone and have a sense of God's presence. I know that I can't heal the children, but to just be there, that helps, and I pray that Jesus will work through me, to use my hands to in some way comfort or do the right thing for the patients.

A doctorally prepared pediatric nurse educator with 14 years of experience in practice described a strong sense of congruence between nursing and ministry:

> My nursing is my service to God. I believe that this is what I am supposed to be doing; this is my ministry. For me nursing and spirituality are intertwined.

I deal with people in their hour of greatest need; whether it's rocking a dying child or helping to support a family. People need more than physical care; they need love and acceptance. And this is when your mission, your ministry, can be a healing presence.

Paula, a master's-prepared medical–surgical nurse, perceived ministry as a key role in nursing practice:

We are ministering when we sit and counsel with patients; you are ministering to them when you are talking spiritual beliefs. This is part of our mission; we nurses wear so many different hats. We go from teacher, to being ministers, to doing the technical things of our trade like catheters and IVs. But the ministry part is a special gift; it is central to caring and to nursing.

And Martha, a critical care nurse, described how she learned the importance of spiritual ministry to those living with HIV/AIDS:

I've found that ministering to [people with HIV], to be open, to listen to them, has led to some very humbling experiences for me, and [they] have also been some of my most rewarding experiences. Once I learned that it was OK to cry with the patients; to scream with them. It was OK to just sit there and say nothing because I just didn't know what to say. I learned to just sit there and hold their hand; they will let you know if they want to talk. They don't want anything a lot of times. All they want is a touch or just to know that you are there; they don't want anything else.

Finally, Shannon, in describing her ministry to intensive care unit (ICU) patients, spoke about her approach to critical care, which included a reluctance to impose her personal faith beliefs on patients:

I try to figure out where a patient or their family is in terms of spirituality, and if there are needs there and they don't know how to bring it up. So, when something good comes up in a conversation, I'll say something like, "Well, you really have been blessed, haven't you?" And about 98 percent of the time that gives them the permission to let me know about their spirituality. I discovered that this way I can get to their spiritual side without being real threatening; it's just a word choice. . . . I've always been real sensitive to the fact that I have no right to impose my faith on anybody else, but to give folks a chance to articulate their own. If they're not clear on what they believe, sometimes just talking it out with a caring listener puts those issues in perspective. . . . There have been a number of times when folks have asked for a prayer after a conversation like that.

In sum, the spiritual mission of nursing might well be encapsulated in the challenge of Brother Roger of Taizé (1991) who asked, "Who will give the best of their creative gifts so that suffering throughout the world may be alleviated, in places where there is sickness, or hunger, or appalling housing conditions?" (p. 13). Brother Roger advised, "Perhaps you could place these Gospel words on the wall of your home; they come straight from the heart of Christ: 'Whatever you do to the least of my brothers and sisters, you are doing to me,' Matthew 25:40" (p. 13).

Messengers of Good Faith

A baccalaureate-prepared pediatric oncology nurse, Maria, described her perceived nursing vocation as related to the comments of a priest–chaplain at her hospital orientation. Maria explained:

> In our orientation Fr. O'Connor told us that we were "messengers of good faith." I really feel that is right but don't always see it happening on the units. The advanced technology has taken us somewhat away from the patients. But this is the kind of nurse I want to be, a nurse with a sense of vocation, of "good faith." . . . The spirituality, the strength of these children and their families amazes me; going through chemo and all that really affects their lives. I, being Catholic, attribute that strength to God. I need to support them with my faith.

Anna, a long-term hospice nurse, also spoke about the importance of spiritually supporting patients and families without imposing one's own beliefs:

> The idea of spiritual care is particularly important in the hospice setting. The spiritual component is just as important to hospice personnel as the physical component is. At every team meeting the spirituality of the patients is discussed; it is very holistic. . . . But we can't just go in and force our spirituality or our belief system on any patient. We need to meet patients wherever they are.

In their roles as messengers of good faith, nurses walk "among the hurting" attempting to "heal" and to "comfort"; they need to proclaim the love of God for His people. In her deeply moving book, *May I Have This Dance?*, Joyce Rupp (1992) reminded us that "[t]he Spirit of God dances among us, calls us to appreciate and enjoy life, and invites us to participate in the Divine Song that makes melody in the heart of all of creation" (p. 95).

No one is ignored; no one is excluded from the call to loving participation in the "Divine Song."

The Almost Sacred

The term *sacred* is defined variously as relating to "the service or worship of a deity"; "a thing worthy of religious veneration, or Holy"; or "something associated with religion or the religious" (*Merriam-Webster's Seventh New Collegiate Dictionary*, 1976, p. 757). A number of practicing nurses who shared spiritual thoughts or experiences used the word *sacred* in relating to some dimension of their interaction with patients. This is exemplified in the comments of Anne Marie and Karen.

A master's-prepared psychiatric–mental health nurse presently working at a research institution, Anne Marie noted that her choice of nursing had been strongly motivated by an "idealistic desire to help people." She reported:

> I considered other careers along the way but nursing gives you an opportunity to make a difference in people's lives. In nursing you deal with the "almost sacred." I know that sounds like strong words but nursing almost touches on the religious. Our work with patients is a real gift. The deep experiences and talks I have had with patients are the closest thing to a spiritual experience.

These are the times when you make these deeper connections with people that are spiritual; that is Christ within. Although you don't always recognize it or define it as God's presence within. I have been personally touched by those times.

And Karen, a doctorally prepared medical–surgical nurse, spoke about her approach to patient spiritual care as being a sacred trust:

I try to look and see if there is a way that patients are signaling me that they need spiritual support. I look to see if maybe they have a Bible laying out and if they're in pain or not sleeping, and I say, "I see you have your Bible here; is there a favorite passage you'd like me to read?" I might also ask, "What kinds of things are important to you?" to see if they might want to go to church or to talk to a chaplain.

I know that my calling as a Christian is to share the Gospel, the good news of Christ; this is a sacred trust. But also, the patient is a captive there and I struggle with getting the balance of "OK, how much am I injecting my values?" So that's why I look for clues to see what's important in their lives; so if it's meditation or listening to music, or whatever, I can pick up on that but if they do mention something to do with the Lord then I can either talk about Scripture or call a chaplain without hitting the person over the head with denominational religion. . . . We have to separate religion and spirituality. Religion is a lot different from spirituality and may be tied up with a lot of rules and prejudices and judgments, but spirituality is about how God reaches out to us and how we respond to that.

Frequently, practicing nurses noted that, although they might not be affiliated with the same religious denomination as a patient, there was, nevertheless, a common sense of spirituality to which they could relate. This provided a starting point from which the nurse could then assess the patient's spiritual needs or concerns.

Touching the Hand of God

The sacredness of a nurse's spiritual ministry was recognized clearly in instances of care for those facing life-threatening illness. In discussing ministry to the terminally ill, Niklas and Stefanics (1975) admitted that this may represent a time when the patient, faced with the reality of his or her own mortality, is open to the presence and the love of God. They suggested that the one ministering actually "walks with the dying person through the valley of the shadow of death" (p. 115). Thus, ministers need to be secure in their own relationship with God and in the understanding of their role in spiritual care.

Christian, a doctorally prepared nurse with 18 years of experience in hospice care, which had recently included a significant amount of care for those with HIV or AIDS, related his nursing vocation to work in the area of death and dying:

In nursing we have many opportunities to minister but we sometimes miss the opportunity to do this. But when facing death you really face the concept of spirituality, your own and your patients'. AIDS patients really articulate their spirituality in their coping. When you work with people who are dying, you touch the hand of God. . . . Spirituality is an area of nursing that would provide a really wonderful expanded role; for me, [spirituality] is primary.

Peg, a master's-prepared medical–surgical nurse with more than 20 years of experience, also described such a perception of closeness to God in caring for seriously ill patients:

> I remember working with some really critically ill patients, and really sensing the presence of God and their spiritual closeness. And especially at night when the hospital is quieter and more lonely, I felt that they [the patients] just wanted me to be there and to understand what they were going through. They may have only a few days to live but I could hold their hand and give them that presence of God's love and caring.

Sensing the Vibrations

Joyce, a master's-prepared nursing administrator with approximately 24 years of experience in medical–surgical and intensive care nursing, understood the concept of nursing as a Sacred Calling. She commented, "Spirituality, for me, is to allow both nurses and patients to self-actualize; to love, that is what brings about healing. That is what makes nursing, caring." Joyce observed that when she entered a nursing unit, she considered that part of her role as a clinical nursing administrator was in sensing the vibrations:

> When I walk on a ward, I can sense the vibrations, whether there's a lot of sickness, whether there's a lot of anxiety, a "darkness," and I think that those vibrations are part of spirituality. And I think that the more we love the more we send out our own vibrations of peace and we can lower the anxiety. As we love people we can bring them light; we can make them feel "lighter" and happier. I think that nurses need to do this to their stressful environments, to promote a wholesome, healthy, healing environment. . . . We are all connected in God.

A Healing Ministry

Jesus taught about the concept of ministry through His example of preaching, teaching, and especially of healing the ill and infirm. McGonigle (1993) pointed out that "Jesus sealed the truth of His ministry by the total gift of Himself for the Salvation of all those whom He came to serve" (p. 658). Many Christian health caregivers feel most appropriate in envisioning their work as a spiritual ministry when they relate their activities to Jesus' healing ministry.

This is well exemplified in the comments of Emily, a master's-prepared critical care nurse with 15 years of experience:

> Nurses, I believe, minister to patients, just as I believe that certified clergy do, as Christ did in his healing ministry. I look at the person in totality, the holistic approach. Sometimes it's just by being there, by listening. We talk about God and the love of God, and that He looks at the whole person, not just the last things you did. I have had many patients ask me to pray with them. . . . Nursing is a calling, a healing ministry. You can read and study but it has to be something that is within you, something you are called to do spiritually. . . . Especially in working with dying or critically ill patients you call on your spirituality. Sometimes if someone is suffering a lot you even pray that they will die but it's OK because of faith in God. We say,

"I see an angel on the foot of the bed." . . . "Growing up" in critical care you can become focused on the technology but you need to go beyond that. You can cry with the family; I have cried with so many patients and families.

Finally, Emily observed that there was a "definite need for staff nurses to 'marry-up' with chaplains and begin to talk about their spiritual experiences."

The comments from the Spirituality and Nursing study group represent only a few selected examples of the nurses' perceptions of their chosen profession as representing a Sacred Calling. As observed earlier, virtually all of the group members viewed some dimension of vocation or spiritual ministry as integral to their profession. Although this perception might be articulated through different concepts or anecdotes, the essential theme of nursing as a Sacred Calling pervaded the discussions.

Nonverbalized Theology

The second concept supporting the construct of the nurse as anonymous minister is described as Nonverbalized Theology. Repeatedly, discussions revealed individual nurses' "God-relationships" and "God-understanding" as being supported by such practices as the reading of Scripture, attendance at formal religious worship services, and personal prayer and meditation. None of the group, however, reported having formally studied theology, although several nurses suggested that it was something they had thought about and might consider doing in the future.

For Christians, theology is the study of "Divinely revealed religious truths. Its theme is the being and nature of God and His creatures and the whole complex of the Divine dispensation from the fall of Adam to the Redemption through Christ" (Livingstone, 1990, p. 509). Gerald O'Collins (1981), in his classic text *Fundamental Theology*, noted that the common understanding of the theological discipline is "faith seeking understanding" (p. 5). Although O'Collins accepted that we must come to the study of theology from a position of personal faith, he posited that the discipline "can help believers to describe, explain, interpret, and account for their faith" (p. 10). O'Collins added, "[Christians] know that they believe in the God revealed in Jesus Christ. Theology makes it easier or even possible to say just what it is they believe. With this help they can state their faith to both themselves and others" (p. 11).

Most of the nurses interviewed were articulate in describing their own faith beliefs, especially in terms of the Christian admonition to care for brothers and sisters in need. Many, however, admitted that they generally did not spend a lot of time speaking or consciously thinking about the dimension of spiritual ministry incorporated into their nursing practice; it was simply considered part of the caring activity central to the profession.

The concept of Nonverbalized Theology was suggested by Paula, a doctorally prepared medical–surgical nurse administrator with 22 years of experience. Paula asserted that nurses "minister" spiritually throughout their professional careers, although the underlying theology may never be verbalized:

Ministry is not a discreet function; a separate task. It is embedded in the careful giving of the meds, the wiping of the brow, the asking of the right questions, the acknowledgment of the patients' humanness, and what they are experiencing in their sickness. I can be there, to be a person of the love of God. You want to alleviate suffering, convey hope, bring love. It is in giving your care in a caring way; but there is no theology being verbalized; it's a nonverbalized theology. It's in our nursing that we recognize the spiritual side of ourselves and others.

Judith, a doctorally prepared cardiovascular nurse, supported the position:

I believe that nurses have been doing, and still do, spiritual care a whole lot but we just haven't called it that. . . . Before we didn't verbalize our theology or spirituality but now at least we have an official "nursing diagnosis" for "spiritual distress." I think that gives us a big opening for spiritual assessment of our patients. . . .

Nursing is a ministry but you don't have to speak Scriptures every time you see a patient. When you do spiritual care it can be like Jesus; He just didn't go in and do teaching; He went in and took care of the needs of people first. He fed them and healed them. So when you go in to a patient, take care of their physical needs before you do spiritual care; I believe that nursing is a combination between the art of caring and science. . . . We need to be sensitive. You can turn somebody off by coming on too strong; but you never turn them off by loving them. You always draw them to the Lord; by letting His love flow through you to them. That is the "Cup of Cold Water"; "you did it unto me."

Peter, a master's-prepared psychiatric–mental health nurse with 25 years of experience, also envisioned the concept of Nonverbalized Theology as supporting his clinical nursing practice:

We are oriented to look at patients holistically, as having a biological, psychological, and spiritual dimension. So, if you're dealing holistically with a patient, and if your underlying theology is that man is made in the image and likeness of God, and you have the perspective of an Incarnational theology, then this is how you approach the patient, even if not on a conscious or verbal level. I am an instrument through which God is present to this person, and in this person is the suffering, or the joyful, Christ. Christ is always present to the other person through you and you encounter Christ in that patient. So even if this theology is not always spoken, or conscious in your mind, but is your underlying theology, then, in holistic nursing, you are relating to the patient's spiritual needs as well as his physiological and psychological; you can't compartmentalize man.

In content analyzing the discussion data, six key concepts articulated by the nurses were identified as being reflective of the overall theme of Nonverbalized Theology: United in Suffering, Proddings of the Holy Spirit, The Day the Lord Has Made, Crying for More, Needing Ventilation, and Praying a Lot.

United in Suffering

Frequently during the discussions, nurse practitioners movingly demonstrated a non-verbalized theological concept of community by revealing a deep sense of empathy with and understanding of their patients' pain. Without sharing specific details, some of the nurses reported that personal experiences of pain and suffering had helped them become more sensitive caregivers; their interpretation was that having "been there" helped them better identify, at least broadly, with the concerns and anxieties of their patients. This is supported by Henri Nouwen's (1979) concept of the wounded healer, which he explained this way: "Making one's own wounds a source of healing . . . does not call for a sharing of superficial personal pains but a constant willingness to see one's own pain and suffering as rising from the depth of the human condition which all men share" (p. 88).

> Sharon, a doctorally prepared gerontologic nurse with 19 years of experience, observed:

> The older I get, the more confident I feel in sharing spiritual issues with my patients; we are all united in suffering, all children of God. I may not talk about my own pain, my own theology, a lot but I feel comfortable praying with my patients or assisting with a person's rituals. I understand where they're coming from if they're hurting. At this point in my career I am secure in my spirituality. . . . Some nurses are afraid of saying the wrong thing. I think it is a fear of confronting their own spirituality in dealing with patients. . . . Spirituality is that sense of community where God is most, through the presence of other people; Grace in our lives comes through other people.

> The concept that we are all united in suffering is well reflected in 1 Corinthians 12:12–26:

> As a body is one though it has many parts, and all the parts of the body though many, are one body, so also Christ. For in one Spirit we were all baptized into one body, whether Jews or Greeks, slaves or free persons, and we were all given to drink of one Spirit; . . . The eye cannot say to the hand, "I do not need you," nor again the head to the feet, "I do not need you." Indeed the parts of the body that seem to be weaker are all the more necessary, and those parts of the body that we consider less honorable, we surround with greater honor and our less presentable parts are treated with great propriety. . . . But God has so constructed the body . . . that the parts may have the same concern for one another. If one part suffers, all the parts suffer with it.

Proddings of the Holy Spirit

In Christian theology the Holy Spirit is understood as "the Third Person of the Trinity, distinct from, but consubstantial, co-equal and co-eternal with the Father and the Son, and in the fullest sense God" (Livingstone, 1990, p. 245). Farrelly (1993) suggested that in the early Church the "dynamism of Christian life" was ascribed to the Holy Spirit as the vehicle of God's love given to His people (p. 496). In John's Gospel, the "personal character" of the Holy Spirit is demonstrated. "'I will ask the Father and He will give you another advocate to be with you always, the Spirit of Truth'; John 14:16–17" (Farrelly, 1993, p. 499). A number of the nurse respondents spoke of the importance of the Holy Spirit's guidance in their work with patients, staff, or students. Maggie, a nursing administrator for over 11 years, who described herself as a Southern Baptist and born-again Christian, noted that, although she would never impose her spirituality on a patient, she was "comfortable discussing her own beliefs," if this seemed warranted. Maggie believed that there was definitely a "spiritual care" role for nurses "if you take the time to go a little deeper." She advised that the nurse has to observe and listen carefully to what a patient may be seeking, prior to any spiritual intervention, however. Her suggestion was, "Be attuned to the proddings of the Holy

Spirit." Maggie reported, "I have prayed with patients. The times I have felt good about a spiritual interaction [with a patient], I knew I was ministering."

Maggie described a specific instance in which she recognized the guidance of the Holy Spirit in her nursing ministry:

> I was working with a mom whose little girl was having some diagnostic tests and they didn't know what was going on and she was really worried. And when they were getting ready to transfer her, the mom came to me and said, "Are you a Christian?" And I said, "Yes, I am," and she said, "I thought you were. And I wanted you to know that you were an answer to prayer; because I prayed for a guardian angel during this hospital experience, because we didn't know what was going on and you were there for me, from the first day to the last.

Maggie concluded, "In those types of experiences I give credit to God; to the Holy Spirit. It was not me; I was just His instrument."

In commenting on the characterization of the Holy Spirit in St. John's Gospel, the ecumenical community of the Brothers of Taizé (Taizé Community, 1992) explained that we are not expected to actually see or experience the Spirit who dwells in us. "What is asked . . . is that we believe in the Holy Spirit, that we trust in Him, that we abandon ourselves to Him. Far from being another demand made on us, this call to faith sets us free" (p. 75).

The Day the Lord Has Made

Several nurses spoke of their gratitude for the spiritual ministry involved in their nursing practice. They saw it as a gift from God to whom they now gave thanks, as directed in Psalm 118:

> Give thanks to the Lord for He is good; His mercy endures forever. . . . The Lord is with me; He is my helper. . . . The Lord is my strength and my song. . . . This is the day the Lord has made; let us rejoice and be glad in it.

Margaret, a practical nurse with 16 years of experience who worked more recently with HIV and AIDS patients, asserted strongly:

> I may not discuss religion a lot but I couldn't do this work without my faith. I ask God to help me and then I can be calm. Prayer is important to me and seeing God in the smallest of things; in the miracles of flowers and birds. To deal with AIDS I have to do this. . . . I am so grateful to God for all that He has given me. I look at the trees in the morning and say, "this is the day the Lord has made." That's what will get you through.

Evelyn, an LPN with extensive experience working with mentally and physically challenged adults, also described her perception that each day was a day to give thanks for serving the Lord. "There is no separation of my day-to-day nursing and my spirituality. I live with it 24 hours a day; prayer in the morning, prayer at night. Each day is a gift of God. I'm not always conscious of it. I think it's like living prayer. It's all the time." Evelyn related her conscious awareness of the spiritual dimension of nursing to when she did hands-on care:

> I don't get to do as much "hands on" as I would like but when I do it's such a gift. I'm so grateful. There is something so holy. You say, "This person is

completely dependent upon my hands and my compassion to be cared for." It's seeing Christ there.

Crying for More

Repeatedly, nurses' comments reflected their perceptions of patients' spiritual hunger for God, their need for spiritual care and healing, even if not articulated in theological terminology. In his classic book *Reaching Out* (1975), Henri Nouwen observed that increased sophistication of the healing professions has resulted in depersonalizing the "interpersonal aspects" of the work (p. 92). Caregivers often are forced, by the demands of their jobs, to "keep some emotional distance to prevent over-involvement with . . . patients" (p. 73). Thus, Nouwen advised that "the healer has to keep striving for a spirituality . . . by which the space can be created in which healer and patient can reach out to each other as fellow travelers sharing the same broken human condition" (p. 93).

Anna, a doctorally prepared nurse educator who has worked with students in the clinical medical–surgical area for more than 28 years, expressed concern about patients' spiritual needs not being met:

> People have psychological and emotional needs, but deep down they have real spiritual needs; they are crying for more. . . . I think it's a real gap in our nursing practice; we get so caught up with the technology, there's no time for theology. There are times in life, especially when you're ill, when you really need spiritual support. . . . I try to get the students to see the whole person. They often don't get to that; especially the values, beliefs, religion. If we're going to look at the whole person, you have to include spirituality.

In the preface to her classic spiritual allegory *Hinds' Feet on High Places*, Hannah Hurnard (1975) reminded us that, as the Song of Songs expresses, there is in each human heart a cry for more, a desire for a deeper union with God. "He has made us for Himself, and our hearts can never know rest and perfect satisfaction until they find it in Him" (p. 11).

Needing Ventilation

Related to the concept of patients' spiritual "cry for more," is that of a need to verbalize spiritual and theological concerns and anxieties in the presence of a caring and supportive listener. Allowing a patient to tell his or her story was a concept that emerged frequently in discussions. Emotional pain, often long held at arm's length, may emerge vividly when the physiologic component of one's persona has been wounded. Defenses may be at an all-time low; this is a time when important healing can begin. Nouwen (1992) asserted that old wounds can only be healed by allowing them out of the dark corners of "forgetfulness." Caregivers must "offer the space in which the wounding memories of the past can be reached and brought back into the light without fear" (p. 23).

Karen, an ICU nurse with 30 years of experience, spoke at length about her intensive care unit patients' need to talk about their old anxieties and fears, especially related to the topics of illness and death. She recounted that when physicians suggest the administration of tranquilizing medication to calm patient anxieties, she reminds the staff that the patients "need ventilation, not sedation!" Karen, as ICU head nurse, directs her staff nurses to "sit down and hold their patients' hands: Be open to listen; it's a humbling and rewarding experience." Karen advises, "It's OK to say nothing!" And she encourages the staff to do continual assessments of their patients' spiritual needs. She also teaches that "It's OK to cry with patients; crying is not a weakness. This may validate the patient's legitimacy in ventilating anxiety through tears."

During periods of illness or physical debilitation, a patient's latent emotional stresses may surface, generating responses such as anxiety and feelings of loneliness and alienation. It is important, as demonstrated by the nurses' anecdotes, that these stress responses be ventilated.

Praying a Lot

Prayer is as unique as the individual who prays. Whether one's prayer is of petition, adoration, reparation, or thanksgiving, both the form and the content may vary greatly. A few generalizations about prayer, however, can be offered.

The term *prayer* means "a petition or request": "Although the word may be used to mean a petition made to anyone at all, its customary use is . . . more particular, made to God or some holy person reigning with God" (Wright, 1993, p. 764). Some methods of prayer identified by Jesuit John Wright (1993) include "vocal prayer," which employs a specific word formula; "mental prayer," which is more of a conversation with God; "discursive prayer," which is led by one's reason; "affective prayer," in which love, joy, or other emotions may predominate; "meditation," in which one considers different aspects of God's activity; "contemplation," which involves a "simple gazing" lovingly upon God; "centering prayer," in which one contemplates God at the center of one's being; "mystical prayer," which is led by God's grace; and finally, "private" and "communal prayer," the latter consisting of a group of worshippers praying together (pp. 773–775).

In relation to the theme of Nonverbalized Theology, the majority of practicing nurses admitted that prayer, in some form, was an important part of their lives. Mark, a baccalaureate-prepared eight-year nursing veteran working with HIV/AIDS patients, reported that his personal faith was critical to his nursing practice:

> I have strong faith. I truly believe that God puts you where He wants you. God tests us as Christians and as nurses. You become friends with your patients; it hurts to lose them. I pray a lot; I can't do what I do without a lot of prayer. . . . Some AIDS patients feel guilty and not worthy of healing; they are afraid that God won't hear their prayers. I tell them that God does not punish illness. I tell them to pray.

And a long-term critical care nurse spoke about prayer in the midst of technology:

> Critical care nurses have to deal with a lot of technology; but the beauty of technology is that after a while it becomes so rote that you can do it without thinking. Once you've got the moves down, I think it is quite possible for you, in the midst of a "Code," while you are pulling up drugs, to pray for that patient, to pray for whoever is making the decisions, to pray for the families who have to cope with whatever happens.

Although most of the nurses interviewed admitted that they did not often speak about theology or spirituality with nursing colleagues, it was definitely an underlying theme related to their practice. Frequently, at the end of the discussions, nurses offered such comments as, "At first, I didn't think I had much to say, but I really enjoyed talking about these spiritual things"; or "I do give spiritual care but I don't often take the time to think about it, or talk about it." The latter seems an excellent reflection of the overall theme of Nonverbalized Theology.

Nursing Liturgy

The third and final concept supporting the research-derived construct of the nurse as an anonymous minister is labeled Nursing Liturgy. Anecdotes describing creative nursing behaviors involving worship related to spiritual care of patients and families abound in the transcripts of the Spirituality and Nursing discussions. The term *liturgy* is broadly understood as relating to rites or rituals associated with public worship; the word *liturgy* is derived from the Greek, *leitourgia*, meaning "the work of the people" (*The Liturgy Documents*, 1991, p. xiv). In its early pre-Christian use, the term was understood to mean any public activities undertaken to promote communal well-being (Collins, 1990, p. 592). Christian usage focused the word's meaning on "the public worship of the Church" (p. 592).

Nursing Liturgy is conceptualized here as consisting of communal, worship-related, spiritual care activities carried out by nurses in the context of their professional practice. In its broadest meaning, the term *communal* may include worshipful interactions of the nurse–patient dyad only; that is, a nurse and patient praying together. The latter activity constitutes liturgy, for, as noted in Scripture, "Wherever two or three come together in My Name, I am there among them" (Matthew 18:20). Key concepts reflective of the Nursing Liturgy theme include Healing Rituals, Experiencing the Divine, Touching the Core, Being Present, Midwifing the Dying, and Privileged Moments.

Healing Rituals

The term *ritual* is derived from the Latin word *ritus*, meaning "structure." "Ritual is understood as a social, symbolic process which has the potential for communicating, creating, criticizing, and even transforming meaning" (Kelleher, 1990, p. 906). Madigan (1993) noted that "Religious rituals, like social rituals, are intended to be formative and expressive of personal and communal identity" (p. 832). Madigan asserted that, essentially, "Religious rituals are symbolic actions that unify the doer with the sacred" (p. 832).

In relating instances of what they perceived to be "spiritual care," many nurses described poignant worship-associated "rituals" that provided healing to both patients and caregivers; several discussants labeled these "graced moments."

Cathy, a pediatric nurse clinician with 15 years of experience, much of it in the area of pediatric critical care, told a touching story of the "liturgy" that she and two other staff members created to mark the passing of an anencephalic newborn.

> The baby, a "preemie," had lived for a couple of weeks, but there were so many congenital anomalies that there was no hope; so the family signed the papers to terminate life support. The parents just couldn't be there, though, so we decided to plan something. It was a very young neonatologist, it was really hard on him, and myself, and the peds ICU head nurse. We came into the NICU [neonatal intensive care unit] at about 5 am on a Saturday, when there weren't a lot of staff around. We took the baby into a separate little

isolation room and discontinued the vent and the IVs, all the life support systems. And then we prayed and we sang hymns and we just held her and loved her until she died. It was her special ritual to go to God, and we shared it with her; that baby gave a lot to us, too.

Julia, a master's-prepared nurse educator with 22 years of experience in medical–surgical and ICU nursing, described a nursing ritual she had created for her students on completion of their clinical experience:

At the end of the semester I wanted to do something special for the students, to acknowledge their gifts and their talents in caring for patients. It was to provide some type of rite of passage that they were finished with their clinical. I called it an "anointing of the hands"; it was a "blessing with oil." I would explain that oil is healing and say something specific to each student about her gifts as I rubbed the oil on her hands. As I was massaging the oil into the palms of their hands, I would describe their giftedness and their talents in terms of who they were. I would bless them in the name of the Lord. After I had been with them for 15 weeks, I could make the prayer specific to each one. It was acknowledging the sacredness within them. Some students would cry.

Megan, a doctorally prepared nursing administrator with 27 years of experience in hospital care, described what she labeled a "para-liturgical" service, during which she also conducted an "anointing of the hands." In this liturgy, she anointed and blessed with oil the hands of her hospital's medical interns at their closing assembly of the year. Megan prayed over each young physician as she did the anointing. She reported that many were close to tears during the experience.

The symbol of anointing has always had a special place in the care of the sick. Oil is used sacramentally as a sign of healing and provides comfort for those who are ill and their loved ones. The concept of anointing the sick is found repeatedly in Scripture, for example, Mark 6:13. "And they cast out many demons, and anointed with oil many that were sick and healed them." Cunningham (1990) suggested that any "anointing" of a person may result in "a change in the person physically [health, strength, fertility] or in the relationship one has with the community" (p. 21).

Several of the nurse educators teaching in schools of nursing reported that they began their classes with a ritual of prayer or spiritual meditation. Frequently these rituals were nondenominational in order to include all of the students present. One nursing faculty member explained, "At the beginning of each class I give about a 2-minute spiritual reflection. One day, when we started into some questions about an exam without doing it, the students stopped me and said, 'Aren't we going to pray today?'"

Experiencing the Divine

The majority of practicing nurses indicated having at some time experienced God through interactions with their patients. For some the experience was conscious and ongoing; for others "critical incidents" highlighted a sense of experiencing the divine in a patient. This varied to some degree according to age and nursing experience, with more than a few nurses explaining that the longer they practiced their profession, the more "tuned in" they became to the presence of God within; this occurred in regard to both themselves and their patients. One nurse observed, "I feel like this kind of caring, this kind of experiencing and caring for God in your patients, is like going to church; it's a worship experience."

Julia, with her 22 years of experience in nursing practice, commented, "Nurses are always involved in spiritual care but they don't talk about it; they don't put a label on it" (as reflected in the theme Nonverbalized Theology). She went on to identify some nursing encounters that she perceived as reflecting spiritual experiences in nurse–patient interactions:

> I remember the first time that I ever experienced the divine in another person, in the woundedness of an individual. It just happened. It was an unattractive little old man who was drooling and unable to feed himself. His name was Tom. He seemed repulsive to me. He wasn't pleasant to look at and couldn't even respond to you. But I was caring for him and all of a sudden I thought, "Oh, this is what is meant by Christ within. Christ is present within this man who I initially saw as repulsive." . . . This was a graced moment for me. It was like a quiet kind of awakening; it was parallel to a faith experience!

Touching the Core

As a dimension of the dominant theme of Nursing Liturgy, several nurses spoke about the unique nature of the relationships developed in providing spiritual care for those who are ill. This was true whether the interactions consisted of formal spiritually oriented rites or rituals or more informal types of behaviors, such as praying with patients or discussing spiritual needs or concerns. Repeatedly the concept of depth in nurse–patient interactions related to spirituality emerged from discussion data; nurses spoke of the special opportunity to relate to patients intimately at a time when they are particularly open and vulnerable. This was perceived as a rewarding experience for the caregiver as well as for the patient.

Kinast (1990) asserted that in spiritual ministry to the sick "the deepest and richest human experiences are those which are shared between persons" (p. 9); that is, those in which the minister is able to touch the heart of another person.

Barbara, a doctorally prepared nurse educator with 23 years of experience in the area of pediatrics, commented that "Nursing is much more important than what you are doing [technically] to people; healing takes place just by being with people, by touching their spirituality. A gift to us as nurses is to be able to touch the core of someone."

Barbara's concept of touching the (spiritual) core, or holy place, of another is supported by a description of ministry to those living with HIV infection, in which a caregiver labeled his patient interactions "holy places we share when we have time together" (O'Brien, 1992, p. 99). The caregiver continued, "There is an incredible sweetness in being with these persons [with HIV], even when they are very ill and death is imminent; it gives one the incredible sense of 'holding a sacredness'".

Being Present

Barbara also spoke about the concept of being present, which she perceived as "integral to the spirituality of the nurse–patient relationship." Barbara described being present as the idea of "listening with a loving heart." She affirmed, "I don't know how you can relate to somebody, to be with them in their loneliness, without that dimension."

Holst (1992) highlighted the loneliness of being ill in his discussion of the hospital as "paradox." Although, he noted, privacy is rare, "there can be an eerie loneliness in the midst of all those human contacts" (p. 6). This is, in part, related to the fact that, although advanced technology is devoted to carefully monitoring disease, the person experiencing the disease may be neglected. Technology, Holst (1992) observed, makes us "more preoccupied with the heart as a pump, than with the heart as the seat of emotions" (p. 7).

This paradox is also addressed by James Nelson (1976) who asserted that fundamental to a patient's healing process is the presence of caring persons in the health-care facility. "Caring," Nelson added, "is an active attitude which genuinely conveys to the other person that he or she really does matter. It is different from wanting to care for another in the sense of making that person dependent on us. Rather it involves a profound respect for the otherness of the other" (p. 63). To take the concepts of presence and caring a step further, Henri Nouwen (1991) observed that the basis of caring ministry, the point at which ministry and spirituality touch each other, is compassion (p. 33). "Compassion," Nouwen continued, "is hard because it requires the inner disposition to go with others to the place where they are weak, vulnerable, lonely and broken" (p. 34). This, he added, is not our natural response to suffering; we generally either desire to flee from it or to find a "quick cure" (p. 34). In so doing, however, Nouwen argued "we ignore our greatest gift, which is our ability to enter into solidarity with those who suffer" (p. 34).

Many other project participants highlighted the importance of being present to patients in their suffering.

Pat, a baccalaureate-prepared critical care nurse with three years of experience, observed that in providing spiritual care "You have to have intuition beyond the psychological. We're the ones right there at the bedside. You can be the facilitator, find out what the patient and family need spiritually, just by being present."

Kathryn, a master's-prepared psychiatric–mental health nursing administrator with more than 30 years of experience in nursing, noted that "Taking care of the sick is a ministry in and of itself. The idea of ministering and really being present to people helps me to see them as whole individuals, and my own spirituality leads me to see the individual through the eyes of Christ."

And, Diane, a master's-prepared operating room nurse with 19 years of experience, described her conceptualization of being present to her OR patients by praying for them during surgery. "Especially when open-heart surgery patients are in the OR, on the 'Pump,' and we are literally touching their hearts; that's the time when I especially pray for that patient." Diane added, "I serve God through being present for my patients."

Midwifing the Dying

In his article "Religious Approaches to Dying," Anglican Father David Head (1994) reminded us that "Death is integrated as a concept into religious belief systems, and also the religious belief systems integrate death and life" (p. 306). For many "religious" people the beliefs surrounding death "may be comforting" (p. 305). Their tenets often include such concepts as "the transitory nature of the state of death" and "entry into an unknown mystery that is congruent to human experience" (p. 305).

In ministering to a dying person, the caregiver must understand not only the patients' beliefs and feelings about death, but his or her own as well. Niklas and Stefanics (1975) pointed out that if a caregiver is "not in tune with his feelings [about death], they become a weapon or a barrier preventing the dying person and his family from expressing their feelings, or cause him to lack appreciation of the feelings that are being expressed" (p. 114).

Although a number of nurses spoke about the importance of being present to their patients and their families during the death and dying experience, two actually described themselves as being like midwives helping their patients to be "born into a new life." One was Jan, a master's-prepared medical–surgical clinician with 21 years of nursing experience, a significant portion of which involved working with terminally ill patients. She observed, "I help patients to 'cross-over' in the last few days. Part of our job is being like midwives in assisting people in getting to that next state, to their new life in God. We are not only nurses and spiritual caregivers, we are family."

And Sarah, a peds oncology nurse with extensive experience in dealing with death and dying among children, related a special midwifing experience:

> I just got a letter at Christmastime from a family of a little boy who died about 5 years ago. And it was such a precious experience for me; how I bonded with him and with the family. When he was dying we picked him up and we held him and prayed with him and sang to him, and I felt like a midwife; that was really a gift. Being a midwife; it was like helping him to be born into eternal life. You feel so humbled and so privileged just being a part of it.

Sherrie, a master's-prepared critical care nurse with 15 years of experience, described her privileged experience in working with a family whose baby died shortly after birth:

> This was a gift for me and I hope I helped the family. We spent a lot of time with [the baby] in the 3 days before she died. We dressed her and held her and sang to her. I told the family, "We are all God's angels and some of us He wants back with Him sooner." . . . God had a special role for that baby. In the 3 days' time this baby gave and received more love than you will ever know. . . . It's a gift to us to be with anyone who is so close to being with God, to be with them in this special time of transition from this life to a new life.

Privileged Moments

As noted earlier, gratitude for the opportunity for spiritual encounters with patients emerged frequently as a theme in the Nursing and Spirituality discussions. Our nurse project participants reported a multiplicity of privileged moments related to spiritual care interactions with patients. A number of these are evident in the comments and anecdotes already presented. Especially touching are those related by Mary, Daniel, and Sarah.

Mary, a master's-prepared community health nurse with approximately 16 years of experience, most of it in hospice care, described her perception of spiritual care:

> Nurses should never force their spiritual beliefs on patients. . . . Just sitting with a patient, especially one who is dying, I think that is very much spiritual care. . . . Being a hospice nurse is so humbling; it's such a privilege. As hospice nurses, people really take us into their hearts. We have the opportunity to be with people during that time of life transition. We are connecting with

the very depth of a person who is facing death. And when they actually pass on, that is a very privileged moment to share with them.

Daniel, a 25-year nursing veteran, also spoke about the privilege of working with patients close to death:

> I have always felt so privileged to work with patients in the final chapter of their lives on earth because it is such a rewarding experience. It is the tremendous privilege of being there. You try to do things that the patient is comfortable with. I remember especially the time I was caring for Mark; he was terminal with AIDS and he wanted me to take him upstairs to the bathroom. So I got him up there and then I thought, "Now, how can I get him back down?"; getting him up had been challenging enough! And I just said, "Well, Mark, I think the best thing is if you just get on my back." And I carried him that way, and it was really a privileged moment, like a mystical experience, I guess. It was like carrying Christ, a really powerful experience. . . . In situations like this you see yourself as merely an instrument through which God's love is present in the life of the suffering person. It's a mystery to us but it's through grace that I am here and can do what needs to be done in order to make God's love and compassion present to this person in his time of need. . . . We don't usually think of this consciously but there are times when it raises our consciousness, to be used by God, like when I carried Mark down the stairs.

Finally, Sarah related a poignant story that she described as a special and privileged moment with one of her small oncology patients:

> Timmy was very disfigured with basal cell sarcoma and he hated to have his blood drawn. He usually screamed and his mom cried, so I'd started praying when I drew it; we prayed together. And so one day we prayed, and I got right in and got the blood, and Timmy was very happy. And it was the first time he had really made a connection with me. So he came into the utility room with me to help label the tubes, and he picked one up to put on the label and dropped it; and it shattered all over the floor. And I thought, "Oh God, how could you have let this happen after we all prayed?" But when I talked to the doctor he said that we could do without the blood that day. But Timmy felt really bad, and as a result, I spent a lot of time with him, and when they went to leave, I went over and hugged and kissed him; that was the first time that we really had connected like that. Since that time Timmy, when he comes in, always runs up and we hug and kiss. And, I realized that God was really working in our lives that day, except maybe not in the way I expected; that hug was much more important than the blood getting drawn. When God reveals something like that to you it is a very privileged moment.

▶ The Mysticism of Everyday Nursing

The comments of Mary, Daniel, and Sarah, like those of other nursing practitioners reported in the previous pages, exemplify a concept identified by theologian Karl

Rahner as the "mysticism of everyday life." Rahner contended that "the human person is 'homo mysticus'—one who experiences God because of an orientation to God rooted in the way God has made human nature" (Egan, 1989, p. 8). In Rahner's mind "everyone is at least an anonymous mystic" (p. 8). Egan observed that for Karl Rahner nothing about day-to-day life was "profane": "Wherever there is radical self-forgetting for the sake of the other . . . surrender to the mystery that embraces all life, there is . . . the mysticism of everyday life" (p. 8). Rahner's concept might appropriately be translated to read: the mysticism of everyday nursing.

Throughout this chapter members of the professional nursing community have, through their anecdotes and reflections, demonstrated themselves to be not only "anonymous ministers" but also "anonymous mystics." This is evidenced by the many reports of tender care and compassion provided for patients. Although contemporary nurses, whether practitioners, educators, administrators, or researchers, generally do not consciously think of themselves as either mystics or ministers, the data, as exemplified in their attitudes and behaviors, warrant the use of both labels. These findings indeed explain why at least one author has called nursing "the finest art" (Donahue, 1985), why nurse authors Joanne Widerquist and Ruth Davidhizar have described nursing as "ministry" (1994), and why mysticism and ministry may truly be considered integral dimensions of everyday nursing.

▶ References

Angking, D. (2012). Preparing for nursing ministry. *Journal of Christian Nursing, 29*(1), 59.

Becker, A. L. (2009). Ethical considerations of teaching spirituality in the academy. *Nursing Ethics, 16*(6), 697–706.

Benbow, D. (2013). Professional boundaries: When does the nurse-patient relationship end? *Journal of Nursing Regulation, 4*(2), 30–33.

Burnard, P. (1988). Search for meaning. *Nursing Times, 84*(37), 34–36.

Collins, M. (1990). Liturgy. In J. Komonchak, M. Collins, & D. Lane (Eds.), *The new dictionary of theology (NDT)* (pp. 591–601). Collegeville, MN: The Liturgical Press.

Cunningham, J. L. (1990). Anointing. In J. Komonchak, M. Collins, & D. Lane (Eds.), *The new dictionary of theology (NDT)* (pp. 21–23). Collegeville, MN: The Liturgical Press.

Devenny, B., & Duffy, K. (2014). Person-centered reflective practice. *Nursing Standard, 28*(28), 37–43.

Dinc, L., & Gastmans, C. (2013). Trust in nurse-patient relationships: A literature review. *Nursing Ethics, 20*(5), 501–516.

Donahue, M. P. (1985). *Nursing: The finest art, an illustrated history*. St. Louis, MO: C. V. Mosby.

Dunn, L. (2008). Spirituality and nursing: Personal responsibility. *Journal of Rural Nursing and Health Care, 8*(1), 3–4.

Egan, H. D. (1989, February). The mysticism of everyday life. *Studies in Formative Spirituality, 10*(1), 7–25.

Farrelly, M. J. (1993). Holy Spirit. In M. Downey (Ed.), *The new dictionary of Catholic spirituality (NDCS)* (pp. 492–503). Collegeville, MN: The Liturgical Press.

Griffith, R. (2013). Professional boundaries in the nurse-patient relationship. *British Journal of Nursing, 22*(18), 1087–1088.

Hart, J. (2010). The Center for Spirituality & Healing at the University of Minnesota. *Alternative and Complementary Therapies, 16*(1), 50–54.

Head, D. (1994). Religious approaches to dying. In I. Corless, B. Germino, & M. Pittman (Eds.), *Dying, death, and bereavement* (pp. 229–314). Sudbury, MA: Jones & Bartlett Learning.

Holland, P. D. (1990). Vocation. In J. Komonchak, M. Collins, & D. Lane (Eds.), *The new dictionary of theology (NDT)* (pp. 1087–1092). Collegeville, MN: The Liturgical Press.

Holst, L. E. (1992). *Hospital ministry.* New York, NY: Crossroad.

Hurnard, H. (1975). *Hinds' feet on high places.* Wheaton, IL: Tyndale House.

Kelleher, M. M. (1990). Ritual. In J. Komonchak, M. Collins, & D. Lane (Eds.), *The new dictionary of theology (NDT)* (pp. 906–907). Collegeville, MN: The Liturgical Press.

Kinast, R. L. (1990). Caring for God's covenant of freedom: A theology of pastoral care. In H. Hayes & C. Van der Poel (Eds.), *Health care ministry* (pp. 7–21). New York, NY: Paulist Press.

Lane, M. R. (2005). Creativity and spirituality in nursing: Implementing art in healing. *Holistic Nursing Practice, 19*(3), 122–125.

Ledger, S. D. (2005). The duty of nurses to meet patients' spiritual and/or religious needs. *British Journal of Nursing, 14*(4), 220–225.

The liturgy documents: A parish resource. (1991). Chicago, IL: Liturgy Training Publications.

Livingstone, E. A. (1990). *The concise Oxford dictionary of the Christian church.* New York, NY: Oxford University Press.

Madigan, S. (1993). Ritual. In M. Downey (Ed.), *The new dictionary of Catholic spirituality (NDCS)* (pp. 832–833). Collegeville, MN: The Liturgical Press.

McCabe, G. (2008). Mind, body, emotions and spirit: Reaching to the ancestors for healing. *Counseling Psychology Quarterly, 21*(2), 143–152.

McGonigle, T. (1993). Ministry. In M. Downey (Ed.), *The new dictionary of Catholic spirituality (NDCS)* (pp. 658–659). Collegeville, MN: The Liturgical Press.

Merriam-Webster's seventh new collegiate dictionary. (1976). Springfield, MA: Merriam-Webster.

Myers, J. (2009). Spiritual calling. *Nursing Standard, 23*(40), 22.

Nelson, J. (1976). *Rediscovering the person in medical care.* Minneapolis, MN: Augsburg.

Niklas, G., & Stefanics, C. (1975). *Ministry to the hospitalized.* New York, NY: Paulist Press.

Nouwen, H. J. M. (1975). *Reaching out.* New York, NY: Doubleday.

Nouwen, H. J. M. (1979). *The wounded healer.* Garden City, NY: Image Books.

Nouwen, H. J. M. (1991). *Creative ministry.* New York, NY: Image Books.

Nouwen, H. J. M. (1992). *The living reminder: Service and prayer in memory of Jesus Christ.* New York, NY: HarperCollins.

O'Brien, M. E. (1992). *Living with HIV: Experiment in courage.* Westport, CT: Auburn House.

O'Collins, G. (1981). *Fundamental theology.* New York, NY: Paulist Press.

O'Connell, L. J. (1993). Vocation. In M. Downey (Ed.), *The new dictionary of Catholic spirituality (NDCS)* (pp. 1009–1010). Collegeville, MN: The Liturgical Press.

Pesut, B. (2008). Spirituality and spiritual care in nursing fundamentals textbooks. *Journal of Nursing Education, 47*(4), 167–173.

Pipe, T., Hansen, P., Hentz, J., & Hartsell, Z. (2010). Rediscovering the art of healing by creating the tree of life poster. *Journal of Gerontological Nursing, 36*(6), 47–54.

Rademacher, W. (1991). *Lay ministry: A theological, spiritual and pastoral handbook.* New York, NY: Crossroad.

Ray, M. A. (1994, May–June). Communal moral experience as the starting point for research in health care ethics. *Nursing Outlook, 43*(3), 104–109.

Reblin, M., Otis-Green, S., Ellington, L., & Clayton, M. F. (2014). Strategies to support spirituality in healthcare communication. *Journal of Holistic Nursing, 32*(4), 269–277.

Robb, I. H. (1912). *Nursing ethics: For hospital and private use.* Cleveland: E.D. Koeckert Publishing.

Roger of Taizé. (1991). *No greater love.* Collegeville, MN: The Liturgical Press.

Rupp, J. (1992). *May I have this dance?* Notre Dame, IN: Ave Maria Press.

Shores, C. (2010). Spiritual perspectives of nursing students. *Nursing Education Perspectives, 31*(1), 8–11.

Taizé Community. (1992). *Listening with the heart.* Collegeville, MN: The Liturgical Press.

Tiew, L., & Creedy, D. (2010). Integration of spirituality in nursing practice: A literature review. *Singapore Nursing Journal, 37*(1), 15–22.

Tyler, I., & Raynor, J. (2006). Spirituality in the natural sciences and nursing: An interdisciplinary perspective. *ABNF (Association of Black Nursing Faculty) Journal, 17*(2), 63–66.

van Leeuwen, R., Tiesinga, L., Jochemsen, H., & Post, D. (2007). Aspects of spirituality concerning illness. *Scandinavian Journal of Caring Science, 21*, 482–489.

Widerquist, J., & Davidhizar, R. (1994). The ministry of nursing. *Journal of Advanced Nursing, 19*, 647–652.

Wright, J. H. (1993). Prayer. In M. Downey (Ed.), *The new dictionary of Catholic spirituality (NDCS)* (pp. 764–775). Collegeville, MN: The Liturgical Press.

Wright, S., & Neuberger, J. (2012). Why spirituality is essential for nurses. *Nursing Standard, 26*(40), 19–21.

CHAPTER 6

Spiritual Care: The Nurse's Role

And remember every nurse should be one who is to be depended upon . . . she must have a respect for her own calling, because God's precious gift of life is often literally placed in her hands.

Florence Nightingale, 1859

I look at nursing's role definitely as a calling to serve the sick. Because I think any nurse has to give 100% of herself or himself into the profession and to truly be a professional, they have to look at it beyond being an ordinary type of job; to include spiritual as well as physical and psychosocial care. I think it is truly a caring profession; nurses need to give of themselves sometimes when they are not feeling up to giving of themselves.

Annemarie, School Health Nurse

In years past, spiritual care was generally not considered a dimension of nursing therapeutics. With the advent of the holistic health movement, however, together with the notion of holistic nursing, assessment of an ill person's spiritual needs, and in some cases the practice of spiritual care, became recognized as legitimate activities within the domain of nursing. In light of the current interest in the nurse's role in patients' spiritual care, the present chapter explores the practice of spiritual care as nursing intervention; the attention given to patients' spiritual needs and concerns within the grand theories of nursing; some basic tenets of key Eastern and Western religious traditions; and the nurse's use of spiritual and religious resources such as prayer, Scripture, and sacred music. Referral to a formally designated pastoral caregiver is an acceptable option for the nurse not personally comfortable with the practice of spiritual care.

▶ The Nurse's Role in Spiritual Care

Clinical and research professionals sometimes question whether indeed the nurse has a relevant role in providing spiritual care to patients in his or her charge. The topic was addressed briefly in terms of nursing assessment of spiritual needs. The point bears repeating, however, that identification of the nurse's role in providing spiritual care is in no way meant to devalue the role of the hospital chaplain or the pastor ministering to the ill in the community. Rather, the nurse and pastoral care provider can work together to assess the spiritual needs of the ill person and support a comprehensive plan of spiritual care. Although not all nurses may feel comfortable providing spiritual care in all situations, the nurse should always be sensitive to the spiritual needs of his or her patients. With the advent of the holistic health-care concept, it is suggested that the "nursing profession must expand its awareness and competence in the spiritual dimension" (Nelson, 1984, p. 26).

Nursing textbooks, particularly those addressing fundamentals of nursing and medical–surgical nursing, reveal that the nurse's role in both assessment of patients' spiritual needs and the provision of spiritual care is a significant component of overall nursing. Several fundamental texts contain chapters with titles such as "Spirituality," "Spiritual Health," and "Spirituality and Religion" (Kozier, Erb, Blais, & Wilkinson, 1995; Potter & Perry, 1997; Taylor, Lillis, & LeMone, 1997). These chapters include such topics as spiritual health, spiritual problems, assessment of patients' spiritual needs, religious practices, spirituality and family needs, spirituality and the nursing process, and nursing diagnosis of spiritual distress. Many medical–surgical nursing texts also contain discussions of the nurse's role in spiritual care of the patient. Topics included are spirituality and nursing practice, spiritual care, assessment of patients' spiritual needs, nursing diagnoses, religious beliefs and practices, death-related spiritual beliefs, and spiritual beliefs in coping with acute and chronic illness (Black & Matassarin-Jacobs, 1997; Ignatavicius, Workman, & Mishler, 1995; Phipps, Cassmeyer, Sands, & Lehman, 1995; Smeltzer & Bare, 1996). In discussing the psychosocial dimensions of medical–surgical nursing, Edmision (1997) stated unequivocally that "meeting the spiritual needs of clients has become a recognized part of nursing care" (p. 68).

In the periodical nursing literature also, spiritual care is identified as a recognized element of holistic practice (Bruner, 1985; Labun, 1988; Sims, 1987) and is viewed as central to quality care (Clark, Cross, Dean, & Lowry, 1991; Simsen, 1988). A number of spiritual care models (Ceronsky, 1993; Karns, 1991) and creative approaches to spiritual care (Praill, 1995) have been advanced. Julia Lane (1987) suggested that the spiritual care of patients be addressed in three parts: first, by identifying the characteristics of spiritual care in relation to the essential nature of the human person; second, by identifying spiritual care interventions; and finally, by viewing nursing as a vocation (p. 332). Emblen and Halstead (1993) identified five spiritual care interventions appropriate to nursing: "listening to the patient express key concerns; praying with the patient; reading favorite portions of religious readings; spending time with the patient; and making a referral to a chaplain" (pp. 181–182). Dennis (1991), in a study of 10 nurses who reported providing spiritual support from a nonreligious perspective, also found the concepts of listening and spending time with patients to be important components of spiritual care. Recent research has demonstrated that there is a need for educational strategies to prepare nurses for spiritual caregiving (Greenstreet, 1999);

spiritual care infiltrates all aspects of nursing care (Carroll, 2001); there are cultural aspects involved in spiritual care (Sellers, 2001); and nurses themselves derive much satisfaction from providing spiritual care to their patients (Kumar, 2004; Narayanasamy & Owens, 2001; Nolan, 2000; Stephenson & Wilson, 2004; Treloar, 2001). From a review of the literature, three key competencies of spiritual care were identified, including "awareness of the use of self; spiritual dimensions of the nursing process; and assurance and quality of expertise" (van Leeuwen & Cusveller, 2004, p. 234).

Explorations into the nature and role of spiritual care in nursing were conducted by Ellis and Narayanasamy (2009) and Pearce (2009). Tanyi, McKenzie, and Chapek (2009) investigated the incorporation of spiritual care into practice by nurse practitioners and other health-care professionals. Spiritual care was defined by Hummell, Galek, Murphy, Tannenbaum, and Flannelly (2008). Nurses' understanding of spiritual care was explored by P. Kemp (2009); Chung, Wong, and Chan (2007); Swift, Calcutawalla, and Elliott (2007); and R. Moore (2007).

How can the nurse not grounded in a religious tradition or spiritual philosophy practice spiritual care? Should such a nurse attempt to intervene relative to the spiritual needs of an ill person? Ultimately the response must lie with the individual nurse.

As noted earlier, all nurses are responsible for being aware of and sensitive to their patients' spiritual needs as a dimension of holistic health care. It is suggested that nurses may even "be called upon to pray with or for patients as a part of holistic care" (Narayanasamy & Narayanasamy, 2008, p. 394), and in a discussion of "ethical principles of spirituality," Cheryl Lantz (2007) observed that nurses are "ethically obligated to provide spiritual care to clients" (p. 36). It has also been noted, however, that the lack of a clear definition of spirituality may hinder nurses from providing adequate spiritual care (Denholm, 2008, pp. 451–452).

The minimizing or neglect of this aspect of patient care may have serious implications for the overall illness adaptation. The nurse must consider spiritual needs as part of a comprehensive nursing assessment. What may vary, however, is the degree to which individual nurses carry out therapeutic intervention in response to spiritual needs. Many nurses do feel both comfortable and confident in engaging in such spiritual care activities as praying with patients, sharing the reading of Scripture passages, and listening to and counseling a patient about spiritual concerns. These activities may be appropriately carried out by a nurse if acceptable to the patient and family. For the nurse who does not feel adequately prepared to be involved in the practice of spiritual care, the appropriate course of action is referral to another nurse comfortable with providing spiritual intervention or to a formally trained pastoral caregiver.

Related to the nurse's role as anonymous minister, the majority of spiritual care provided as a component of nursing activity is unrecognized and unacknowledged. Spiritual care is rarely documented on patients' charts (Broten, 1997, p. 29). Nevertheless, current nursing research and clinical evaluations continue to identify the value placed on the nurse's role in providing spiritual care, by both patients and families.

A number of 21st-century professional articles confirm the importance of the role of spirituality in nursing practice. Nursing leader Phillip Kemp (2009) points out that spiritual care is so central to nursing practice that it is incorporated in "the way in which [a nurse] behave[s], talk[s], care[s], guide[s] or treat[s] people" (p. 334). Spiritual care, it is asserted, "is widely recognized in nursing theory," and "involves a complexity of social processes, of which developing caring relationships is core" (Carr, 2008, p. 686). Nevertheless, it is also recognized that spiritual care is not always understood and sometimes "dwells on the periphery of the profession" (Carr, 2010, p. 1379). Nursing leader Anna-Marie Stevens (2011) suggests that there can be "a role for spirituality in palliative care leadership" (p. 315), and nurse educator Donia Baldacchino reported the introduction of an experience in spiritual care for nursing students in order to expose them to the practice (2010).

The contemporary nurse's role in providing spiritual care to patients also seems to be cemented by a proliferation of journal articles discussing related issues such as: "Who can give spiritual care?" (Kevern, 2012); nurses' perceptions of spiritual care (McSherry & Jamieson, 2013; McSherry & Jamieson, 2011); a health services framework of spiritual care (Daaleman, 2012); perspectives of spiritual care among nurse managers (Battey, 2012); "creating conditions for good nursing by attending to the spiritual" (Biro, 2012, p. 1002); research on spiritual care in nursing (Cockell & McSherry, 2012); and studying "the lived experience of giving spiritual care" (Deal & Grassley, 2012). A spiritual care values model to guide what is described as one having a "careful nursing perspective" was published by nurse educator Therese Connell Meehan (2012, p. 990).

The importance of the nurse's role in spiritual care is also reflected in journal articles discussing the importance of education on patients' spiritual needs and spiritual care interventions in undergraduate nursing programs. Some examples include: "the efficacy of integrating spirituality into undergraduate nursing curricula" (Yilmaz & Gurler, 2014, p. 929); introducing spirituality into a baccalaureate nursing program (Yuan & Porr, 2014, p. 240); use of simulation techniques to teach students spiritual care (Costello, Atinaja-Faller, & Hedberg, 2012); undergraduate nursing educators teaching spiritual care (Cone & Giske, 2012); nursing students learning spiritual care (Giske & Cone, 2012); undergraduate nursing students learn to care spiritually (Giske, 2012); and nurse educators promote inclusive spiritual care (Barss, 2012).

Pediatric nurse practitioner Mary Sweat (2012) observes that part of spiritual care may be simply providing a "quiet place" for the patient and suggests four premises to support the idea; these ask the nurse to "respect privacy," "create an environment that promotes respect," "respect individual preferences," and "respect yourself" (p. 180). Wright and Neuberger (2012) offer "a seven point manifesto" for integrating spirituality into nursing care. The positions include:

1. Spiritual care is not a luxury . . . but goes to the heart of care.
2. Educational programs that nurses undertake must provide an in-depth understanding of what people mean by spirituality.
3. Imaginative educational programs for nurses relating to spiritual care [should be offered].
4. The workplaces of nurses should ideally provide all patients with access to spiritual support.
5. Spirituality has a direct effect on health and well-being.
6. Spiritual care . . . is essential for the ongoing training of all nurses.
7. Spiritual care is also a part of enhancing the healing environment (p. 21).

▶ Spiritual Care and Religious Tradition

In order to engage in the assessment of spiritual needs and the provision of spiritual care for patients whose personal spirituality is intimately interwoven with religious beliefs and practices, the nurse should have some basic knowledge about the traditions of the major world religions. Obviously, the nurse may not herself subscribe to the religious tenets and practices of a particular patient; however, a broad understanding of the patient's religious culture will assist in identifying spiritual problems and in making referrals to an appropriate pastoral caregiver. The spiritual care of the atheist, who denies the existence of God, and the agnostic, who questions the existence of God, may consist of listening to and providing emotional support for the patient.

It is neither the intent nor within the scope of this text to present a comprehensive review of world religions. The following discussion is intended only as an overview of key tenets of the religious groups described. This delineation of selected spiritual and religious beliefs and practices may, however, provide the nurse with a starting point in interaction with patients of different faiths. The best strategy in conducting a spiritual assessment is to attempt to learn from the patient or a family member which religious beliefs and practices are most important, especially those pertinent to health and illness issues.

Two major categories of religious tradition are generally considered to be Western spiritual philosophy and Eastern spirituality. The three key Western religions are Judaism, Christianity, and Islam; all are founded on a monotheistic theology. Major Eastern traditions include Buddhism, Hinduism, and Confucianism, the tenets of which differ, especially in regard to the worship of God or of a multiplicity of gods.

Native American religions, of which there are many, generally look to the earth and the spirits of nature for comfort, sustenance, and support. Most Native American religions share a common view of the cycle of life and death and use ritual ceremonies to mark life transitions (Taylor, Lillis, & LeMone, 1997).

Western Religious Traditions

Within the Western religions of Judaism, Christianity, and Islam, the one supreme being is named Yahweh, God, or Allah.

Judaism is described as one of the oldest religions "still practiced in western civilization" and "the foundation on which both Christianity and Islam were built" (Taylor, Lillis, & LeMone, 1997, p. 885). The major religious Jewish groups are Orthodox, Conservative, and Reform; a more recently identified fourth Jewish tradition, which emerged out of a conservative mind-set, is Reconstructionist Judaism (Pawlikowski, 1990, p. 543). The groups differ significantly in regard to religious beliefs and practices. Orthodox Jews follow the traditional religious practices, including careful observance of the Talmudic laws; the Conservative and Reform movements interpret the laws more broadly (Charnes & Moore, 1992). All Jewish traditions emphasize the practice of good deeds or mitzvahs each day (Nutkiewicz, 1993, p. 561). Although daily religious rituals are central to the faith of most Jewish persons, health is so valued that "almost all religious injunctions may be lifted to save a life or to relieve suffering" (Charnes & Moore, 1992, p. 66). Jewish people tend to believe that the occurrence of illness is not an accident but rather a time given one to reflect on life and the future (Beck & Goldberg, 1996, p. 16). The keeping of a kosher dietary regimen, if not injurious to health, is very important to many Jewish patients' coping with an illness experience (Fine, 1995), as is the keeping of Shabbat or Sabbath, which is observed from sunset on Friday evening to sunset on Saturday. "It is suggested that home visits should not be scheduled on the Sabbath [*Shabbos,* from sundown Friday to sundown Saturday] for this is a day set apart for God, to honor him and use for prayer, studying scripture and special family time" (Salladay & Bitting, 2012, p. 15). Death, for the Jewish believer, is viewed as part of life; it is important to document the precise hour when death occurs in order to establish the time of mourning, shiva, and the annual "honoring of the dead, Yahrzeit" (Beck & Goldberg, 1996, p. 18).

Christianity, the largest of the world religions, consists of three main divisions: Roman Catholicism, Eastern Orthodox religions, and the Protestant faiths.

Roman Catholicism identifies that group of Christians who remain in communion with Rome, and who profess allegiance to the doctrines, traditions, philosophies, and practices supported by the pope, as religious leader of the Church. Roman Catholics are trinitarian in theology and place great importance on the seven sacraments: Baptism, Reconciliation (Confession), Holy Eucharist, Confirmation, Matrimony, Holy Orders, and Anointing of the Sick (formerly called "Extreme Unction"); participation in the holy sacrifice of the Mass is the central element of worship.

The Eastern Orthodox tradition, which represents a group of churches whose international leaders are located in Eastern Europe, differs from the Roman Church on both theological issues and aspects of ritual and worship. These churches respect the primacy of the patriarch of Constantinople and include reverence for the Holy Trinity as a central spiritual tenet of the faith. Veneration of holy icons is an important devotion leading ultimately to worship of God the Father, God the Son, and God the Holy Spirit. Currently the term *Eastern Orthodox Church* refers to four ancient patriarchates (Constantinople, Alexandria, Antioch, and Jerusalem), as well as a number of other churches such as those of Russia and Romania, Cyprus, Greece, Egypt, and Syria (Farrugia, 1990, p. 306).

The term *Protestant* generally refers to the churches that originated during the 16th-century Reformation (Gros, 1990). Some characteristics of original Protestantism are "the acceptance of the Bible as the only source of revealed truth, the doctrine of justification by faith alone, and the universal priesthood of all believers" (Livingstone, 1990). Protestant Christians generally regard Baptism and Holy Communion as important sacraments, although denominations may differ on associated rituals. Some of the major Protestant denominations are Adventist, Baptist, Church of the Brethren, Church of the Nazarene, Episcopal (Anglican), Friends (Quakers), Lutheran, Mennonite, Methodist, and Presbyterian.

Christianity is based on the worship of God and promotion of the Kingdom of God through the living out of the Gospel message of Jesus of Nazareth. For the Christian patient, the nurse will need to be sensitive to a multiplicity of religious beliefs and rituals associated with such health-related events as birth, childbearing, organ donation, and death. For example, infant Baptism is required by Roman Catholics and Episcopalians, and Last Rites or the Sacrament of the Sick is optional for some Protestant groups, but traditional for Eastern Orthodox Christians (Krekeler & Yancey, 1993). In a study of Christian patients' attitudes toward spiritual care, Conco (1995) found that three key themes emerged from interview data. Christian patients described the spiritual care they received as "enabling transcendence for higher meaning and purpose," which helped the patients find meaning in their illness and suffering; "enabling hope," which included the belief that the patients could find a better future; and "establishing connectedness," a theme that spoke to the support provided by the caregiver in terms of such activities as touching, listening, and being present to the patient (pp. 271–272).

Other Western churches of which the practicing nurse should be aware include Christian Science, Church of Jesus Christ of Latter Day Saints (Mormons), Jehovah's Witnesses, and Unitarian Universalist Association of Churches (Taylor, Lillis, & LeMone, 1997, p. 886).

Islam is frequently viewed as having been founded by the prophet Muhammed in the seventh century, with the revelation of the Holy Qur'an. Muslims themselves, however, do not regard Islam as a new religion; "they believe that Allah is the same God who revealed His will to Abraham, Moses, Jesus and Muhammed" (Esposito, 1990). A key tenet of Islam is Tauhid, which means faith in the total Lordship of Allah as ruler of heaven and earth; allied with this concept is the understanding that one's life must be centered on this belief (Abdil-Haqq Muhammad, 1995). Important religious practices for Muslims include the ritual prayer, prayed five times each day (preceded by ritual washing) while facing Mecca (the east); honoring Ramadan, the month of fasting from sunup to sundown, which occurs in the ninth lunar month of the Islamic calendar; and the experience of a hajj, a pilgrimage to Mecca, once in one's lifetime, if possible. Spiritual care for a hospitalized Muslim patient should be focused on providing the time (about 15 minutes) and the setting (a quiet, private place) for the five-times-daily ritual prayer (C. Kemp, 1996, p. 88). Most hospitals have access to the services of a Muslim spiritual leader, an imam, if requested by the patient (Rassool, 2000).

A Muslim registered nurse, Selia, spoke about some of the needs of Muslim patients who have entered into the health-care system:

> A Muslim patient, what they need during their sickness is similar to what a Christian patient needs: they need a faith in God; they need someone to listen to them; someone to talk about God with them; to know the support coming from God. We have some people in Islam, Muslim women, like who you might say is a "nun," and they are very prayerful and we might ask them to visit and to pray for someone who is sick. We also have in Islam, an imam, who is the spiritual leader of the mosque; he can be called to visit and pray with patients.

Selia also spoke of the importance of faith in helping her own sister accept a diagnosis of cancer. "The staff nurse helped her see that the cancer was not a punishment from God. The nurse sat with her and prayed with her in Arabic and after this she was able to accept her chemotherapy. The 'spiritual' was the most important thing in helping my sister accept her cancer and her treatment." Selia noted that if a patient was not physically able to pray facing Mecca during an illness or treatment, "They can pray while they are lying in bed; they can pray in their minds, even if they are not able to talk. Nurses should encourage Muslim patients to pray to accept their disease because it will help them to cope." She added, "One does not mourn if a family member dies from an illness; they accept this as the will of Allah and one does not contradict this."

Selia continued, "Although a Muslim patient who is very ill is not required to pray five times each day, Muslim hospitals usually prepare prayer rooms; one for women and one for men, who are able to move about. During Ramadan, a patient is not required to fast. The Qur'an says that the sick person, after he gets well, can fast then. She explained, however, that some patients "insist on fasting because they think it is like a prayer; it is something from God."

Finally, Selia spoke of the importance in Islam of visiting the ill:

> The Prophet Mohammed, in the Holy Qur'an, it is written in his own words, that each Muslim should visit patients who are sick and support them and pray with them. It is a must for each Muslim to pray; to ask Allah to help that patient and to help all patients all over the world, whatever their religion.

Eastern Religious Traditions

The major Eastern traditions—Buddhism, Hinduism, and Confucianism—incorporate beliefs about God that differ significantly from those of religions of the Western tradition.

Buddhism derives its beliefs and practices from the life and teachings of the Buddha, the "enlightened one," who lived in India some 2500 years ago (Borelli, 1990). Myriad Buddhist traditions are associated with the cultures of particular geographical communities, such as Tibetan Buddhism or Chinese Buddhism. Wherever Buddhists are found, there are usually monasteries of monks, and sometimes nuns, who preserve the Buddhist teachings and liturgies. Buddhists believe that suffering can be ended by following the eightfold path: "right understanding, right intention, right speech, right action, right livelihood, right effort, right mindfulness and right contemplation" (Borelli, 1990, p. 146). Buddhists do not revere any particular sacraments.

Hinduism does not embrace one particular body of beliefs and practices; the name Hindu is derived from the geographical region of the Indus river valley and the subcontinent, Hindustan, where many of those who practice Hinduism reside (Cenkner, 1990). Key concepts in Hinduism relate to reincarnation or rebirth and the idea of karma, or "the law by which one's personal deeds determine one's present and future status in this life and in future lives" (Cenkner, 1990, p. 467). Hindus who have lived well do not fear death; it is seen as the preparation for reincarnation into another life.

Confucianism is an Eastern tradition derived primarily from the personal philosophy of the ancient Chinese scholar Confucius. Inherent in Confucian thought is belief in the importance of maintaining harmony and balance in the body. Two potentially conflicting forces are thought to occur in the world, the "yin" and the "yang"; it is critical that these dimensions of function be kept in balance in order to achieve and maintain a good and productive life.

▶ Nursing Theory and Spiritual Care

In the ideal world of nursing, clinical practice would be based on and directed by well-validated nursing theory; this includes the practice of spiritual care. Nursing theory, however, is still relatively new, having been developed primarily over the past three decades. And in a number of the grand theories of nursing, the spiritual needs of the ill person are given only minimal attention. As more grand nursing theory, as well as theory of the middle range, is generated, scholars anticipate that spirituality will be an important concept of interest. One example is the work of Judith Allen Shelly and Arline Miller, *Called to Care: A Christian Theology of Nursing* (1999).

Speaking from the practitioner's perspective, hospital charge nurse Andrew Oldnall (1995) decried the fact that many nurse theorists have either omitted discussion of the concept of spirituality from their models or have "referred to it only implicitly" (p. 417). There has, however, been a recent reawakening to the importance of the spiritual nature of the human person among contemporary nurse theorists. Barbara Barnum (1995) posited three reasons for what she describes as a "spiritual resurgence" in nursing; these include "a major shift in the normative world view," "a spiritual focus in the growing self-help movement," and "a renewed drive on the part of traditional religious groups and individuals within nursing" (p. 24). Barnum's suggestion that the "self-help movement" has been a catalyst for nursing's current interest in spirituality may be related to the holistic health-care concept, a central premise of the holistic approach being patient autonomy and participation in therapeutic planning.

In examining the writings of some of the key nurse theorists of past and present, one finds significant variability in terms of interest in spirituality or the spiritual needs of the ill person. One of the earliest theorists, Virginia Henderson, writing with Harmer in 1955, observed that "sickness may threaten the patient's faith in the ultimate 'goodness' of life. He cannot believe in a God that lets terrible things happen; or he may fear he has lost favor in the sight of God, considering illness a punishment for real or imagined sins" (p. 74). In her later work, Henderson (1966) identified as 1 of 14 "Components of Basic Nursing Care" provision for "Worship according to one's faith" (p. 17); she did not, however, explore this precept in any detail. Faye Abdellah (Abdellah & Levine, 1979), in "Criterion Measures of Patient Care," also included a patient care component related to personal faith "to facilitate progress toward achievement of personal spiritual goals"; Abdellah, like Henderson, viewed attention to the patient's spiritual needs as a key component of nursing care.

Joyce Travelbee (1971), in her theory of illness as a "self-actualizing experience," was more explicit in her concern with both the patient's and the nurse's spirituality, observing, "It is believed the spiritual values a person holds will determine, to a great extent, his perception of illness. The spiritual values of the nurse or her philosophical beliefs about illness and suffering will determine the degree to which he or she will be able to help ill persons find meaning, or no meaning, in these situations" (p. 16). Travelbee further asserted that a patient's religious beliefs will greatly influence the experience of, and the ability to cope with, suffering (p. 64). She admitted, however, that the degree to which a person actually practices his or her religion is a mediating factor in relation to coping with distress and suffering (p. 71).

Nurse theorist Betty Neuman's systems model is a conceptual framework that addresses the spiritual dimension and needs of the ill person. In Neuman's model, the patient system is assessed holistically from five perspectives: physiologic, psychological, developmental, sociocultural, and spiritual (Sohier, 1997, p. 112). For Neuman, the spiritual dimension of a person supports and permeates all other systems (Fawcett, 1989, p. 172). In her earlier work, Betty Neuman placed less emphasis on the spiritual; the spiritual aspects of her theory were first significantly displayed in her 1989 understanding of the patient system (Meleis, 1991, p. 294). In the third edition of the theorist's book *The Neuman Systems Model*, Neuman's "spiritual variable" is described as the pivot on which the framework centers and as having important implications for patients from a variety of world cultures (Curran, 1995, p. 581).

Callista Roy's adaptation model, which focuses on the adaptive needs of the ill person and family, includes a self-concept adaptive mode that emphasizes the psychological and spiritual characteristics of an individual. This model addresses the "self-consistency, self-ideal and moral-ethical-spiritual self" of a patient (Phillips, 1997, p. 177). Religion or religious practice is considered one of the significant cultural influences on a patient's adaptation. Although Roy identified the concept of religion as primarily associated with the major organized traditions of Eastern and Western society, she noted that this cultural category may also include "spiritual beliefs, practices and philosophies that are not necessarily attached to institutional forms of religion" (Sato, 1984, p. 69). Callista Roy views religion as an important variable in the adaptive process, as she perceives religiosity or religious practice as potentially influencing all dimensions of a person's life view and functional capacity, especially in terms of attitudes and behaviors related to health and illness.

Two other nursing theories that indirectly address the concept of the patient's spiritual nature in terms of phenomenological and humanistic approaches are the models of Parse (1981) and Paterson and Zderad (1976). Parse accepted the transcendent nature of humanity. "Nursing is unfolding in simultaneous mutual interchange with the world transcending with greater diversity and complexity" (p. 172). Paterson and Zderad viewed the human person as "an incarnate being, always becoming, in relation with men and things in a world of time and space" (p. 19).

And finally, nurse theorist Jean Watson (1985) explained the nature of personhood by placing significant emphasis on the existence of the "human soul [spirit or higher sense of self] that is greater than the physical, mental and emotional existence of a person at any given point in time" (p. 45). Sarter (1992) asserted that Jean Watson is the only nurse theorist who explicitly describes the concept of the soul (p. 152).

In examining the writings of the select group of nursing theorists mentioned, one finds key words related to patients' spiritual needs, including faith, worship, spiritual goals, spiritual values, transcendence, human soul, higher authority, and organized religion. Identifying the patient's understanding of these concepts is important for a nurse undertaking the practice of spiritual care.

▶ Nursing Intervention: The Practice of Spiritual Care

Admittedly, a nurse may not know precisely which nursing therapeutics to employ when faced with a patient experiencing spiritual need. Simple guidelines presented in an earlier publication may provide some basic ground rules for spiritual care:

> The nurse must attempt to respect and understand a patient's religious beliefs and practices, even if very different from his or her own. The nurse must take time to allow the patient to express religious, ethical, or philosophical views, as well as any fears and anxieties related to the patient's spiritual belief system. The nurse must be spiritually supportive, assisting the patient whenever it is within the realm of his or her understanding or expertise, and recognize the need to seek outside spiritual or ministerial counseling, either personally or for the patient, when the situation warrants. (O'Brien, 1982, p. 108)

Nurses should keep two important principles of spiritual intervention in mind when ministering to those who are ill. First, because each person has a unique spirituality, the provision of spiritual care cannot be derived from a procedure book of orders; and second, to intervene in the spiritual needs of others, the nurse must first understand his or her own spirituality or relationship to God (Fish & Shelly, 1979, p. 68).

In his best-selling book, *Care of the Soul*, Thomas Moore (1992) observed that spiritual caring forces one to transcend the self and to "recover a sense of the sacredness of each individual life" (p. 19). Moore asserted that spiritual care of the soul incorporates the mystery of suffering and does not deny life's problems (pp. 19–20). Ultimately, Moore contended that spiritual care "requires craft (techne), skill, attention and art" (p. 285).

A number of factors, both positive and negative, have been identified that can affect the practice of spiritual care by nursing staff. In a study of 110 nurses, nursing professor Moon Fai Chan (2009) learned that "the greater the nurse's [positive] spiritual care perceptions, the more frequently spiritual care is included in that nurse's practice" (p. 2128). Chan's tool measuring "perceptions" of spiritual care included such topics as the importance of spiritual care to the sick, the strength that can be drawn from spiritual care, and the relevance of spiritual care as an "important dimension of nursing" (p. 2132). Family practice physicians and nurse practitioners were studied to determine how spiritual care was carried out "in spite of documented barriers" (Tanyi, McKenzie, & Chapek, 2009, p. 690). Five key themes emerged from this phenomenological research: "(1) discerning instances for overt spiritual assessment; (2) displaying a genuine and caring attitude; (3) encouraging the use of existing spiritual practices; (4) documenting spiritual care for continuity of care; (5) managing perceived barriers to spiritual care" (p. 690).

▶ Nursing Intervention in Spiritual Distress

A patient's experience of spiritual suffering, or spiritual distress, may pose unique challenges for nursing intervention (Kahn & Steeves, 1994). Spiritual distress may be experienced by any ill person questioning the reason for his or her suffering (Harrison, 1993). Defining characteristics of spiritual distress include questioning one's relationship with God, attempting to identify religious idols, guilt feelings, and a variety of somatic symptoms (Heliker, 1992, p. 16); questioning the meaning and purpose of life; expressing anger toward God; refusing to participate in usual religious practices; regarding illness as God's punishment; and seeking spiritual assistance, other than usual spiritual or religious support (Tucker, Canobbio, Paquette, & Wells, 1996, p. 52).

The nurse does not need religious training to meet the needs of a patient in spiritual distress (DiMeo, 1991, p. 22); nurses continually engage in the process of assessing, planning, intervening, and evaluating (the nursing process) related to physical and emotional nursing diagnoses. In assessing spiritual need, the nurse must determine whether he or she may provide the spiritual care, such as listening and counseling, or whether referral should be made to a chaplain or formally trained minister of the patient's denomination (Duff, 1994).

Counseling a person in spiritual distress can constitute a growth experience for the nurse while also providing support for the patient (Burnard, 1988). This was validated in the observations of Gail, a 16-year veteran of nursing interviewed by the author:

> Spiritual care, listening, advising is so important, because people are hurting so much. They suffer a lot and the main thing is to listen and let them tell you their pain. I can't tell them there's a cure and they know that; they lean on God, because there is no other answer. Sometimes chaplains come up

and do a "quickie": "I'll keep you in my prayers." But sometimes the patient just needs somebody to sit and listen to her, and be with her. . . . I have seen and listened to much more spiritual distress in patients than I would ever have imagined, and I think it has made me grow spiritually. It's helped me to think about Christ's forsakenness. Suffering in itself can be a prayer.

Spiritual care interventions were identified in response to a nursing diagnosis of spiritual distress in a 41-year-old AIDS patient who demonstrated symptoms of fear of death and questioning belief in God. These nursing therapeutics included assisting the client to explore the spiritual meaning of coping with the HIV experience, providing support for the expression of feelings, and allowing the patient to proceed through the grief process related to physical and psychosocial losses (O'Brien & Pheifer, 1993, p. 314).

The success of spiritual interventions such as prayer in patients with spiritual distress, related to a number of disease/illness conditions, has been documented in the literature. Some examples are: "seeking comfort through prayer" among coronary artery bypass graft patients (Hawley & Irurita, 1998); prayer as a health strategy in managing HIV-related symptoms (Coleman, Nokes, Corless, Kirksey, Nicholas, & Tsai, 2006); and the benefits of prayer for cancer survivors (Levine, Aviv, Yoon, Ewing, & Au, 2009; Ross, Hall, Fairley, Taylor, & Howard, 2008). The importance of spirituality in coping with the distress of early Alzheimer's disease was documented by Beuscher and Grando (2009).

Findings from an online survey of 4,054 nurses in the United Kingdom revealed that "nurses recognize that attending to the spiritual needs of patients enhances the overall quality of nursing care" (McSherry & Jamieson, 2011, p. 1757). In addition, two nursing authors contend that spiritual care includes considering the "soul" of the patient being served: Stephen Wright (2011) asserts that spiritual care is "an essential feature of high-quality patient care" (p. 18) in "The Heart and Soul of Nursing," as does Fenske (2011), an advanced practice nurse who used "multiple theoretical frameworks to make meaning of her severely developmentally disabled son's untimely death" (p. 229) in "Soul Mate: Exploring the Concept of Soul."

The Problem of Suffering

Perhaps the most difficult challenge a practicing nurse may face in attempting to carry out the theological mandate of caring is addressing a patient's suffering. Washholtz, Pearce, and Koenig (2007) explored the relationship between spirituality and the suffering of chronic pain in order to understand why "some people rely on their faith to cope with pain" (p. 311). These authors concluded that "spiritual and religious coping may affect a number of physiological, psychological, neurological and emotional domains that influence pain perception and tolerance" (p. 316). Nurse theorist Katie Eriksson (2007) has asserted that "the mission of caring is the alleviation of human suffering and the serving of life and health" (p. 8). And a team of palliative care providers report that addressing the "spiritual issues in suffering . . . is recognized as a very important component of palliative care" (Hinshaw, Carnahan, Breck, Mosoiu, & Mosoiu, 2011, p. 7).

In some cases, the nurse's therapeutic toolbox will contain instruments to alleviate the suffering, at least for a time. In other situations, the pain, whether physical, emotional, or spiritual, seems to take on a life of its own; no techniques or supplies in the nurse's armamentarium prove effective. At such an impasse the nurse, like the chaplain, must wrestle with the imponderable "why." And for the caregiver with a strong religious foundation, be it of the Judeo-Christian tradition or some other belief system, the "why" of suffering may take on a powerful spiritual élan. Why does an all-powerful God allow an infant to be born with multiple congenital anomalies? Why does a loving and compassionate God not intervene to alleviate a teenage cancer patient's intractable pain? Why does a merciful God not use his strength to heal a terminally ill mother whose death will leave orphaned children?

The nurse may also be called on to respond to patients' and family members' inability to understand or accept the reason for an injury or illness. Joyce Travelbee (1971) focused specifically on this point when she defined the purpose of nursing as being "to assist an individual, family or community to prevent or cope with the experiences of illness and suffering, and, if necessary, to find meaning in their experiences" (p. 16). Often, however, it is difficult to articulate a profound existential meaning in an illness experience; thus, the nurse must indeed draw on Moore's thesis of accepting suffering as mystery and of not attempting to offer a patient or family false hope or an unreal prognosis.

Several years ago, the author spent a summer as a chaplain intern at a research medical center whose treatment was directed primarily to those with life-threatening illness. Most of the patients were coping with the potential for a relatively imminent death or at least a shortened life; many were burdened with pain and suffering, both physical and spiritual. For the patients, the families, the staff, and the chaplains, the "why" question always seemed to be lurking in the background. Sometimes it was spoken aloud; at other times it could be read in the eyes of the patients and those who loved and cared for them. The following excerpt from the author's chaplaincy journal describes a mother's distress over the suffering of her son:

> This morning Catherine, the mother of a teenage son, Michael, who was facing mutilating surgery in hope of slowing the progress of advanced rhabdomyosarcoma, came to me in great spiritual pain; she said: "I need you to answer a question: Why? Why my beautiful, generous, loving son? Why not me; I've lived a full life? Why is the God I pray to letting this happen to him? I don't understand." I tried to respond to Catherine's question with some thoughts about the mystery of God's ways; mostly I just listened. Catherine spoke for over an hour, pouring out all of the pain in her heart, all of the love for her son, stopping only once to remind me gently, "You still haven't answered my question: Why?"

At the end of our meeting Catherine said, "Thank you for spending this time with me; it's helped more than I can ever tell you." She did not raise the "why" question again; I breathed a sigh of relief.

When this experience was shared with other medical center chaplains, one observed, "I'm sure that mother knew in her heart there was no answer to the question, 'why?'; she just needed someone to be with her while she asked it."

Most patients and families who suffer, especially those with spiritual foundations, understand that in the realm of the Holy Mystery, the why question has no answers that we, as humans, can comprehend. Rather, what they ask of us as caregivers is, like Catherine, that we be there with them while they ask the questions, that we accept with them the mystery of human suffering, and that we offer no false illusions. This is the essence, the heart of spiritual caregiving.

Suffering as a concept has been defined as "any experience that impinges on an individual's or a community's sense of well-being" (Sparks, 1993, p. 950). Sparks added that suffering may be "physical, psychological, interpersonal or spiritual," though he commented that generally it is a combination of all four (p. 950). Suffering is usually understood as a state rather than an incident. It is described not "by sharp pains and moments of terror but by an almost unbearable duration and inescapability" (Maes, 1990, p. 29). Suffering defines an ongoing and consistent state of distress, not merely a brief encounter with painful stimuli. Many of those who are chronically ill well understand the notion of an ongoing state of distress; they may experience, at any one time, a combination of physical, emotional, and spiritual suffering related to an illness condition.

A dimension of suffering frequently encountered in the health-care setting and explored in the theological literature relates to the question of "why"; what or who is responsible for the suffering? Suffering, religious faith, and illness have long been associated concepts (Hufford, 1987). The "why" query is highlighted in the classic biblical story of Job. "They [Job's friends] sat down upon the ground with him seven days and seven nights, but none of them spoke a word to him, for they saw how great was his suffering" (Job, 2:13). Job was, seemingly, a good man, and yet he suffered great physical trials, which both he and his friends questioned. In his anger and frustration Job cried out to God, "Why?" According to the Scripture, God never answered Job's question but simply asked him to have faith, which ultimately Job accepted. Theologians agree that the story of Job, often quoted in relation to suffering, leaves the "why" question unanswered and supports the need for absolute faith in God (Baird, 1994; Bergant, 1990; Kidner, 1983).

Robert, a young man who had been living with cancer for more than five years, described a kind of "Job-like" anger at God. Like Job, Robert ultimately was able to trust in his long-standing faith relationship with his creator:

> When I found out I had cancer I was depressed and really mad at God. But then, because I was so scared, I started to pray. And, you know, I learned about praying and about how you really can talk to God. God has always been with me and he'll be with this too. I just have to trust his love.

Robert's conclusion is supported by theologian Kathleen O'Conner's commentary on the "Job Story." O'Conner (1990) observed that the book of Job is not really about suffering but about one's relationship to God while experiencing suffering (p. 104). She asserted, like Robert, that the lesson to be learned is to pray, to ask God for answers, and then to accept and trust.

In discussing religious interpretations of sickness-related suffering, Emeth and Greenhut (1991) decried explanations claiming that illness is a form of God's punishment or that God gives illness and suffering to those He loves (p. 63). While obviously God allows suffering and may use a suffering experience to draw an ill person to Him, most contemporary theologians would argue that a loving God could not purposely choose to hurt or cause pain. This thinking was reflected by Eriksson (1994) who warned against attempting to find "premature" or "quick-fix" explanations for suffering, asserting that to do so might block an individual from discovering his or her own phenomenological understanding of the meaning of a suffering experience (p. 7). As Eriksson observed, "Suffering in itself has no meaning, but people could, having lived through it, realize that it was in fact meaningful to do so" (p. 7).

In a pastor's response to the suffering experience, especially as related to illness, Rabbi Harold Kushner, author of the best-selling book *When Bad Things Happen to Good People* (1981), asserted, "The God I believe in does not send us the problem; He gives us the strength to cope with the problem" (p. 127). Rabbi Kushner's position is reflected in the comments of Paul, a middle-aged cancer patient:

> God doesn't design diseases; He is a God of love. Why does God allow His people to suffer from sickness? I don't know! But I do know He holds us up. We are His. We belong to Him and He will sustain us. We may walk the way of suffering but we will not be alone.

For the individual who denies or is uncertain about the existence of God, the condition of human suffering is more difficult to manage. Nurses need to be aware of the secular humanist philosophy of such a person. In the case of a patient who professes to be either an atheist or an agnostic, the listening, loving presence of a caring nurse may provide spiritual support and comfort in an experience of suffering.

The most difficult suffering for a nurse to work with is that which is unrelieved. Hospice physician Ira Byock (1994), in discussing persistent suffering, admitted that he sometimes asks himself the question, "how complete is my commitment?" (p. 8). Sister Rosemary Donley (1991) believes that part of the nurse's mission is to "be with people who suffer, to give meaning to the reality of suffering"; it is in these activities, Donley asserted, that the "spiritual dimension" of nursing lies (p. 180).

▶ Spiritual and Religious Resources

In order to provide spiritual care to patients from a variety of religious traditions, the nurse must have some familiarity with the available resources, particularly pastoral care, prayer, Scripture, religious rituals, devotional articles, and sacred music. The importance of nurses' understanding the meaning of spiritual and religious resources for patients from a variety of ethnic and religious groups was identified through hospital-based interviews and panel discussions (Davidson, Boyer, Casey, Matzel, & Walden, 2008).

Pastoral Care

Pastoral care describes the interventions carried out by religious ministers in response to the spiritual or religious needs of others. The activities of the pastoral caregiver, "including sacramental and social ministries, can be as informal as conversational encounters and as formal as highly structured ritual events" (Studzinski, 1993, p. 722). Howard Clinebell (1991), identified five specific pastoral care functions: "healing, sustaining, guiding, reconciling, and nurturing" (p. 43). Such spiritual care interventions may promote significant healing on the part of ill persons.

Shelly and Fish (1988) noted the importance of the clergy as a resource in spiritual care of the ill; they asserted that spiritual care given by clergy and nurses should be complementary (p. 138). For such complementarity to exist, three conditions are suggested: mutuality of goals in the caregiving, a delineation of role responsibilities, and communication (p. 138). The activities of the minister or pastoral caregiver offer an important religious comfort dimension by providing the patient with familiar symbols and experiences (Atkinson & Fortunato, 1996, p. 99). A pastoral advisor understands the patient's religious belief system and can plan care to be congruent with the individual's religious heritage (Krekeler & Yancey, 1993, p. 1010).

In making a pastoral care referral, the nurse may contact a priest, minister, rabbi, imam, or other spiritual advisor of the patient's acquaintance and tradition, or refer the patient to a health-care facility's department of pastoral care. To facilitate a pastoral care visit, the nurse may prepare a place close to the patient for the spiritual minister to sit, provide privacy to the degree possible in the setting, and cover the bedside table with a white cover if a sacrament such as Anointing of the Sick is to be administered (Taylor, Lillis, & LeMone, 1997, p. 896).

A renal failure patient, Catherine, spoke about the importance of pastoral ministry in helping her cope with the acute onset of her disease:

> When I first went on dialysis and was in the hospital, I was sick as a dog. I had pneumonia plus the kidney failure and I thought I might die. But the response that I got from my minister and the church was just fantastic. The minister prayed for me, and I had everybody wanting to know how's my dialysis going, and I got a list of 35 people from the church, especially the deacons, who were willing to drive me anyplace I need to go.

Prayer

The word *prayer* is generally understood as a request or a petition to obtain some good outcome. There are a number of other kinds of prayer, such as prayers of thanksgiving, as well as specific methods of prayer, including vocal prayer, contemplation, and centering prayer.

Spiritual writer Carlo Carretto (1978) observed that "we can never define what prayer is . . . prayer is communicating with the mystery" (p. 75). Prayer is envisioned as the spiritual action one takes to bring an individual "into connection with God" (Johnson, 1992, p. 148). Prayer, whether formal or informal, may be central to healing the sick (Normille, 1992, p. 74). Healing prayer has been described as bringing oneself and a situation of disease before God, "with at least one other person to listen, discern, speak and respond, so that healing in relation to or with God can take place" (Bacon, 1995, p. 15).

Although prayer may be engaged in individually by a patient, and often is, it is important to remember that illness, especially acute illness, may create a "barrier to personal prayer" (Shelly & Fish, 1995, pp. 9–10). In such instances a nurse's prayer for and with the patient can be an important spiritual care intervention. Shelly and Fish remind the nurse that his or her prayer should reflect what the patient would pray for if capable of doing so; they advised, "The most helpful prayer is usually a short, simple statement to God of the patient's hopes, fears and needs, and a recognition of God's ability to meet the patient in his [or her] situation" (p. 11). Prayer as a nursing intervention was described by a practicing nurse as "possible in any setting, as long as we ask people's permission" (Mason, 1995, p. 7). Mason believes that prayer can be an important source of peace and comfort for an ill person (p. 7).

In a 1995 editorial in the *Journal of Christian Nursing*, editor Judith Shelly posed the rhetorical question, "Is prayer unprofessional?" In answering, decidedly in the negative, Shelly cited an address by Florence Nightingale to students at the Nightingale School of Nursing. Nightingale commented, in part, "Did you ever think how Christ was a nurse; and stood by the bedside, and with His own hands, nursed and did for the suffering?" (p. 3). In supporting prayer as an appropriate dimension of holistic nursing, Lewis (1996) also drew on the wisdom of Florence Nightingale as mentor and guide. "Nightingale recognized that the use of prayer attuned the inward man to the universal laws of God . . . and . . . contended that prayer could be applied to daily life for health, wholeness and healing" (p. 309). The importance of the healing power of prayer in holistic nursing was supported by Narayanasamy and Narayanasamy (2008), DiJospeh and Cavendish (2005), and Ameling (2000).

Two chronically ill persons experiencing bouts of acute exacerbation of their conditions described the comfort personal prayer afforded them. Agnes, a maintenance hemodialysis patient who was hospitalized at the time, reported, "I believe in a hereafter, and in a God someplace, and that makes you feel like, OK, I can go on. If I feel bad, I can lay in bed and talk to Him, when I don't want to talk to anybody else about my feelings. That's it. That's what religion is all about." Nicholas, an AIDS patient suffering from acute symptoms of cytomegalovirus, admitted, "Sometimes when I'm having a bad day, you know, Why is this happening to me? I say to God, 'could you give me a little hand here?' And usually what happens is I get overwhelmed with gratitude, and I get a sense that God's saying, 'You can handle it, Nicholas; I'm right here.' Sometimes His words actually come to me. I mean, I don't hear a booming voice, but I hear real words in my heart."

A family member of an AIDS patient who had recently died in the ICU after a bout with *Pneumocystis carinii* pneumonia, described the importance of a nurse's prayer in the unit:

> I was particularly touched when [she] prayed for Jonathan in the hospital. I didn't say it at the time but when she prayed aloud it was like I was burning inside. And I prayed too. She really had a way with words and I hoped to emulate that.

As advised by Shelly and Fish, the nurse praying aloud for a patient should try to pray as the patient would. An example is a prayer said by the author while in chaplaincy training. Michael, a 36-year-old hospitalized patient suffering from an anaplastic astrocytoma, had described himself as a born-again Christian. Michael loved to talk to and about Jesus in a very direct and simple manner; however, it was difficult for him to articulate a prayer, so he asked that it be done for him. The prayer, recorded in a clinical pastoral education report, is as follows:

> Lord Jesus, put your arms around Michael as he prepares for his chemo treatment. Let him know that he is not walking on this path alone, that you are right there by his side; you are holding him up and supporting him with your strength. Let him know that you are holding his hand. Remind Michael that his name is written on the palm of your hand. [Michael frequently responded, "Amen" or "Thank you, Jesus."] Michael knows you, Jesus, and knows that you are His Lord. Help him to feel your love and care during this illness. Bless the doctors and the nurses who are giving Michael his treatments, that their hands may be Your Hands as they care for him on this journey. God, our Father, you know what Michael needs in these days, and you know the prayers that are in his heart. Bless his prayer, protect him, guide him and comfort him, we ask this in the name of your son, our Lord Jesus. Amen.

Michael responded to the prayer by saying, "Thank you, your coming here and ministering means a lot to me."

Scripture

Scripture, or the "word of God," is written material that represents venerated and guiding principles for many religious traditions. For the Jewish community, the Hebrew Scripture as contained in the Torah represents God's word and laws for his people. For a Christian, both Old (or "First") and New Testaments contained in the Bible are revered. The Old Testament, shared with the Jewish religion, contains "the story of God's work in the world from creation to the period of the second temple (built in 515 bce)"; the second, or "New Testament . . . begins with the story of Jesus, and contains documents and letters and visions of the early Christian community in the 1st century ce" (Nowell, 1993, p. 857). *Merriam-Webster's New Collegiate Dictionary* (1976) defines the term *scripture*, not only as "the books of the Old and New Testaments," but also, broadly, as "the sacred writings of a religion" (p. 775). Thus, other scriptural materials, comforting for patients of the appropriate denominations, might include the Holy Qur'an (for Muslims) or the Book of Mormon (for members of the Church of Jesus Christ of Latter Day Saints).

Shelly and Fish (1988) cautioned that a "principle of appropriate timing" should govern the nurse's use of Scripture (p. 121). If a patient is angry or depressed, or experiencing severe discomfort, such as that accompanying acute pain, the seemingly glib quoting, even of an apparently comforting Scripture passage, may seem like "rubbing salt into the wounds" of the sufferer. If, however, it seems that a patient might benefit from a Scripture passage, the nurse can always ask permission in a noncontrolling manner, leaving the patient free to refuse without discomfort. Related to nurses' sensitivity to timing in the use of Scripture, a study of the spiritual caring behaviors of 303 nurses (Hall & Lanig, 1993) revealed that of three types of interventions (conversing, praying, and reading Scripture), nurses were least likely to read Scripture to their patients (p. 736). Ultimately, Piles (1990) suggested that prior to a nurse initiating the sharing of Scripture with patients, he or she should have acquired some sense of when the use of Scripture is an "appropriate intervention" (p. 39).

When a nurse feels comfortable sharing a passage of Scripture with a patient or family member, the reading can represent an important and valid dimension of spiritual care. Following are some suggested Scripture passages and their underlying messages:

> For comfort in times of fear and anxiety—Psalm 23; Philippians 4:4–7; 1 Peter 5:7; Romans 8:38–39
> For fear of approaching death—Psalm 23; John 14:17
> For one in need of healing—Isaiah 53:4–6
> For one seeking God's care and protection—Isaiah 43:2; Isaiah 40:28–31; Psalm 25; Psalm 121; Psalm 139:11–19; Deuteronomy 8:2–3; Jeremiah 29:11; Matthew 10:26–33; Luke 12:22–31
> For one seeking God's mercy and forgiveness—Isaiah 1:18; Isaiah 53:5–6; Hebrews 4:14–16; 1 John 1:9
> For one who is fatigued by illness or life stress—Isaiah 40:31

Religious Rituals

"One must observe the proper rites".... "What is a rite?" asked the little prince. "These are actions too often neglected," said the fox.

—**Antoine de Saint-Exupéry**, *The Little Prince*

The concept of rite or ritual may be understood theologically as "a social, symbolic process which has the potential for communicating, creating, criticizing and even transforming meaning" (Kelleher, 1990, p. 906). Religious rituals are sets of behaviors that reflect and honor spiritual or religious beliefs on the part of the participant. There can be a profoundly healing value in participation in religious ritual, especially for the acutely ill person (Texter & Mariscotti, 1994). Thus, the use of or support for religious rituals meaningful to a patient should be an integral part of spiritual care intervention provided by a nurse. Some important religious rituals in relation to health and healing have been identified by Young and Koopsen (2011) as including such activities as prayer, meditation, visualization, guided imagery, dance, and storytelling.

A number of religious rituals may be appropriate for an ill person, whether at home or in the hospital setting. For the Muslim patient whose theology is anchored in the five pillars of Islam, formal prayer (salat) is prayed five times daily, facing the east (Mecca). To support the Muslim's daily prayer requirement, a nurse may provide a prayer rug facing the east, situated in a place of privacy, as well as facilities for the ritual washing of hands and face. Advice from an imam may have to be sought regarding fasting if a Muslim falls ill during the holy period of Ramadan. Some other important Muslim rituals are those associated with birth and death. At the birth of an infant the husband stands near his wife's head; when the infant is born, the new father whispers a prayer from the Qur'an in the child's ear. Usually a dying Muslim chooses to lie facing Mecca (the east); he or she may also wish to confess prior sins and to recite the words, "There is no God but Allah, and Muhammed is His prophet."

The Orthodox Jewish patient is required to pray three times each day. A male patient, if able, may wish to wear a yarmulke (skull cap) and prayer shawl, as well as phylacteries (symbols of the Ten Commandments) when praying (Charnes & Moore, 1992, p. 66). On the eighth day after birth, a Jewish male child must be circumcised. Circumcision may be done in the hospital, if necessary, or in the home by a mohel or Jewish rabbi trained in the procedure. When a Jewish patient is dying, family and friends consider it a religious duty to visit and pray with the dying person and his or her family. In the case of an Orthodox Jew, the nursing personnel may not need to perform postmortem care, as a group from the patient's synagogue, the "burial society," will come to care for the body.

For the Christian person who is ill, the sacraments, as mentioned earlier, as well as prayers particular to each denomination, may be an important part of the healing process. Some years ago, a Roman Catholic could only receive Anointing, then called Extreme Unction, when death was perceived to be imminent. Current Church teaching allows the Catholic patient to request the Anointing in the revised ritual of the Sacrament of the Sick at any point during an illness experience. Receiving Holy Communion at that time, or at any time during one's illness, is an important religious ritual for the Catholic and also for many Protestant patients.

Infant Baptism is also an important Roman Catholic ritual. Ordinarily it is carried out in the parish church several weeks after mother and baby have left the hospital. If, however, an infant is in danger of death, any nurse may perform an emergency Baptism by pouring a small amount of water on the child's head and reciting simultaneously, "I baptize you in the name of the Father and of the Son and of the Holy Spirit." Many other Christians practice infant Baptism; some of these church groups include the Episcopal, Lutheran, Methodist, and Presbyterian denominations. Baptismal rites may vary slightly. For example, in the Methodist tradition, "the one baptizing should put his or her hands in the water and then place the wet hand on the baby's head and repeat the baptismal words. In the Lutheran rite, the water is poured on the head three times, while saying the baptismal words" (Reeb & McFarland, 1995, p. 27).

Rosemarie, an operating room nurse for more than 20 years, described a situation in which she felt that she was providing spiritual care by supporting a patient's religious ritual belief, even though she was of a different faith.

> In this situation I was a fairly new nurse, and the patient came in [to the OR suite], and I just had a sense that this patient was going to die. The patient was very ill; he was elderly and had a bowel obstruction. He had come in the middle of the night for emergency surgery. The man was Catholic, and I thought, "well if this man is this bad, then he needs to see a priest." I felt strongly about supporting that and the surgeon got angry with me for not taking the patient in. I literally stepped in front of the gurney, and didn't let the patient get rolled into the OR until the priest came and he was able to give his last confession. That patient died on the table!? . . . It was scary for me. I don't know why I felt so strongly; normally I wouldn't go up against an authoritative role like the surgeon. I don't know what drove me to do it but it was based on my own religious beliefs. . . . The wife of the patient was so grateful that I insisted on waiting for the priest; the family never got to see him alive again.

Devotional Articles

Frequently the first clue to an ill patient's religious beliefs and practices is the presence or use of religious or devotional articles. A Jewish person, especially one of the Orthodox tradition, may use a prayer shawl and phylacteries during times of prayer. A Muslim may choose to read passages from the Holy Qur'an, or to pray with prayer beads, which identify the 99 names of Allah. A Christian patient, as well as reading sacred books such as the Bible or the Book of Mormon, will often display devotional items such as relics, medals, crosses, statues, and holy pictures with symbolic meaning for the person. For example, an ill Mexican American of the Christian tradition will frequently carry a medal or picture of Santo Niño de Atocha, a religious personage believed to be instrumental in healing the sick. Other religious symbols an ill person might display include sacred threads tied around the neck of a Hindu, Native American medicine bags, or mustard seeds used by Mediterranean groups to ward off the "evil eye" (Morris & Primomo, 1995, p. 111).

A medical–surgical nurse caring for acutely ill patients validated the notion that the visible presence of patients' devotional articles signaled religious belief and practice. "Usually we get a cue; if you see a Bible or a prayer book, or if they have a cross or a rosary, you think the patient probably has an interest in spiritual matters."

Sacred Music

Music, especially music reflecting an interest in the transcendent, expresses the depth of feeling of one's spirit. Music is a part of all cultures and religious traditions, especially as a central dimension of religious worship (Hurd, 1993, p. 675). Music is frequently used by individuals to relieve stress, and music therapy may be used as an adjunct to healing (Keegan, 1994, p. 169). In a nursing study exploring the use of music in the postoperative recovery period, researchers learned that experimental group patients reported that the music served to relax them, as well as serving as a distracter from pain and discomfort (Heiser, Chiles, Fudge, & Gray, 1997).

Karen Sutherland (2005) observed that "the first recorded use of music as an instrument of healing is in the Bible" and cited the story of the young shepherd David who was "summoned to play his music to heal King Saul's emotional and spiritual distress" (p. 29). "The therapy was so successful," Sutherland adds, "Saul requested that David remain in his service (1 Samuel 16:14–23)" (p. 29). The story of a contemporary David is reported in *The Nurse with an Alabaster Jar: A Biblical Approach to Nursing*. The author was told an anecdote about a hospitalized elderly end-stage emphysema patient who was experiencing severely compromised breathing. While she received prescribed nebulizer treatments periodically throughout the day, her breathing and her anxiety became more and more pronounced toward the end of each afternoon. Thus, "a young respiratory therapist, who had been working with the patient, asked the head nurse if he could try an intervention with music; he was a folk guitarist. The head nurse, desperate for any kind of relief for her patient, agreed. The respiratory therapist brought his guitar to the unit and began to play gently for the patient during the periods when her breathing became extremely labored. Everyone, including the head nurse, was amazed at how this gentle 'folk guitar therapy' eased the rapid, labored breathing of the anxious patient" (O'Brien, 2006, p. 104).

Religious music ranges from religious rock, folk, or country-western music, which may appeal to younger patients, to the traditional religious hymns and classical religious pieces such as Handel's *Messiah*, often preferred by the older generation. Playing a recording of religious music, or even softly singing a hymn with a patient, may be incorporated into spiritual care (Folta, 1993, p. 29), if nurse and patient find it meaningful. Music has been identified as a "therapeutic intervention for healing" by Young and Koopsen (2011, p. 175).

Anna, a 13-year-old Ewing's sarcoma patient from a Christian missionary family, loved the traditional hymns of her church. Anna was very ill and experiencing severe pain from her disease; she also required periodic painful bone marrow exams to determine the side effects of her chemotherapy. Anna's mother and the nursing staff decided that singing hymns would be a good way to distract her during the procedure. It was deeply moving to hear the gentle singing of "Abide with me, fast falls the eventide" coming from the pediatric clinic treatment room during Anna's "bone marrows."

If a nurse believes that a patient of any religious tradition might find comfort and support in sacred music, yet the ill person has little experience with religious music, one suggestion might be the beautiful ecumenical chants of Taizé, known throughout the world. The community of Taizé, founded by Lutheran Brother Roger Shutz, has become a center of ecumenical prayer and reconciliation for people from all countries and of all religious traditions. The simple and beautiful chants were created so that Taizé visitors of all cultures and religious persuasions might be able to sing together as one choir. Recordings of the Taizé chants, which include a short scripture verse or brief prayer, with refrains such as "Alleluia," "Bless the Lord," and "Stay with us O Lord," are available at most religious bookstores.

This chapter describes the importance of the nurse's role in spiritual care. Many contemporary nurses find assessment, and in some cases intervention, relative to patients' spiritual needs to be a treasured part of their clinical practice. It is nevertheless important to reiterate that not all nurses will feel competent or comfortable undertaking nursing therapeutics in the area of spiritual care. These nurses should, however, be sensitive to the importance of nursing assessment of patients' spiritual needs; referral to a pastoral caregiver for support or intervention is always an acceptable option.

▶ References

Abdellah, F. G., & Levine, E. (1979). *Better patient care through nursing research.* New York, NY: Macmillan.

Abdil-Haqq Muhammad, K. (1995, June). What Muslims believe and why. *Muslim Community News*, 1–2.

Ameling, A. (2000). Prayer: An ancient healing practice becomes new again. *Holistic Nursing Practice, 14*(3), 40–48.

Atkinson, L. J., & Fortunato, N. M. (1996). *Berry & Kohn's operating room technique.* St. Louis, MO: C. V. Mosby-Yearbook.

Bacon, J. (1995). Healing prayer: The risks and the rewards. *Journal of Christian Nursing, 12*(1), 14–17.

Baird, R. H. (1994). On bad luck: Job and Jesus. *Journal of Religion and Health, 33*(4), 305–312.

Baldacchino, D. (2010). Caring in Lourdes: An innovation in students' clinical placement. *British Journal of Nursing, 19*(6), 358–366.

Barnum, B. S. (1995, Spring). Spirituality in nursing. *Nursing Leadership Forum, 1*(1), 24–30.

Barss, K. S. (2012). Building bridges: An interpretive phenomenological analysis of nurse educators clinical experience with the T.R.U.S.T. model for inclusive spiritual care. *International Journal of Nursing Education Scholarship, 9*(1), 1–17.

Battey, B. W. (2010). Perspectives on spiritual care for nurse managers. *Journal of Nursing Management, 20*(8), 1012–1020.

Beck, S. E., & Goldberg, E. K. (1996). Jewish beliefs, values and practices: Implications for culturally sensitive nursing care. *Advanced Practice Nursing Quarterly, 2*(2), 15–22.

Bergant, D. (1990). The book of Job (introduction). In D. Senior, M. Getty, C. Stuhlmueller, & J. Collins (Eds.), *The Catholic study Bible* (pp. 611–612). New York, NY: Oxford University Press.

Beuscher, L., & Grando, V. (2009). Using spirituality to cope with early-stage Alzheimer's disease. *Western Journal of Nursing Research, 31*(1), 583–598.

Biro, A.L. (2012). Creating conditions for good nursing by attending to the spiritual. *Journal of Nursing Management, 20*(8), 1002–1011.

Black, J. M., & Matassarin-Jacobs, E. (1997). *Medical–surgical nursing: Clinical management for continuity of care* (5th ed.). Philadelphia, PA: W. B. Saunders.

Borelli, J. (1990). Buddhism. In J. A. Komonchak, M. Collins, & D. A. Lane (Eds.), *The new dictionary of theology* (pp. 144–147). Collegeville, MN: The Liturgical Press.

Broten, P. (1997). Spiritual care documentation: Where is it? *Journal of Christian Nursing, 14*(2), 29–31.

Bruner, L. (1985). The spiritual dimension of holistic care. *Imprint, 31*(4), 44–45.

Burnard, P. (1988). Spiritual distress and the nursing response: Theoretical considerations and counseling skills. *Journal of Advanced Nursing, 12*(3), 377–382.

Byock, I. R. (1994). When suffering persists. *Journal of Palliative Care, 10*(2), 8–13.

Carr, T. (2008). Mapping the processes and qualities of spiritual nursing care. *Qualitative Health Research, 18*(5), 686–700.

Carr, T. (2010). Facing existential realities: Exploring barriers and challenges to spiritual nursing care. *Qualitative Health Research, 20*(10), 1379–1392.

Carretto, C. (1978). *Summoned by love*. Maryknoll, NY: Orbis Books.

Carroll, B. (2001). A phenomenological exploration of the nature of spirituality and spiritual care. *Mortality, 6*(1), 81–98.

Cenkner, W. (1990). Hinduism. In J. A. Komonchak, M. Collins, & D. A. Lane (Eds.), *The new dictionary of theology* (pp. 466–469). Collegeville, MN: The Liturgical Press.

Ceronsky, C. (1993). Creative models of spiritual care. *Health Progress, 74*(4), 58–61.

Chan, M. F. (2009). Factors affecting staff in practicing spiritual care. *Journal of Clinical Nursing, 19*, 2128–2136.

Charnes, L., & Moore, P. (1992). Meeting patients' spiritual needs: The Jewish perspective. *Holistic Nurse Practitioner, 6*(3), 64–72.

Chung, L. Y., Wong, F. K., & Chan, M. F. (2007). Relationship of nurses' spirituality to their understanding and practice of spiritual care. *Journal of Advanced Nursing, 58*(2), 158–170.

Clark, C. F., Cross, J. R., Dean, D. M., & Lowry, L. W. (1991). Spirituality: Integral to quality care. *Holistic Nursing Practice, 5*(3), 67–76.

Clinebell, H. (1991). *Basic types of pastoral care and counseling*. Nashville, TN: Abington Press.

Cockell, N., & McSherry, W. (2010). Spiritual care in nursing: An overview of published international research. *Journal of Nursing Management, 20*(8), 958–969.

Coleman, C., Nokes, K., Corless, I., Kirksey, K., Nicholas, P., & Tsai, Y. (2006). Prayer as a complementary health strategy for managing HIV-related symptoms among ethnically diverse patients. *Holistic Nursing Practice, 20*(2), 65–72.

Conco, D. (1995). Christian patients' views of spiritual care. *Western Journal of Nursing Research, 17*(3), 266–276.

Cone, P. H., & Giske, T. (2012). Teaching spiritual care: A grounded theory study among undergraduate nurse educators. *Journal of Clinical Nursing, 22*(13/14), 1951–1960.

Costello, M., Atinaja-Faller, J., & Hedberg, M. (2012). The use of simulation to instruct students on the provision of spiritual care. *Journal of Holistic Nursing, 30*(4), 277–281.

Curran, G. (1995). The spiritual variable, a world view. In B. Newman (Ed.), *The Neuman systems model* (3rd ed., pp. 581–589). Stamford, CT: Appleton & Lange.

Daaleman, T. P. (2012). A health services framework for spiritual care. *Journal of Nursing Management, 20*(8), 1021–1028.

Davidson, J., Boyer, M., Casey, D., Matzel, S., & Walden, D. (2008). Gap analysis of cultural and religious needs of hospitalized patients. *Critical Care Nursing Quarterly, 31*(2), 119–126.

Deal, B., & Grassley, J. S. (2012). The lived experience of giving spiritual care: A phenomenological study of nephrology nurses. *Nephrology Nursing Journal, 39*(6), 471–496.

Denholm, B. (2008). Staff nurses and prayer. *AORN Journal, 88*(3), 451–455.

Dennis, P. (1991). Components of spiritual nursing care from the nurse's perspective. *Journal of Holistic Nursing, 9*(1), 27–42.

DiJoseph, J., & Cavendish, R. (2005). Expanding the dialogue on prayer relevant to holistic care. *Holistic Nursing Practice, 19*(4), 147–154.

DiMeo, E. (1991). Patient's advocate: Rx for spiritual distress. *RN, 54*(3), 22–24.

Donley, R. (1991). Spiritual dimensions of health care. *Nursing and Health Care, 12*(4), 178–183.

Duff, V. (1994). Spiritual distress: Deciding to care. *Journal of Christian Nursing, 11*(1), 29–31.

Edmision, K. W. (1997). Psychosocial dimensions of medical–surgical nursing. In J. M. Black & E. Matassarin-Jacobs (Eds.), *Medical–surgical nursing: Clinical management for continuity of care* (5th ed., pp. 50–74). Philadelphia, PA: W. B. Saunders.

Ellis, H. K., & Narayanasamy, A. (2009). An investigation into the role of spirituality in nursing. *British Journal of Nursing, 18*(14), 886–890.

Emblen, J., & Halstead, L. (1993). Spiritual needs and interventions: Comparing the views of patients, nurses and chaplains. *Clinical Nurse Specialist, 7*(4), 175–182.

Emeth, E. V., & Greenhut, J. H. (1991). *The wholeness handbook.* New York, NY: Continuum.

Eriksson, K. (1994). Theories of caring as health. In D. A. Gaut & A. Boykin (Eds.), *Caring as healing: Renewal through hope* (pp. 3–20). New York, NY: National League for Nursing Process.

Eriksson, K. (2007). Becoming through suffering on the path to health and holiness. *International Journal of Human Caring, 11*(2), 8–16.

Esposito, J. L. (1990). Islam. In J. A. Komonchak, M. Collins, & D. A. Lane (Eds.), *The new dictionary of theology* (pp. 527–529). Collegeville, MN: The Liturgical Press.

Farrugia, E. G. (1990). Oriental orthodoxy. In J. A. Komonchak, M. Collins, & D. A. Lane (Eds.), *The new dictionary of theology* (pp. 306–310). Collegeville, MN: The Liturgical Press.

Fawcett, J. (1989). *Analysis and evaluation of conceptual models of nursing* (2nd ed.). Philadelphia, PA: F. A. Davis.

Fenske, J. M. (2011). Soul mate: Exploring the concept of soul. *Journal of Holistic Nursing, 29*(3), 229–232.

Fine, J. (1995). Long-term care in the Jewish tradition. *The Nursing Spectrum, 5*(22), 2.

Fish, S., & Shelly, J. A. (1979). *Spiritual care: The nurse's role.* Downer's Grove, IL: InterVarsity Press.

Folta, R. H. (1993). Music: Arousing the human spirit. *Journal of Christian Nursing, 10*(2), 27–29.

Giske, T. (2012), How undergraduate nursing students learn to care for patients spiritually. *Journal of Nursing Management, 20*(8), 1049–1057.

Giske, T., & Cone, P. H. (2012). Opening up to learning spiritual care of patients: A grounded theory study of nursing students. *Journal of Clinical Nursing, 21*(13/14), 2006–2015.

Greenstreet, W. M. (1999). Teaching spirituality in nursing: A literature review. *Nurse Education Today, 19*(8), 649–658.

Gros, J. (1990). Protestantism. In J. A. Komonchak, M. Collins, & D. A. Lane (Eds.), *The new dictionary of theology* (pp. 811–815). Collegeville, MN: The Liturgical Press.

Hall, C., & Lanig, H. (1993). Spiritual caring behaviors as reported by Christian nurses. *Western Journal of Nursing Research, 15*(6), 730–741.

Harmer, B., & Henderson, V. (1955). *Textbook of the principles and practice of nursing* (5th ed.). New York, NY: Macmillan.

Harrison, J. (1993). Spirituality and nursing practice. *Journal of Clinical Nursing, 2*(3), 211–217.

Hawley, G., & Irurita, V. (1998). Seeking comfort through prayer. *International Journal of Nursing Practice, 4*(1), 9–18.

Heiser, R., Chiles, K., Fudge, M., & Gray, S. (1997). The use of music during the immediate postoperative recovery period. *Association of Operating Room Nurses Journal, 65*(4), 777–785.

Heliker, D. (1992). Re-evaluation of a nursing diagnosis: Spiritual distress. *Nursing Forum, 27*(4), 15–20.

Henderson, V. (1966). *The nature of nursing: A definition and its implications for practice, research and education.* New York, NY: Macmillan.

Hinshaw, D., Carnahan, J., Breck, J., Mosoiu, N., & Mosoiu, D. (2011). Spiritual issues in suffering: Creating a dialogue between clergy and palliative care providers. *Progress in Palliative Care, 19*(1), 7–14.

Hufford, D. J. (1987). The love of God's mysterious will: Suffering and the popular theology of healing. *Listening, 22*(2), 115–126.

Hummel, L., Galek, K., Murphy, K. M., Tannenbaum, H. P., & Flannelly, L. T. (2008). Defining spiritual care: An exploratory study. *Journal of Health Care Chaplaincy, 15*, 40–51.

Hurd, B. (1993). Music. In M. Downey (Ed.), *The new dictionary of Catholic spirituality* (pp. 674–677). Collegeville, MN: The Liturgical Press.

Ignatavicius, D. D., Workman, M. L., & Mishler, M. A. (1995). *Medical–surgical nursing: A nursing process approach.* Philadelphia, PA: W. B. Saunders.

Johnson, R. P. (1992). *Body, mind, spirit: Tapping the healing power within you.* Liguori, MO: Liguori Publications.

Kahn, D. L., & Steeves, R. H. (1994). Witnesses to suffering: Nursing knowledge, voice and vision. *Nursing Outlook, 42*(6), 260–264.

Karns, P. S. (1991). Building a foundation for spiritual care. *Journal of Christian Nursing, 8*(3), 11–13.

Keegan, L. (1994). *The nurse as healer.* Albany, NY: Delmar.

Kelleher, M. M. (1990). Ritual. In J. A. Komonchak, M. Collins, & D. A. Lane (Eds.), *The new dictionary of theology* (pp. 906–907). Collegeville, MN: The Liturgical Press.

Kemp, C. (1996). Islamic cultures: Health care beliefs and practices. *American Journal of Health Behavior, 20*(3), 83–89.

Kemp, P. (2009). Spirituality in health care: What can you do? *British Journal of Healthcare Assistants, 3*(7), 333–335.

Kevern, P. (2012). Who can give spiritual care? The management of spiritually sensitive interactions between nurses and patients. *Journal of Nursing Management, 20*(8), 981–989.

Kidner, D. (1983). Poetry and wisdom literature. In D. Alexander & P. Alexander (Eds.), *Eerdmans' handbook to the Bible* (pp. 316–369). Grand Rapids, MI: W. B. Eerdmans.

Kozier, B., Erb, G., Blais, K., & Wilkinson, J. (1995). *Fundamentals of nursing: Concepts, process and practice* (5th ed.). Menlo Park, CA: Addison-Wesley.

Krekeler, K., & Yancey, V. (1993). Spiritual health. In P. A. Potter & A. G. Perry (Eds.), *Fundamentals of nursing: Concepts, process and practice* (3rd ed., pp. 1000–1013). St. Louis, MO: C. V. Mosby.

Kumar, K. (2004). Spiritual care: What's worldview got to do with it? *Journal of Christian Nursing, 21*(1), 24–27.

Kushner, H. (1981). *When bad things happen to good people.* New York, NY: Avon.

Labun, E. (1988). Spiritual care: An element in nurse care planning. *Journal of Advanced Nursing, 13*(3), 314–320.

Lane, J. A. (1987). The care of the human spirit. *Journal of Professional Nursing, 3*(6), 332–337.

Lantz, C. (2007). Teaching spiritual care in a public institution: Legal implications, standards of practice and ethical obligations. *Journal of Nursing Education, 46*(1), 33–38.

Levine, E., Aviv, C., Yoon, G., Ewing, C., & Au, A. (2009). The benefits of prayer on mood and well-being of breast cancer survivors. *Support Care Cancer, 17*, 295–306.

Lewis, P. J. (1996). A review of prayer within the role of the holistic nurse. *Journal of Holistic Nursing, 14*(4), 308–315.

Livingstone, E. A. (1990). *The concise Oxford dictionary of the Christian church.* New York, NY: Oxford University Press.

Maes, J. (1990). *Suffering: A caregiver's guide.* Nashville, TN: Abington.

Mason, C. H. (1995). Prayer as a nursing intervention. *Journal of Christian Nursing, 12*(1), 4–8.

McSherry, W., & Jamieson, S. (2011). An online survey of nurses' perceptions of spirituality and spiritual care. *Journal of Clinical Nursing, 20*, 1757–1767.

McSherry, W., & Jamieson, S. (2013). The qualitative findings from an online survey investigating nurses' perceptions of spirituality and spiritual care. *Journal of Clinical Nursing, 22*(21/22), 3170–3182.

Meleis, A. I. (1991). *Theoretical nursing, development and progress* (2nd ed.). Philadelphia, PA: J. B. Lippincott.

Meehan, T. C. (2012). Spirituality and spiritual care from a careful nursing perspective. *Journal of Nursing Management, 20*(8), 990–1001.

Merriam-Webster's new collegiate dictionary (7th ed.). (1976). Springfield, MA: Merriam-Webster.

Moore, R. (2007). Higher connection. *Nursing Standard, 22*(12), 20–21.

Moore, T. (1992). *Care of the soul.* New York, NY: HarperCollins.

Morris, D. L., & Primomo, J. (1995). Nursing practice with young and middle-aged adults. In W. J. Phipps, V. L. Cassmeyer, J. K. Sands, & M. K. Lehman (Eds.), *Medical–surgical nursing: Concepts and clinical practice* (5th ed., pp. 45–64). St. Louis, MO: C. V. Mosby.

Narayanasamy, A., & Narayanasamy, M. (2008). The healing power of prayer and its implications for nursing. *British Journal of Nursing, 17*(6), 394–398.

Narayanasamy, A., & Owens, J. (2001). A critical incident study of nurses' responses to the spiritual needs of their patients. *Journal of Advanced Nursing, 33*(4), 446–455.

Nelson, B. (1984). Who should give spiritual care? *Journal of Christian Nursing, 1*(2), 20–26.

Nightingale, F. (1859). *Notes on nursing: What it is and what it is not.* London, UK: Hamson, Bookseller to the Queen.

Nolan, P. (2000). Learning from the past, not living in it. *Nursing Review, 17*(4), 92–95.

Normille, P. (1992). *Visiting the sick: A guide for parish ministers.* Cincinnati, OH: St. Anthony Messenger Press.

Nowell, I. (1993). Scripture. In M. Downey (Ed.), *The new dictionary of Catholic spirituality* (pp. 854–863). Collegeville, MN: The Liturgical Press.

Nutkiewicz, M. (1993). Jewish spirituality. In M. Downey (Ed.), *The new dictionary of Catholic spirituality* (pp. 561–565). Collegeville, MN: The Liturgical Press.

O'Brien, M. E. (1982). The need for spiritual integrity. In H. Yura & M. Walsh (Eds.), *Human needs and the nursing process* (Vol. 2, pp. 85–115). Norwalk, CT: Appleton-Century-Crofts.

O'Brien, M. E. (2006). *The nurse with an alabaster jar: A biblical approach to nursing.* Madison, WI: NCF Press.

O'Brien, M. E., & Pheifer, W. G. (1993). Physical and psychosocial nursing care for patients with HIV infection. *Nursing Clinics of North America, 28*(2), 303–315.

O'Conner, K. M. (1990). *The wisdom literature.* Collegeville, MN: The Liturgical Press.

Oldnall, A. S. (1995). On the absence of spirituality in nursing theories and models. *Journal of Advanced Nursing, 21*(3), 417–418.

Parse, R. R. (1981). *Man, living, health: A theory for nursing.* New York, NY: Wiley.

Paterson, J. G., & Zderad, L. T. (1976). *Humanistic nursing.* New York, NY: Wiley.

Pawlikowski, J. (1990). Judaism. In J. Komonchak, M. Collins, & D. A. Lane (Eds.), *The new dictionary of theology* (pp. 543–548). Collegeville, MN: The Liturgical Press.

Pearce, L. (2009). Delivering spiritual care. *Nursing Standard, 23*(28), 22–23.

Phillips, K. D. (1997). Roy's adaptation model in nursing practice. In M. R. Alligood & A. Marriner-Tomey (Eds.), *Nursing theory: Utilization and application* (pp. 175–198). St. Louis, MO: Mosby-Yearbook.

Phipps, W. J., Cassmeyer, V. L., Sands, J. K., & Lehman, M. K. (1995). *Medical–surgical nursing: Concepts and clinical practice* (5th ed.). St. Louis, MO: C. V. Mosby.

Piles, C. L. (1990). Providing spiritual care. *Nurse Educator, 15*(1), 36–41.

Potter, P. A., & Perry, A. G. (1997). *Fundamentals of nursing: Concepts, process and practice* (4th ed.). St. Louis, MO: C. V. Mosby.

Praill, D. (1995). Approaches to spiritual care. *Nursing Times, 91*(34), 55–57.

Rassool, G. H. (2000). The crescent and Islam: Healing, nursing and the spiritual dimension. *Journal of Advanced Nursing, 32*(6), 1476–1484.

Reeb, R. H., & McFarland, S. T. (1995). Emergency baptism. *Journal of Christian Nursing, 12*(2), 26–27.

Ross, L., Hall, I., Fairley, T., Taylor, Y., & Howard, D. (2008). Prayer and self-reported health among cancer survivors in the United States, National Health Interview Survey, 2002. *The Journal of Alternative and Complimentary Medicine, 14*(8), 931–938.

Salladay, S., & Bitting, M. (2012). Caring for familiar strangers. *Journal of Christian Nursing, 29*(1), 15.

Sarter, B. (1992). Philosophical sources of nursing theory. In L. H. Nicoll (Ed.), *Perspectives on nursing theory* (2nd ed., pp. 147–156). Philadelphia, PA: J. B. Lippincott.

Sato, M. K. (1984). Major factors influencing adaptation. In C. Roy (Ed.), *Introduction to nursing: An adaptation model* (2nd ed., pp. 64–87). Englewood Cliffs, NJ: Prentice-Hall.

Sellers, S. C. (2001). The spiritual care meanings of adults residing in the Midwest. *Nursing Science Quarterly, 14*(3), 239–248.

Shelly, J. A. (1995). Is prayer unprofessional? (Editorial). *Journal of Christian Nursing, 12*(1), 3.

Shelly, J. A., & Fish, S. (1988). *Spiritual care: The nurse's role* (3rd ed.). Downer's Grove, IL: InterVarsity Press.

Shelly, J. A., & Fish, S. (1995). Praying with patients. *Journal of Christian Nursing, 12*(1), 9–13.

Shelly, J. A., & Miller, A. (1999). *Called to care: A Christian theology of nursing.* Downer's Grove, IL: InterVarsity Press.

Sims, C. (1987). Spiritual care as a part of holistic nursing. *Imprint, 34*(4), 63–65.

Simsen, B. (1988). Nursing the spirit. *Nursing Times, 84*(37), 32–33.

Smeltzer, S. C., & Bare, B. G. (1996). *Brunner and Suddarth's textbook of medical–surgical nursing* (8th ed.). Philadelphia, PA: J. B. Lippincott.

Sohier, R. (1997). Neuman's systems model in nursing. In M. R. Alligood & A. Marriner-Tomey (Eds.), *Nursing theory: Utilization and application* (pp. 109–127). St. Louis, MO: Mosby-Yearbook.

Sparks, R. (1993). Suffering. In M. Downey (Ed.), *The new dictionary of Catholic spirituality* (pp. 950–953). Collegeville, MN: The Liturgical Press.

Stephenson, C., & Wilson, K. (2004). Does spiritual care really help? A study of patient perceptions. *Journal of Christian Nursing, 21*(2), 26–29.

Stevens, A. (2011). A role for spirituality in palliative care leadership. *International Journal of Palliative Care Nursing, 17*(7), 315.

Studzinski, R. (1993). Pastoral care and counseling. In M. Downey (Ed.), *The new dictionary of Catholic spirituality* (pp. 722–723). Collegeville, MN: The Liturgical Press.

Sutherland, K. (2005). Can music help heal us? The first recorded use of music as an instrument of healing is in the Bible. *Journal of Christian Nursing, 22*(3), 29–31.

Sweat, M. (2012). Is respecting the "quiet place" giving spiritual care? *Journal of Christian Nursing, 29*(3), 180.

Swift, C., Calcutawalla, S., & Elliott, R. (2007). Nursing attitudes toward recording of religious and spiritual data. *British Journal of Nursing, 16*(20), 1279–1282.

Tanyi, R. A., McKenzie, M., & Chapek, C. (2009). How family practice physicians, nurse practitioners, and physician's assistants incorporate spiritual care in practice. *Journal of the American Academy of Nurse Practitioners, 21*, 690–697.

Taylor, C., Lillis, C., & LeMone, P. (1997). *Fundamentals of nursing: The art and science of nursing care* (3rd ed.). Philadelphia, PA: J. B. Lippincott.

Texter, L. A., & Mariscotti, J. M. (1994). From chaos to new life: Ritual enactment in the passage from illness to health. *Journal of Religion and Health, 33*(4), 325–332.

Travelbee, J. (1971). *Interpersonal aspects of nursing* (2nd ed.). Philadelphia, PA: F. A. Davis.

Treloar, L. L. (2001). Spiritual care: Safe, appropriate, ethical. *Journal of Christian Nursing, 18*(2), 16–20.

Tucker, S., Canobbio, M., Paquette, E., & Wells, M. (1996). *Patient care standards: Collaborative planning guides.* St. Louis, MO: C. V. Mosby.

van Leeuwen, R., & Cusveller, B. (2004). Nursing competencies for spiritual care. *Journal of Advanced Nursing, 48*(3), 234–246.

Washholtz, A., Pearce, M., & Koenig, H. (2007). Exploring the relationship between spirituality, coping and pain. *Journal of Behavioral Medicine, 30*, 311–318.

Watson, J. (1985). *Nursing: Human science and human care.* Norwalk, CT: Appleton-Century-Crofts.

Wright, S. (2011). The heart and soul of nursing. *Nursing Standard, 25*(30), 18–19.

Wright, S., & Neuberger, J. (2012). Why spirituality is essential for nurses. *Nursing Standard, 26*(40), 19–21.

Yilmaz, M., & Gurler, H. (2014). The efficacy of integrating spirituality into undergraduate nursing curricula. *Nursing Ethics, 21*(8), 929–945.

Young, C., & Koopsen, C. (2011). *Spirituality, health, and healing: An integrative approach* (2nd ed.). Sudbury, MA: Jones & Bartlett Learning.

Yuan, H., & Porr, C. (2014). Integrating spiritual care into a baccalaureate nursing program in China. *Journal of Holistic Nursing, 32*(3), 240–243.

CHAPTER 7

Spiritual Needs of the Patient with an Acute Illness

Waiting for tomorrow ... asks for ... a deep faith in the value and meaning of life, and a strong hope which breaks through the boundaries of death.

Henri Nouwen, *The Wounded Healer*, 1979

> For your patients who are suffering physically, you have to give compassion; trying to empathize [with] how they are feeling ... and always wanting to do the right thing for the patient, relieve their pain or discomfort, or try to, if you can't do anything else, just listen to them. I think that aspect of empathy and compassion sets nurses apart from other healthcare providers, the caring aspect.
>
> Katie, Team Leader on a Medical–Surgical Unit

The spiritual needs of the adult patient suffering from an acute illness vary greatly depending on such factors as age, religious tradition, and the seriousness of the condition. These and other variables are explored in this chapter, which describes the spiritual needs of patients experiencing conditions including congestive heart failure, septicemia, pneumonia, myasthenia gravis (myasthenic crisis), toxoplasmosis, acute renal failure, and acute pain. Data documenting the importance of personal spirituality and religious support were obtained through the author's interviews of and interaction with patients, family members, and nurse caregivers of patients with acute illness.

Currently the spiritual care practices of nurses caring for acutely ill patients are being explored in relation to ease or difficulty of providing such care. The most significant barriers reported in a study of 271 acute care nurses included: "belief that patients' spirituality is private, insufficient time, difficulty distinguishing proselytizing from spiritual care and difficulty meeting spiritual needs when spiritual beliefs are different from their own" (Gallison, Xu, Jurgens, & Boyle, 2013, p. 95). Specific barriers to spiritual care carried out in a hospital setting were identified as: "the difficulty in defining spirituality; the lack of clear guidelines for the nurse's role in providing spiritual care; nurses' lack of time to provide spiritual care; and a lack of training and education on spirituality" (Rushton, 2014, p. 370).

Some of the acutely ill patient populations among whom spiritual care needs have recently been examined are: coronary care patients (Abu-El-Noor & Abu-El-Noor, 2014); coronary syndrome patients (Jahani, Rajeh, Heravi-Karimooj, Vaismoradi, & Jasper, 2014); intensive care unit patients (Turan & Karamanoglu, 2012); palliative care patients (Ronaldson, Hayes, Aggar, Green, & Carey, 2012); and medical-surgical hospital patients (Barber, 2013).

▶ The Case of Acute Illness

Nursing texts distinguish between acute and chronic illnesses, differentiating the two phenomena as distinct entities. Taylor, Lillis, and LeMone (1997) described acute illness as "a rapidly occurring illness that runs its course, allowing the person to return to his or her previous level of functioning" (p. 1451), whereas Potter and Perry (1997) defined it as "characterized by symptoms that are of relatively short duration, are usually severe, and affect the functioning of the client in all dimensions" (p. 1475). These conceptualizations are appropriate to describe a multiplicity of illness conditions such as pneumonia, influenza, bronchitis, gastritis, herpes zoster ("shingles"), and a host of other self-limiting disease processes. With an uncomplicated acute illness, an individual may pass rapidly through the stages of initial symptom development, treatment and "sick role" behavior, and recovery.

However, a number of "chronic" disease conditions may begin or end with an acute illness phase or manifest acute symptoms during periods of exacerbation over the course of the illness trajectory. One example is that of chronic renal failure (CRF), which may, if undiagnosed, initially manifest in a state of acute renal failure, necessitating emergency dialytic therapy and, in some cases, critical care nursing. Human immunodeficiency virus (HIV) infection, another condition currently being categorized as chronic, may be initially diagnosed by the acute onset of an opportunistic infection such as *Pneumocystis carinii* pneumonia (PCP) or cytomegalovirus. Patients suffering from various types of carcinoma may experience acute illness symptoms related to a therapeutic regimen incorporating radical surgery and/or chemotherapy.

During periods of acute illness, whether self-limiting or associated with a chronic disease, the patient may experience significant physical discomfort and anxiety, especially if symptoms are severe or life threatening. Patients with self-limiting illness may need comfort and support in coping with the sequelae of an infectious process, such as the acute pain accompanying a bout with herpes zoster ("shingles"). Individuals experiencing acute exacerbations of a potentially life-threatening chronic illness may need help in coping with the prognosis as well as the diagnosis of their condition. For the acute renal failure patient faced with the possibility of a future of dependency on medical technology, quality of life may become questionable; in a few cases, patients have elected to die rather than continue living supported by continuous dialytic therapy (O'Brien, 1982b). Thus the need for spiritual care and assessment of spiritual concerns are important aspects of holistic nursing care during periods of acute illness.

▶ Spiritual Needs in Acute Illness

Spiritual beliefs and, for some, religious practices, may become more important during illness than at any other time in a person's life (Kozier, Erb, Blais, & Wilkinson, 1995, p. 314). While an individual is enjoying good mental and physical health, spiritual or religious practices may be relegated, in terms of both time and energy, to a small portion of one's life activities. With the onset of acute illness, however, especially if associated with the exacerbation of a chronic condition, some significant life changes may occur both physically and emotionally. First, the ill person is usually forced to dramatically curtail physical activities, especially those associated with formal work or professional involvement. This may leave the individual with a great deal of uncommitted time to ponder the meaning of life and the illness experience. Such a time of forced physical "retreat" may effect considerable emotional change in one's assessment of past and future attitudes and behaviors.

Meeting patients' spiritual needs in institutional settings such as the hospital or long-term care facility often poses unique challenges for nursing staff (Minnix, 2008). Developing a positive relationship between the nursing department and staff chaplains is an important facilitator for the provision of spiritual care (Weaver, Koenig, & Flannelly, 2008); the caring presence of nurses can be critical to the spiritual well-being of many hospitalized patients (Pipe et al., 2008). It is suggested that hospitals can, in fact, become "healing spaces" if appropriate attention to the spiritual needs of patients and families is considered and attended to (Sternberg, 2009). In discussing the spiritual needs of hospitalized patients, March and Caple (2012) pointed out that hospital-based clergy often reported "assisting patients to cope with not only their religious/spiritual concerns but also with feelings of loneliness, despair, anger, frustration, guilt and shame, physical pain and suffering, and with issues surrounding family discord" (p. 1). In essence, the clergy were coping with an expanded definition of spiritual needs for the acutely ill hospitalized patient.

It is also important for nurses to be attuned to the spiritual needs of acutely ill patients who may be at or near the end of their lives. In relation to a nurse's responsibility to either provide or facilitate the provision of spiritual care to these patients, one nursing study evaluated the relationship between nurses' personal religiosity and attitudes toward end-of-life care. Findings revealed that there was a significant positive association between the nurse's own religious beliefs and practices and his or her view of the importance of end-of-life care (Bjarnason, 2010, p. 78).

The remarks of a 32-year-old male patient reflected such an experience during an episode of acute renal failure. "It enlightened me as to just how fast I was really going. It made me reevaluate my life. Now I can place my needs before my wants. It hasn't been so difficult in looking at the good advantages. This thing has made me think a lot about the way I used to live, and put different values on things" (O'Brien, 1983, p. 146). A 47-year-old male renal failure patient who had also suffered a serious bout of acute illness at the time of disease onset, commented in a similar vein. "This illness definitely made me think; get my mind together. I know all things happen for the good. It turned me around spiritually and mentally. Now I listen better. I try to be more patient, and I have more to learn from others" (O'Brien, 1983, p. 146).

Of the 126 renal failure patients studied, 93 individuals (approximately 74 percent of the total group) reported that religious or spiritual beliefs were, to some degree, responsible for their ability to accept their disease and its prognosis.

Despite a possible positive effect, however, the onset of a sudden and unanticipated acute illness may pose serious emotional and spiritual problems related to fear of possible death or disability. Psychological depression may occur as a result of severe physical symptoms such as acute pain and fatigue. Some patients question God's will and even express anger toward God for allowing the illness to occur. At this point, especially, the nurse must be alert and astute in assessing the spiritual concerns and needs of an acutely ill patient. Although a diagnosis of spiritual distress may be masked by the physical and emotional symptoms of an illness, the patient's remarks can provide a hint as to the presence of spiritual symptoms in need of attention. For example, comments such as "God help me," or "I wonder where God is in all of this?" can give the nurse an opening for informal spiritual assessment.

In essence, meeting the spiritual needs of the acutely ill may encompass basic concepts of spiritual care such as listening, being present, praying or reading Scripture (if acceptable to the patient and comfortable for the nurse), and/or making a referral to a chaplain or other pastoral caregiver. These activities, however, must be handled sensitively, related to the severity of patient symptoms such as pain, nausea, or fatigue. Appropriate spiritual care behaviors for the acutely ill person might include sitting quietly at the patient's bedside for a brief period, saying a short prayer aloud or offering a silent prayer, or sharing a comforting Scripture passage that may help to focus the patient away from the present suffering.

Interestingly the contemporary nursing literature seems to use the terminology "serious illness" rather than "acute illness" when describing patients' spiritual needs. One example of this is an article that identifies the types of spiritual care provided for persons during serious illness. Some of the caregiving activities reported were: "help relationship with God," "help you feel at peace with God," "help you attend religious/spiritual services," "help you with prayer," "help to better understand (one's) faith," and "help by asking others to pray for you" (Hanson et al., 2008, p. 911). Another paper focused on the spiritual needs of patients with serious illness at an urban public hospital. The authors contend that providers of spiritual care need to consider "difficult life events such as estrangement, homelessness, substance abuse, and imprisonment (which may have) shaped patients' approaches to serious illness" (Dzul-Church, Cimino, Adler, Wong, & Anderson, 2010, p. 695).

Nurses must assess the spiritual needs of seriously/terminally ill patients in clinical practice in order to "incorporate spiritual care into their clinical practice" (Smyth & Allen, 2011, p. 337; Hayden, 2011). Clinical conditions such as heart failure or the final stage of cardiac disease warrant assessment of spiritual needs to "improve life satisfaction" (Westlake, Dyo, Vollman, & Heywood, 2008, p. 257). A similar case is made for victims of serious illness related to hematological malignancies or "those individuals surviving the confrontation with death caused by a life threatening illness" (McGrath, 2004, p. 227).

Spiritual care is considered an intrinsic feature of palliative care for those with critical or terminal illnesses (Amoah, 2011). Amoah asserts that "spirituality should be considered on an equal footing with other key themes in palliative care, like relieving pain and advance care planning" (p. 353). Finally, spiritual care is identified as important for acutely ill or terminally ill persons as they may be "at special risk of spiritual crisis" (Agrimson & Taft, 2008, p. 454). "Spiritual crisis," explain Agrimson and Taft, may be described as "a unique form of grieving or loss, marked by a profound questioning of or lack of meaning in life" (p. 454).

▶ Spiritual Health in Acute Illness

Even though an acutely ill person may be facing a potentially life-threatening situation, the concept of spiritual health is not only possible, but may be the key factor in his or her coping successfully with the physiologic deficit. In discussing the spiritual health of the acutely ill patient, Peterson and Potter (1997) suggested that "the strength of a client's spirituality influences how he or she copes with sudden illness, and how quickly he or she can move to recovery" (p. 443).

Spiritual health can be defined as "a state of well-being and equilibrium in that part of a person's essence and existence which transcends the realm of the natural and relates to the ultimate good. Spiritual health is recognized by the presence of an interior state of peace and joy; freedom from abnormal anxiety, guilt, or a feeling of sinfulness; and a sense of security and direction in the pursuit of one's life goals and activities" (O'Brien, 1982a, p. 98). Spiritual health is also understood as relating to the ability to identify and describe one's purpose in life (Chapman, 1986; Levin & Schiller, 1987). Health-care researchers found a significant correlation between spiritual health and an individual's subjective evaluation of overall physical health (Michello, 1988), and that spiritual health can be predictive of how a person confronts his or her personal mortality (Hart, 1994). In emphasizing the value of the concept, Seidl (1993) argued that, as spiritual health organizes the values, meaning, and purpose in one's life, it also motivates an individual to "optimize" personal health so that he or she can serve God and community (p. 48). This places the notion of spiritual health in a religious context, which indeed is appropriate for many persons. An individual who professes no particular religious beliefs, however, may also be in a state of spiritual health. The terms *spiritual* and *religious* are not synonymous. Spirituality may, however, undergird religious practice, and thus, both concepts become relevant to a discussion of spiritual health (Fahlberg & Fahlberg, 1991).

An acutely ill person who is spiritually healthy can find comfort and strength in his or her spiritual or religious philosophy of life. This is reflected in the comments of Evan, HIV-positive for three years, who had recently experienced an acute episode of an opportunistic infection, *Pneumocystis carinii* pneumonia. "It's the spiritual dimension of religion that I want to practice. I meditate a lot. I sing the refrain from 'Day by Day.' Remember that? That's what I want to do; love Him more dearly. That's the most important thing in my life right now, with this disease" (O'Brien, 1992, pp. 47–48).

For the atheist or the agnostic who may be struggling to find a state of spiritual health, coping with the acute symptoms of an illness may be expressed very differently and, for some, may be much more difficult. Atheism, denial of the existence of God, or agnosticism, uncertainty about the existence of God, may leave a person diagnosed with serious illness struggling to find meaning and purpose in the experience. Burnard (1988) pointed out that patients with such beliefs also have spiritual needs, however, and nurses must be creative and compassionate in carrying out assessment and interventions.

Kent, an HIV-positive patient with cytomegalovirus, described his belief system as basically universal. "I believe in a superior force or being. It's an energy that I tap into. It's everywhere and it speaks to everything. I call on it when I need some reinforcement and encouragement in dealing with the stress of this illness" (O'Brien, 1992, p. 48).

Gerry, still in the process of recovering from a bout with toxoplasmosis, poignantly expressed the distress of his personal struggle to find spiritual health. "I don't think I believe in God. But it is hard not to believe in God because I am so afraid of death.

If there is no God, then death is really going to be the 'death' that I am afraid of, which is nothingness" (O'Brien, 1992, p. 48).

For an acutely ill patient such as Evan, the nurse might anticipate spiritual needs related to traditional religious belief and practice as reflected in his comment about wanting to love God more dearly. For patients such as Kent and Gerry, however, whose belief systems are either humanistic or currently in a state of crisis, spiritual care must be creative and tailored to assist the patient in relation to his or her faith or lack of faith.

The comments of those living with acute sequelae of HIV and acquired immunodeficiency syndrome (AIDS) demonstrate that spiritual health correlates importantly with one's ability to cope with an illness experience. The patients themselves recognized that their spiritual or religious beliefs or lack thereof were significantly related to their adaptation to living with their illness conditions.

As well as being associated with the acute illness conditions and the acute phases of chronic illness, serious physiologic and psychological challenges requiring spiritual support are also present in such experiences as the perioperative journey, the critical care experience, the emergency room experience, and the experience of pain; these are reflected in the following sections.

▶ Spiritual Needs of the Perioperative Patient

The term *perioperative* refers to the period encompassing the preoperative, intraoperative, and postoperative experiences for a surgical patient. Specifically, the preoperative phase begins with the plan to carry out surgery and ends with the actual transfer of the patient to the operating room (OR); the intraoperative phase covers the period of the actual surgical procedure; and the postoperative phase begins with the transfer of the patient out of the OR to recovery, and continues through the healing process to the time of discharge from the physician's care. The perioperative client may be found in a hospital, a community-based surgery center, or, for minor procedures, a physician's office.

The perioperative patient and family may pose significant challenges to the nursing staff related to the anxiety experienced prior to, during, and immediately after the surgery; yet, the perioperative nurse often has little time to develop a relationship with the patient due to the fast-paced nature of the nursing (Dearing, 1997). Some of the most frequently identified causes for fear in the preoperative period are "fear of the unknown," "fear of pain or death," and "fear of changes in body image and self-concept" (Taylor et al., 1997, pp. 676–677); fear of the unknown may encompass the other fears. Fear of the unknown may also include fear of the postoperative diagnosis, especially if the surgical procedure is focused on an exploration to determine the possible presence of a malignancy. Fear of surgical death or of a painful postoperative death lurks in the minds of most patients and families during the intraoperative period. Even if the surgery has been described as a "simple procedure," preoperative patients often express fear of "going under the knife" or going under anesthesia, especially if general anesthesia is used.

A dimension of the perioperative nurse's role is to provide comfort and support to patients and families, especially during the pre- and post-operative periods (Fairchild, 1996). Meeker and Rothrock (1995) described the perioperative nurse's role as including a "continuous awareness of the dignity of persons and their physical, emotional, cultural, ethnic, and spiritual needs." In a 1994 statement, the Association of Operating Room Nurses asserted that "the perioperative nurse designs, coordinates, and delivers care to meet the identified physiologic, psychologic, sociocultural and spiritual needs of patients whose protective reflexes or self-care abilities are potentially compromised because they are having invasive procedures. The nursing activities address the needs and responses of patients and their families or significant others" (cited in Atkinson & Fortunato, 1996, p. 22).

The perioperative nurse can identify a patient's spiritual beliefs through use of the nursing history and thus can provide spiritual care through "acceptance, participation in prayer, or referral to clergy or chaplain" (Taylor et al., 1997, p. 678). Although some nurses may feel that raising spiritual issues may be threatening to the patient, Burns (1996) asserted that regardless of religious tradition, discussing spiritual concerns is therapeutic during the perioperative period (p. 361). Burns believes that simply asking if a perioperative patient's pastor is aware of impending surgery is a supportive approach (p. 361).

The model of perioperative nursing developed by Phippen, Wells, and Martinelli (1994) contains the earlier identified assumption of the appropriateness of holistic health care, including attention to the patient's spiritual nature (p. 3). The individual's spiritual component is viewed as the "animating" principle of life, and this spiritual dimension of the patient is influenced by underlying "religious and philosophical beliefs" (p. 4). If the nurse diagnoses "spiritual distress" manifested by symptoms of fear of death, anger at God, or disruption of spiritual practices on the part of a perioperative patient, appropriate spiritual care interventions may be carried out. The strategy suggested by Phippen et al. involves an exploration of the type of spiritual or religious practices to which the patient relates (e.g., spiritual reading or a visit with a chaplain); the nurse may then intervene by providing materials or making an appropriate referral (p. 66).

In a study of perioperative nurses' perceptions of caring practices, McNamara (1995) found that spiritual care was viewed as primarily including those activities and behaviors that "comforted patients or increased their feelings of security" (p. 385). The perioperative nurses interviewed in McNamara's study asserted the importance of avoiding judgmental attitudes about patients' religious beliefs and practices. Listening and being aware of the patient's religious tradition was considered essential to spiritual care. Several nurses reported praying with patients; others made referral to a pastor of the patient's choice (p. 385). In a discussion of the meaning of spirituality to perioperative nurses and their patients, Rothrock (1994) advocated supporting hope as a "healing force." Heiser, Chiles, Fudge, and Gray (1997) advocated that perioperative nurses use music therapy in the immediate postoperative recovery period as a contemporary spiritual intervention strategy.

Carol, a nurse anesthetist with 18 years of experience in perioperative nursing, explained the importance of spiritual care in the immediate preoperative period:

> I try to talk to patients when they arrive in the OR suite. They are just scared to death. I might be the last person to talk to them before they go to sleep. I talk to them outside the OR while the surgeons are changing clothes. We usually have a few minutes of privacy. I listen to their concerns. I listen to hear if they say anything like, "I'm in God's hands," and then I just take it

from there. I say it's OK to put all your trust in God; He'll be with you in there [the OR]. Especially if a person is in for cancer surgery, I reassure them of God's love and care during the surgery. This is when people are at their most vulnerable; they feel like they are losing all control of their lives. They don't know what the surgery will bring and their future is in the balance. This is the most logical time to think of God, to think, "Am I ready to die?" This is the time they really need some spiritual care . . . I pray silently while the patient is under anesthesia; if they're having a hard time, I ask God to give them strength.

Diane, a master's-prepared operating room nurse with 19 years of experience, spoke of spiritual care as "being with" the patient during the intraoperative phase; she also incorporates touch in her caring. "I think there isn't a patient that has gone to sleep here that I haven't held their hand while they're being put to sleep. That is spiritual care as far as I'm concerned. You stand beside them and hold their hand and talk to them. I consider all that part of spiritual care." Diane also admitted that she prayed for patients during surgery, while performing her duties as a scrub nurse or circulating nurse. "I especially pray for the 'open hearts.' When they go on and off that pump, believe me, I'm praying like crazy. When open heart surgery patients are in the OR and on the pump, and we are literally touching their hearts; that's the time when I especially pray for that patient." Diane added, "I serve God through being present for my patients."

Opportunities for spiritual care of the perioperative patient in the postoperative period may vary significantly depending on the nature of the surgical procedure. Many patients currently experiencing less complex surgeries, classified as "same day surgery," are in and out of the hospital very quickly. Nevertheless, a gentle touch or a word of comfort or support may still be possible during the recovery room stay. This is also a time when anxious family members or friends greatly welcome a kind word of encouragement from the nursing staff. For the patient immediately postoperative from a complex surgical procedure, such as a coronary artery bypass graft (CABG) who may emerge from the OR on mechanical ventilation, the intensive care unit (ICU) will be the setting where spiritual intervention is needed and much appreciated by both patients and families.

▶ Spiritual Needs of the ICU Patient

In the contemporary critical care unit, with its ever more complex therapeutic technology, the persona of the patient may seem lost in the myriad tubes, wires, and sophisticated monitoring devices. Obviously, a central responsibility of the critical care nurse is to skillfully employ the technology at hand in the service of intensive patient care. If the nurse is to provide truly holistic care to the critically ill patient, however, attention to the needs of the mind and the spirit must accompany the delivery of high-quality physical care. Dossey, Guzzetta, and Kenner (1992) in the introduction to their text *Critical Care Nursing: Body, Mind, Spirit*, admitted that their subtitle may seem inappropriate to some readers who might regard the emphasis on mind and spirit as irrelevant to contemporary science. The authors argued, however, that sensitivity to the patient's emotional and spiritual needs is an essential dimension of the subfield of critical care nursing. They suggested that during a period of critical illness "patients frequently search for how to create new perceptions for their life as well as to find wholeness and spirituality" and that they "need guidance in their transformation" (p. 11). Dossey et al. explained that the critical care nurse, therefore, needs to be sensitive to a variety of factors in order to help patients deal with spiritual issues, including the pluralism of spiritual beliefs and religious practices that patients may adhere to, the difference between spiritual and religious concepts, and the nurse's own possible personal confusion in regard to spiritual or religious values (p. 12). Meeting the spiritual and/or religious needs of acutely ill patients such as those suffering from heart failure (Westlake et al., 2008) can greatly alleviate anxiety over the illness condition.

Critical care units (CCUs) or ICUs, first created in the early 1960s, were developed to sustain individuals who might not otherwise survive a serious physiologic deficit or complex surgical procedure, such as acute myocardial infarction or a coronary artery bypass graft. The critical care patient in the ICU is considered physiologically unstable and at great risk for developing life-threatening complications (Kidd, 1997). Like acutely ill patients in general, ICU patients may include persons experiencing bouts of severe symptomatology related to a chronic illness, such as myasthenic crisis in a myasthenia gravis patient, or a sudden onset acute illness or trauma, as in the case of patients diagnosed with meningococcal meningitis or multiple fractures sustained in an accident.

Among the current variety of specialized critical care units are neonatal ICUs (NICUs), pediatric ICUs (PICUs), surgical ICUs (SICUs), medical ICUs (MICUs), neurologic and neurosurgical ICUs, and coronary care units (CCUs). These contemporary critical care units, as centers for advanced health-care technology, are host to many medical "machines" such as cardiac, hemodynamic, and intracranial pressure monitors, ventilators, and defibrillators, the sight of which may be anxiety provoking to patients and their families. Another particularly frightening aspect of the ICU environment is the potential for observing crisis intervention in another patient (Hopkins, 1993, p. 1564); a patient or family member might unexpectedly be witness to an emergency intubation or a "code blue" occurring close to their own assigned space in the unit.

Virtually all cognitively aware adult patients report significant stress associated with the ICU experience. As well as those discussed already, other identified stressors include "social isolation, enforced immobility, pain from procedures, poor communication with staff, excessive noise and lack of sleep" (Dracup, 1995, pp. 12–13). Lack of personal autonomy (Walleck, 1989) and a feeling of utter helplessness (Niklas & Stefanics, 1975, p. 75) are perhaps the most devastating emotions that the ICU patient experiences. This may result in an overwhelming sense of depersonalization as a result of such factors as "powerlessness, emotional/touch deprivation, loss of privacy, invasion of personal space, and transfer anxiety" (Clochesy, 1988, p. 193). Thus, concepts such as prayer and spirituality are becoming more and more sought after as dimensions of care by critically ill patients and their families (Holt-Ashley, 2000).

Related to the stress of critical illness, with its painful sequelae, as well as the sometimes persistent fear of death and the added stressor of hospitalization in a critical care unit, Busch (1994) recognized that the experience may either enhance or challenge a patient's spiritual or religious beliefs (p. 16). A first step in providing spiritual care for the critically ill patient, then, is to carry out an assessment of the person's spiritual and/or religious beliefs, practices, and current needs. Some pertinent information about spiritual or religious history may be obtained from the patient's chart and from the family; hopefully, information about current spiritual needs will emerge through personal interaction between patient and nurse.

Because of the patient's possible isolation from usual religious practices, such as attending worship services or reading Scripture or other spiritual books, and because of the fear and anxiety about his or her illness condition, the nurse may diagnose spiritual distress in the ICU patient. Twibell, Wieseke, Marine, and Schoger (1996) identified some defining characteristics of a spiritual distress diagnosis for a critically ill patient, including a request of spiritual guidance or support, the verbalization of distress over not being able to carry out usual religious practices, expression of "spiritual emptiness," questioning the credibility of one's belief system, and expressing anger or frustration over the meaning of the present illness experience (p. 249). Following such a diagnosis, the nurse may intervene or may elect to contact a chaplain or other pastoral care provider. Bell (1993) advised that if the nurse chooses to pray with the critically ill patient, using "the patient's own words" in relation to illness-related needs may be comforting (p. 27).

Gillman, Gable-Rodriguez, Sutherland, and Whitacre (1996) identified some basic postures in providing spiritual care in a critical care setting: "inclusion," meaning that the nurse should try to imagine what the ICU experience must actually be like for the patient; "confirmation," that the nurse should support the patient's personal spiritual goals; and "mutuality," a spirit of cooperation between nurse and patient in seeking healing (p. 13). Stromberg (1992) described the role of the spiritual care provider in a coronary care unit as encompassing three tasks: listening empathetically, confronting reality, and being a "fellow pilgrim" on the patient's current spiritual journey (p. 127). Listening and "being there" are central to spiritual care in the ICU. The concept of presence, "enhanced by empathetic listening," reflects the nurse's sense of "genuineness, trust and positive regard," which will allow the patient freedom to express his or her spiritual needs or concerns (Shaffer, 1991, p. 45). Beverly Hall (1997), in discussing the nurse's role as spiritual caregiver in life-threatening illness, observed that "what patients need from us is not psychology or theology but caring and presence while they seek answers" (p. 93). As well as providing a listening presence for the critically ill patient in the ICU, and praying with him or her if acceptable to the patient, nurses should refer patients to clergy when appropriate (Bardanouve, 1994; Bucher, Wimbush, Hardie, & Hayes, 1997; Reed, 1991; Shelly & Fish, 1995).

A sometimes neglected yet no less important dimension of spiritual care for the ICU patient that should be included in the nurse's role is that of providing care and support to the patient's family (Chesla & Stannard, 1997). The ICU hospitalization of one of its members may create great anxiety on the part of the rest of the family (Rukholm, Bailey, & Coutu-Wakulczyk, 1991); thus, spending even a brief period of time with family visitors is an important dimension of spiritual care (DiSarcina, 1991, p. 23).

ICU nurse Joyce Hahn related a poignant anecdote about taking the times allocated for her mealtime and break in order to sit with a dying patient's husband. After his beloved wife's death, the husband returned with a lovely poem he had written for their nurse. The meditation included the thought that he had experienced an "angel clothed in white" and ended with the words, "It was one of God's children, a nurse from the ICU" (Hahn, 2001, p. 32).

In discussing spirituality in the CCU, Gloria Nussbaum (2003), MSN, points out that nurses must be available to provide spiritual care when it is needed, noting that "The critical care unit is most vulnerable because the intensity of the illness is so great. Conscious or unconscious, the patient needs human touch and consolation which transcends technology. Indifference to this is all but negligence on the part of the nurse" (p. 214). Spiritual care is provided in the ICU by "giving mental support, facilitating religious rituals, communicating with patients and patients' families, assessing the spiritual needs of patients and showing respect" (Lundberg & Kerdonfag, 2010, p. 1121). A program titled "Embrace Hope," which included spiritual care, was created to support neurological critical care patients and their families in another unit (Yeager et al., 2010).

The concept of spiritual assessment in intensive and cardiac care nursing is advocated in order to "formulate a care plan of spiritual care that provides a powerful inner resource to critically ill patients in acute clinical environments" (Timmins & Kelly, 2008, p. 124). As a result, spiritual care such as that provided for a critically ill elderly woman with "rapidly advancing small cell lung cancer" can be given; the result was described by the coordinator of a cardiac critical medical care unit as "spirituality shining through in a magnet moment" (Monroe, 2011, p. 98).

For the majority of critical care patients, regardless of professional credentials or life history, the ICU experience is new and exceedingly traumatic. This concept was clearly exemplified in the case of an ordained minister who was hospitalized in the same ICU where he himself ministered to others. Pastor Norton, who was a longtime myasthenia gravis patient, was brought to the unit late one evening in myasthenic crisis; he was immediately intubated and placed on mechanical ventilation. He remained on ventilatory support for approximately two weeks. Shortly after his critical care experience, Pastor Norton admitted that although the physical and technical care had been excellent, he had in fact felt isolated during the intubation period and longed for more caring "touch." There were times, the minister admitted, when he would have liked a nurse simply to come and sit by the bed, take his hand, and be with him. As he reflected on the experience, Pastor Norton's conclusion about the lack of "spiritual care" related to his personal identity as a minister; he speculated that the staff probably felt shy about attempting to comfort or support him spiritually, thinking that he already possessed a vast store of resources to draw on. With honesty and humility, Pastor Norton confessed that despite his own strong faith, he had experienced significant feelings of anxiety, loneliness, and helplessness during his stay in the intensive care unit.

An older female patient, Mrs. McCarthy, who was experiencing an exacerbation of a chronic endocrine disorder, and who had also been intubated for several weeks, admitted to feelings of devastating helplessness while on mechanical ventilation, as had Pastor Norton. Mrs. McCarthy, who reported after extubation that her nursing care had been fine, confessed that while on the ventilator she had fantasized that because of the physical deterioration of her body, an ICU staff member, questioning the quality of her life, might "pull the plug" while she was sleeping. This was very threatening to her as she was looking forward to the high school graduations of two of her grandchildren. Obviously, the ICU nursing staff expressed shock when told of this fear. Mrs. McCarthy's frightening fantasy, however, was a reminder of the fragility of the ICU patient's emotional state, and of the constant need for reassurance and support.

In the case of a confused or comatose patient, caregivers should provide spiritual care and support directly toward the family of the person receiving intensive care. One such case was that of a 67-year-old patient, Mr. Lundquist, who was critically ill as the result of a rampant septicemia following bowel surgery; he was mechanically ventilated and his physiologic functioning was being maintained by the continual use of pharmacologic agents (the use of multiple "pressors"). As his illness progressed,

Mr. Lundquist was only minimally responsive to verbal or tactile stimuli. Mr. Lundquist's family, including his wife and several adult children, spent many hours in the critical care waiting room, as well as at the bedside. Their pastor visited frequently and helped them begin the process, on the physician's advice, of facing the patient's imminent death. The adult children's concern, which was verbalized on several occasions to the nursing staff, especially as new therapeutic procedures were initiated, was, "how long would Dad want to live like this?" They were very concerned about their father's suffering. Mr. Lundquist's wife and children reported that he had never discussed his wishes in regard to the use of "extraordinary measures" to prolong life. A nurse researcher working with patients and families in the ICU was able to spend time at Mr. Lundquist's bedside and also be with the family in order to provide a caring presence when such issues as the "DNR" (Do Not Resuscitate) option were discussed. The family expressed gratitude for this supportive nursing presence in a note sent after Mr. Lundquist's death.

Critical care nurses often comment on the need for the practice of spiritual care in the ICU. Margaret, a relatively new ICU staff nurse, observed:

> My patients are all very sick, and communication is a key issue. When I talk to them about religious things, they often exhibit strengths related to how they are handling their illness. For some of these patients it's really tough, like with young bone marrow transplants in the MICU flunking the second transplant, and they're not going to live and they know it and the family knows it. They really need spiritual support. The physicians get to leave the room but it's the nurses who have to stay and be with the patients while they suffer . . . I'm trying to work on the nonpharmacologic approach to decreasing anxiety. Patients may be anxious because of unmet spiritual needs, so we're trying to use music, listening, visitors, communication . . . just being open to whatever the patients' spiritual needs are, whether they're religious like associated with a church or just their own spirituality.

Coleen, a 22-year veteran of ICU nursing, spoke about critically ill patients' fear of death:

> I've worked in critical care for many, many years and I can't even count the number of patients who have said to me, "Am I going to die?" This is the biggest opening for spiritual care that anybody could present. Usually what I say back is, "Do you mean if or when?" Then we can get down to what's really bothering them. The only answer you can give is "I don't know"; it also depends on where the nurse is spiritually herself. If you're Christian and the patient is, you can give them a parable like the man who built his house on rock and it will not be blown away, or if the patient is Jewish, something "Old Testament." You can pray out loud with the patient or silently, and just help them be at peace . . . Most people will let you know if they have a religious background and want you to pray or read the Scripture with them. Sometimes you just have to go with the Holy Spirit, and hope you say what the Holy Spirit wants you to say.

Coleen related a personal prayer experience in the ICU:

> I've been reading about some scientific research where nurses were praying for cardiac surgical patients; an experimental group who got prayers and a control group that didn't, and the experimental group didn't have any

complications and did a lot better than the control group. I had a hint of that last year when one of the unit nurses I was working with said, "Watch my patient; I'll be right back." There wasn't anything to do so I just started to pray for the patient. When his nurse came back she said, "Coleen, what did you do? His O_2 sat [oxygen saturation] has never been this good!"

Coleen concluded with advice about spiritual intervention in the ICU:

You want to be careful to respect the religious practice of the patient. You don't want to shock anybody by a religious practice that might seem strange or different, or inappropriate in their eyes. When we are going to do spiritual care for patients I think that it is better to be on the conservative side until they give us clues as to what they want or need, if it's prayer or whatever. If you have the love of God in you, they are going to respond to that regardless of what their religious affiliation is.

Judith, a master's-prepared nurse with 24 years of experience in critical care nursing, shared her perception of the change in attitude toward the provision of spiritual care by the ICU nurse:

When I first went into critical care I did it because of the focus on the technical aspect, but shortly into my career I really kept looking for the person; that you are not just taking care of the equipment, but that there is a person there in the bed. I believe there's been a change, especially in the last five to eight years. Patients are not afraid to share how they feel spiritually. It used to be, years ago, I remember, that the nurse never talked about God or church or praying with a patient. The minister came and prayed with the patient and everybody else left the room. What I've seen over these last few years is nurses being less anxious and more comfortable in their own spirituality; then they can comfort others . . . Sometimes you are really busy in ICU and you don't have much time to talk to the patient about spirituality but you can find out where they are with it and maybe call the chaplain. You can get the ball rolling for the chaplain to come in. We are the ones right there at the bedside, especially in critical care. You can sense what the patient needs and pick up on it . . .

I'm not Catholic, but this past week I had a Catholic patient who was really anxious, and one of the other nurses was Catholic so she went and they had a talk. She gave the patient a little "Lady of Perpetual Help" charm [medal], pinned it on her, blessed her with some holy oil, and shared prayer with her . . . I think that is a prime example of a nurse attending to a patient's spiritual needs. We shouldn't ever foster one religion over another, and sometimes we don't know what a person believes really, but just to be there with them. Death is really hard in the ICU so just sitting with a family, I am sometimes at a loss for words but just to be there, I think is part of caring.

An excerpt from the author's research journal, maintained during the course of a five-year study of the nursing needs of persons living with HIV and AIDS, presents a final example of spiritual care that a practicing nurse might carry out in the ICU setting.

It was a clear, crisp Friday morning in autumn, my favorite season, as I headed off to a local medical center, but my heart was heavy. I had just received a phone call from Luke, the friend of Jonathan, an AIDS patient with whom

I had been working. Luke apologized for calling early but, he said, "Jonathan asked that I get in touch with you. He was admitted to ICU during the night and they're putting him on the ventilator; it doesn't look good."

As I drove to the hospital I tried to imagine, or perhaps to not imagine, what condition I would find Jonathan in. I couldn't help but reminisce about when we had first met some 2 years previously; it was shortly after he had been diagnosed with HIV infection. I was searching for persons living with HIV to participate in a five-year NIH-supported study of coping strategies, and Jonathan had agreed to speak with me. His enthusiasm for the study matched his enthusiasm for life: it was infectious. During the past months we had laughed and worried and cried over the strange twists and turns which the human immunodeficiency virus had introduced into his life, but always, underneath it all, Jonathan maintained a serenity and a joy that were exquisite to behold.

When I arrived in the intensive care unit, Jonathan had already been placed on the ventilator and was barely conscious; Luke was standing at his bedside. After filling me in on the events of the past few hours, Luke looked across the bed and said, "Mary Elizabeth, would you do something for Jonathan?" I immediately responded, "Of course," wondering, considering the setting, what it could be. I assumed Luke's request was for some nursing task, a comfort measure perhaps, yet Jonathan appeared to be resting peacefully, at least as peacefully as one can when attached to a ventilator, IVs, and the multiple system monitoring devices usual to the ICU environment. Luke, who was an aeronautical engineer, explained, "Religion is not something that is very big with me; as a scientist I have difficulty with the mystery, but for Jonathan it's important. He didn't go to church a lot but faith in God was a real part of his life. Would you say a prayer for him?"

My first reaction was something akin to panic [this occurred prior to my chaplaincy training]; where is a chaplain? I thought. As a nurse I'm not "credentialed" in prayer. But I quickly realized that since it was I, the nurse, whom Luke had asked, surely God would compensate for my perceived weakness in the prayer department.

I cannot recall the exact prayer that I prayed that morning in the medical center intensive care unit. I remember that I reached out and took one of Jonathan's hands; I also grasped Luke's hand, so that we three could be connected, as a small worship community in our makeshift chapel. The words were simple, I think. I asked God to put His arms around Jonathan and hold him close, to give him strength and comfort, to let him know how deeply he was loved and cherished as one of God's own. The musical accompaniment was provided by the rhythmic hum of the ventilator as it coaxed and supported Jonathan's labored breathing; the choir, the hushed whispers of the nurses and technicians as they quietly worked in the background. Together, hand in hand, amidst the tubes and lines and wires apropos of contemporary intensive care, our small community celebrated a liturgy. When we had finished Luke's eyes filled with tears and he whispered, "Thank you"; my eyes also filled with tears and I silently prayed "Thank you" to the God of love who carries us in His arms when we feel most fragile.

The experience with Jonathan and Luke taught me that we, as nurses, are indeed called to a lived reality of God's love which may be manifested in terms of spiritual care, as well as physical and emotional support. I recognized the importance of allowing myself to be "used" as God's instrument in the midst of feelings of personal inadequacy. Although I did not feel competent to minister spiritually, through prayer, at the time, the Spirit provided the courage and the words. Luke told me several days later, after Jonathan's death, that he felt peace after we prayed together; that this was a turning point, and that he had now begun to think about his own spiritual life and how he might understand God. I believe that not only the praying together, but also our joining hands, as a worshipping community, was an important dimension of our ICU liturgy. Through the intimate touch of palm against palm, we became aware of our connectedness both as a human family and as the spiritual family of God. We were thus able to support and strengthen each other, even as we sought the support and strength of our Creator.

▶ Spiritual Needs of the Emergency Room Patient

An emergency is defined as "any sudden illness or injury that is perceived to be a crisis threatening the physical or psychological well-being of a person or a group" (Lazure & DeMartinis, 1997, p. 2501). Although most large hospitals house emergency departments to care for those persons and groups, it is well known that a number of individuals seek care at an emergency room for nonlife-threatening, and even routine, problems. This occurs most frequently in large urban inner-city areas, where indigent and homeless individuals have no other available and accessible source of medical care.

The goal of emergency departments is to provide care for "the acutely sick and injured" (Santacaterina & Stein-Spencer, 1990, p. 3). Most hospital emergency rooms (ERs) are also involved in prehospital care, provided prior to arrival at the health-care facility; for example, care provided at an emergency scene by emergency medical technicians (EMTs) and carried on during ambulance transport. Sophisticated telemetry systems may connect the EMTs with the hospital emergency room staff physicians and nurses (Robinson, 1992).

The Emergency Nurses Association defines *emergency nursing care* as "assessment, diagnosis and treatment of perceived, actual or potential, sudden, or urgent physiologic or psychosocial problems that are primarily episodic or acute. These may require medical care or life support measures, client and significant other education, appropriate referral, and knowledge of legal limitations" (Lazure & DeMartinis, 1997, p. 2503). A key role of the emergency department nurse is that of triage, or initial nursing assessment of the patient's condition in order to determine priority care needs (Blair & Hall, 1994, pp. 21–23). Following triage, the patient may be assigned to one of several types of ER space such as "major trauma or arrest room, minor suture room, gynecologic examination room, psychiatric room, family room, or general examination room" (MacPhail, 1992, p. 7).

The Emergency Nurses Association has articulated comparative standards for working with individual patients. Standard 1, Assessment, states, "The emergency nurse initiates accurate and ongoing assessment of physical, psychological and social problems of patients within the emergency care system" (Emergency Nurses

Association, 1995, p. 16). The consideration of the ER patient's psychological and social problems, as well as physical assessment and triage, as part of the emergency nurse's role, is underscored in a list of ER nurse activities. This is identified in a contemporary fundamentals of nursing text, which includes caring for the patient with severe anxiety (Long, 1993, p. 1540). The current philosophy of emergency care has become so broad as to consider an emergency "whatever the patient or family considers it to be" (Miller, 1996, p. 2000).

Spiritual care and support may be an important need for both patient and family in an emergency situation, especially if the admitting diagnosis contains a life-threatening dimension. In 1993, Eileen Corcoran (1993), president of the Emergency Nurses Association, posed the question, "Is it reasonable to believe that the emergency room nurse's role includes addressing spiritual needs of patients and their families?" (p. 183). In posing her rhetorical question in the *Journal of Emergency Nursing*, Corcoran admitted that a significant amount of the ER nurse's time must be spent on meeting the patient's physical needs, but she argued that this does not relieve the ER nurse from attention to spiritual needs. Some suggestions Corcoran offered for spiritual care intervention by emergency nurses include establishing a trusting relationship with the patient; maintaining a supportive environment, including providing privacy for patient and family if necessary and identifying religious resources such as the availability of on-call clergy; and finally, recognizing the role of the nurse in "healing the whole person" (p. 184).

Anecdotal reports in the nursing literature document ER patients questioning God's will. See "Has God forsaken the emergency department?" (Schlintz, 1987) and "Would God listen to me now?" (Schlintz, 1988). Guthrie (1985), an ER nurse, also recorded the distress of ER patients. Three contemporary ER nurses spoke of the need for and experiences in spiritual care in their setting.

Pat, a 19-year ER nursing veteran, worried:

In the ER you really see the need for spiritual care but sometimes you are moving and working; you feel you are not able to provide much. With death, you always ask, "Would you like us to call a chaplain?" But there are a lot of other needs to minister to, like thinking from a staff nurse's point, dealing with abuse cases, especially the kids.

Ann, with 8 years of ER experience, expressed gratitude for her own spirituality:

Having my own spiritual base really helped me because I've done so much work in the ER and trauma. You see so much death and dying. You only have a few minutes with the patient before you see them die, and you have to support them in that little bit of time. You also deal with supporting the families; they need a lot of spiritual care. It makes you look at life differently; it makes you a different person . . . Sometimes the chaplains don't get there at the time of a crisis and you are the only one giving support. I can think of many times when I have been the only one there to talk with a family who had just lost a patient . . .

Nurses need to know how to do ministry especially in the crisis times. I see nursing as a ministry, no question about it. Taking care of these patients in the ER is a ministry in and of itself. There are individuals who incorporate that into their nursing. There are some nurses who may not consciously think about it all the time, but they allow themselves to be used by God . . . I think that nurses have to work at being truly spiritual people. I think that my own spirituality leads me to being a more feeling individual, to see a client through their own eyes instead of mine.

Helen, head nurse of an emergency department for five years, spoke of spiritual care interventions she had carried out in the ER:

My coping comes out of a belief that there is a God and that He is loving and generous and forgiving. I always believe that He allows things for a reason and that we can learn from it, the trials and tribulations. For my patients it's the idea that I am given the gift of taking care of them in the ER, to get them through this crisis. I spend a lot of time talking and listening to them. I touch their hand. I believe there are energies from God that we are not necessarily aware of. I think nursing supports the person in giving this kind of spiritual care.

Finally, Helen spoke about her ER nursing staff:

I am very proud of the spiritual care they give; that is one of our strong points. Sometimes we need to get someone in on the patient, and we call pastoral care to come and sit with the family. It works well in our ER. You need a sense of your own spirituality to function well and take care of patients. I think ideally you address the patients' needs by knowing what you believe in yourself.

▶ Spiritual Needs of the Patient in Pain

Although no common definition of pain exists, many nurse clinicians still rely on the pragmatic description first articulated in 1968 by McCaffery. "Pain is whatever the experiencing person says it is, existing whenever the experiencing person says it does" (p. 95). A more contemporary, yet also practical, definition identifies pain as "the state in which an individual experiences and reports the presence of severe discomfort or an uncomfortable sensation" (Gunta, 1993, p. 1538). Pain is broadly understood as a word used to reflect a "subjective perception of distress"; the concept may be divided into three major categories: acute pain, chronic pain, and the pain of malignancy (Gildenberg & DeVaul, 1985, pp. 4–5). Acute pain is described as that which "follows acute injury, disease or surgical intervention, and has a rapid onset, varying in intensity [mild to severe], and lasting for a brief time" (Potter, 1997, p. 1160). Chronic pain has been characterized as pain that "persists longer than three months," "cannot be eliminated," "often becomes diffuse," "may originally have been acute," and has an "insidious onset" (Watt-Watson & Long, 1993, p. 167). The chronic pain of malignancy is identified as pain that lasts for more than 6 months, "after tissue damage has healed or in the absence of evident tissue damage" (Gunta, 1993, p. 1541).

Pain, whether acute, chronic, or related to a malignancy, is influenced by a multiplicity of physiologic, psychological, sociocultural, and spiritual factors. Therapeutic interventions for the relief of pain include pharmacologic (e.g., analgesic drugs) and physiologic (e.g., acupuncture, acupressure, cutaneous stimulation, surgery) measures, as well as nonpharmacologic measures such as biofeedback, meditation, relaxation, and guided imagery.

Potter (1997) advised that in attempting to provide relief for those in pain, the nurse must remember that the patient interprets and experiences both pain and comfort in light of his or her own "physiological, social, spiritual, psychological, and cultural characteristics" (p. 1154). The National Institute of Nursing Research report, submitted by the priority expert panel on symptom management of acute pain, while including spiritual factors as influential in pain perception and response, also identified the religious ethic as a mediating variable (National Institute of Nursing Research, 1994, p. 30).

Any pain diagnosis may, as noted, be influenced by or contain within its boundaries a spiritual dimension; thus, a nursing diagnosis of spiritual distress may be identified in a patient experiencing chronic pain such as that of malignancy. In a study to explore the management of "spiritual distress in patients with advanced cancer pain," Georgensen and Dungan (1996) identified a list of questions to be used in the assessment of spiritual distress, including, "Has your illness affected your faith/belief system?" "Do you pray? What do you think the power of prayer means?" "Is God or other power important to you?" "How can I assist you in maintaining spiritual strength?" and "Are there religious rituals that are important to you now?" (p. 379). Some defining characteristics for the diagnosis of spiritual distress in patients with advanced cancer pain were anger at God, expressions of helplessness, questioning the meaning and purpose in life, grief, and concerns regarding religious beliefs (p. 381).

Religious beliefs can be particularly important to the pain experience as they may provide support and strength through such activities as prayer (Springhouse Corporation, 1985, p. 21). Religious or spiritual beliefs may also provide the person in pain with a vehicle for finding meaning in suffering, or for "offering" the pain experience to God, in expiation for one's failings or the failings of others. Some individuals, however, may also view pain or suffering as a punishment from God, for example, the concept of *castigo* (punishment) in the Mexican-American culture. A nurse or pastor familiar with contemporary theology may be helpful in counseling a patient with this negative perception of God and of the pain experience (Kumasaka, 1996).

As well as recommending or participating in prayer (if acceptable to the patient in pain) and seeking counsel of a chaplain, another therapeutic spiritual care activity that the nurse may recommend and teach is the use of spiritual imagery (Ferszt & Taylor, 1988). A suggestion that the patient imagine God as a loving parent holding him or her in His arms and gently loving and caring may do much to comfort the person in pain. Some other spiritual care strategies for alleviating patients' pain include listening with a caring manner to the individual's fears and anxieties related to the pain experience, and facilitating the participation of family members or other significant persons who may be a primary source of support (Turk & Feldman, 1992; Warner, 1992). As it is appropriately observed, "spiritual views can have a substantial impact on patients' understanding of pain and decisions about pain management" (Unruh, 2007, p. 67).

Ultimately, as described in spiritual care of acutely ill patients in general, sometimes simply the nurse's presence is an important spiritual intervention. Molly, an advanced cancer patient, although medicated with self-administered analgesics, was experiencing acute pain during her final hospitalization at a clinical research facility. Molly had consistently refused the ministrations of a pastoral caregiver with the excuse that she was too tired and in too much pain to be bothered. One day a chaplain desperate to provide some support for Molly asked gently if she might just sit by her bed and pray silently; the chaplain promised not to talk. Molly acquiesced. She seemed to drowse during most of the chaplain's visit, but opened her eyes periodically to see if the pastoral caregiver was still there. A few days later, as Molly was dying, she asked the staff to call the chaplain to be with her. Molly told the staff, "She's the only one who knows what to say!"

Spiritual care is an important dimension of holistic care for the person with an acute illness or an acute exacerbation of a chronic condition. Spiritual care is also essential for persons experiencing a serious physical or psychosocial challenge related to a perioperative experience, a critical care experience, an emergency room experience, or a pain experience. Often the nurse must employ creative strategies to intervene spiritually for persons who may be experiencing a crisis of faith as well as a serious illness. Ultimately, however, spiritual care is appropriate and acceptable for the nurse working with acutely ill patients.

▶ References

Abu-El-Noor, M., & Abu-El-Noor, A. (2014). Importance of spiritual care for cardiac patients admitted to coronary care units in the Gaza strip. *Journal of Holistic Nursing, 32*(2), 104–105.

Agrimson, L., & Taft, L. (2008). Spiritual crisis: A concept analysis. *Journal of Advanced Nursing, 65*(2), 454–461.

Amoah, C. (2011). The central importance of spirituality in palliative care. *International Journal of Palliative Care Nursing, 117*(7), 353–358.

Atkinson, L. J., & Fortunato, N. M. (1996). *Berry & Kohn's operating room technique.* St. Louis, MO: Mosby-Yearbook.

Barber, C. (2013). Spirituality 7: Spiritual support in a ward or in a care home. *British Journal of Healthcare Assistants, 7*(6), 278–281.

Bardanouve, V. E. (1994). Spiritual ministry in the ICU. *Journal of Christian Nursing, 11*(4), 38–39.

Bell, N. (1993). Caring: The essence of critical care nursing. In N. M. Holloway (Ed.), *Nursing the critically ill adult* (4th ed., pp. 14–29). New York, NY: Addison-Wesley.

Bjarnason, D. (2010). Nurse religiosity and end-of-life care. *Journal of Research in Nursing, 17*(1), 78–91.

Blair, F., & Hall, M. (1994). The Klein nursing process: Assessment and priority setting. In A. Klein, G. Lee, A. Manton, & P. Parker (Eds.), *Emergency nursing core curriculum* (4th ed., pp. 3–23). Philadelphia, PA: W. B. Saunders.

Bucher, L., Wimbush, F., Hardie, J., & Hayes, E. (1997). Near death experiences: Critical care nurses' attitudes and interventions. *Dimensions of Critical Care Nursing, 16*(4), 194–201.

Burnard, P. (1988). The spiritual needs of atheists and agnostics. *The Professional Nurse, 4*(3), 130–132.

Burns, L. (1996). Preoperative nursing management. In S. C. Smeltzer & B. G. Bare (Eds.), *Brunner and Sudarth's textbook of medical–surgical nursing* (8th ed., pp. 357–367). Philadelphia, PA: J. B. Lippincott.

Busch, K. D. (1994). Psychosocial concepts and the patient's experience with critical illness. In C. M. Hudak, B. M. Gallo, & J. J. Benz (Eds.), *Critical care nursing: A holistic approach* (pp. 8–22). Philadelphia, PA: J. B. Lippincott.

Chapman, L. S. (1986, Summer). Spiritual health: A component missing from health promotion. *American Journal of Health Promotion, 1*(1), 38–41.

Chesla, C., & Stannard, D. (1997). Breakdown in the nursing care of families in the ICU. *American Journal of Critical Care, 6*(1), 64–71.

Clochesy, J. M. (1988). *Essentials of critical care nursing.* Rockville, MD: Aspen Systems.

Corcoran, E. (1993). Spirituality: An important aspect of emergency nursing. *Journal of Emergency Nursing, 19*(3), 183–184.

Dearing, L. (1997). Caring for the perioperative client. In P. A. Potter & A. G. Perry (Eds.), *Fundamentals of nursing: Concepts, process and practice* (pp. 1379–1427). St. Louis, MO: C. V. Mosby.

DiSarcina, A. (1991). Spiritual care at a code. *Journal of Christian Nursing, 8*(3), 20–23.

Dossey, B. M., Guzzetta, C. E., & Kenner, C. V. (Eds.). (1992). Body, mind, spirit. In *Critical care nursing: Body, mind, spirit* (pp. 10–16). Philadelphia, PA: J. B. Lippincott.

Dracup, K. (1995). Key aspects of caring for the acutely ill. In S. G. Funk, E. M. Tornquist, M. T. Champagne, & R. A. Wise (Eds.), *Key aspects of caring for the acutely ill* (pp. 8–22). New York, NY: Springer.

Duzl-Church, V., Cimino, J., Adler, S., Wong, P., & Anderson, W. (2010). I'm sitting here by myself . . . experiences of patients with serious illness at an urban public hospital. *Journal of Palliative Care Medicine, 13*(6), 695–701.

Emergency Nurses Association. (1995). *Standards of emergency nursing practice* (3rd ed.). St. Louis, MO: Mosby-Yearbook.

Fahlberg, L. L., & Fahlberg, L. A. (1991). Exploring spirituality and consciousness with an expanded science. *American Journal of Health Promotion, 5*(4), 273–281.

Fairchild, S. S. (1996). *Perioperative nursing: Principles and practice* (2nd ed.). Boston, MA: Little, Brown and Company.

Ferszt, G. G., & Taylor, P. B. (1988). When your patient needs spiritual comfort. *Nursing '88, 18*(4), 48–49.

Gallison, B. S., Xu, Y., Jurgens, C. Y. & Boyle, S. M. (2013). Acute care nurses' spiritual practices. *Journal of Holistic Nursing, 31*(2), 95–103.

Georgensen, J., & Dungan, J. M. (1996). Managing spiritual distress in patients with advanced cancer pain. *Cancer Nursing, 19*(5), 376–383.

Gildenberg, P. L., & DeVaul, R. A. (1985). *The chronic pain patient: Evaluation and management.* New York, NY: Karger.

Gillman, J., Gable-Rodriguez, J., Sutherland, M., & Whitacre, J. (1996). Pastoral care in a critical care setting. *Critical Care and Nursing Quarterly, 19*(1), 10–20.

Gunta, K. E. (1993). Chronic pain. In J. M. Thompson, G. K. McFarland, J. E. Hirsch, & S. N. Tucker (Eds.), *Mosby's clinical nursing* (3rd ed., pp. 1538–1543). St. Louis, MO: C. V. Mosby.

Guthrie, J. (1985). E.R.: One nurse's struggle with problem patients and self-righteousness. *Journal of Christian Nursing, 2*(4), 20–21.

Hahn, J. (2001). Ministry in ICU. *Journal of Christian Nursing, 18*(2), 31–32.

Hall, B. A. (1997). Spirituality in terminal illness. *Journal of Holistic Nursing, 15*(1), 82–96.

Hanson, L., Dobbs, D., Usher, B., Williams, S., Rawlings, J., & Daaleman, T. (2008).

Providers and types of spiritual care during serious illness. *Journal of Palliative Medicine, 11*(6), 907–914.

Hart, C. W. (1994). Spiritual health, illness, and death. *Journal of Religion and Health, 33*(1), 17–22.

Hayden, D. (2011). Spirituality in end-of-life care: Attending the person on their journey. *British Journal of Community Nursing, 16*(11), 546–551.

Heiser, R., Chiles, K., Fudge, M., & Gray, S. (1997). The use of music during the immediate postoperative recovery period. *Association of Operating Room Nurses Journal, 65*(4), 777–785.

Holt-Ashley, M. (2000). Nurses pray: Use of prayer and spirituality as a complimentary therapy in the intensive care setting. *AACN Clinical Issues: Advanced Practice in Acute and Critical Care, 11*(1), 60–67.

Hopkins, M. (1993). Care of the patient in a critical care unit. In B. Long, W. J. Phipps, & V. L. Cassmeyer (Eds.), *Medical–surgical nursing: A nursing process approach* (3rd ed., pp. 1564–1585). St. Louis, MO: C. V. Mosby.

Jahani, R., Rejeh, N., Heravi-Karimooj, M., Vaismoradi, M., & Jasper, M. (2014). Spiritual well-being of Iranian patients with acute coronary syndromes: A cross-sectional descriptive study. *Journal of Research in Nursing, 19*(6), 518–527.

Kidd, P. S. (1997). Caring for the critically ill patient: Patient, family and nursing considerations. In P. S. Kidd & K. D. Wagner (Eds.), *High acuity nursing* (2nd ed., pp. 3–24). Stamford, CT: Appleton & Lange.

Kozier, B., Erb, G., Blais, K., & Wilkinson, J. (1995). *Fundamentals of nursing: Concepts, process and practice* (5th ed.). Menlo Park, CA: Addison-Wesley.

Kumasaka, L. (1996). My pain is God's will. *American Journal of Nursing, 96*(6), 45–47.

Lazure, L. A., & DeMartinis, J. E. (1997). Basic concepts of emergency care. In J. H. Black & E. Mahassarin-Jacobs (Eds.), *Medical–surgical nursing: Clinical management for continuity of care* (5th ed., pp. 2501–2516). Philadelphia, PA: W. B. Saunders.

Levin, J. S., & Schiller, P. L. (1987). Is there a religious factor in health? *Journal of Religion and Health, 26*(1), 9–36.

Long, B. C. (1993). Problems encountered in emergencies and disasters. In B. Long, W. J. Phipps, & V. L. Cassmeyer (Eds.), *Medical–surgical nursing: A nursing process approach* (3rd ed., pp. 1537–1560). St. Louis, MO: C. V. Mosby.

Lundberg, P., & Kerdonfag, P. (2010). Spiritual care provided by Thai nurses in intensive care units. *Journal of Clinical Nursing, 19*, 1121–1128.

MacPhail, E. (1992). Overview of emergency nursing and emergency care. In S. Sheehy (Ed.), *Emergency nursing principles and practice* (pp. 1–8). St. Louis, MO: Mosby-Yearbook.

March, P., & Caple, C. (2012, June). Spiritual needs of hospitalized patients. *Cinahl Information Systems, 14*(2), 1–2.

McCaffery, M. (1968). *Nursing practice theories related to cognition, bodily pain, and man–environment interaction.* Los Angeles, CA: University of California at Los Angeles.

McGrath, P. (2004). Reflections on serious illness as spiritual journey by survivors of haematological malignancies. *European Journal of Cancer Care, 13*, 227–237.

McNamara, S. (1995). Perioperative nurses' perceptions of caring practices. *Association of Operating Room Nurses Journal, 61*(2), 377–388.

Meeker, M. H., & Rothrock, J. C. (1995). *Alexander's care of the patient in surgery* (10th ed.). St. Louis, MO: C. V. Mosby.

Michello, J. A. (1988). Spiritual and emotional determinants of health. *Journal of Religion and Health, 27*(1), 62–70.

Miller, K. (1996). Emergency nursing. In S. C. Smeltzer & B. B. Bare (Eds.), *Brunner and Suddarth's textbook of medical–surgical nursing* (8th ed., pp. 2000–2018). Philadelphia, PA: J. B. Lippincott.

Minnix, L. (2008). Maintaining spirituality in institutional settings. *Generations, 32*(2), 65–67.

Monroe, C. (2011). Spirituality shines through in a magnet moment. *Critical Care Nurse, 31*(4), 98–99.

National Institute of Nursing Research. (1994). *Symptom management: Acute pain, a report of the NINR priority expert panel.* Bethesda, MD: Author.

Niklas, G. R., & Stefanics, C. (1975). *Ministry to the hospitalized.* New York, NY: Paulist Press.

Nouwen, H. J. M. (1979). *The wounded healer.* Garden City, NY: Image Books.

Nussbaum, G. (2003). Spirituality in critical care: Patient comfort and satisfaction. *Critical Care Nursing Quarterly, 26*(3), 214–220.

O'Brien, M. E. (1982a). The need for spiritual integrity. In H. Yura & M. B. Walsh (Eds.), *Human needs and the nursing process* (Vol. 2, pp. 85–115). Norwalk, CT: Appleton-Century-Crofts.

O'Brien, M. E. (1982b). Religious faith and adjustment to long-term hemodialysis. *Journal of Religion and Health, 21*(1), 68–80.

O'Brien, M. E. (1983). *The courage to survive: The life career of the chronic dialysis patient.* New York, NY: Grune & Stratton.

O'Brien, M. E. (1992). *Living with HIV: Experiment in courage.* Westport, CT: Auburn House.

Peterson, V., & Potter, P. A. (1997). Spiritual health. In P. A. Potter & A. G. Perry (Eds.), *Fundamentals of nursing: Concepts, process and practice* (4th ed., pp. 441–456). St. Louis, MO: C. V. Mosby.

Phippen, M. L., Wells, M. P., & Martinelli, A. M. (1994). A conceptual model for peri-operative nursing practice. In M. L. Phippen & M. D. Wells (Eds.), *Perioperative nursing practice* (pp. 3–67). Philadelphia, PA: W. B. Saunders.

Pipe, T. B., Kelly, A., LeBrun, G., Schmidt, D., Atherton, P., & Robinson, C. (2008). A prospective descriptive study exploring hope, spiritual well-being, and quality of life in hospitalized patients. *Medsurg Nursing, 17*(4), 247–257.

Potter, P. A. (1997). Comfort. In P. A. Potter & A. G. Perry (Eds.), *Fundamentals of nursing: Concepts, process and practice* (4th ed., pp. 1153–1190). St. Louis, MO: C. V. Mosby.

Potter, P. A., & Perry, A. G. (1997). *Fundamentals of nursing: Concepts, process and practice* (4th ed.). St. Louis, MO: C. V. Mosby.

Reed, P. (1991). Preferences for spiritually related nursing interventions among terminally ill and non-terminally ill hospitalized adults and well adults. *Applied Nursing Research, 4*(3), 122–128.

Robinson, K. (1992). Pre-hospital care. In S. Sheehy (Ed.), *Emergency nursing: Principles and practice* (3rd ed., pp. 9–18). St. Louis, MO: Mosby-Yearbook.

Ronaldson, S., Hayes, L., Aggar, C., Green, J., & Carey, M. (2012). Spirituality and spiritual caring: Nurses' perspectives and practice in palliative and acute care environments. *Journal of Clinical Nursing, 21*(15/16), 2126–2135.

Rothrock, J. C. (1994). The meaning of spirituality to perioperative nurses and their patients. *Association of Operating Room Nurses Journal, 60*(6), 894–895.

Rukholm, E. E., Bailey, P. H., & Coutu-Wakulczyk, G. (1991). Family needs and anxiety in ICU: Cultural differences in Northeastern Ontario. *The Canadian Journal of Nursing Research, 23*(3), 67–81.

Rushton, L. (2014). What are the barriers to spiritual care in a hospital setting? *British Journal of Nursing, 23*(7), 370–374.

Santacaterina, S., & Stein-Spencer, L. (1990). Emergency medicine services. In S. Kidd & J. Kaiser (Eds.), *Emergency nursing: A physiologic and clinical perspective* (pp. 3–12). Philadelphia, PA: W. B. Saunders.

Schlintz, V. (1987). Has God forsaken the emergency department? *Journal of Christian Nursing, 4*(1), 18–19.

Schlintz, V. (1988). Would God listen to me now? *Journal of Christian Nursing, 5*(2), 14–16.

Seidl, L. G. (1993, September). The value of spiritual health. *Health Progress, 10*(1), 48–50.

Shaffer, J. (1991). Spiritual distress and critical illness. *Critical Care Nurse, 11*(10), 42–45.

Shelly, J. A., & Fish, S. (1995). Praying with patients. *Journal of Christian Nursing, 12*(1), 9–13.

Smeltzer, S. C., & Bare, B. G. (1996). *Brunner and Suddarth's textbook of medical–surgical nursing* (8th ed.). Philadelphia, PA: J. B. Lippincott.

Smyth, T., & Allen, S. (2011). Nurses' experiences assessing spirituality of terminally ill patients in acute clinical practice. *International Journal of Palliative Nursing, 17*(7), 337–343.

Springhouse Corporation. (1985). *Nursing now series: Pain.* Springhouse, PA: Author.

Sternberg, E. M. (2009). *Healing spaces: The science of place and well-being.* Cambridge, MA: Harvard University Press.

Stromberg, R. (1992). The voices on coronary care: A confrontation with vulnerability. In L. E. Holst (Ed.), *Hospital ministry: The role of the chaplain today* (pp. 127–138). New York, NY: Crossroad.

Taylor, C., Lillis, C., & LeMone, P. (1997). *Fundamentals of nursing: The art and science of nursing care* (3rd ed.). Philadelphia, PA: J. B. Lippincott.

Timmons, F., & Kelly, J. (2008). Spiritual assessment in intensive and cardiac care nursing. *Nursing in Critical Care, 13*(3), 124–131.

Turk, D. C., & Feldman, C. S. (1992). Facilitating the use of noninvasive pain management strategies with the terminally ill. *The Hospice Journal, 8*(1), 193–214.

Turan, T., & Karamanoglu, A. Y. (2012). Determining intensive care unit nurses' perceptions and practice levels of spiritual care. *Nursing in Critical Care, 18*(2), 70–78.

Twibell, R., Wieseke, A., Marine, M., & Schoger, J. (1996). Spiritual and coping needs of critically ill patients: Validation of nursing diagnosis. *Dimensions of Critical Care Nursing, 15*(5), 245–253.

Unruh, A. (2007). Spirituality, religion and pain. *Canadian Journal of Nursing Research, 39*(2), 66–86.

Walleck, C. A. (1989). Spinal cord injury. In K. T. Von Rueden & C. Walleck (Eds.), *Advanced critical care nursing* (pp. 181–203). Rockville, MD: Aspen Systems.

Warner, J. E. (1992). Involvement of families in pain control of terminally ill patients. *The Hospice Journal, 8*(1), 155–170.

Watt-Watson, J. H., & Long, B. C. (1993). Pain. In B. Long, W. J. Phipps, & V. L. Cassmeyer (Eds.), *Medical–surgical nursing: A nursing process approach* (3rd ed., pp. 163–179). St. Louis, MO: C. V. Mosby.

Weaver, A. J., Koenig, H. G., & Flannelly, L. T. (2008). Nurses and healthcare chaplains: Natural allies. *Journal of Health Care Chaplaincy, 14*(2), 91–98.

Westlake, C., Dyo, M., Vollman, M., & Heywood, J. T. (2008). Spirituality and suffering of patients with heart failure. *Progress in Palliative Care, 16*(5–6), 257–265.

Yeager, S., Doust, C., Epting, S., Iannantuono, B., Indian, C., Lenhart, B. . . . Thomas, K. (2010). Embrace hope: An end-of-life intervention to support neurological critical care patients and their families. *Critical Care Nurse, 30*(1), 47–58.

CHAPTER 8

Spiritual Needs of the Chronically Ill Person

Those who wait for the Lord shall renew their strength, they shall mount up with wings as eagles, they shall run and not be weary, walk and not faint.

Isaiah 40:31

Virtually all of our cancer patients are in some way or another in a psychological, emotional, or spiritual crisis at some point, and they all address it in different ways . . . and of course, one of the things you run into is, like, "Why should I get treatment? I trust God." Then I like to explain to them that God does help those who help themselves, not in those words specifically. On occasion you seek outside help [for someone] who is really just beyond what you can do. But most times people just need to talk, get it off their chest. If I were in their place I would want a nurse there.

Sarah, Oncology Research Nurse

For the chronically ill individual, personal spirituality and/or religious beliefs and practices often constitute an important, even critical, dimension of coping with the life changes necessitated by the illness experience. This was clearly recognized in the author's longitudinal research with persons facing long-term adaptation to such illnesses as chronic renal failure (CRF) and human immunodeficiency virus (HIV) infection. The corporate élan of both groups was reflected in the titles of books reporting their coping strategies: *The Courage to Survive: The Life Career of the Chronic Dialysis Patient* (O'Brien, 1983) and *Living with HIV: Experiment in Courage* (O'Brien, 1992). For the CRF and HIV-positive study participants, as for many persons living with serious, life-threatening chronic illnesses, it is exquisitely courageous to go on about the business of living, knowing that each new day may possess myriad physical or emotional threats to one's quality of life. For many persons living with chronic illness, transcendent belief and experience provide the impetus to live and to love in the midst of significant pain and suffering. As one 8-year survivor of an HIV-positive diagnosis put it:

> God is the one reliable constant in my life. When I'm feeling unsure about everything else, I know that God is with me. I feel it. It's not a "head thing." It's in my heart. I almost think I'm being arrogant but it really is indescribable, the feeling of the presence of God; it's like the hymn puts it: "Standing on Solid Rock."
>
> (O'Brien, 1995, p. 129)

A topic currently under study is that of "spirituality self-care," especially as it relates to quality of life among persons diagnosed with chronic illness (White, 2013, p. 23). In research with 142 outpatients it was found that "spiritual self-care practices helped manage the chronic illness, specifically heart failure and quality of life" (p. 23). Other chronic illness conditions in which spiritual support was found to be particularly important included cancer (Egan, McKechnie, Jobson, Herbison, & Richards, 2013; Nixon, Narayanasamy, & Penny, 2013; and Blanchard, Dunlap, & Fitchett, 2012); mental health conditions such as dementia (Odbehr, Kvigne, Hauge, & Danbolt, 2014); and acute psychiatric inpatient conditions (Raffay, 2014). It has been reported that "people with mental health needs are increasingly identifying spirituality as a vital part of their recovery" (Elliott, 2011, p. 4). This chapter documents spiritual needs in chronic illness as identified in interviews with persons living with such conditions as cancer (including Burkitt's lymphoma), chronic renal failure, depression, and multiple chronic sequelae of HIV infection and acquired immunodeficiency syndrome (AIDS). The patients' spiritual needs are further explained through analysis of interview data elicited from families and professional nurse caregivers. In addition, practicing nurses report and describe specific instances of spiritual care in a variety of settings.

▶ The Case of Chronic Illness

Any experience of illness may bring about a degree of disruption in a person's life. Usual patterns of life activity are temporarily, or in some cases permanently, changed or modified to cope with the situation. The need for a major life change occurs more frequently in patients facing chronic illness. Corbin (1996) defined chronic illness as "a medical condition or health problem with associated symptoms or disabilities that require long-term management" (p. 318). Taylor, Lillis, and LeMone (1997) described chronic illness as having the following characteristics: results in "permanent change," "causes or is caused by irreversible alterations in normal anatomy and physiology," "requires special client education for rehabilitation," and "requires a long period of care or support" (p. 61). Currently, chronic illness is considered the "primary health problem in the United States," with some 50 percent of the population experiencing one or more conditions (Ignatavicius, Workman, & Mishler, 1995, p. 213).

Chronic illness symptoms may range from mild to severe, and often fluctuate between periods of exacerbation and remission (LeMone & Burke, 1996, p. 44). Medical sociologists point out that in cases of chronic illness, frequently the fulfillment of previous roles and responsibilities becomes impossible, and significant reorganization of an individual's patterns of behavior is required. Major changes may occur in social relationships and future life plans, as well as in personal self-concept and self-esteem (Turk & Rudy, 1986, p. 309). The family, especially, may be significantly disrupted by the chronic illness of one of its members, especially when well family members are intimately involved with the care and support of the ill person. Both current and prior nursing research suggest that spiritual well-being is, for many chronically ill persons, a key factor in successful long-term adaptation to the illness condition (Landis, 1996).

▶ Spiritual Care of the Chronically Ill Patient

If, as the literature suggests, an individual's spiritual well-being is central to coping with the physical and psychosocial sequelae of chronic illness, what interventions may a nurse initiate in the provision of spiritual care for a chronically ill patient? And, in what setting(s) will spiritual care for the chronically ill person need to be provided?

The chronically ill person, although most frequently living at home, may also be found in a hospital or clinic setting; the latter in times of illness exacerbation or during the carrying out of diagnostic or therapeutic procedures. The kind of spiritual care provided by the nurse will be influenced by the setting and also by the type and degree of the patient's disability. Physical disability, such as being unable to ambulate freely, may necessitate a creative strategy to facilitate participation in religious rituals, if desired by the client. Spiritual care may also be directed toward the emotional sequelae of chronic illness, which may affect overall spiritual well-being, such as "low self-esteem, feelings of isolation, powerlessness, hopelessness, and anger" (Soeken & Carson, 1987, p. 606). Spiritual interventions that a nurse can initiate in response are an affirmation of God's love and care for each person, encouragement to participate in rituals shared with others, and support for an individual's hope in God's protection (pp. 608–609).

In discussing a "spirituality for the long haul," Muldoon and King (1991) observed that the challenge for the chronically ill person is to integrate the illness experience into his or her self-concept (p. 102). Central to accomplishing this is the support of one's spiritual philosophy undergirding the ultimate meaning and purpose in life. For 181 chronic obstructive pulmonary disease (COPD) patients, a "high sense" of spirituality was associated with "low stress" and "high quality of life" as reported by nonhospitalized patients (Delgado, 2007, p. 229). This finding is supported by the idea that individuals may "make sense of chronic illness" by finding spiritual meaning in their suffering (Greenstreet, 2006, p. 938). Greenstreet presents a conceptual model that incorporates a spiritual perspective on "making sense of chronic illness in relation to coping skills" (p. 938).

Spiritual care interventions for the chronically ill are similar to those proposed for the acutely ill patient. They include listening to and being with the patient, which may facilitate the integration of spirituality into coping behaviors; praying with a patient, if the patient so desires; reading Scripture, if appropriate; providing spiritual books or other devotional materials; and referring the patient to a clergy member. These spiritual interventions need to be adapted, however, to particular illness conditions and their sequelae, such as mental illness and physical disability, and to specific settings, such as those involving home health care and homelessness, which are discussed later in this chapter. Obviously, careful attention to the patient's religious tradition should precede any spiritual interventions as well as the assessment of spiritual needs.

▶ Spiritual Needs in Chronic Illness

All individuals have spiritual needs, regardless of religious belief or personal philosophy of life. The experience of illness, especially of a long-term chronic illness, may be a time when spiritual needs previously unnoticed or neglected become apparent (Baldacchino & Draper, 2001). It has been reported that individuals with chronic illness "have identified spirituality as a resource that promotes quality of life" (Adegbola, 2007, p. 42). Spiritual needs may manifest in a multiplicity of symptoms, depending on the person's particular theology, religious tradition, or philosophical understanding of the meaning and purpose of life. For the adherent of one of the monotheistic Western religious groups, Judaism, Christianity, or Islam, spiritual needs are generally associated with one's relationship to God. Shelly and Fish (1988) identified God in the believer's life to be the source of "meaning and purpose, love and relatedness and forgiveness" (p. 38); they asserted that an absence of belief in any one of these factors will result in spiritual need (p. 39). Spiritual needs may also include hope and creativity (Highfield & Cason, 1983, p. 188), as well as reassurance and self-esteem (Cassidy, 1992).

Although assessment of a patient's spiritual needs may be more readily carried out by a practicing nurse, it is often at the stage of intervention that difficulties arise. Although most nurses profess to practice holistic patient care, Forbis (1988) asserted that "they often avoid dealing pragmatically with the spiritual realm" (p. 158). In interviewing nurses prior to designing a course on spiritual care, Ellis (1986) found that many nurses were uncomfortable discussing spiritual issues with patients and were decidedly uneasy about praying with their patients (p. 76). Nurses need to develop an understanding of and comfort with their own spiritual beliefs in order to be at ease discussing spiritual matters with others (Burnard, 1988; McSherry, 1996).

In a study of nurses' perceptions of patients' spiritual needs, Boutell and Bozeht (1988) identified the concepts of faith (in religious beliefs), peace (inner strength), hope, and trust (in the importance of religious practices) (p. 174). Additional needs, those of courage and love, were reflected in nursing research data elicited from CRF and AIDS patients (O'Brien, 1983, 1992, 1995). The spiritual needs of hope, trust, courage, faith, peace, and love on the part of chronically ill persons are explored in the following pages; examples of these characteristics are drawn from the comments of individuals experiencing such illness conditions as cancer, HIV infection and AIDS, and CRF.

Hope

And now, O Lord, what do I wait for? My hope is in you.

—**Psalm** 39:7

Hope, as a general term, relates to an anticipation that something desired will occur. Hope, or the act of hoping, defined theologically for a member of a monotheistic religious tradition, is the "focusing of attention, affectivity and commitment to action toward the future goal of fulfillment in God, the realization of the reign of God" (Hellwig, 1993, p. 506). Shelly and Fish (1988) pointed out that placing one's hope in God does not mean an immediate end to suffering or anxiety; rather, hoping relates to trust in God's support during a crisis (p. 44). Both clinical anecdotes and research have documented the fact that when a patient loses hope and the will to live, death may result (Ross, 1994, p. 440). Thus, supporting and nurturing hope is described as a "vital ingredient" in a nurse's plan of spiritual care (Gewe, 1994; Le Peau, 1996; Thompson, 1994).

Phillip, a young adult cancer patient who described himself as a born-again Christian, manifested a beautifully direct sense of hope as he faced his illness:

> I put all my hope in Jesus, in the Cross. I have my daily minute with Him. I mean, it's about an hour, but I call it my "minute." I try to always have the special "minutes." I pray to Jesus; He is with me. Jesus is my hope.

Because of his disease, an anaplastic astrocytoma, Phillip's speech patterns were sometimes difficult to follow; by listening carefully, however, one could understand his meaning; his eyes were very expressive as he spoke about his relationship with Jesus. On a page in his Bible, Phillip had written "Born again in Jesus"; he explained, "That's when I accepted Him, and now He's always with me."

Trust

I trust in you, O Lord, I say, "You are my God."

—**Psalm** 31:14

The concept of trust indicates having confidence in something or someone. Theologically, the term is considered to be a relational one, "describing the quality of a relationship among two or more persons" (Schreiter, 1993, p. 982). The Hebrew word for trust, which occurs frequently in the Old Testament, "refers most often to trust in God" (p. 982). Possessing the ability to trust in others is considered "essential to spiritual health" (Simsen, 1988, p. 33).

In discussing adaptation to chronic illness, nursing scholar Ruth Stoll (1989) noted that "a dynamic spiritual belief system enables us to trust that somehow tomorrow will not be beyond our capacities" (p. 195). Trusting, for the ill person who is a believer, will give a sense of security that God's healing power will be operative in his or her life (Johnson, 1992, p. 92). It is important to recognize, however, that the "healing" that occurs may be of a spiritual or emotional nature, rather than a physical healing.

A recently married and newly diagnosed Burkitt's lymphoma patient, David, spoke eloquently to the concept of trust:

> Well, this is not what I had expected at this time in my life but this is the Cross, the folly of the Cross they say, so I put it in the hands of the "man upstairs." I mean I'm really with Him and He's with me, you know . . . I have to tell you, though, even with my faith, we're all human, and I was really scared in the beginning. When they first brought me in to the hospital, they rolled me into that ICU, through the doors, and I saw all that equipment and those monitors, I thought: "Whoa! Is this the Cross?" But you know that God is going to be walking beside you.

David's life had, he admitted, been "turned upside down" by his diagnosis and hospitalization, and yet he described a sense of comfort in knowing that this, for him, was God's will. He laughingly commented that this kind of attitude would, he knew, be considered "folly" by some; for David it was, quite simply, a matter of trust.

Courage

I took courage for the hand of the Lord, my God, was upon me.

—**Ezra** 7:28

Courage, or emotional strength, is described not as the absence of fear, but rather as "the ability to transcend one's fears, to choose to actively face what needs to be" (Stoll, 1989, p. 196).

Martha, an adult woman in midlife diagnosed with CRF and experiencing maintenance hemodialysis, spoke openly about the need for courage to face a life dependent on technology:

You have to get yourself together and face the thing; be courageous about it because nobody is going to do it for you. I think adjusting to kidney failure and dialysis is very difficult because I can't answer why. Why did this happen to me? But my faith says that all things have a reason, and God won't put anything on us that we can't bear . . . But it's still difficult because chronic illnesses may be with you a long time before they lead to dying; you have to have some courage about it.

We, as nurses, long to do something for those with whom we work: to heal, to cure, to alleviate the suffering of our courageous patients and their families. Yet frequently we must accept that such accomplishments are beyond our power; we must learn to accept that our desire to comfort and our empathy are, of themselves, an important dimension of nursing care.

Faith

Daughter, your faith has made you well.

—**Luke** 8:48

Faith means belief or trust in someone or something. From a theological perspective, faith is the basis of our personal relationship with God "on whose strength and absolute sureness we can literally stake our lives" (Fatula, 1993, p. 379). Faith is identified as "a prerequisite for spiritual growth" (Carson, 1989, p. 28), and faith in God is often a critical element in surviving a loss (Sandin, 1996) or coping with an illness experience (Ross, 1994). A holistic nursing philosophy suggests that religious faith may give one the strength to "combat disease and facilitate healing" (Kennison, 1987, p. 29).

An example of the support provided by personal faith in coping with an advanced cancer diagnosis was reflected in Matthew's perception of his condition:

I can't question how I got this disease or what God's plan is for me. But I know my faith will get me through. At a time like this, faith is the key. My faith makes me strong. Chemo is tough but God's in that too. I don't know; I just know my faith will get me to the place I need to be.

Peace

May the Lord give strength to His people, may the Lord bless His people with peace.

—**Psalm** 29:11

Peace is a sense of being undisturbed, a feeling of freedom from anxiety and fear. Theologically, peace is described as being derived from "a right relationship with God, which entails forgiveness, reconciliation and union" (Dwyer, 1990, p. 749). In a study of spiritual well-being (SWB), researcher David Moberg (1979) found that, according to most respondents' perceptions, two significant indicators of SWB were "peace with God" and "inner peace" (p. 9).

Two chronic renal failure patients on maintenance hemodialysis described the peace their religious faith afforded them in relation to their disease and treatment regimens. Carolyn, who had been on dialysis for over 3 years, asserted:

> Well, I think if I didn't believe in God and have the religious beliefs I have, I don't think I'd be able to survive this. I don't think I'd have any peace. I think I probably would have attempted suicide at one time or another. But my faith helps me be optimistic about it; it really helps.

And Elizabeth, a two-year veteran of dialytic therapy, reported that the illness experience had a positive effect on her personal spirituality:

> My faith has really strengthened. I'm still a good old "knee-slapping" Baptist. I still love my pastor and I enjoy going to church on Sunday. I pray a lot, but I don't want to ask too much. I'm at peace. If healing is for me, then it will come to me. I just take the attitude that I don't worry about it. God will provide.

Love

How precious is your steadfast love, O God.

—**Psalm** 36:7

To love means to care for or to treasure someone or something. Love, from a religious perspective, relates to "God's benevolent love"; thus, "by association, God's love encompasses human love for God, human love for neighbor, human love for creation, and self-love" (Dreyer, 1993, p. 613). Shelly and Fish (1988) asserted that God's love will be with one, unconditionally, during a crisis such as illness (pp. 46–47), and that His supportive love is best reflected in the Old Testament Scripture, Isaiah 43:2–3:

> When you pass through raging waters, I will be with you; in the river you shall not drown. When you walk through fire, you shall not be burned; the flames shall not consume you. For I am the Lord, your God, the Holy One of Israel, your savior.

Mary Grace, a cancer patient, described the importance of God's love as manifested by her church:

> Well the one thing that helps you deal with this is that you know that your church is behind you. The pastor, he remembers to call you and the church members come to visit and the deacons bring me my Communion to the house. All those things make me feel good; they make me feel loved.

Tom, a 37-year-old lymphoma patient and a practicing attorney who described his personal spirituality as "secular humanism," also admitted the need for love in coping with his diagnosis:

> I'm not sure about the "God thing"—I mean whether God exists or not. But I believe in human goodness and the responsibility we have to each other and to the universe. I don't lean on any religion to help me live with this disease, but I do rely on my family and friends who love me. That's what gets me through the day, knowing I'm loved.

Cancer, HIV/AIDS, and CRF are three chronic illness syndromes from which many individuals currently suffer. Examples of data-based spiritual needs of the oncology patient, the HIV-positive patient, and the CRF patient can serve to guide spiritual care therapeutics for persons suffering from other chronic illnesses that a nurse may encounter.

▶ Spiritual Needs of the Cancer Patient

The term *cancer* is a broad label that covers a family of diseases characterized by uncontrollable growth of mutated cells that may disseminate to various parts of the body. Cancerous growths originate in various tissues or organs, differ in size and appearance, develop in a variety of ways, and respond differently to therapeutic interventions (Petty, 1997, p. 533). Roughly 20 percent of all deaths in the United States are attributable to some form of the approximately 12 major and 50 minor types of cancer (LeMone & Burke, 1996, p. 306). Because of the serious, life-threatening nature of most cancer diagnoses, the spiritual needs of the patient may be significant. A study of 45 adult cancer patients (with diagnoses such as breast cancer, lung cancer, and leukemia) revealed that religious belief was a source of strength and comfort in coping with the illness (Moschella, Pressman, Pressman, & Weissman, 1997). Moschella et al. found that patients diagnosed with cancer reported an increase in faith, more time spent in prayer, and greater frequency of church attendance, despite the fact that their religious belief systems provided no theological explanation for suffering (p. 17). Findings from research with 114 adult cancer patients indicated a positive association between high levels of spiritual well-being and lower levels of anxiety (Kaczorowski, 1989). Spiritual well-being, as evaluated in a study of 175 breast cancer patients, was demonstrated to be highest in those women who were classified as intrinsically religious, that is, those who internalized their religious belief as a core motivator in life (Mickley, Soeken, & Belcher, 1992). Highfield (1992) found the spiritual health of 23 primary lung cancer patients to be high when normed according to the current literature on spirituality and cancer. Highfield posited some reasons: the study participants' reliance on spiritual resources, and a greater degree of spiritual development, related either to age or the terminal diagnosis (p. 7).

Research on the attitudes and beliefs about spiritual care among Oncology Nursing Society members revealed that the community held the nurse's role of providing spiritual care in high regard (Taylor, Highfield, & Amenta, 1994). The study of 181 members of the Oncology Nursing Society reported spiritual care behaviors such as talking with patients about spiritual or religious matters; referring patients to other spiritual caregivers such as chaplains or clergy; praying with or for a patient; supporting a patient's family; facilitating the use of religious or devotional resources;

and being with and touching the patient, with a supportive and nonjudgmental attitude (Taylor, Amenta, & Highfield, 1995, p. 36). Recent nursing research has also demonstrated the increasing role of spiritual caring among oncology nurses (Thomas & Retsas, 1999); the importance of the nurse's sensitivity to diverse cultural and religious traditions (Lackey, Gates, & Brown, 2001); and nurses' recognition of the uniqueness of individualized spiritual experience for oncology patients (Halstead & Hull, 2001; MacDonald, 2001). In a qualitative study exploring oncology nurses' coping processes, the concepts of caritas, religiosity, and spirituality were considered and found to "have a protective function that facilitates coping as the nurse has something to turn to" (Ekedahl & Wengstrom, 2010, p. 530). The study data also suggested that "religious coping dominated by basic trust where prayer is used as a coping strategy may support the nurse" (p. 530).

Some additional research on the spiritual needs of cancer patients includes the work of McClain, Rosenfeld, and Breitbart (2003) in "Effect of Spiritual Well-Being on End-of-Life Despair in Terminally Ill Cancer Patients" and in "Spiritual Care Nursing: What Cancer Patients and Family Caregivers Want" (Taylor & Mamier, 2005). In attempting to map the "processes and qualities of spiritual care" with oncology patients, Carr (2009) conducted open-ended interviews with patients, nurses, and families that revealed that "developing caring relationships" was core in the nurse–patient interactions, and that the nurse should possess four qualities: "receptivity, humanity, competency, and positivity" (p. 686). Other studies highlighting the importance of spiritual well-being in cancer patients were conducted by Lopez, McCaffrey, Griffin, and Fitzpatrick (2009); and Schneider (2007).

Spiritual care for Mrs. Anna Smithfield, an advanced ovarian cancer patient participating in an experimental chemotherapy protocol, consisted primarily of listening and supporting the patient's existing spiritual and religious beliefs and traditions. Mrs. Smithfield's religious tradition was Methodist; her nurse, Beth, was Roman Catholic. At their first meeting, Beth and Mrs. Smithfield discussed their denominational differences; they agreed, however, that as Christians they really had more similarities in belief than differences. Mrs. Smithfield was receiving spiritual support from her pastor and church members. What she needed to talk to Beth about was her fear of leaving her husband of 26 years alone. She was also saddened over the fact that her young grandchildren would never get to know her as "grandmother." For Beth, the primary spiritual care intervention was to sit with Mrs. Smithfield, to listen, and to talk with her about her family; they also prayed together. Beth made a point to drop in when Mr. Smithfield visited, because the patient had expressed the wish that he meet her nurse; this provided Beth the opportunity to be available for Mr. Smithfield who also needed spiritual support in his anxiety over his wife's prognosis.

▶ Spiritual Needs of the HIV-Infected Person

HIV infection, identified in 1983 under the acronym LAV (lymphadenopathy associated virus), and in 1984 as HTLV III (human T-cell lymphotropic virus) has progressed through many phases and mutations over the last 33–34 years; numerous therapeutic protocols have been tested on both the virus and related opportunistic infections with varying degrees of efficacy. Although HIV infection in the United States was originally a disease of white gay men, the condition later became more prevalent in the black and Hispanic communities (Ungvarski & Matassarin-Jacobs, 1997). The clinical course of HIV infection is directed by the immune system response, with the development of opportunistic infection symptoms such as fever, malaise, sweating, headache, weight loss, sore throat, and rashes, among others (Lisanti & Zwolski, 1997). HIV infection may progress to a stage officially categorized as AIDS related to a variety of immune system parameters and symptomatology. More recent pharmacologic therapies have significantly slowed the progression of the human immunodeficiency virus and its related disease conditions. Many of those infected with HIV are living longer and with better quality of life than in the past.

Nevertheless, the anxiety and stigma often associated with HIV infection remain as concerning for some 21st-century patients as in the early days of the condition.

In the past countless psychosocial concerns related to both the seriousness and stigma of HIV infection were identified in the nursing research literature; spiritual and religious needs were central among these (Belcher, Dettmore, & Holzemer, 1989; Carson, Soeken, Shanty, & Terry, 1990; Mellors, Riley, & Erlen, 1997; O'Brien, 1992, 1995; O'Brien & Pheifer, 1993; Warner-Robbins & Christiana, 1989). There was also a plethora of early books published on the topics of spirituality, religion, and pastoral care for people living with HIV and AIDS. Some examples that may continue to prove useful as resources for the nurse in providing spiritual care are *The Gospel Imperative in the Midst of AIDS* (Iles, 1989); *The Church with AIDS* (Russell, 1990); *Ministry to Persons with AIDS* (Perelli, 1991); *Embracing the Mystery: A Prayerful Response to AIDS* (Sandys, 1993); *AIDS, Ethics and Religion: Embracing a World of Suffering* (Overberg, 1994). Nevertheless, nursing literature of the time suggested that spirituality remained a neglected area of concern in the assessment of HIV patients' needs (Newshan, 1998; Sherman, 2001). Presently, that neglect continues to be a concern. Today, as in the past, spiritual care of the person living with HIV or AIDS may take many forms depending on the stage and current symptomatology of the illness. It is important to keep in mind that some HIV-positive persons who have become alienated from their churches may not be receiving formal religious ministry because of the stigma of the disease (Perelli, 1991). That, however, is a situation that can be remedied, if the patient and church desire. Some suggestions for spiritual care for the HIV-positive person that may be carried out by a nurse include listening to the patient's "stories" surrounding the illness (Crowther, 1991); offering small gestures of friendship, which may be missing in the alienated patient's life (AIDS Ministry Program, 1991); providing empathy and emotional support (Sunderland & Shelp, 1987); allowing the patient to take the lead in the offering of prayer (Christensen, 1991); and presenting the patient with a nonjudgmental attitude (W. J. Smith, 1988). For the HIV-positive individual who is physically and cognitively well enough to participate, activities such as creating and appreciating religious art or poetry may provide healing for the heart (Roche, 1992).

John Michael, who had lost many friends to AIDS and who had been living with an HIV diagnosis for over six years, began to write poetry as a way of coping with his illness. A nurse researcher provided spiritual support by listening to and appreciating John Michael's poetry. Reading the poetry often provided an opening to discuss spiritual issues related to both living and dying with HIV. One poem, entitled "The Touch of the Maestro," reveals the impact of the HIV experience on John Michael's personal spirituality. In the piece, the poet muses on how HIV disease has alerted him to the fragility of the human condition and has brought into focus the importance of transcendent issues; this is reflected in the final stanza:

> Never again, will I find satisfaction from a mundane ordinary success.
> There is only one reward that needs to be filled,
> That is the plucking of the instrument that is my heart, which now only sings at the touch of the Maestro.
> (O'Brien, 1995, p. 126, reprintzed with permission of the poem's author)

▶ Spiritual Needs of the Chronic Renal Failure Patient

Matassarin-Jacobs (1997) defined CRF as irreversible and "progressive reduction of functioning renal tissue such that the remaining kidney mass can no longer maintain the body's internal environment" (p. 1641). CRF may result from any one of a variety of diseases such as polycystic kidney disease, glomerulonephritis, and pyelonephritis; CRF may also accompany other illness conditions such as diabetes mellitus or hypertension. CRF, if undetected and untreated, generally progresses unilaterally through three stages: diminished renal function, renal insufficiency, and uremia. As a patient progresses toward the critical uremic stage, with symptoms of greatly decreased urine output, fatigue, nausea, and general malaise, dialytic therapy is usually considered. The four major modes of dialysis currently in use are hemodialysis, peritoneal dialysis, continuous ambulatory peritoneal dialysis (CAPD), and continuous cyclic peritoneal dialysis (CCPD). Hemodialysis employs a machine with a "semipermeable filtering membrane [artificial kidney] that removes accumulated waste products from the blood" (Kilpatrick, 1997, p. 1298). The peritoneal dialysis methods cleanse the blood by filling the abdominal cavity with dialysate (electrolyte solution) and using the peritoneum as a filter for waste not excreted by the kidneys. Any method of dialytic therapy, combined with the diagnosis of renal failure, may prove extremely stressful for the CRF patient and family (Flaherty & O'Brien, 1992; Korniewicz & O'Brien, 1994; O'Brien, 1990; O'Brien, Donley, Flaherty, & Johnstone, 1986).

Among the psychosocial sequelae of CRF and its treatment modality, perhaps the least studied yet possibly most important factor relates to the patient's spiritual or religious needs. In a nursing study of hemodialysis patients' needs, according to family perception, one of those most frequently identified was the patients' desire to feel "cared for" by their nurses (C. D. Wagner, 1996). A paper exploring successful aging among chronic renal disease patients included the concept of spirituality within the study framework as a "foundational coping process": "the process describes a person's view and feelings regarding a higher power and the extent of spiritual awareness" (Blevins & Troutman, 2011, p. 257). These authors advised that the identified theory of successful aging, which included spirituality, could be "utilized to assist nurses with enhancing and promoting successful aging" among CRF patients (p. 260). For CRF patients "who live totally dependent upon [technology] for their continued existence, the need for truly caring nursing staff is key. For these patients, also, the quality of life may become questionable"; thus, a multiplicity of spiritual or ethical concerns can result for patients and families (O'Brien, 1983, p. 35).

One early study of religious faith and long-term adaptation to CRF revealed that 78 percent of the 126 maintenance hemodialysis patients studied believed that religious beliefs were to some degree associated with their ability to cope with CRF and the related treatment regimen (O'Brien, 1983). Open-ended questioning of the same group of study respondents produced comments such as, "I knew everything would be alright [after cardiac arrest] because I asked God to carry me through. I know that He's got His arms around me." Another patient, after reporting that faith had been very important in coping with the illness, asserted, "A lot of people couldn't have gone through what I went through without faith in God" (O'Brien, 1982, p. 76).

For the CRF patient, often it is the therapeutic regimen, especially if consisting of maintenance hemodialysis carried out in a dialysis center, that is the most trying. One new hemodialysis patient admitted that the treatment regimen was the most difficult part of the CRF experience. "I pray to God all the time to help me stay on my treatment and to do what I have to do." The remarks of several other hemodialysis patients reflected a similar theme. "Without my religious faith, I couldn't make it"; "Religious faith really helps you go on"; "Without faith I don't know what I'd do"; and "If it hadn't been for my religion, I wouldn't even be here now" (O'Brien, 1983, p. 37).

Spiritual nursing care for the CRF maintenance dialysis patient should incorporate some element of spiritual or religious support that facilitates coping with the altered quality of life imposed by the disease and its treatment regimen. Virtually all dialysis patients report moderate to severe symptoms of fatigue and general malaise that periodically interfere with social and professional or work activities. As Joseph, a young businessman, described:

> You have to pull yourself up and do for yourself. You can't keep waiting for everybody else. Sometimes when I get up in the morning I feel bad, but I just get up and go to my business and make myself keep busy. You have to accept the fact that your kidneys are gone but you can still do things. A lot of it's in your own head, how you feel about it, how you accept it. (O'Brien, 1983, p. 40)

For a CRF patient who adheres to the theology of Reform Judaism, such as Joseph, a dimension of spiritual care might consist in exploring how his religious tradition views God's role in trials such as chronic illness. Joseph stated that "how you feel about" the illness influences "how you accept it." A comforting Scripture for Joseph might be Isaiah 43:2 ("When you pass through raging waters") or Jeremiah 29:11–12 ("For I know well the plans I have in mind for you, says the Lord, plans for your welfare, not for woe. Plans to give you a future full of hope."). Such a reading might provide the opportunity to discuss the need for hope in light of the CRF diagnosis and therapeutic regimen.

▶ Spiritual Needs of the Mentally Challenged

The Person with Mental Illness

Mental health and mental illness are relative terms, existing along a continuum of attitude and behavior; the label mental illness covers a vast array of diagnostic categories, ranging from mild conditions, such as situational anxiety and depression, to the frank psychosis of schizophrenic disorders. The concepts are culturally determined also. What may be considered pathologic in one society, such as the trancelike states entered into during some West Indian religious rituals, is normal according to the perception of that particular community. In order to determine functional mental status, some factors to be evaluated include "level of consciousness, orientation, memory, mood and affect, intellectual performance, judgement and insight and language and communication" (Bruegge, 1997, p. 715). Problems in any of these areas may reflect a deficit in one's mental health, whether of a temporary or a more lasting nature.

Mental health viewed from a Christian perspective is defined as "a state of dynamic equilibrium characterized by hope, joy and peace, in which positive self-regard is developed through love, relationship, forgiveness and meaning and purpose resulting from a vital relationship with God, and a responsible interdependence with others" (Shelly & John, 1983, p. 27). In exploring mental health for the person who does not embrace a monotheistic spirituality, this definition may be modified in terms of relationship with a deity.

The standards of psychiatric mental health nursing identify spiritual variables as important to the nurse, who is advised to be attentive to the "interpersonal, systemic, sociocultural, spiritual or environmental circumstances or events which affect the mental and emotional well-being of an individual, family or community" (American Nurses Association, 1994, as cited in Carson, 1997, p. 144). Nurses who work with those categorized as mentally ill admit that assessing spiritual needs for the psychiatric patient is a difficult task. Frequently, the patient's manifestation of spiritual concerns is considered to be "part of the client's pathology" (Mickley, Carson, & Soeken, 1995; Peterson & Nelson, 1987, p. 34). Assessing the psychiatric patient's spiritual needs may be confounded by the individual's altered thought processes (Varcarolis, 1994; Walgrove, 1996), including religious delusions and hallucinations (Fontaine, 1995b, p. 305). Judith Shelly (1983) pointed out, however, that it is precisely the fact that so many psychiatric clients do manifest religiously oriented delusions or distortions in thinking that highlights the presence of spiritual need (p. 55). Shelly observed, "Clients tend to distort only those things that are intensely meaningful to them" (p. 56). It is important, in providing spiritual care to the mentally disturbed, that a nurse understand how a patient's religious or spiritual beliefs may interact with illness symptoms. For example, in the case of an individual who perceives suffering as a penance for past sins, prayer may be "as much a part" of the healing as therapy (Shoemaker, 1996, p. 298). Another facet of mental illness, which may be supported by prayer, is that of loss of faith in God or a distancing from God, which is "a common occurrence during depressive episodes" (Fontaine, 1995a, p. 243). Suggesting the use of prayer to a client needs to be done judiciously, related to the individual's personal spiritual and religious tradition; for the client with a theistic worldview, however, prayer is identified as "one of the main spiritual tools for seeking God's help" (Walsh & Carson, 1996, p. 498). The lack of attention to spiritual care in some instances of mental health nursing has been associated with reliance on a medical model of care (Greasley, Chiu, & Gartland, 2001). It is suggested, nevertheless, that spiritual needs must be included in effective mental health nursing practice (Fry, 1998; Weaver, Flannelly, Koenig, & Larson, 1998).

To assist the nurse in distinguishing a psychiatric client's spiritual needs from those directly related to his or her mental health condition, John (1983) suggested a series of questions relating to such issues as whether a person's religious belief or behavior seems to contribute to the illness, whether religious concerns reflect a pathologic inner conflict, whether religious beliefs and behavior bring comfort or distress, and whether religion is used merely as a context for psychotic delusions (pp. 81–83). In the case of a religiously oriented delusion, the role of the person providing spiritual care is to "support the person but not the delusion" (W. Wagner, 1992, p. 156). A case example offered by Wagner is that of a psychiatric patient who asserted that because he has not done God's will, God has "taken away his brain"; the patient questioned whether God will give it back. In this situation, Wagner contended, the spiritual caregiver should focus not on the delusion or any interpretations, but rather "support the reality of God's continued love and care" for the patient (p. 156). As noted throughout this discussion, a different strategy of spiritual support will need to be provided for the psychiatric client who is not from a monotheistic religious tradition.

An example of a nursing diagnosis associated with a moderately serious condition such as mood disorder is "spiritual distress related to no purpose or joy in life; lack of connectedness to others; misperceived guilt" (Fontaine, 1995a, p. 253). Assessment of decreased spiritual well-being, associated with depression in older women, is also a diagnosis amenable to nursing intervention (Morris, 1996).

Angela McBride (1996) emphasized caring as a key dimension of the psychiatric–mental health nurse's role (p. 7); caring includes sensitivity to the values, beliefs, and practices of an individual, which is identified as the "first step" toward nursing competence in the provision of spiritual care for the patient with a mental health deficit (Campinha-Bacote, 1995, p. 24). In a study of 50 psychiatric–mental health nurses, the nurses' personal spiritual perspectives were found to be notably high (Pullen, Tuck, & Mix, 1996, p. 85). Spiritual interventions reported by the mental health nurses included "being with," or spending time with, the client; "doing for," or employing personal and environmental resources to care for the client; "encouraging the client to look inward for strength"; and "encouraging the client to look outward for people and objects that could be resources" (Tuck, Pullen, & Lynn, 1997, p. 351). The research of Awara and Fasey (2008) supports the value of providing spiritual care to the psychiatric outpatient population; and Wilding, Muir-Cochrane, and May's (2006) study of spirituality and mental health nursing concluded that mentally ill patients "wanted to discuss their experiences of spirituality" (p. 144). Spiritual care approaches for the dementia patient were identified by Bephage (2008).

An article published by the American Psychiatric Association entitled "Psychiatrists Urge More Direct Focus on Patients' Spirituality" noted, "Many patients have spiritual needs that when addressed in psychiatric treatment help unearth important existential issues and strengthen the therapeutic relationship" (Bender, 2004). A 2012 edition of a text on contemporary psychiatric nursing practice contains an entire chapter devoted to "Cultural and Spiritual Issues Related to Mental Health Care." The author, nursing professor Mary Ann Boyd, points out that "both spirituality and religion are factors that influence beliefs about mental illness" as well as having an "impact on treatment and recovery" (p. 24). Boyd asserts that "religion and spirituality can provide support and strength in dealing with mental illnesses and emotional problems" (p. 26). Some examples of spiritual interventions appropriate for nurses include "guided imagery" and "when appropriate, prayer" (p. 26).

Spirituality is considered the "heart of caring" (Aaron, 2008) and the strength of "whole person care" (Diggins, 2012) for patients dealing with mental health challenges. While it can admittedly be challenging for health-care professionals to sort out the meaning of spiritual concerns and beliefs articulated by some mentally challenged patients, it can also be challenging for the patients. This is reflected in the following comment by a patient: "Well if we talk about our belief systems to a mental health professional, we find that our medication dose is substantially increased" (Gilbert, Kaur, & Parkes, 2010, p. 29). Spirituality can be incorporated into mental health practice, however, in a number of creative ways. One example is described in the paper "Integrating Spirituality into Mental Health Rehabilitation" (Lloyd & O'Connor, 2007). Another model is presented by Janice Clarke (2010), who urges a holistic approach to mental health, employing a threefold conceptualization that consists of "soul (which contains the mind), spirit and body" (p. 649). "All three aspects," Clarke notes, "are connected in a constant dynamic cycle" (p. 649).

The challenge of incorporating a patient's spiritual beliefs into a mental health nursing assessment is addressed by Ruth Elliott (2011), who proposes some potential strategies to overcome a nurse's personal bias or prejudice. Elliott suggests the use of "recognized assessment methods to assess someone's spiritual beliefs" (p. 10) but admits that these have limitations and recommends further research on the topic. Perhaps one of the most difficult clinical conditions for which to assess spiritual beliefs is that of the patient with dementia. While the dementia patient may have the same spiritual needs as any ill person, complicating factors need to be considered, such as "expanding experience of discontinuation, which means not knowing places, names and faces, as well as declining memories" (Jolly, 2011, p. 388). However, in a study of dementia patients who scored "12 or more on the Mini Mental State Examination," 29 study participants "rated their beliefs as strong and considered practices associated with their beliefs to be very important" (Jolly et al., 2010, p. 311). The research team recommended that "service providers should integrate questions about spirituality and faith into their routine assessments and structure care plans to accommodate identified spiritual needs" (p. 311).

Specific spiritual care interventions for the psychiatric client will vary greatly, depending not only on the patient's identified needs, but also on personal spiritual and religious history. For this patient population, especially, the nurse will need to employ the art, as well as the science, of nursing.

Mathias Johnson was a 66-year-old patient suffering from moderate depression associated with a multiplicity of physical ailments, as well as financial and situational stressors. Mr. Johnson's chart identified him as Baptist, although he admitted that he was not a frequent church attender. After spending about 15 minutes visiting with Mr. Johnson, during which time he spoke briefly about faith, his nurse Beth asked if he would like her to say a prayer before leaving. Mr. Johnson nodded in the affirmative. Beth took Mr. Johnson's hand and offered a brief prayer, asking God to give Mr. Johnson strength and comfort during his illness; she also prayed that God would let the patient feel his love and care. As Beth was concluding the prayer, she noticed that tears were streaming down Mr. Johnson's face; she handed him a tissue without comment. After taking a few deep breaths, Mr. Johnson looked up and said with a smile, "Thank you, I really needed that!"

Attempting to analyze and understand the spiritual needs of a mentally ill patient, especially a depressed individual, is extremely challenging to the nurse. Much time may be spent in simply encouraging the patient to verbalize his or her concerns. During the interaction, however, the nurse can communicate a sense of care and empathy, sometimes opening the door to the possibility of therapeutic intervention in the area of spiritual need.

The Cognitively Impaired Client

Cognitive functioning affects both physical and psychosocial dimensions of an individual's life. Although cognition is "primarily an intellectual and perceptual process, [it is] closely integrated with . . . emotional and spiritual values" (Arnold, 1996, p. 977). The cognitively disabled person may have been diagnosed from infancy with some degree or type of mental retardation; cognitive processes may have been injured during childhood or early to middle adulthood as a result of illness or traumatic injury; or a cognitive disability may have its onset only in the elder years, in cases such as senile dementia.

In the past, the religious community has raised some concern about the role of the cognitively disabled individual in the church or worship setting. Some have questioned whether a person who is not cognitively functional can have a relationship with God, much less understand the meaning of religious practices. Reverend John Swinton (1997), a minister and former psychiatric–mental health nurse, admitted that theological confusion still exists about the spiritual and religious capabilities of persons with profound cognitive disabilities, and that some believe that to allow "sacramental participation without intellectual comprehension is dishonoring to God" (p. 21). Swinton argued, however, that "faith is not an intellectual exercise but relational reality," and that relationship to God is for any of us a mystery beyond intellectual understanding (pp. 21–22). True affective understanding of God, Swinton concluded, occurs at a much more interior level than that of intellectual comprehension (p. 23). Swinton's position is supported by ethicist Stanley Hauerwas (1995), who pointed out that, although including cognitively handicapped persons in worship services may not be easy, the extent to which they may bring about the unexpected is a reminder that "the God we worship is not easily domesticated" (p. 60). Hauerwas contended that "in worship the church is made vulnerable to a God who would rule this world not by coercion but by the unpredictability of love" (p. 60).

In a video entitled *We Are One Flock*, produced by the National Catholic Office for Persons with Disabilities (1990), a young woman with Down syndrome is shown assisting with the distribution of the Holy Eucharist during Mass. Her comments after the service reflect the validity of her active participation in the Eucharistic liturgy. "My idea about God is you feel it in your heart. When you really love God and you know He's around you, you feel it in your heart. And I feel it when I'm singing and when I'm ministering, and that brings me close to God, really close when I'm ministering."

A magnificent example of spiritual care for the profoundly cognitively impaired is that carried out in L'Arche (the Ark) communities founded by French Canadian philosopher Jean Vanier. Vanier (1975) began his work during a visit to the small town of Trosly, France, when he moved into a house with two mentally handicapped men. Gradually, other mentally challenged persons began to come, together with volunteers to live with and care for them. New L' Arche communities started to flourish under Vanier's spiritual philosophy of responsibility to care for one's brothers and sisters; this caring was to be done as in a family, where all are accepted and equal as God's children. Henri Nouwen (1988), who spent his later years living in a L' Arche community in Canada, wrote, "Today, L' Arche is a word that inspires thousands of people all over the world . . . its vision is a source of hope" (p. 13).

Evelyn, a veteran of 30 years in nursing, reported that she had worked for the past 13 years in an intermediate care facility (ICF), for the profoundly mentally retarded. Evelyn described her first encounter with the ICF patients:

The youngest was about 12 and that's around the age my children were. They looked strange, and they acted strange. I didn't have any experience in this field of nursing. And I said, "I will never be able to do this!" I questioned God. I said, "Why? I just can't see the value of their lives. This is just too sad." . . . Every day I would walk home from work and every day I would cry, because I felt like I wouldn't ever be able to help them. I wouldn't ever have any impact on their lives. But then one day something just started to happen, and I started to realize how they were God's children and they began to have an impact on my life. And then, I began to see that each one has their own personality. They became special to me. And I started to think that even if they live on earth for only 20 or 30 years, they are going to live in heaven forever . . .

Now they serve such purpose in my life, I couldn't imagine living my life without them. They have become so unique. Now I try to give them spiritual care. I try to anticipate their needs; I try to communicate with them and they do communicate, even if it is nonverbal . . .

I don't get to do as much "hands on" as I would like to but when I do it's such a gift. I'm so grateful. There is something so holy. You say, "this person is completely dependent upon my hands and my compassion to be cared for." They depend solely upon you. If you let yourself be used by God, this is what spiritual care means to me.

Another ICF nurse, Sarah, commented that her Jewish faith supported her spiritual care of cognitively impaired patients. "I don't believe that God is sitting up somewhere looking down on us, but I believe He is all around us. I believe that the Spirit of goodness and giving all around us is God; that's how I live spirituality." Sarah spoke about her interaction with the ICF patients. "I talk to them as people, even the very lowest cognitively functioning person is still a person, so I try to explain things to them. I also try to see that they get the best possible care that we can give. I think there is a 'spirituality of touch' in the holding and the caring. I know we can't change their abilities, but we can make sure the quality of their lives is as good as possible." Sarah concluded, "I think that the patients understand a lot more than we think sometimes. I think we can bring our spirituality and our God to them, even though we think it is beyond their intellectual functioning ability. I think my caring brings them spirituality."

Marti, another nurse who had worked with cognitively impaired young adults for many years, added, "I feel very humble in working with the MRDD [mentally retarded, developmentally disabled] population. I know their intelligence and cognitive functioning isn't where ours is, but they have a perception of reality that is childlike and Godlike all at the same time. I think touching them and loving them is spiritual care."

▶ Spiritual Needs in Physical Disability and Rehabilitation

Who are those persons on whom our society imposes the label "disabled"? Theologian Michael Downey (1993) believes that, excluding those who may temporarily require special attention such as infants and young children, the very elderly, and persons incapacitated for a time due to illness or accident, the term *disabled* generally describes individuals who are to some degree permanently impaired (p. 273). Downey (1993) defined the disabled as those persons "whose capacities of mind or body are diminished in any way during the pre, peri or post-natal period or at some later period in the course of psychosomatic development, so as to necessitate particular attention or special assistance in meeting basic human needs" (p. 273).

It should be pointed out that among 21st-century persons living with physical challenges there is some disagreement about the use of the term *disabled*. Some individuals feel that the disability label is pejorative and do not wish it used to describe their conditions; these persons prefer to call themselves *differently abled* or *other-abled*. However, there is another school of thought among some persons with physical deficits who feel that the concept of "disability" is not negative but rather an important descriptor in defining and clarifying their functional abilities. In attempting to determine the spiritual needs of one who is physically challenged it is important for a nurse to discern how that individual wishes to be viewed and labeled. For the following discussion of physical deficits and rehabilitation the classic term *disability* is being used.

Disability may affect all dimensions of an individual's life: physical, social, emotional, and spiritual. The goal of rehabilitation is to return to the disabled person as much pre-illness functioning in each of those life arenas as possible. Ultimately the goal of the rehabilitation process is to help an individual regain as much independence as possible. In analyzing the "anatomy of illness," Schreiter (1988) posited that experiencing illness for a disabled person is like taking a long journey to an unknown country: "disabled persons leave behind their accustomed ways of relating to their bodies, their friends, their workplaces, their families" (p. 7). J. L. McBride and Armstrong (1995) suggested, additionally, that while no standardized tests currently exist to measure "spiritual damage," "something does happen to the spiritual development of a person who is traumatized" (p. 7). Theologian Donald Senior (1995) pointed out that although an authentic response would be to bear the illness in a "spirit of Faith," persons with disabilities need spiritual support in the process of achieving fullness of life (p. 17). Even though Congress passed the Americans with Disabilities Act (ADA) in 1990, making it illegal to discriminate against the handicapped, individuals who make up our churches have not always internalized a supportive attitude for the disabled (Krafft, 1988).

In a book discussing the "psychospiritual aspects of rehabilitation," Carolyn Vash (1994) observed that "disability is a symbol we all fear"; this, she asserted, is why religion has not well supported the disabled (p. 49). Vash demonstrated through numerous examples from history that disabled individuals such as Helen Keller can use adversity to achieve significant life goals. The rehabilitation nurse may refer to such role models in providing spiritual care.

The concept of spiritual care is an appropriate dimension of rehabilitation nursing, which is concerned with the promotion of client wholeness (Solimine & Hoeman, 1996, p. 628). Some suggested spiritual interventions for a disabled patient experiencing rehabilitation are recommending a spiritual counselor; providing prayer materials, as denominationally appropriate; and introducing imagery, music, or meditative prayer to the client (Solimine & Hoeman, 1996, p. 636). In regard to the latter activity, Solimine and Hoeman suggested that through prayer, disabled individuals are able to give over their situation to God and "trade their weakness for God's strength" (p. 631). Accardi (1990) suggested three other pastoral care interventions for the disabled: listening to the patient's "spiritually significant stories," that is, walking with the patient on his or her spiritual journey; "indwelling the stories," or expressing the empathy and compassion that results from entering into another's pain; and "linking the stories" with biblical references that may help the person find meaning in, or the ability to transcend, the disability (p. 91).

For the rehabilitation patient not associated with a religious tradition that employs devotional practices, Boucher (1989) suggested that spiritual care may draw on such basic needs as "the need to belong, to feel attachment to a person or group, to reach out beyond oneself, to have a meaningful life, and to be creative" (p. 46). In general, spiritual care of the disabled person must focus on the acceptance of present life circumstances as a basis for future growth and accomplishment (Saylor, 1991). Some related activities include maximizing the client's wellness and assisting him or her to move out of the sick role, supporting the client's present talents and abilities, teaching the client to conserve energy and to avoid focusing on deficits, and promoting activities that enhance self-esteem (Davidhizar & Shearer, 1997, pp. 132–133).

An article entitled "Dance of Disability and Spirituality" presents the findings of in-depth interviews with 13 adults with physical disabilities. In general, the study participants "described disability and spirituality as essential, interactive dimensions of their lives . . . all but one participant expressed strong beliefs related to a higher being and all participants stressed the influence of these beliefs on their lives as a person with disability" (Boswell, Hamer, Knight, Glacoff, & McChesney, 2007, p. 35). The researchers concluded that "the interaction of spirituality and disability unfolded in the lives of these participants as a dance in which both partners influence the direction and rhythm of the steps. This interaction was characterized by five major themes: purpose, awareness, connections, creativity and acceptance" (p. 39). And, in a 2011 study exploring the needs of people with learning disabilities, clinical psychologist Claire Wilson found that spirituality was a "neglected topic across the lifespan for people with a learning disability" (p. 31). Through a series of questions, Wilson found that parents, service managers, and faith-based professionals believed that concern for a patient's spiritual needs was "a legitimate topic for health care professionals to inquire about during clinical contacts" (p. 31).

The rehabilitation nurse may employ usual spiritual assessment skills to determine the religious beliefs and practices and spiritual support system of the patient prior to the occurrence of the disability (Davis, 1994, p. 298). The point, of course, is to help the disabled patient return to former spiritual and religious practices to the degree possible. Because the rehabilitation nurse may have more time to provide spiritual care than a nurse in an acute illness setting, Clifford and Gruca (1987) suggested setting aside time to discuss spiritual needs and concerns with the client, reading meditations or poetry to the client, or playing spiritual music (p. 332).

Two nurses who worked in a rehabilitation setting with partially disabled persons described their perceptions of spiritual care. One reported:

> For me, rehabilitation nursing of patients has to do with spiritual care, with establishing the quality of their lives. One patient considers himself rehabilitated because he can walk from his house to his car; now he can get out. To him that establishes his need to be connected to people.

A second nurse added:

> Spiritual care is about quality of life, and quality of life is whatever the patient wants to make it. I have a patient who is very disabled. He can't

walk, so they got him a wheelchair with a motor on it, so he can get around and do his church work . . . that's what makes his quality of life. (O'Brien, 1983, p. 41)

▶ Spiritual Needs of the Client in the Community

Nursing care of the client in the community is carried out in the overall context of community health nursing, which is identified as "a synthesis of nursing practice and public health practice applied to promoting and preserving the health of populations" (American Nurses Association, 1980, cited in Nies & Swanson, 1997, p. 10). The American Nurses Association (ANA) definition goes on to explain that the primary responsibility of community health nursing is to the community as a whole or aggregate nursing (Nies & Swanson, 1997). In discussing the role of the community health nurse in providing spiritual care to clients, Burkhardt and Nagai-Jacobson (1985) advised that three questions may guide the initial assessment of need: Does the client's formal religious tradition or denomination provide a good structure for spiritual care? Does the way in which the client speaks or does not speak of God reveal spiritual concerns or needs? and Do the client's religious contacts seem to provide strength and comfort? (p. 194). The answers to such questions can then lead the nurse to a more detailed spiritual assessment and plans for intervention, if needed.

This section focuses on one specific dimension of community health nursing: spiritual needs of the home health-care client.

The Home Health-Care Client

McNamara (1982) defined *home health care* as "that component of comprehensive health care where services are provided to individuals and families in their places of residence for the purpose of promoting, maintaining or restoring health or minimizing the effects of illness and disability" (p. 61). Some examples of clients receiving home health care include acutely ill patients, especially those suffering from AIDS; terminally ill clients; the frail elderly; and at-risk women and children (Lyon, Bolla, & Nies, 1997, pp. 798–799). A primary component of home health care is nursing care, which is one of the largest contemporary nursing practice areas. Home health-care nurses help clients manage their prescribed plans of care and also help them cope with the social and environmental factors that may influence the course of illness and treatment (T. Smith, 1997).

Dealing with illness in the home, the client or family has to coordinate the meeting of a multiplicity of needs that may require such items as medications, medical supplies, special diet, or physical therapy equipment; the nurse can serve as advisor in obtaining necessary therapeutic materials (Humphrey, 1994, p. 1). Some home health-care clients are acutely ill, some have chronic debilitating health problems, and many are elderly. An individual must be seriously ill, homebound, and "in need of skilled nursing services" to receive home health care (Smeltzer & Bare, 1996, p. 18). A significant role identified for the home health nurse is that of client advocate (LeMone & Burke, 1996, p. 54); this title lends itself well to the inclusion of spiritual care as an appropriate activity in home health nursing.

Spiritual assessment and, if appropriate, the provision of spiritual care, are important activities for the home health nurse, as "hope and faith" have been identified as playing a major role in the home care client's adaptation to illness or disability (Rice, 1996, p. 47). Jaffe and Skidmore-Roth (1993) suggested several issues to be addressed in a spiritual assessment of the home health-care patient: religious beliefs and practice, how one's belief (or lack of belief) in a supreme being relates to illness, specific people who provide spiritual support, religious symbols of importance (e.g., a Bible or Sabbath candles), religious restrictions (dietary, medical treatment), requirements for church attendance, and religious leaders (pp. 42–43). Bauer and Barron (1995) noted that spiritual nursing interventions are particularly important for the elderly client who lives alone in the community with no religiously based support system available; the community health nurse may be the only visitor who is able and willing to discuss spiritual issues with such a client. In their research with elderly community-based clients, Bauer and Barron found that older individuals especially wanted nurses to be respectful, caring, and sensitive to their religious beliefs and traditions.

Dorothy, a community health nurse for more than 17 years, described the caring relationship she developed in providing spiritual care to clients:

> In my clinical practice in community health, it's like the "I–thou" relationship, where you give of your own spiritual energy to the people you're working with. You have to respect their beliefs and where they are spiritually, and then go from there. Some people will ask you to pray with them, if they're having a hard time, or they'll say, "think of me," and I think they just want you to send them some energy. Sometimes a patient has something very deep, like being away from their church, and you need to call in a priest or a minister. But that's part of the nurse's job, especially the community health nurse.

Megan, another nurse, with an MSN in community health nursing and 23 years of experience, added:

> You have to be attuned to what the client is saying. Sometimes they don't say it in spiritual words or religious words, but really the thing they need is some spiritual care. You have to listen with your heart to what is behind the words they say.

Personal spirituality and/or religious beliefs and practices may constitute an important mediating variable for the individual coping with a chronic illness. For the chronically ill patient, such concepts as hope, trust, courage, and love may take on new and deeper meaning following the illness onset. Nurses may support and facilitate the presence of positive attitudes and attributes in a patient's life through a variety of spiritual care interventions. As well as providing spiritual care for the hospitalized patient, contemporary nurses need to be sensitive to the spiritual needs and concerns of persons with a variety of other chronic conditions and in a variety of settings.

▶ References

Aaron, M. (2008). Spirituality, the heart of caring. *A Life in the Day, Pavilion Journals, 12*(4), 23–26.

Accardi, R. F. (1990). Rehabilitation: Dreams lost, dreams found. In H. Hayes & C. J. van der Poel (Eds.), *Health care ministry: A handbook for chaplains* (pp. 88–92). New York, NY: Paulist Press.

Adegbola, M. (2007). Spirituality and quality of life in chronic illness. *The Journal of Theory Construction & Testing, 10*(2), 42–46.

AIDS Ministry Program, the Archdiocese of St. Paul and Minneapolis. (1991). *For those we love: A spiritual perspective on AIDS.* Cleveland, OH: The Pilgrim Press.

American Nurses Association. (1980). *A conceptual model of community health nursing* (ANA publication #CHI0). Kansas City, MO: Author.

American Nurses Association. (1994). *A statement on psychiatric–mental health clinical nursing practice and standards of psychiatric–mental health clinical nursing practice.* Washington, DC: Author.

Arnold, E. N. (1996). The journey clouded by cognitive disorders. In V. B. Carson & E. N. Arnold (Eds.), *Mental health nursing: The nurse–patient journey* (pp. 977–1019). Philadelphia, PA: W. B. Saunders.

Awara, M., & Fasey, C. (2008). Is spirituality worth exploring in psychiatric outpatient clinics? *Journal of Mental Health, 17*(2), 183–191.

Baldacchino, D., & Draper, P. (2001). Spiritual coping strategies: A review of the nursing research literature. *Journal of Advanced Nursing, 34*(6), 833–841.

Bauer, T., & Barron, C. R. (1995). Nursing interventions for spiritual care. *Journal of Holistic Nursing, 13*(3), 268–279.

Belcher, A. E., Dettmore, D., & Holzemer, S. P. (1989). Spirituality and sense of well-being in persons with AIDS. *Holistic Nurse Practice, 3*(4), 16–25.

Bender, E. (2004). Psychiatrists urge more direct focus on patients' spirituality. *Psychiatric News, 39*(12), 30.

Bephage, G. (2008). Care approaches to spirituality and dementia. *Nursing & Residential Care, 10*(3), 134–137.

Blanchard, J., Dunlap, D., & Fitchett, G. (2012). Screening for spiritual distress in the oncology inpatient: A quality improvement pilot project between nurses and chaplains. *Journal of Nursing Management, 20*(8), 1076–1084.

Blevins, C., & Troutman, M. (2011). Successful aging theory and the patient with chronic renal disease: Application in the clinical setting. *Nephrology Nursing Journal, 38*(3), 255–270.

Boswell, B., Hamer, M., Knight, S., Glacoff, M., & McChesney, J. (2007). Dance of disability and spirituality. *Journal of Rehabilitation, 73*(4), 33–40.

Boucher, R. J. (1989). Nursing process. In S. S. Dittmar (Ed.), *Rehabilitation nursing: Process and application* (pp. 45–62). St. Louis, MO: C. V. Mosby.

Boutell, K. A., & Bozeht, F. W. (1988). Nurses' assessment of patients' spirituality: Continuing education implications. *Journal of Continuing Education in Nursing, 21*(4), 172–176.

Boyd, M. A. (2012). Cultural and spiritual issues related to mental health care. In M. A. Boyd (Ed.), *Psychiatric nursing, contemporary practice* (5th ed., pp. 21–28). Philadelphia, PA: Lippincott, Williams & Wilkins.

Bruegge, M. V. (1997). Assessment of clients with neurologic disorders. In J. M. Black & E. Matassmarin-Jacobs (Eds.), *Medical–surgical nursing: Clinical management for continuity of care* (5th ed., pp. 709–742). Philadelphia, PA: W. B. Saunders.

Burkhardt, M. A., & Nagai-Jacobson, M. G. (1985). Dealing with spiritual concerns of clients in the community. *Journal of Community Health Nursing, 2*(4), 191–198.

Burnard, P. (1988, December). Discussing spiritual issues with clients. *Health Visitor, 61,* 371–372.

Campinha-Bacote, J. (1995). Spiritual competence: A model of psychiatric care. *Journal of Christian Nursing, 12*(3), 22–44.

Carr, T. (2009). Mapping the processes and qualities of spiritual nursing care. *Qualitative Health Research, 18*(5), 686–700.

Carson, V. B. (1989). Spiritual development across the lifespan. In V. B. Carson (Ed.), *Spiritual dimensions of nursing practice* (pp. 24–51). Philadelphia, PA: W. B. Saunders.

Carson, V. B. (1997). Spirituality and patient care. In A. W. Burgess (Ed.), *Psychiatric nursing: Promoting mental health* (pp. 143–149). Stamford, CT: Appleton & Lange.

Carson, V. B., Soeken, K. L., Shanty, J., & Terry, L. (1990). Hope and spiritual well-being: Essentials for living with AIDS. *Perspective in Psychiatric Care, 26*(2), 28–34.

Cassidy, J. (1992, April). What keeps people well? A new paradigm for pastoral care. *Health Progress, 73*(3), 34–36.

Christensen, M. J. (1991). *The Samaritans imperative: Compassionate ministry to people living with AIDS.* Nashville, TN: Abington Press.

Clarke, J. (2010). Body and soul in mental health care. *Mental Health, Religion and Culture, 13*(6), 649–657.

Clifford, M., & Gruca, J. (1987). Facilitating spiritual care in the rehabilitation setting. *Rehabilitation Nursing, 12*(6), 331–333.

Corbin, J. (1996). Chronic illness. In S. C. Smeltzer & B. G. Bare (Eds.), *Brunner and Suddarth's textbook of medical–surgical nursing* (8th ed., pp. 317–324). Philadelphia, PA: J. B. Lippincott.

Crowther, C. E. (1991). *AIDS: A Christian handbook.* London, UK: Epworth Press.

Davidhizar, R., & Shearer, R. (1997). Helping the client with chronic disability achieve high level wellness. *Rehabilitation Nursing, 22*(3), 131–134.

Davis, M. C. (1994). The rehabilitation nurse's role in spiritual care. *Rehabilitation Nursing, 19*(5), 298–301.

Delgado, C. (2007). Sense of coherence, spirituality, stress and quality of life in chronic illness. *Journal of Nursing Scholarship, 39*(3), 229–234.

Diggins, K. (2012). Hope yields health: Offering whole person care. *Journal of Christian Nursing, 29*(1), 11–12.

Downey, M. (Ed.). (1993). Disability: The disabled. In M. Downey (Ed.), *The new dictionary of Catholic spirituality* (pp. 273–274). Collegeville, MN: The Liturgical Press.

Dreyer, E. (1993). Love. In M. Downey (Ed.), *The new dictionary of Catholic spirituality* (pp. 612–622). Collegeville, MN: The Liturgical Press.

Dwyer, J. A. (1990). Peace. In J. A. Komonchak, M. Collins, & D. A. Lane (Eds.), *The new dictionary of theology* (pp. 748–753). Collegeville, MN: The Liturgical Press.

Egan, R., McKechnie, R., Jobson, J., Herbison, P., & Richards, R. (2013). Perspectives on psychosocial and spiritual cancer support services in New Zealand. *Journal of Psychosocial Oncology, 31*(1), 659–674.

Ekedahl, M., & Wengstrom, Y. (2010). Caritas, spirituality and religiosity in nurses' coping. *European Journal of Cancer Care, 19*, 530–537.

Elliott, R. (2011). Spirituality, mental health nursing and assessment. *Journal of Community Nursing, 25*(3), 4–10.

Ellis, C. (1986, April). Course prepares nurses to meet patients' spiritual needs. *Health Progress, 9*(1), 76–77.

Fatula, M. A. (1993). Faith. In M. Downey (Ed.), *The new dictionary of Catholic spirituality* (pp. 379–390). Collegeville, MN: The Liturgical Press.

Flaherty, M. J., & O'Brien, M. E. (1992). Family styles of coping in end-stage renal disease. *ANNA Journal, 19*(4), 345–350.

Fontaine, K. L. (1995a). Mood disorders. In K. L. Fontaine & J. S. Fletcher (Eds.), *Essentials of mental health nursing* (3rd ed., pp. 236–258). New York, NY: Addison-Wesley.

Fontaine, K. L. (1995b). Schizophrenic disorders. In K. L. Fontaine & J. S. Fletcher (Eds.), *Essentials of mental health nursing* (3rd ed., pp. 300–321). New York, NY: Addison-Wesley.

Forbis, P. A. (1988). Meeting patients' spiritual needs. *Geriatric Nursing, 9*(3), 158–159.

Fry, A. (1998). Spirituality communication and mental health nursing: The tacit interdiction. *Australian New Zealand Journal of Mental Health Nursing, 7*(1), 25–32.

Gewe, A. (1994). Hope: Moving from theory to practice. *Journal of Christian Nursing, 11*(4), 18–21.

Gilbert, P., Kaur, N., & Parkes, M. (2010, October). Let's get spiritual. *Mental Health Today, 20*(6), 28–33.

Greasley, P., Chiu, L. F., & Gartland, M. (2001). The concept of spiritual care in mental health nursing. *Journal of Advanced Nursing, 33*(5), 629–637.

Greenstreet, W. (2006). From spirituality to coping strategy: Making sense of chronic illness. *British Journal of Nursing, 15*(17), 938–942.

Halstead, M. T., & Hull, M. (2001). Struggling with paradoxes: The process of spiritual development in women with cancer. *Oncology Nursing Forum, 28*(10), 1534–1544.

Hauerwas, S. (1995). The church and mentally handicapped persons: A continuing challenge to the imagination. In M. Bishop (Ed.), *Religion as a disability: Essays in scripture, theology and ethics* (pp. 46–64). Kansas City, MO: Shead & Ward.

Hellwig, M. K. (1993). Hope. In M. Downey (Ed.), *The new dictionary of Catholic spirituality* (pp. 506–515). Collegeville, MN: The Liturgical Press.

Highfield, M. F. (1992). Spiritual health of oncology patients. *Cancer Nursing, 15*(1), 1–8.

Highfield, M. F., & Cason, C. (1983). Spiritual needs of patients: Are they recognized? *Cancer Nursing, 6*(6), 187–192.

Humphrey, C. J. (1994). *Home care nursing handbook.* Gaithersburg, MD: Aspen.

Ignatavicius, D. D., Workman, M. L., & Mishler, M. A. (1995). *Medical–surgical nursing: A nursing process approach.* Philadelphia, PA: W. B. Saunders.

Iles, R. (Ed.). (1989). *The gospel imperative in the midst of AIDS.* Wilton, CT: Morehouse.

Jaffe, M. S., & Skidmore-Roth, L. (1993). *Home health nursing care plans.* St. Louis, MO: C. V. Mosby.

John, S. D. (1983). Assessing spiritual needs. In J. A. Shelly & S. D. John (Eds.), *Spiritual dimensions of mental health* (pp. 73–84). Downers Grove, IL: InterVarsity Press.

Johnson, R. P. (1992). *Body, mind, spirit: Tapping the healing power within you.* Liguori, MO: Liguori Publications.

Jolly, D. (2011). Dementia care: Spiritual and faith perspectives. *Nursing & Residential Care, 13*(8), 388–391.

Jolly, D., Bnebow, S., Grizzell, M., Willmott, S., Bawn, S., & Kingston, P. (2010). Spirituality and faith in dementia. *Dementia, 9,* 311–325.

Kaczorowski, J. M. (1989). Spiritual well-being and anxiety in adults diagnosed with cancer. *The Hospice Journal, 5*(3), 105–116.

Kennison, M. M. (1987). Faith: An untapped health resource. *Journal of Psychosocial Nursing, 25*(10), 28–30.

Kilpatrick, J. A. (1997). Urinary elimination. In P. A. Potter & A. G. Perry (Eds.), *Fundamentals of nursing: Concepts, process and practice* (4th ed., pp. 1293–1334). St. Louis, MO: C. V. Mosby.

Korniewicz, D., & O'Brien, M. E. (1994). Evaluation of a hemodialysis patient education and support program. *ANNA Journal, 21*(1), 33–38.

Krafft, J. (1988). *The ministry to persons with disabilities.* Collegeville, MN: The Liturgical Press.

Lackey, N. R., Gates, M. F., & Brown, G. (2001). African American women's experiences with the initial discovery, diagnosis and treatment of breast cancer. *Oncology Nursing Forum, 28*(3), 519–527.

Landis, B. J. (1996). Uncertainty, spiritual well-being and psychosocial adjustment to chronic illness. *Issues in Mental Health Nursing, 17*(1), 217–231.

LeMone, P., & Burke, K. M. (1996). *Medical–surgical nursing: Critical thinking in client care.* New York, NY: Addison-Wesley.

Le Peau, P. J. (1996). Finding hope when everything's up for grabs. *Journal of Christian Nursing, 13*(1), 16–19.

Lisanti, P., & Zwolski, K. (1997). Understanding the devastation of AIDS. *American Journal of Nursing, 97*(7), 26–34.

Lloyd, C., & O'Connor, C. (2007). Integrating spirituality into mental health rehabilitation. *International Journal of Therapy and Rehabilitation, 14*(4), 168–172.

Lopez, A. J., McCaffrey, R., Griffin, M. T., & Fitzpatrick, J. J. (2009). Spiritual well-being and practices among women with gynecologic cancer. *Oncology Nursing Forum, 36*(3), 300–305.

Lyon, J. C., Bolla, C. D., & Nies, M. A. (1997). The home visit and home health care. In J. M. Swanson & M. A. Nies (Eds.), *Community health nursing: Promoting the health of aggregates* (pp. 798–821). Philadelphia, PA: W. B. Saunders.

MacDonald, B. H. (2001). Quality of life in cancer care: Patients' experiences and nurses' contributions. *European Journal of Oncology Nursing, 5*(1), 32–41.

Matassarin-Jacobs, E. (1997). Nursing care of clients with renal disorders. In J. M. Black & E. Matassarin-Jacobs (Eds.), *Medical–surgical nursing: Clinical management for continuity of care* (5th ed., pp. 1625–1681). Philadelphia, PA: W. B. Saunders.

McBride, A. B. (1996). Psychiatric–mental health nursing in the twenty-first century. In A. B. McBride & J. K. Austin (Eds.), *Psychiatric–mental health nursing* (pp. 1–10). Philadelphia, PA: W. B. Saunders.

McBride, J. L., & Armstrong, G. (1995). The spiritual dynamics of chronic post traumatic stress disorder. *Journal of Religion and Health, 34*(1), 5–16.

McClain, C., Rosenfeld, B., & Breitbart, W. (2003). Effect of spiritual well-being on end-of-life despair in terminally ill cancer patients. *The Lancet, 361*(9369), 1603.

McNamara, E. (1982). Hospitals discover comprehensive home care. *Hospital, 56*(1), 60–66.

McSherry, W. (1996). Raising the spirits. *Nursing Times, 92*(3), 49–50.

Mellors, M. P., Riley, T. A., & Erlen, J. A. (1997). HIV, self-transcendence, and quality of life. *Journal of the Association of Nurses in AIDS Care, 8*(2), 59–69.

Mickley, J. R., Carson, V. B., & Soeken, K. L. (1995). Religion and adult mental health: State of the science in nursing. *Issues in Mental Health Nursing, 16*(1), 345–360.

Mickley, J. R., Soeken, K., & Belcher, A. (1992). Spiritual well-being, religiousness and hope among women with breast cancer. *Image Journal of Nursing Scholarship, 24*(4), 267–272.

Moberg, D. O. (Ed.). (1979). The development of social indicators of spiritual well-being for quality of life research. In *Spiritual well-being: Sociological perspectives* (pp. 1–13). Washington, DC: University Press of America.

Morris, L. E. (1996). A spiritual well-being model: Use with older women who experience depression. *Issues in Mental Health Nursing, 17*(1), 439–455.

Moschella, V. D., Pressman, K. R., Pressman, P., & Weissman, D. E. (1997). The problem of theodicy and religious response to cancer. *Journal of Religion and Health, 36*(1), 17–20.

Muldoon, M. H., & King, J. N. (1991). A spirituality for the long haul: Response to chronic illness. *Journal of Religion and Health, 30*(2), 99–108.

National Catholic Office for Persons with Disabilities. (1990). *We are one flock.* Washington, DC: Author.

Newshan, G. (1998). Transcending the physical: Spiritual aspects of pain in patients with HIV and/or cancer. *Journal of Advanced Nursing, 28*(6), 1236–1241.

Nies, M. A., & Swanson, J. M. (1997). Health: A community view. In J. M. Swanson & M. A. Nies (Eds.), *Community health nursing: Promoting the health of aggregates* (pp. 4–15). Philadelphia, PA: W. B. Saunders.

Nixon, A., Narayanasamy, A., & Penny, V. (2013). An investigation into the spiritual needs of neuro-oncology patients from a nurse perspective. *BMC Nursing, 12*(2), 1–11.

Nouwen, H. (1988). *The road to daybreak: A spiritual journey.* New York, NY: Doubleday.

O'Brien, M. E. (1982). Religious faith and adjustment to long-term hemodialysis. *Journal of Religion and Health, 21*(1), 68–80.

O'Brien, M. E. (1983). *The courage to survive: The life career of the chronic dialysis patient.* New York, NY: Grune & Stratton.

O'Brien, M. E. (1990). Compliance behavior and long-term maintenance dialysis. *American Journal of Kidney Disease, 15*(3), 209–214.

O'Brien, M. E. (1992). *Living with HIV: Experiment in courage.* Westport, CT: Auburn House.

O'Brien, M. E. (1995). *The AIDS challenge: Breaking through the boundaries.* Westport, CT: Auburn House.

O'Brien, M. E., Donley, R., Flaherty, M., & Johnstone, B. (1986). Therapeutic options in end-stage renal disease: A preliminary report. *ANNA Journal, 13*(6), 313–318.

O'Brien, M. E., & Pheifer, W. G. (1993). Physical and psychosocial nursing care for patients with HIV infection. *Nursing Clinics of North America, 28*(2), 303–315.

Odbehr, L., Kvigne, K., Hauge, S., & Danbolt, L. (2014). A qualitative study of nurses' attitudes toward and accommodations of patients' expressions of religiosity and faith in dementia care. *Journal of Advanced Nursing, 71*(2), 359–369.

Overberg, K. R. (Ed.). (1994). *AIDS, ethics and religion: Embracing a world of suffering.* Maryknoll, NY: Orbis Books.

Perelli, R. J. (1991). *Ministry to persons with AIDS.* Minneapolis, MN: Augsburg.

Peterson, E. A., & Nelson, K. (1987). How to meet your client's spiritual needs. *Journal of Psychosocial Nursing, 25*(5), 34–39.

Petty, J. (1997). Basic concepts of neoplastic disorders. In J. M. Black & E. Matassarin-Jacobs (Eds.), *Medical–surgical nursing: Clinical management for continuity of care* (5th ed., pp. 533–590). Philadelphia, PA: W. B. Saunders.

Pullen, L., Tuck, I., & Mix, K. (1996). Mental health nurses' spiritual perspectives. *Journal of Holistic Nursing, 14*(2), 85–97.

Raffay, J. (2014). How staff and patient experience shapes our perception of spiritual care in a psychiatric setting. *Journal of Nursing Management, 22*(7), 940–950.

Rice, R. (Ed.). (1996). Developing the plan of care and documentation. In *Home health nursing practice, concepts and application* (pp. 41–60). St. Louis, MO: C. V. Mosby.

Roche, J. (1992, March). Spiritual care of the person with AIDS. *Health Progress, 73*(2), 78–81.

Ross, L. A. (1994). Spiritual aspects of nursing. *Journal of Advanced Nursing, 9*(1), 437–440.

Russell, L. M. (Ed.). (1990). *The church with AIDS.* Louisville, KY: Westminister/John Knox Press.

Sandin, F. C. (1996). Walking through fire: Fostering faith in times of loss. *Journal of Christian Nursing, 13*(1), 23–26.

Sandys, S. (Ed.). (1993). *Embracing the mystery: A prayerful response to AIDS.* Collegeville, MN: The Liturgical Press.

Saylor, D. E. (1991). Pastoral care of the rehabilitation patient. *Rehabilitation Nursing, 16*(3), 138–140.

Schneider, M. A. (2007). Broadening our perspective on spirituality and coping among women with breast cancer and their families: Implications for practice. *Indian Journal of Palliative Care, 13*(2), 25–31.

Schreiter, R. J. (1988). The faces of suffering. *New Theology Review, 1*(4), 3–14.

Schreiter, R. (1993). Trust. In M. Downey (Ed.), *The new dictionary of Catholic spirituality* (pp. 982–983). Collegeville, MN: The Liturgical Press.

Senior, D. (1995). Beware of the Canaanite woman: Disability and the Bible. In M. Bishop (Ed.), *Religion and disability: Essays in scripture, theology and ethics* (pp. 1–26). Kansas City, MO: Sheed & Ward.

Shelly, J. A. (1983). What are spiritual needs? In J. A. Shelly & S. D. John (Eds.), *Spiritual dimensions of mental health* (pp. 55–60). Downers Grove, IL: InterVarsity Press.

Shelly, J. A., & Fish, S. (1988). *Spiritual care: The nurse's role* (3rd ed.). Downers Grove, IL: InterVarsity Press.

Shelly, J. A., & John, S. D. (1983). *Spiritual dimensions of mental health.* Downers Grove, IL: InterVarsity Press.

Sherman, D. W. (2001). The perceptions and experiences of patients with AIDS: Implications regarding quality of life and palliative care. *Journal of Hospice and Palliative Nursing, 3*(1), 7–16.

Shoemaker, N. (1996). Getting to know the traveler: Mental health assessment. In V. B. Carson & E. N. Arnold (Eds.), *Mental health nursing: The nurse–patient journey* (pp. 273–302). Philadelphia, PA: W. B. Saunders.

Simsen, B. (1988). Nursing the spirit. *Nursing Times, 84*(37), 32–33.

Smeltzer, S. C., & Bare, B. G. (1996). *Brunner and Suddarth's textbook of medical–surgical nursing* (8th ed., pp. 17–24). Philadelphia, PA: J. B. Lippincott.

Smith, T. (1997). Restorative and home health care. In P. A. Potter & A. G. Perry (Eds.), *Fundamentals of nursing: Concepts, process and practice* (4th ed., pp. 79–95). St. Louis, MO: C. V. Mosby.

Smith, W. J. (1988). *AIDS: Issues in pastoral care.* New York, NY: Paulist Press.

Soeken, K. L., & Carson, V. B. (1987). Responding to the spiritual needs of the chronically ill. *Nursing Clinics of North America, 22*(3), 603–611.

Solimine, M. A., & Hoeman, S. P. (1996). Spirituality: A rehabilitation perspective. In S. P. Hoeman (Ed.), *Rehabilitation nursing: Process and application* (2nd ed., pp. 628–643). St. Louis, MO: C. V. Mosby.

Stoll, R. I. (1989). Spirituality and chronic illness. In V. B. Carson (Ed.), *Spiritual dimensions of nursing practice* (pp. 180–216). Philadelphia, PA: W. B. Saunders.

Sunderland, R. H., & Shelp, E. E. (1987). *AIDS: A manual for pastoral care.* Philadelphia, PA: The Westminister Press.

Swinton, J. (1997). Restoring the image: Spirituality, faith and cognitive disability. *Journal of Religion and Health, 36*(1), 21–27.

Taylor, C., Lillis, C., & LeMone, P. (1997). *Fundamentals of nursing: The art and science of nursing care* (3rd ed.). Philadelphia, PA: J. B. Lippincott.

Taylor, E. J., Amenta, M., & Highfield, M. (1995). Spiritual care practices of oncology nurses. *Oncology Nursing Forum, 22*(1), 31–39.

Taylor, E. J., Highfield, M., & Amenta, M. (1994). Attitudes and beliefs regarding spiritual care. *Cancer Nursing, 17*(6), 479–487.

Taylor, E. J., & Mamier, I. (2005). Spiritual care nursing: What cancer patients and family caregivers want. *Journal of Advanced Nursing, 49*(3), 260–267.

Thomas, J., & Retsas, A. (1999). Transacting self-preservation: A grounded theory of the spiritual dimensions of people with terminal cancer. *International Journal of Nursing Studies, 36*(3), 191–201.

Thompson, M. (1994). Nurturing hope: A vital ingredient in nursing. *Journal of Christian Nursing, 11*(4), 11–17.

Tuck, I., Pullen, L., & Lynn, C. (1997). Spiritual interventions provided by mental health nurses. *Western Journal of Nursing Research, 19*(3), 351–363.

Turk, D., & Rudy, T. (1986). Living with chronic disease: The importance of cognitive appraisal. In J. S. McHugh & T. Vallis (Eds.), *Illness behavior: A multidisciplinary model* (pp. 309–320). New York, NY: Plenum Press.

Ungvarski, P. J., & Matassarin-Jacobs, E. (1997). Nursing care of clients with altered immune systems. In J. M. Black & E. Matassarin-Jacobs (Eds.), *Medical–surgical nursing: Clinical management for continuity of care* (5th ed., pp. 614–651). Philadelphia, PA: W. B. Saunders Company.

Vanier, J. (1975). *Be not afraid.* New York, NY: Paulist Press.

Varcarolis, E. M. (Ed.). (1994). Alterations in mood: Grief and depression. In *Foundation of psychiatric-mental health nursing* (2nd ed., pp. 415–464). Philadelphia, PA: W. B. Saunders.

Vash, C. L. (1994). *Personality and adversity: Psychospiritual aspects of rehabilitation.* New York, NY: Springer.

Wagner, C. D. (1996). Family needs of chronic hemodialysis patients: A comparison of perceptions of nurses and families. *ANNA Journal, 23*(1), 19–26.

Wagner, W. (1992). The voices on psychiatry: Inner tumult and the quest for meaning. In L. E. Holst (Ed.), *Hospital ministry: The role of the chaplain today* (pp. 151–162). New York, NY: Crossroad.

Walgrove, N. J. (1996). Unique attributes of successful travelers: Personal strengths for the journey. In V. B. Carson & E. N. Arnold (Eds.), *Mental health nursing: The nurse–patient journey* (pp. 175–190). Philadelphia, PA: W. B. Saunders.

Walsh, M. B., & Carson, V. B. (1996). Mind, body, spirit therapies. In V. B. Carson & E. N. Arnold (Eds.), *Mental health nursing: The nurse–patient journey* (pp. 487–502). Philadelphia, PA: W. B. Saunders.

Warner-Robbins, C. G., & Christiana, N. M. (1989). The spiritual needs of persons with AIDS. *Family Community Health, 12*(2), 43–51.

Weaver, A. J., Flannelly, L. T., Flannelly, K. J., Koenig, H. G., & Larson, D. B. (1998). An analysis of research on religious and spiritual variables in three major mental health nursing journals, 1991–1995. *Issues in Mental Health Nursing, 19*(3), 263–276.

White, M. L. (2013). Spirituality self-care effects on quality of life for patients diagnosed with chronic illness. *Self-Care, Dependent-Care and Nursing, 20*(1), 23–32.

Wilding, C., Muir-Cochrane, E., & May, E. (2006). Treading lightly: Spirituality issues in mental health nursing. *International Journal of Mental Health Nursing, 15,* 144–152.

Wilson, C. (2011). Is there a case for community learning disability teams considering the spiritual needs of people with learning disabilities? *Tizard Learning Disability Review, 16*(3), 31–40.

CHAPTER 9

Spiritual Needs of Children and Families

We are made by relationships with other people.

Carlo Carretto, *Summoned by Love*, 1978

We've sent dying children home on palliative care, and that is very challenging, knowing that you're stopping all your care. But it may be best for their future illness trajectory. I think that at times like this, viewing nursing as a vocation, we had to put our own emotions aside and help the family make the best decision. . I think your personal faith comes in a lot in that situation . . . I think that if you view nursing as a vocation, you're able to have more open conversations with the family; about what all this means spiritually and help them make the decisions they need to make.

Tara, Team Leader on a Pediatric Unit

In this chapter, the spiritual needs of the ill child are identified and described through reports of the author's interactions with children living with such illnesses as cancer, including leukemia and lymphoma, and human immunodeficiency virus (HIV) infection. The spiritual needs of family members of both ill children and ill adults are also documented in data elicited through formal and informal interviews and observations. Patient and family data are supplemented through interviews with nurses caring for ill children and their families. The first part of the chapter is directed toward the spiritual needs of the ill child in a variety of settings; the latter part explores the spiritual needs of the family, beginning with those of the new and expanding family at the time of childbirth and concluding with a discussion of family needs in terminal illness.

▶ Spiritual Needs of the Child

Perhaps no therapeutic intervention calls on the nurse's creative skills as much as that of providing spiritual care to an ill child. Children are unique and challenging in their varied developmental stages (Kenny, 1999); as frequently noted, a child is much more than a small adult. Children, especially ill children, tend to be astoundingly straightforward in expressing their questions and concerns. They expect no less from their caregivers. Honesty and directness, to the degree possible and appropriate, is the most therapeutic approach for a nurse in the provision of spiritual care to an ill child.

It is suggested that children are "born with 'spiritual competence', an inner quality or power for faith development, thus assessment and intervention techniques must be developed unique to the population" (Mueller, 2010, p. 197). Spiritual care must be considered from a child's earliest days in a neonatal intensive care unit (Caldeira & Hall, 2012), through school-age years (Quinlivan, 2014) up to adolescence (Spurr, Berry, & Walker, 2013). Spiritual needs of ill children, such as those critically ill with cancer, should be specifically addressed focusing on such issues as "assessing spiritual needs; assisting the child to express feelings; guiding the child in strengthening relationships; helping the child to be remembered; assisting the child to find meaning; and aiding the child to find hope" (Peterson, 2013, p. 1243).

Spirituality and the Child

Children! They are such a joy and such a mystery in our lives! Who can ever express sufficiently all that they are able to communicate, through gifts unknown to themselves . . . ? They make us understand something of the living God by the trust they show us.

—**Roger of Taizé**, 1990

The term *child* is broadly understood to refer to a young person from the developmental stage following infancy to the onset of adolescence; that is, from approximately 1 to 12 years of age. Moran (1997) identified the formal stages of growth and development as newborn (birth to 1 month), infancy (1 month to 1 year), toddlerhood (1 to 3 years), preschool age (3 to 6 years), school age (6 to 11 or 12 years), and adolescence (11 or 12 to 21 years of age) (p. 28). A child's trajectory of physical and psychological growth is accompanied by a parallel process of moral development (Kohlberg, 1984) and spiritual or faith development (Fowler, 1981).

In describing a child's moral development, Lawrence Kohlberg (1984) posited three phases of morality: the preconventional level (early childhood), the conventional level (later childhood to adolescence), and the postconventional level (adulthood). In brief, Kohlberg's schema suggests that the child progresses from an initial stage of simple acceptance of right and wrong, as identified through punishment or non-punishment for an act; to the school-age phase of more abstract understanding of morality; and later, to the adolescent/adult stage, encompassing a societal view of right and wrong.

James Fowler (1981) proposed a paradigm of spiritual development across the life span, labeled "stages of faith development." Of Fowler's seven faith stages, three may be associated with the child's parallel physical and psychological development. Stage 2, intuitive–projective faith, is the period when the preschool child is influenced by the example of adults. During this period, God is often imagined as appearing similar to adult figures with whom the child interacts, and the child may imitate the religious practices of the family without really understanding the meaning. Many preschoolers, around age 5 or 6, can create their own prayers, and a number attend church services with the family. Stage 3, mythic–literal faith, occurs during the school-age period, as the child begins to internalize religious beliefs. The child understands and accepts a more sophisticated God from a monotheistic tradition and develops a conscience. Early school-age children pray and trust that prayers will be answered. Religious stories are often appreciated during this period, especially those describing biblical or religious heroes. Stage 4, synthetic–conventional faith, is developed during the adolescent period. The teen may begin to question some or all of the religious beliefs and practices of the family. Faith experiences occur outside of the home, and the adolescent begins to claim his or her own faith identity. Some teens become very involved in their faith and religious experience during the adolescent years; they may interact with other young people of similar religious belief as a significant peer group.

Burkhardt (1991) believes that children "live in their spirits more than adults," because they are less inhibited and more intuitive about spiritual matters (p. 34); she noted that while understanding the work of the developmental theorists is important, one should adopt a broad definition of spirituality in working with children (p. 34). Spirituality related themes suggested by Burkhardt (1991) include the child's capacity for searching for meaning in life; a sense of relationship to "self, others, nature, and God or Universal Force"; and spirituality, viewed as the "deepest core" of the child's being (p. 34). The comments of Anne Marie, a doctorally prepared pediatric nurse practitioner, reflect Burkhardt's perception related to a child's intuition:

> Working with children you have to have a very clear sense of your own spirituality, because they are very sensitive to the spiritual in others. You have to have a spirituality that projects total acceptance because, if not, the kids can read right through it; anything that's a facade or put on, they know it in a heartbeat . . . In my nursing with children and families I have learned a lot about spiritual needs. I think some nurses are uncomfortable with spiritual care, to go into a 9-year-old's room and ask if he wants to talk about something religious. You just need to be open and give them the chance. They're not afraid of the hard questions, like "what's it like to die?" or "will I die?"; but you have to not be afraid to let them ask. Children will give you spiritual clues; you just have to pick up on them.

In exploring the spirituality of 40 children, ages 4 to 12, David Heller (1985) discovered differences in prayer styles among children from Jewish, Catholic, Protestant, and Hindu traditions. For example, whereas Baptist children reported being comfortable with silent devotion, both Catholic and Jewish children perceived prayer as associated with more formal religious ritual; Hindu children preferred chanting (p. 14). Psychologist Robert Coles (1990) offered poignant examples of differing religious beliefs of school-age children in his book *The Spiritual Life of Children*. Coles identified four spiritual themes from his conversations with children of different traditions: Christian salvation, Islamic surrender, Jewish righteousness, and secular soul-searching. Mary, a 9-year-old Christian with whom Coles conversed, explained that Jesus "died so we will live forever" (p. 203). Rita, a 10-year-old Muslim, asserted, "God is the one who made us, and He'll be the one to decide where we go" (p. 233). Joseph, a 12-year-old Jewish boy, explained, "We have the book, our Bible; it tells us what we should believe . . . a Jew is someone who lives the law" (p. 253). Finally, in examining the concept of secular soul-searching, Robert Coles spoke with 12-year-old Eric, who reported that although he did not belong to any church, he did sometimes "wonder" about things such as the existence of God (pp. 281–283).

The Ill Child and Religious Practice

"Children," Young and Koopsen (2011) point out "unlike adults, do not make clear distinctions between spirituality and religion" (p. 285). Children do, however "draw on previous experiences of life, including religious and spiritual beliefs . . . to cope with crises" (McSherry & Smith, 2006, p. 17). For a child of any religious tradition who is experiencing illness, the ability to participate in religious devotions or practices, such as prayer, may provide a source of comfort and stability. Religious practices and beliefs can affect a child's health; illness may be interpreted in light of a child's religious understanding (Spector & Spertac, 1990, p. 58). The presence in a sickroom of devotional articles such as holy pictures, statues, crucifixes, crosses, or Bibles may provide a sense of security and stability during the disruption of usual life activities. For the preschooler who has a concrete concept of God as protector and father, simple bedtime prayers, such as "Now I lay me down to sleep, I pray the Lord my soul to keep," may help the child to feel more at ease during the night. The reading of a religious story or looking at images from a children's picture Bible can be comforting. If mealtime grace is usual in the family, this may be carried out in the sickroom. A preschooler, ill during a religious holiday such as Christmas, Easter, or Hanukkah, should be encouraged to participate in as many of the associated rituals as possible, to help maintain some sense of normalcy in the child's life.

In the case of an ill school-age child, use of a Bible or prayer book, if part of one's tradition, can be encouraged. A Jewish child may want to experience the lighting of Sabbath candles on Friday evening and have traditional passages from Hebrew Scripture read to him or her. The early school-age child can be encouraged to pray, but will, as noted earlier, expect to have prayers answered, so some counseling may need to be done around that issue. The older school-age child will have learned that prayers are not always directly answered; thus a discussion about the meaning of prayer will be helpful. Some school-age children find it important when ill to continue to participate in certain religious practices such as reception of the sacraments (Holy Eucharist and the Sacrament of Reconciliation), also. Special religious anniversaries, such as Christmas, Easter, Rosh Hashanah, Yom Kippur, Hanukkah, and Ramadan, may be very important to the school-age child, especially if participation in the associated worship rituals is usual in the family. Some reflections of the religious meaning of the celebrations may be brought into the child's sickroom, for example, the setting up of a small Christmas crèche or a menorah. These spiritual symbols can help the child cope with the frightening nature of an illness experience.

The ill adolescent may need spiritual counseling about the relationship of his or her sickness to the religious or spiritual meaning of life. During this developmental period, when the teen may question many of the tenets of organized religion, the young person might well question "why me?" in relation to an illness. The adolescent who has a strong commitment to his or her church and has experienced consistent participation in activities such as weekly Sunday school, church youth group, youth choir, or Bible study group may experience significant anxiety over not being able to participate in these activities, which are social as well as religious. Visits from an adolescent's peers in such a church group can provide support and comfort, as well as distracting the teen from the illness experience. Adolescence is also a time when young people cherish privacy. Teens often choose to keep their deepest and most treasured feelings to themselves. Thus, adolescents may "reject formal worship services, but engage in individual worship in the privacy of their rooms" (Wong, 1997, p. 472).

It is important, even in illness, to allow for such periods of privacy, to the degree possible, for an adolescent patient.

In a study of hope and spiritual well-being in adolescent cancer patients, Hendricks-Ferguson (2008) found higher levels of spiritual well-being and religious well-being in the earlier time periods after diagnosis; it was suggested that health-care professionals assess and plan spiritual care interventions for this patient population (p. 397).

Sometimes a very ill adolescent will request a church-associated ritual. Evelyna was a hospitalized 16-year-old from a Latin American country whose lymphoma was terminal. As a Catholic, Evelyna requested the sacrament of the Eucharist each day. One afternoon, after the chaplain, Sister Elizabeth, had administered the sacrament and offered a prayer, Evelyna looked up and said, "Sister, will you lay hands on me?" Because the "laying on of hands" is not a common practice in the Roman Catholic tradition, Sister Elizabeth was not certain what Evelyna desired, but wanted to honor her request. Several members of the family were present, so the chaplain asked that all gather around the bed with her and place their hands on Evelyna while God's blessing was sought. Especially in the case of an ill child, nurses and chaplains often have the opportunity to create small religious rituals appropriate to the sickroom setting and yet helpful in meeting the spiritual needs of the patient and the family.

Assessment of the Ill Child's Spiritual and Religious Needs

As to the question of whether a child is capable of having a serious relationship with God, Judith Shelly (1982) noted that "stories abound of very young children who made serious and lasting commitments to God" (p. 12). Obviously a child's spiritual interests and concerns will vary greatly depending on age and the religious or denominational tradition of the family. Some broad measurement items reflective of religious tradition contained in a "family assessment interview" (Wong, 1997, p. 90) include identification of usual religious beliefs and practices, whether the family associates with a particular denomination or church, how religious beliefs influence the family's perception of illness, whether the family relies on religious healers or remedies for illness, and who provides religious support for the family (e.g., clergy, relatives, or healers). Pediatric head nurse Judith Van Heukelem-Still (1984) wrote that, in assessing the spiritual needs of children, it is important not only to ask questions but also to observe the child for unusual behaviors such as nightmares or withdrawal from social activities (p. 5). She pointed out that the kind of visitors and cards a child receives may give some hint of whether spiritual influences and support are present (p. 5).

Spiritual assessment questions that Van Heukelem (1982) identified for an ill child focused on such topics as how the child behaves when frightened, who provides support in times of trouble, and what the child's understanding is of God and prayer (p. 89). A nursing diagnosis of spiritual distress can be identified for the ill child. Some defining characteristics of the diagnosis might relate to the child or family's lack of spiritual support or spiritual strength (Marlow & Redding, 1988, p. 78). Nursing interventions for a child reflecting spiritual distress may begin by encouraging the child to verbalize his or her feelings to a caring adult. Elkins and Cavendish (2004) assert that "developing a plan for pediatric spiritual care" should include attention to "the child's spirituality, religion, culture, developmental stage, age-appropriate spiritual care activities, and the needs of the family" (p. 179).

Some of the needs of ill children identified by nursing professor Carolyn Mueller (2010) as important in assessment of spiritual needs include "assistance in dealing with feelings of fearfulness, anxiousness or for coping with pain or other physical symptoms . . . and help exploring such questions as 'Why me?' 'What is the meaning and purpose of suffering?' and 'When or how will death occur'" (p. 200). Peter, a six-year-old lymphoma patient, confronted his pediatric nurse practitioner one day with the question, "What will heaven be like?" His nurse, who really had no idea what kind of response Peter was hoping for, responded that "Heaven is where God lives and heaven will be beautiful, with green grass and flowers and big trees to climb with lots of leafy branches to sit on and a swing." Peter was comforted; his nurse's assessment of what information was needed at that point seemed accurate.

Spiritual Needs of the Acutely Ill Child

Pediatric nursing care, as defined by the American Nurses Association and the Society of Pediatric Nurses (1996), "focuses on helping children and their families and communities achieve their optimum health potentials" (cited in Ashwill, Droske, & Imhof, 1997, p. 11). Spiritual care of the pediatric patient is directed toward helping the child and family achieve and maintain the greatest degree of spiritual health possible, in light of the present illness experience. As noted, in terms of assessment of spiritual need, the defining characteristics of spiritual health will vary according to the child's age, religious tradition, and the severity of the illness. Pediatric chaplain George Handzo (1990) advised that, regardless of religious background, one must be direct and frank in talking about spirituality with an ill child. "Children think a lot about faith and have more ability in theological reflection than most adults give them credit for" (p. 17). Chaplain Handzo asserted that children have essentially the "same faith needs as adults"; they need to view God as one who will care for and support them, especially in times of crisis such as that of illness (p. 18).

The child experiencing an acute illness, even if being cared for at home, may suffer psychosocial sequelae such as loneliness related to isolation from a peer group and interruption of school and school-related social activities (Melamed & Bush, 1985). For the older school-age child or adolescent, missing classes may cause not only a sense of alienation from peers, but also anxiety about future goals related to college and career. The adolescent may worry about "keeping up" with classes, even in the case of a relatively temporary condition. The ill teen whose schoolwork has been interrupted may feel some anger at God or at religious beliefs and question "Why me?" Spiritual counseling at such a time will allow the adolescent to verbalize frustration and potentially achieve a degree of peace and patience, a sense that ultimately all will be well.

Sixty children with advanced cancer, ages 6 to 17, were asked to respond to a spiritual quality-of-life interview; "seventy-eight percent of the interviewees reported that they did something to 'feel close to God.' Children prayed for a 'sense of normalcy' (59%) and relational concerns (31%)" (Kamper, VanCleve, & Savedra, 2010, p. 301). Kamper, VanCleve, and Savedra point out that "Children's care will be enhanced when given the opportunity to express their spiritual and relational concerns" (p. 301).

For the young child who is acutely ill, spiritual care may be directed toward interaction with a parent or parents. Hashim was a six-year-old Muslim child with acute lymphocytic leukemia; his father Mr. Mukti stayed with him almost continuously during a hospitalization, while his mother cared for the family's other children. On a first visit, the unit's chaplain, Elizabeth, asked Mr. Mukti if it would be acceptable, even though she was a Christian, to say a prayer for Hashim, who was receiving chemotherapy. Mr. Mukti responded, "Oh, yes, yes, we all worship the same God; you call him God; we say Allah! But He is the same God." This, and subsequent interactions with Hashim and Mr. Mukti gave Elizabeth the opportunity to discuss and learn more about Islam and the spiritual needs of a Muslim patient. One of Elizabeth's colleagues taught her a Muslim greeting in Arabic: *A salaam a le kum* (Peace be unto you). She asked Mr. Mukti if it would be appropriate for her to greet him and Hashim with the blessing when she visited. Mr. Mukti replied enthusiastically, "Oh, yes, that's wonderful. It means may you be filled with God's blessing. You can say the words when you arrive and when you leave and we will answer asking a blessing for you, *A le kum a salaam.*"

The Hospitalized Child

The hospitalized child is generally experiencing an acute illness or an acute exacerbation of a chronic condition. Such factors as the severity of illness, type of care unit (e.g., pediatric intensive care unit versus general pediatric care unit), previous hospital experience, and family support will influence the child's emotional and spiritual needs. Ashwill and Volz (1997) identified some universal stressors for the hospitalized child, however, including separation from family, fear of pain or physical injury, and fear of the unknown. Although the primary goal of a pediatric hospital unit is care of the ill child, parents, an important resource, also need attention (Hardgrove & Roberts, 1989; Leavitt, 1989). The spiritual care of the child should include spiritual support of the parents. In discussing spiritual ministry in a pediatric unit, Arnold (1992) asserted that pediatric ministry must include the entire family (p. 94). Because, Arnold noted, hospitalization of a child represents a crisis situation, needs are usually identified in spiritual language: "hope, trust, love and acceptance"; such needs may be met through the use of religious resources or simply by developing caring relationships with the child and family (p. 95).

A study of the identified spiritual needs of five hospitalized children revealed key themes emerging from the interview data related to "the role of the child's relationship with family, friends, and healthcare professionals, the impact of the hospital environment on the child, coping with invasive procedures and (the child's religious) beliefs" (Bull & Gillies, 2007, p. 34). The study authors assert that all health-care professionals must recognize that children have spiritual needs that can include religious beliefs, and that it is part of their duty of care to attempt to identify and meet such needs (p. 38). This can best be done by "taking time to talk and listen with each child, [which] enables a health care professional to identify, and therefore try to meet, the needs of children" (p. 38).

Anna was a 13-year-old hospitalized for evaluation and staging of her escalating Ewing's sarcoma with metastasis; there was a question of surgery, which would include a radical amputation of her right leg, including a hemipelvectomy. Anna's disease was progressing rapidly and known sources of chemotherapy had been exhausted. Anna relied on her own and her family's religious resources and demonstrated spiritual peace in her hope and trust in God; this was reinforced by hospital nursing staff and chaplains. Anna resisted the surgery, which physicians agreed had little chance of successfully alleviating the disease process; she decided to place her trust in God, fully aware that a physical cure might not happen. That was okay, Anna assured the staff, because, in her words, she was in a "win–win situation." She explained, "If God heals my body, then it will be wonderful and I can be a missionary and tell people about Him; but if He doesn't, then I will die and be with Jesus, so there's no way I can lose" (O'Brien, 1995, p. 141).

Spiritual Needs of the Chronically Ill Child

Childhood chronic illness is a long-term condition for which there is no cure, and which may affect the child's physical and psychological functioning. Statistics suggest that 10 to 15 percent of the pediatric population is chronically ill (Martin, 1997). Management of a child's chronic illness is complicated because of the necessity of family involvement in the provision of care (Johnson, 1985). A situation of childhood chronic illness may interfere in sibling relationships because parental attention is often heavily focused on the sick child. Although some non-ill siblings cope well, jealousy and emotional distress can occur for the well child (Holiday, 1989); the situation may thus engender feelings of guilt and inadequacy in the chronically ill sibling.

Fulton and Moore (1995) believe that the spiritual well-being of the school-age child with a chronic illness significantly affects the course of illness and treatment (p. 224). They described two nursing approaches to providing spiritual care as "therapeutic play," to generate understanding of the child's perception of spirituality vis-à-vis the illness experience; "bibliotherapy," employing such techniques as storytelling or journaling to help the child explore the meaning of life; and "use of self" in establishing rapport that may comfort the child and decrease anxiety associated with the illness and treatment (Fulton & Moore, 1995, pp. 228–231). The importance of providing devotional material to an older chronically ill child is described by a mother who reported that until her physically and cognitively disabled son's "beloved and much read Children's Bible" had recently fallen apart, he had carried it daily, attached to his walker (Cichon, 1995, p. 24).

Tony, an 18-year-old with recurrent lymphoma, was hospitalized for a course of chemotherapy. Although he talked mostly about sports with the nurses, his chaplain, Elizabeth, noticed a small worn Bible on the bedside stand. Tony's religious prefer-ence was listed on his chart simply as "Christian." As she was leaving the room one day, Elizabeth asked Tony if he would like her to read a passage from Scripture. Tony smiled and said, "Yes, that would be good. You pick something." Elizabeth chose a comforting passage about God's care from Matthew 6:25–30, commonly called the "lilies of the field" passage. "Therefore I tell you, do not worry about your life . . . If God so clothes the grass of the fields . . . how much more will he not provide for you." Tony responded, "When I think like that, there really isn't anything to worry about. I get pretty scared about this cancer sometimes but when I put my thoughts to God, I know it's going to be okay. If God takes care of the birds and the flowers, He'll take care of me."

▶ Spiritual Needs of the Dying Child

It has been asserted that "caring for a child at the end of life stage is one of the greatest challenges a nurse can encounter in practice" (Pearson, 2010, p. 31). The manner in which a nurse cares for a dying child may well "help shape the experience the young patient is about to face" (p. 31). Children, especially dying children, do have a spiritual dimension and it thus becomes very important to address their spiritual, as well as physical and emotional, needs (Hufton, 2006, p. 240). In describing the spirituality of an eight-year-old with terminal leukemia, Jerome (2011) reported that "although her short life was filled with challenges . . . [her] spirituality was an innate essence . . . it supported her in shoring up her resources and bearing the burden of her illness and impending death" (p. 200).

Like other ill children, the dying child's spiritual needs are reflective of age, spiritual or religious background, and degree of physiologic and cognitive functioning. As a rule, the broad needs of dying children model those of dying adults; they desire comfort and freedom from pain, and the security that they will not be alone at the time of death (Martin, 1997, p. 414). These needs, Martin added, will be more acutely manifested in the school-age child and the adolescent (p. 414). Four of the most frequently occurring emotional reactions of dying children are "fear, depression, guilt and anger" (Winkelstein, 1989, p. 231). A school-age child, especially, may experience fear related not so much to the death itself but rather to the dying process. Children of this age may have witnessed the deaths of older family members or friends and are fearful of having to go through the pain and suffering they observed. The preschooler can feel guilty about dying, and leaving parents and siblings; he or she may feel responsible for the illness. The dying adolescent, while also experiencing some degree of fear and guilt, frequently goes through a period of depression and anger over the illness and impending death. As noted earlier, adolescence is the time of questioning spiritual and religious beliefs, as well as being the developmental stage when privacy is valued. Thus the dying adolescent may internalize and hide feelings of anger and depression for some time, resulting in an unexpected eruption of emotion as death nears.

To provide spiritual care to dying children, pediatric chaplain Dane Sommer (1989) advised that the caregiver become "theologically honest" (p. 231); that is, in order to help the child cope with suffering and death, nurses must be able to imagine their own deaths and admit that their personal faith may not provide satisfactory answers to the question, why? An exercise integral to most hospice training programs is imagining one's death and writing a personal obituary. A second requirement for those caring for dying children, identified by Chaplain Sommer, is to be able to "speak the language of children" and "enter into" the child's world (p. 231). The nurse must be sensitive to the age-related developmental stage of the child and also keep in mind that children can "see through" dishonesty and subterfuge quite easily; they find security in truth and directness, even if the information is painful. Caregivers must remember as well that a dying child who has experienced significant contact with the health-care system may be very knowledgeable about his or her disease; such children expect information at a level of sophistication that may seem far beyond that warranted by chronological age. In an article presented in the *American Journal of Hospice and Palliative Medicine*, spirituality was identified as a key need in an empirically developed conceptual model of the needs of children with life-limiting conditions (Donnelly, Huff, Lindsey, McMahon, & Schumacher, 2005).

Pediatric oncologist Kate Faulkner (1997) offered some general suggestions related to caring for a dying child; these include being flexible in one's approach, being sensitive to the use of nonverbal communication, respecting the child's desire for privacy, and being "explicit and literal" in responding to questions about death (p. 69). These maxims are most appropriate for the provision of spiritual care. Regardless of a dying child's age and religious tradition, a nurse needs to employ the art as well as the science of nursing in approaching such difficult topics as spirituality and death. Perhaps the best advice is to let the child take the lead, through questions or comments; the nurse can then attempt to cross over, as it were, to the child's world, to that place where the dying child may feel alone. Thus the nurse can become friend and advocate, as well as spiritual caregiver.

Teresa, a baccalaureate-prepared pediatric oncology nurse, described the difficulty and the rewards of such nursing advocacy:

> In peds oncology, the most stressful time is around a child's death, and it's the most rewarding time also. It's a gifted experience to be with that child and family. It's a lot like being a midwife to send the child to God; but it hurts so much to lose them when you've become their friend and the family's friend. But it's a spiritual experience for the nurse and for the child. Sometimes you pray with them, sometimes you sing hymns with them, and then again, maybe you just hold them.

Teresa, a Christian, explained that, for her, if the dying child was from a religious family, it was sometimes easier to know how to give spiritual care. "I mean, you know there are certain prayers or rituals for a Christian or for a Jewish child." Teresa related a recent experience with a dying eight-year-old who did not believe in God and who asked her what would happen after death. She said, "I told him it would be like walking in a beautiful woods, a beautiful forest where there are all kinds of trees and flowers and birds, and everything will be really peaceful. And, that he will be happy and not ever be sick again."

Pam, a master's-prepared pediatric nurse, also described the rewards of providing spiritual care for dying children:

> I was raised Southern Baptist and that is generally my preference, although I also consider myself a born-again Christian. I would never impose my beliefs on anyone, especially a child, but I feel that I can discuss spiritual needs and assess children's needs, especially for the dying child. I have prayed with children, but sometimes maybe it's just listening and a hug. And in some instances I would call a chaplain . . . I have found the chaplains to be very good—excellent, in fact. It's just that sometimes you are the one who is there, who the child knows and will talk to. This is a special gift for you; it's real rewarding. I think spiritual care is definitely in the pediatric nurse's job description.

Certainly not to be neglected in the case of a dying child are the spiritual needs of the family, those of both parents and healthy siblings. As in caring for the child, a nurse will need to call on all of his or her own spiritual strength and experience in order to journey with a family during the predeath and death experience. Cook (1982) suggested, first, that one accept that the family members are probably "not totally rational" during this time (p. 125). Second, Cook advised that the family be encouraged to "continue to function as a family," and that family communication be fostered (p. 125). A parent of a dying child may express seemingly undue anger over a small "glitch" in the provision of hospital or hospice nursing care; this is related to the terrible frustration associated with the loss of parental control in protecting one's child. Nonjudgmental, caring support expressed by a nurse during such an outburst may go far in alleviating the parent's anxiety. The family may also experience internal disorganization during the terminal illness and death of a child. With the ill child receiving so much attention, well siblings can experience feelings of neglect and rejection. Well siblings may also feel guilty about being healthy while a brother or sister is suffering from catastrophic illness. A supportive nurse who welcomes the verbalization of fears and anxieties on the part of all members of the family can facilitate communication between parents and well children.

Camille, a pediatric oncology nurse with more than 22 years of experience, spoke articulately about the spiritual care and spiritual needs of the family of a dying child:

> I think especially that nurses have to be careful not to be overzealous and impulsive with sharing their own spirituality, like saying, "this is God's will." The parents may be angry at God and not ready to hear that. Families accepting a terminally ill child is something they have to work through at their own pace; you don't want somebody anticipating that for you. Part of the art of nursing, the art of being human, is to determine where a person is spiritually. You want to embrace their needs and provide them empathy, but not overwhelm them . . . You have to remember also that not everyone believes that there is a Divine Force guiding our lives, and so illness of a child can be totally overwhelming. You just have to try and be where that parent is at the time.

The first part of this chapter focused on the spiritual and religious needs of the ill child and the ill adolescent—in acute illness, in chronic illness, during hospitalization, and in the dying process. The discussion concluded with a reminder that in caring for an ill or dying child, one must not forget the spiritual needs of the family. The remainder of the chapter concerns the spiritual needs of the family of the ill adult, as well as those of the family of the ill child.

▶ Spiritual Needs of the Family

The family is an important resource in the provision of spiritual care, not only for the sick child but for the ill adult as well. There are a number of understandings of the term *family* in contemporary society. Generally, the concept evokes an image of the basic nuclear family composed of two legally married parents and one or more offspring. Friedmann (1992) defined family as "two or more persons who are joined together by bonds of sharing and emotional closeness, who identify themselves as being part of the family" (p. 9). Today, however, there is a growing emergence of the single-parent family; for the single, unmarried individual, a number of persons belonging to such associations as church or friendship groups may be loosely described as family. It is important for nurses to also consider families' cultural needs when interacting with them. Such culturally sensitive caring can provide "spiritual support for family members" who may be involved in patient care and/or support, both while the patient is hospitalized and "after the patient returns home" (Neils, 2010, p. 235).

Families may be open, allowing members individuality and flexibility in role behavior, or closed and more rigid in terms of behavioral expectations (Dossey, 1988, p. 308). As social systems, families are said to have structure and function, including assigned roles, interactional patterns, and histories, each of which needs to be acknowledged in the planning of care (Turk & Kerns, 1985, p. 3). Some key functions of the modern family involve providing affection, companionship, security, a sense of purpose, socialization, and moral values (Reeder, Martin, & Koniak-Griffin, 1997, p. 46);

additionally, the provision of shelter and material support and the maintaining of morale fall within the purview of family responsibilities (LeMone & Burke, 1996, p. 37). The family also plays an important role in managing its members' health: primary prevention in supporting a healthy lifestyle, secondary prevention related to decisions to treat illness symptoms, and tertiary prevention manifested by family support of a member's compliance with a prescribed therapeutic regimen (Danielson, Hamel-Bissell, & Winstead-Fry, 1993, p. 11).

A plan for spiritual assessment and spiritual intervention for families was devised by Tanyi (2006); the unique spiritual needs of families of children with disabilities or special needs was highlighted by Speraw (2006). Speraw reported that parents or caregivers of ill children did not perceive nurses as being aware of or interested in their family spiritual needs (p. 213).

The Family, Illness, and Spirituality

Because healthy families generally function as units, it is important to minister to the spiritual needs of the entire family when one member is ill or in need of support (Clinebell, 1991). Families faced with serious short-term or chronic long-term illness of one of the members can benefit greatly from spiritual support provided by friends, church members, or pastoral care providers both from within or outside the health-care system. Emeth and Greenhut (1991) noted that remaining connected with God or with spiritual beliefs "can be difficult in a health crisis" and observed that often one needs to "rely on the faith of others, to get through a difficult period" (p. 210). Thus, the nurse should welcome a family's presence as a resource in the provision of spiritual support; including family members in a religious ritual or prayer service may help them feel comfortable in sharing in the spiritual support and care of the ill person (Peterson & Potter, 1997, p. 452). Research has identified prayer and belief in God as being the most important coping strategies for a family dealing with illness (Friedmann, 1992, p. 331).

The family's particular spiritual or religious tradition and experience will, of course, direct the kind and degree of spiritual care and support that will prove helpful during an illness experience. For the family not of a religious tradition, spiritual care may consist simply of the presence and concern demonstrated by those providing the intervention. For the family whose members are or have been actively involved in a church or faith group, the religious prayers and practices of the community can be extremely comforting. A Jewish family may appreciate reading the Psalms or other passages found in the Jewish canon of Scripture; for the Muslim family, a passage from the Holy Qur'an can provide support and comfort; and for the Christian family, the Gospel messages of Jesus often provide hope and sustenance during times of illness.

The New or Expanding Family: Spiritual Needs in Childbirth and the Postnatal Experience

For the new or expanding family the childbirth experience can be a time of significant emotional stress, especially for the mother-to-be. Certain factors such as cultural background, social support, and maternal confidence may ameliorate the stress and pain associated with the birthing experience (Reeder, Martin, & Koniak-Griffin, 1997, p. 532). Spiritual support may also help in reducing anxiety and facilitating the labor and delivery process. Three maternal–child nurses explored the "provision of spiritual care" by nurses on a maternal–infant unit (Dunn, Handley, & Dunkin, 2009). The study findings revealed important associations between the nurses' personal spirituality and spiritual well-being and the provision of spiritual care on the maternal–infant unit (p. 19).

The childbirth experience itself may incorporate aspects of the family's spiritual or religious tradition. Callister (1995) recounted the story of an Orthodox Jewish mother who gave thanks to God at the time of delivering a first-born son because of the belief that she is now "fulfilling the measure of her creation in obedience to Rabbinical law," and of a Mormon (Church of Jesus Christ of Latter Day Saints) mother who requested a blessing from her husband in the delivery room as she was about to give birth (p. 327). Callister (1995) asserted that nurses should provide the childbearing woman with an experience that respects the spiritual dimensions of her life (p. 330).

A maternal–child health (MCH) nurse may diagnose spiritual distress in a new mother in the case of death of the neonate (Corrine, Bailey, Valentin, Morantus, & Shirley, 1992, p. 141) or following delivery of an infant with a disorder such as a congenital or genetic anomaly. Moderately severe neonatal conditions such as cleft lip and palate, talipes equinovarus (club foot), or hip dysplasia may be more or less distressing, depending on parental experience and expectations. More serious congenital or genetic anomalies, such as trisomy 21 (Down syndrome) or spina bifida, may be exceedingly traumatic for parents and siblings. Disorders such as anencephaly or Tay-Sachs disease have a devastating impact on the family. Obviously, the occurrence of any illness or anomaly in a newborn poses difficult spiritual and ethical questions for the family. Hardee (1994) raised the rhetorical question "Should severely impaired or handicapped newborns be allowed to die?" Findings from conversations with 10 intensive care nursery (ICN) nurses revealed three themes of concern in response to the question: the suffering of the newborn, the nurse's stress in caring for a suffering newborn, and the nurse's feelings of inadequacy in terms of ethical knowledge to confront such dilemmas (p. 28). Ultimately, response to this question will be guided by the nurse's personal spiritual and/or religious belief system.

In the provision of spiritual care to parents faced with a critically or terminally ill newborn, some suggested interventions are to attempt to include the entire extended family in the experience in order to engender support and affirmation for the parent or parents, to assist the family in facing the reality of the situation rather than retreating into denial or fantasy, and to try to create some meaningful and positive interaction with the newborn (Kline, 1991, pp. 89–91).

Spiritual Needs of the Family in Acute Illness

Families of acutely ill patients can be found both at home and in the hospital. Because of the unexpected and often sudden onset of an acute illness, or of an acute exacerbation of a chronic condition, families may be neglected and left to fend for themselves regardless of the setting. In a home care situation, where the family is more directly involved in a therapeutic regimen, spiritual support of extended family members and friends can be available and accessible; in the hospital a more formal type of spiritual care may be required. In the hospital setting, however, many families feel constrained by the institution's restrictions and schedules (Katonah, 1991). Most hospital and clinic waiting rooms abound with anxious family members in need of spiritual support. Some needs identified by the families of acutely ill persons include the desire for competent care, pain management, compassion, and extended family support in coping with the impact of the illness on their lives (Durand, 1993, p. xii). Additional needs perceived by the families of hospitalized acutely ill patients are information about changes in a patient's condition and honest answers to questions (Leavitt, 1989). Lynn-McHale and Smith (1993) described religion as an "additional support for families experiencing crisis" and considered addressing a family's spiritual and religious concerns as facilitating coping in an acute illness experience (p. 318).

Maria, the mother of Anna, a 13-year-old suffering from advanced Ewing's sarcoma with metastasis, spoke at length about the importance of spirituality in terms of personal faith and religious practices such as prayer and hymn singing for herself and for Anna:

> We are a very Christian family. I was saved when I was about 21 and ever since I have lived my life for Jesus. Anna has witnessed for Jesus too. I couldn't get through this without my faith. You know Anna has Ewing's, one of the worst cancers you can get, and now she's relapsed so we just have to take each day at a time, each hour really! But we are putting the treatment in Jesus' hands; we are praying about it . . . Anna has really gotten involved with the Church Youth; she has witnessed with them. They are a real support to her now. They come and pray with her . . . I try to keep Anna up spiritually. Yesterday she had a "bone marrow" and we sang hymns and prayed through it to keep her spirits up. She's got a lot of faith; it's what gives her so much courage.

The Family in the Intensive Care Unit

Clark and Heindenreich (1995) identified spiritual well-being for the acutely ill patient experiencing intensive care as encompassing the support of caregivers, family members and friends, and religion and faith beliefs. The family of an acutely ill patient hospitalized in an intensive care unit (ICU) may spend long hours in waiting rooms, sometimes rarely leaving the hospital setting. This is a time when the arrival of a chaplain or nurse willing to provide spiritual care is generally welcomed unequivocally. Families need to verbalize their anxieties to someone with a caring heart as they attempt to face the severity of a loved one's illness (Niklas & Stefanics, 1975, p. 81). Families of ICU patients often express feelings of "helplessness" and "isolation" (Stromberg, 1992, p. 134) due to restricted visiting hours in a unit; the nurse or chaplain who is able to spend even a brief period of time with the family can become a bridge between the professional/technical aspects of the intensive care environment and the caring dimensions of the health-care facility. Ultimately, spiritual support is reported to be a key dimension of family care in the ICU (Rukholm, Bailey, & Coutu-Wakulczyk, 1991).

Some spiritual care interventions for the family in a critical care setting might include giving information about the patient, environment, and staff, to the degree possible; encouraging the family members to verbalize their anxieties and concerns; suggesting some coping strategies for attempting to keep up with physical needs such as nutrition and sleep; and reinforcing the fact that the family's anxiety is normal in such a situation, with the suggestion of some possible coping strategies to reduce stress (Gillman, Gable-Rodriguez, Sutherland, & Whitacre, 1996, p. 15). The ICU nurse might also include patients' families in bedside discussions whenever acceptable and attempt to include family needs when developing a plan of care (Chesla & Stannard, 1997).

Karen, an ICU head nurse, explained how she had learned the importance of allowing critically ill patients' families to express their stressful emotions:

> My first experience with a family having a really hard time, I said something to the doctor like, "this patient is dying and the family is really upset. Could we have something to help calm them down a little bit?" Well, he got all over my case, and he said "They don't need sedation; they need ventilation." At first I couldn't figure it out, and then I thought, you know, he's right. So, if a family wants to scream and yell and lay on the floor or do whatever they need to do to let it out, let them do it. Let them express that anger and pain in whatever way they have to, at least for the time being. That's part of spiritual care as far as I'm concerned.

Spiritual Needs of the Family in Chronic Illness

Chronic illness may have periods of acute exacerbation, requiring intense medical care and perhaps even hospitalization. Because of the long-term nature of chronic illness, families may become very fatigued and frustrated in the process of providing care. The family of a chronically ill person must continually be alert to changes in the health of their loved one; thus, these families need "ongoing support from friends, health care providers and communities" (Gilliss, Rose, Hallburg, & Martinson, 1989, p. 289). One example is that of the family raising a child with a disability. Following a study of families of a child with a disability (CWD), it was recommended that nurses working with CWD families acknowledge the importance of the parents' spirituality and encourage "parents' religiosity and spirituality in a sensitive and respectful manner" (Parker, Mandleco, Roper, Freeborn, & Dyches, 2011, p. 82).

The syndromes identified as HIV infection and acquired immunodeficiency syndrome (AIDS) are, with the advent of more effective therapeutic regimens, now being described as chronic illnesses, although acute exacerbations of HIV-related cancer or opportunistic infections still occur and may be considered life threatening. Smith (1988) asserted that "AIDS is a family syndrome," which has an impact not only on the person infected with the virus, but also on all of the family members and friends with whom he or she "shares important relationships" (p. 135). The spiritual needs of the families of those living with HIV and AIDS may be complicated by the need for privacy related to the stigma some still associate with the conditions. Stigma and secrecy can isolate a family from usual support systems such as extended family members, friends, and church members (Perelli, 1991, p. 41). One mother commented, however, that in caring for her son, she was forced to tell certain people that he had AIDS, "because I needed their support, as did he, through prayers and physical help" (AIDS Ministry Program, the Archdiocese of Saint Paul and Minneapolis, 1991, p. 40). Despite all of the physical and psychosocial patient considerations associated with an HIV diagnosis, the family is also grieving and needs spiritual or religious support to assist in their own coping (Amos, 1988).

Cancer is another illness syndrome identified as a chronic condition with potentially life-threatening manifestations as well. Danielson, Hamel-Bissell, and Winstead-Fry (1993) believe that a family member's diagnosis of cancer can be "one of the most spiritually disabling events" that a family will ever experience (p. 357). Often, following such a diagnosis, both the patient's and the family's lives are disrupted because of a treatment regimen involving surgery and possible chemotherapy.

The family needs significant support to facilitate coping with the myriad illness-related life changes (Sproull, 1992, p. 125).

In a study of 101 cancer patients and 45 parents of children with cancer, Spilka, Spangler, and Nelson (1983) discovered that spiritual and religious support was more important than psychological counseling; some activities appreciated were prayer, religious or spiritual reading, discussing church-related issues, spiritual counseling, and simply the presence of the spiritual caregiver (pp. 101–102). Raleigh (1992), in a study comparing 45 cancer patients and 45 patients with other chronic illnesses, found that overall the most important sources of hope were family, friends, and religion.

The significance of spirituality among 17 family caregivers of chronic dementia patients was revealed in nursing research conducted by Kaye and Robinson (1994). The investigators learned that the caregiver wives engaged in religious practices such as prayer and spiritual direction in coping with their spouses' illnesses and their own caring activities (p. 218). Based on their findings, the investigators recommended that nurses work with local churches that provide networks for such caregivers (p. 218).

Spiritual Needs of the Family Coping with a Terminal Illness

Here, a brief discussion of family needs in the predeath phase is presented; two case examples are drawn from the author's research with family members of persons in the later stages of AIDS.

In exploring the concept of nurse–family spiritual relationships among 11 hospice nurses and 12 bereaved families, Stiles (1990) identified five behaviors ascribed to nurses: being, doing, knowing, receiving and giving, and welcoming a stranger (p. 235). A nurse's way of being is sitting with and listening to the family; doing includes explaining, reassuring, and comforting; knowing involves sensitivity to the dying process; receiving and giving describes quality time spent between nurse and patient; and welcoming a stranger means inviting the patient's family to help prepare for the death (pp. 237–243). Wright (1997) asserted that listening to and being present to witness a terminally ill patient's and family's suffering is "the soul" of clinical nursing with families (p. 3). A veteran of 20 years of clinical work with families, Wright (1997) maintained that concern about a family's religious and spiritual beliefs has been one of the "most neglected" topics in family care. Yet, she asserted "the experience of suffering becomes transposed to one of spirituality as family members try to make meaning out of their suffering and distress" (p. 5).

Palliative care providers advise that "spiritual assessments should be conducted for all parents as differing support services may be needed. The palliative care team should ensure that parents' spirituality is being incorporated, as appropriate, into their children's routine care" (Knapp et al., 2011, p. 437).

Julia, the mother of 39-year-old Jonathan who was suffering from *Pneumocystis carinii* pneumonia as well as cytomegalovirus retinitis and other complications of advanced AIDS, spoke about the importance of spiritual care for herself and for her son:

> I can't tell everybody about this, but my pastor and some of the church members have been really kind and supportive; that helps so much. You

really need God and the church at a time like this. Jonathan needs the support of prayers too. I've asked the pastor to pray. That's all we can do now but it's so comforting.

And Nora, whose 42-year-old son Matthew was also experiencing symptoms of advanced AIDS, asserted:

It's only God and people's prayers that's getting me through this; they are holding me up. People have been sending prayers in cards and with phone calls. My wonderful priest is praying all the time. I don't know how I could survive without this spiritual support.

Nora admitted that sometimes she became angry with God over Matt's illness and questioned why, but she concluded, "Even when I was screaming at God, because you know, why, and why, and why? Even when I was angry with Him, I knew that God was crying with me" (O'Brien, 1992, p. 67).

Children and families have unique and important spiritual needs in dealing with illness and disability. For the young child as well as for the teen, the support of personal faith and religious practice can significantly mediate the suffering involved with an illness experience. Families of sick children and families of adults who are ill also need and benefit from spiritual care. Although the patient as the center of attention often receives much spiritual support and care, the patient's family members may be neglected or forgotten. Nurses have a prime opportunity to minister spiritually to children and to family members, especially during critical or terminal illness. The nurse must employ art and creativity in attempting to provide spiritual intervention for this fragile population.

▶ References

AIDS Ministry Program, the Archdiocese of Saint Paul and Minneapolis. (1991). *For those we love: A spiritual perspective on AIDS* (2nd ed.). Cleveland, OH: The Pilgrim Press.

American Nurses Association and the Society of Pediatric Nurses. (1996). *Statement of the scope and standards of pediatric clinical practice* (pp. 25–35). Washington, DC: American Nurses Publishing.

Amos, W. E. (1988). *When AIDS comes to church*. Philadelphia, PA: The Westminister Press.

Arnold, J. (1992). The voices on pediatrics: Walking with children and parents. In L. E. Holst (Ed.), *Hospital ministry: The role of the chaplain today* (pp. 93–106). New York, NY: Crossroad.

Ashwill, J. W., Droske, S. C., & Imhof, S. (1997). Introduction to pediatric nursing. In J. W. Ashwill & S. C. Droske (Eds.), *Nursing care of children: Principles and practice* (pp. 2–23). Philadelphia, PA: W. B. Saunders.

Ashwill, J. W., & Volz, D. (1997). The ill child in the hospital and other care settings. In J. W. Ashwill & S. C. Droske (Eds.), *Nursing care of children: Principles and practice* (pp. 346–371). Philadelphia, PA: W. B. Saunders.

Bull, A., & Gillies, M. (2007). Spiritual needs of children with complex healthcare needs in the hospital. *Paediatric Nursing, 19*(9), 34–38.

Burkhardt, M. A. (1991). Spirituality and children: Nursing considerations. *Journal of Holistic Nursing, 9*(2), 31–40.

Caldeira, S., & Hall, J. (2012). Spiritual leadership and spiritual care in neonatology. *Journal of Nursing Management, 20*(8), 1069–1075.

Callister, L. C. (1995). Cultural meanings of childbirth. *Journal of Obstetrics, Gynecology, and Maternity Nursing, 24*(4), 327–331.

Carretto, C. (1978). *Summoned by love*. Maryknoll, NY: Orbis Books.

Chesla, C. A., & Stannard, D. (1997). Breakdown in the nursing care of families in the ICU. *American Journal of Critical Care, 6*(1), 64–71.

Cichon, K. K. (1995). Life with Noah: Growing toward wholeness through parenting a handicapped child. *The Journal of Christian Healing, 17*(4), 18–25.

Clark, C., & Heindenreich, T. (1995). Spiritual care for the critically ill. *American Journal of Critical Care, 4*(1), 77–81.

Clinebell, H. (1991). *Basic types of pastoral care and counseling*. Nashville, TN: Abington Press.

Coles, R. (1990). *The spiritual life of children*. Boston, MA: Houghton Mifflin.

Cook, M. (1982). Ministering to dying children and their families. In J. A. Shelly (Ed.), *The spiritual needs of children* (pp. 117–129). Downers Grove, IL: InterVarsity Press.

Corrine, L., Bailey, V., Valentin, M., Morantus, E., & Shirley, L. (1992). The unheard voices of women: Spiritual interventions in maternal-child health. *American Journal of Maternal Child Nursing, 17*(3), 141–145.

Danielson, C. B., Hamel-Bissell, B., & Winstead-Fry, P. (1993). *Families, health & illness: Perspectives on coping and intervention*. St. Louis, MO: C. V. Mosby.

Donnelly, J., Huff, S., Lindsey, M., McMahon, K., & Schumacher, J. (2005). The needs of children with life-limiting conditions: A healthcare-provider-based model. *American Journal of Hospice and Palliative Care Medicine, 22*(4), 259–267.

Dossey, B. M. (1988). Relationships: Learning the patterns and processes. In B. M. Dossey, L. Keegan, C. E. Guzzetta, & L. G. Kolkmeier (Eds.), *Holistic nursing: A handbook for practice* (pp. 305–330). Rockville, MD: Aspen.

Dunn, L., Handley, M., & Dunkin, J. (2009). The provision of spiritual care by registered nurses on a maternal-infant unit. *Journal of Holistic Nursing, 27*(1), 19–28.

Durand, B. A. (1993). Preface: Determination of need. In S. L. Feetham, S. B. Meister, J. M. Bell, & C. L. Gillis (Eds.), *The nursing of families* (pp. ix–xiii). Newburg Park, CA: Sage.

Elkins, M., & Cavendish, R. (2004). Developing a plan for pediatric spiritual care. *Holistic Nursing Practice, 18*(4), 179–185.

Emeth, E. V., & Greenhut, J. H. (1991). *The wholeness handbook: Care of body, mind and spirit for optimal health*. New York, NY: Continuum.

Faulkner, K. W. (1997). Talking about death with a dying child. *American Journal of Nursing, 97*(6), 64–69.

Fowler, J. (1981). *Stages of faith: The psychology of human development and the quest for meaning*. San Francisco, CA: Harper San Francisco.

Friedmann, M. M. (1992). *Family nursing: Theory and practice*. (3rd ed.). Norwalk, CT: Appleton & Lange.

Fulton, R. A., & Moore, C. M. (1995). Spiritual care of the school age child with a chronic condition. *Journal of Pediatric Nursing, 10*(4), 224–231.

Gilliss, C. L., Rose, D., Hallburg, J. C., & Martinson, I. M. (1989). The family and chronic illness. In C. L. Gilliss, B. M. Highley, B. M. Roberts, & I. M. Martinson (Eds.), *Toward a science of family nursing* (pp. 287–299). New York, NY: Addison-Wesley.

Gillman, J., Gable-Rodriguez, J., Sutherland, M., & Whitacre, J. H. (1996). Pastoral care in a critical care setting. *Critical Care Nursing Quarterly, 19*(1), 10–20.

Handzo, G. F. (1990). Talking about faith with children. *Journal of Christian Nursing, 7*(4), 17–20.

Hardee, L. B. (1994). When a newborn cannot survive: What nurses really believe. *Journal of Christian Nursing, 11*(1), 26–28, 47.

Hardgrove, C., & Roberts, B. M. (1989). The family with a hospitalized child. In C. L. Gilliss, B. M. Highley, B. M. Roberts, & I. M. Martinson (Eds.), *Toward a science of family nursing* (pp. 148–161). New York, NY: Addison-Wesley.

Heller, D. (1985). The children's God. *Psychology Today, 19*(1), 11–17.

Hendricks-Ferguson, V. (2008). Hope and spiritual well-being in adolescents with cancer. *Western Journal of Nursing Research, 30*(3), 385–401.

Holiday, B. (1989). The family with a chronically ill child: An interactional perspective. In C. L. Gilliss, B. M. Highley, B. M. Roberts, & I. M. Martinson (Eds.), *Toward a science of family nursing* (pp. 300–311). New York, NY: Addison-Wesley.

Hufton, E. (2006). Parting gifts: The spiritual needs of children. *Journal of Child Health, 10*(3), 240–250.

Jerome, A. (2011). Comforting children and families who grieve. *School Psychology International, 32*, 194–209.

Johnson, S. B. (1985). The family and the child with chronic illness. In D. C. Turk & R. D. Kerns (Eds.), *Health, illness and families: A life-span perspective* (pp. 110–154). New York, NY: John Wiley & Sons.

Kamper, R., VanCleve, L., & Savedra, M. (2010). Children with advanced cancer: Responses to a spiritual quality of life interview. *Journal for Specialists in Pediatric Nursing, 15*(4), 301–306.

Katonah, J. (1991). Hospitalization: A rite of passage. In L. E. Holst (Ed.), *Hospital ministry: The role of the chaplain today* (pp. 55–67). New York, NY: Crossroad.

Kaye, J., & Robinson, K. M. (1994). Spirituality among caregivers. *Image: Journal of Nursing Scholarship, 26*(3), 218–221.

Kenny, G. (1999). Children's nursing: Assessing children's spirituality, what is the way forward? *British Journal of Nursing, 8*(1), 28; 30–32.

Kline, S. J. (1991). The voices on obstetrics: Participants and partners. In L. E. Holst (Ed.), *Hospital ministry: The role of the chaplain today* (pp. 79–91). New York, NY: Crossroad.

Knapp, C., Madden, V., Wang, H., Curtis, C., Sloyer, P., & Shenkman, E. (2011). Spirituality of parents of children in palliative care. *Journal of Palliative Medicine, 14*(4), 437–443.

Kohlberg, L. (1984). *The psychology of moral development.* San Francisco, CA: Harper & Row.

Leavitt, M. B. (1989). Transition to illness: The family in the hospital. In C. L. Gilliss, B. M. Highley, B. M. Roberts, & I. M. Martinson (Eds.), *Toward a science of family nursing* (pp. 161–186). New York, NY: Addison-Wesley.

LeMone, P., & Burke, K. M. (1996). *Medical–surgical nursing: Critical thinking in client care.* New York, NY: Addison-Wesley.

Lynn-McHale, D. J., & Smith, A. (1993). Comprehensive assessment of families of the critically ill. In G. D. Wegner & R. J. Alexander (Eds.), *Readings in family nursing* (pp. 309–328). Philadelphia, PA: J. B. Lippincott.

Marlow, D. R., & Redding, B. A. (1988). *Textbook of pediatric nursing* (6th ed.). Philadelphia, PA: W. B. Saunders.

Martin, G. T. (1997). The child with a chronic or terminal illness. In J. W. Ashwill & S. C. Droske (Eds.), *Nursing care of children: Principles and practice* (pp. 394–417). Philadelphia, PA: W. B. Saunders.

McSherry, W., & Smith, J. (2006). How do children express their spiritual needs? *Pediatric Nursing, 19*(3), 17–20.

Melamed, B. G., & Bush, J. P. (1985). Family factors in children with acute illness. In D. C. Turk & R. D. Kerns (Eds.), *Health, illness and families: A life-span perspective* (pp. 183–219). New York, NY: John Wiley & Sons.

Moran, M. (1997). Growth and development. In J. W. Ashwill & S. C. Droske (Eds.), *Nursing care of children: Principles and practice* (pp. 26–49). Philadelphia, PA: W. B. Saunders.

Mueller, C. (2010). Spirituality in children: Understanding and developing interventions. *Pediatric Nursing, 36*(4), 197–204.

Neils, P. (2010). The influence of Nightingale rounding by the liaison nurse on surgical patient families with attention to differing cultural needs. *Journal of Holistic Nursing, 28*(4), 235–243.

Niklas, G. R., & Stefanics, C. (1975). *Ministry to the hospitalized.* New York, NY: Paulist Press.

O'Brien, M. E. (1992). *Living with HIV: Experiment in courage.* Westport, CT: Auburn House.

O'Brien, M. E. (1995). The AIDS challenge: *Breaking through the boundaries.* Westport, CT: Auburn House.

Parker, J., Mandleco, B., Roper, S., Freeborn, D., & Dychess, T. (2011). Religiosity, spirituality and marital relationships of parents raising a typically developing child or a child with a disability. *Journal of Family Nursing, 17*(1), 82–104.

Pearson, H. (2010). Managing the emotional aspects of end of life care for children and young people. *Paediatric Nursing, 22*(7), 31–35.

Peterson, C. L. (2013). Spiritual care of the child with cancer at the end of life: A concept analysis. *Journal of Advanced Nursing, 70*(6), 1243–1253.

Perelli, R. (1991). *Ministry to persons with AIDS: A family systems approach.* Minneapolis, MN: Augsburg.

Peterson, V., & Potter, P. A. (1997). Spiritual health. In P. A. Potter & A. G. Perry (Eds.), *Fundamentals of nursing: Concepts, process and practice* (pp. 440–456). St. Louis, MO: C. V. Mosby.

Quinlivan, M. (2014). Supporting the delivery of effective pastoral care. *British Journal of School Nursing, 9*(8), 405–406.

Raleigh, E. D. (1992). Sources of hope in chronic illness. *Oncology Nursing Forum, 19*(2), 443–448.

Reeder, S. J., Martin, L. L., & Koniak-Griffin, D. (1997). *Maternity nursing: Family, newborn and women's health care* (18th ed.). Philadelphia, PA: J. B. Lippincott.

Roger of Taizé. (1990). *His love is a fire.* Collegeville, MN: The Liturgical Press.

Rukholm, E. E., Bailey, P. H., & Coutu-Wakulczyk, G. (1991). Family needs and anxieties in the ICU. *The Canadian Journal of Nursing Research, 23*(3), 67–81.

Shelly, J. A. (Ed.). (1982). Jesus and the children: A mandate to care. In *The spiritual needs of children* (pp. 11–16). Downers Grove, IL: InterVarsity Press.

Smith, W. J. (1988). *AIDS, living and dying with hope: Issues in pastoral care.* New York, NY: Paulist Press.

Sommer, D. R. (1989). The spiritual needs of dying children. *Issues in Comprehensive Pediatric Nursing, 12*(1), 225–233.

Spector, R. E., & Spertac, A. M. (1990). Social and cultural influences on the child. In S. R. Mott, S. R. James, & A. M. Spertac (Eds.), *Nursing care of children and families* (2nd ed., pp. 53–75). New York, NY: Addison-Wesley.

Speraw, S. (2006). Spiritual experiences of parents and caregivers who have children with disabilities or special needs. *Issues in Mental Health Nursing, 27,* 213–230.

Spilka, B., Spangler, J. D., & Nelson, C. B. (1983). Spiritual support in life threatening illness. *Journal of Religion and Health, 22*(2), 98–104.

Sproull, A. (1992). The voices on cancer care: A lens unfocused and narrowed. In L. E. Holst (Ed.), *Hospital ministry: The role of the chaplain today.* New York, NY: Crossroad.

Spur, S., Berry, L., & Walker, K. (2013). The meanings older adults attach to spirituality. *Journal for Specialists in Pediatric Nursing, 18*(3), 221–232.

Stiles, M. K. (1990). The shining stranger: Nurse–family spiritual relationships. *Cancer Nursing, 13*(4), 235–245.

Stromberg, R. (1992). The voices on coronary care: A confrontation with vulnerability. In L. E. Holst (Ed.), *Hospital ministry: The role of the chaplain today.* New York, NY: Crossroad.

Tanyi, R. A. (2006). Spirituality and family nursing: Spiritual assessment and interventions for families. *Journal of Advanced Nursing, 53*(3), 287–294.

Turk, D. C., & Kerns, R. D. (Eds.). (1985). The family in health and illness. In *Health, illness and families: A life-span perspective* (pp. 1–22). New York, NY: John Wiley & Sons.

Van Heukelem, J. (1982). Assessing the spiritual needs of children and their families. In J. A. Shelly (Ed.), *The spiritual needs of children* (pp. 87–97). Downers Grove, IL: InterVarsity Press.

Van Heukelem-Still, J. (1984). How to assess spiritual needs of children and their families. *Journal of Christian Nursing, 1*(1), 4–6.

Winkelstein, M. (1989). Spirituality and the death of a child. In V. B. Carson (Ed.), *Spiritual dimensions of nursing practice* (pp. 217–253). Philadelphia, PA: W. B. Saunders.

Wong, D. L. (1997). *Whaley & Wong's essentials of pediatric nursing* (5th ed.). St. Louis, MO: C. V. Mosby.

Wright, L. M. (1997). Spirituality and suffering: The soul of clinical work with families. *Journal of Family Nursing, 3*(1), 3–14.

Young, C., & Koopsen, C. (2011). *Spirituality, health, and healing: An integrative approach.* Sudbury, MA: Jones & Bartlett Learning.

CHAPTER 10

Spiritual Needs of the Older Adult

There is no such notion as retirement in terms of the purpose of God . . . God calls us to live life with Him as co-creators, co-workers in the reshaping and renewing of human history . . . and that calling is never completed until the day He calls us to live with Him.

Jitsuo Morikawa, 1974, as cited in Seymour, 1995

I treat patients as if they were part of my family. Especially the geriatric folks. People deserve to be treated with dignity and respect and care. Believing that nursing is a vocation impacts that. I just treat everyone with the understanding that they are spiritual beings, and we are all children of God. I have a theory that when we help one another we are helping each other.

Alice, Charge Nurse on a Geriatric Unit

This chapter documents the spiritual needs of the frail or ill older adult. Data identifying spiritual needs were obtained through both structured and unstructured interviews and interactions with three groups of older persons living with illness; the study populations included chronically ill elders who are active, homebound elders, and elders residing in a nursing home. The elders experienced a multiplicity of illness conditions including congestive heart disease, hypertension, arteriosclerosis, arthritis, diabetes, and Alzheimer's disease. Interview data were also elicited from caregivers of the frail elderly. Nursing research has documented the importance of nurses providing spiritual care to elders living both in the community (Castellaw, Wicks, & Martin, 1999) and in nursing homes (Hicks, 1999).

Currently the spiritual needs and spiritual care of older adults are receiving significant attention in the nursing literature. One study exploring the relationship of dignity to spirituality in elders revealed that "spiritual care underpins dignity through uplifting the spirit and (allowing the person to) feel alive and be valued" (Rykkje & Raholm, 2014, p. 17). Among the most fragile older adults are frequently those residing in nursing homes or continuing care retirement communities. For these elders the relationship between transcendence and spiritual well-being has been found to be significant (Haughen, Rannestad, Hammervold, Garasen, & Espnes, 2013). It is suggested that "facilitating patients' self-transcendence, both interpersonally and intrapersonally may increase spiritual well-being among cognitively intact nursing home patients' overall satisfaction" (Haughen et al., 2013, p. 66). Some defining characteristics of pastoral care for older adults in residential care include: "a trusting relationship, spiritual support, emotional support and practical support" (Wilkes, Cioffi, Fleming, & LeMiere, 2011, p. 213).

Perhaps the most challenging elder residential population for whom spiritual care is needed is the group experiencing dementia symptoms. Some current suggestions for spiritual care for dementia residents include: "integrating spiritual care into general care, described as physical touch and responsive intuition . . . being present and sensitive in communication . . . and meeting residents' religious needs" (Odbehr, Kvigne, Hauge, & Danbolt, 2015, p. 1). Other spiritual care intervention for dementia patients suggested are: "reflective practice and meaningful engagement with the person with dementia so as to facilitate shared understanding," "supporting the spiritual and religious beliefs of the person," and employing "an individualized or person-centered approach to care" (Daly & Fahey-McCarthy, 2014, p. 787). Also important are such activities as facilitating a patient's attendance at church services and supporting them in private prayer (Higgins, 2013, p. 25). The concepts of both spirituality and religiosity need to be considered in providing care for one suffering from dementia (Jolley & Moreland, 2011).

▶ The Older Adult

Who are the elderly? Who are those individuals whom society labels "seniors," or "older adults"? Definitions based on chronological age are changing as a result of the increasing longevity and functional ability of contemporary men and women. In a study to determine the preferred group descriptor of older Americans, the terms *mature*, *older*, and *senior* were the most frequently chosen adjectives; *aged* and *old* were the most disliked terms (Finley, 1989, p. 6). Past demographic profiles have identified persons as older adults if they had passed the age of 65. Individuals between 65 and 74 years of age were described as "young old"; those over 74 were identified as the "older elderly." In 1997, however, Roen suggested that the "young old" subgroup "may soon include people as old as 84" (p. 348).

Today, popular thinking seems to embrace the concept that, barring serious physical or emotional challenges, the majority of older adults are both cognitively and physiologically about 10 years younger than their chronological age indicates. Thus, a 21st-century 75-year-old is comparable to a 65-year-old of the past century. The theoretical understanding for this perception is based on two characteristics of contemporary society, first, the general publics' increased interest in and concern with healthy nutrition (for example the avoidance of high-cholesterol foods); second, the fact that today's elders are more active both physically and cognitively, which has the potential to keep both body and mind functioning better and longer than in the past.

Older adults are the most rapidly growing segment of the population. In 1991, the U.S. census identified 31 million Americans older than age 65; Holland and McCurren (1997) estimated that the number will increase "to approximately 33.5 million by the year 2005" (p. 81). Twenty percent of the U.S. population will be older than 65 by the year 2020; this group is anticipated to account for 70 percent of those who need "primary, acute, home and long-term nursing care" (Rice, Beck, & Stevenson, 1997, p. 27).

Tournier (1983) described the movement from adulthood to older age as one of the great turning points in life. Admittedly, certain potentially negative physiologic and psychosocial changes accompany the aging process. Although each person ages differently, some common characteristics are physical changes in hair, skin, and teeth; impaired vision and hearing; lessened appetite; skeletal changes related to arthritis or osteoporosis; and lowered energy levels, among others. As a result of these physiologic modifications, the older adult may experience social isolation, financial concern associated with the inability to work, and anxiety and depression related to worry about future health and health-care issues. Despite this rather bleak chronology of negative factors associated with the aging process, Taylor, Lillis, and LeMone (1997) believe that the older adult can continue to carry out the usual activities of middle age as long as the pace is modified and rest periods are included (p. 59).

Heriot (1995) warned that for too long our society has viewed aging in depressing terms rather than seeking out the positive developmental processes that can occur despite the negative physical changes (p. 349). Some developmental tasks for the elder include the creation of a new self-image as an older person, learning to adjust to and find meaning in life despite physical impairments or decreasing energy levels, adapting to a simpler lifestyle necessitated by lowered or fixed income, and seeking to promote and maintain a high quality of life as an older adult (Lueckenotte, 1997, p. 573). It is possible for the older adult to move past his or her physical deficits and "find a sense of identity and worth in relationships, and in intellectual, artistic and spiritual pursuits" (Maltby, 1990, p. 101). As well as enjoying relationships with family and friends, some other strategies for aging well are cultivating a positive attitude toward life, choosing activities one enjoys, and maintaining a health regimen of diet and exercise (Hogstel, 1995).

More and more older adults, especially in the younger-old category, are remaining in the workforce or initiating second or third careers; many are also involved in full-time volunteer activities. Chronological age, of itself, should not be considered a disqualifier for maintaining a responsible place in society (Stagg, 1981, p. 11). Ultimately, Finch (1993) posited, the aging process may become a time of peace and joy during which the elder, no longer struggling with the challenges of career or ego, may be able to enjoy the beauties of loved ones and of nature in "wise tranquility" (p. 11). Wisdom is a spiritual gift that the older adult has to give to the world, a gift much needed in contemporary society.

▶ The Spirituality of Aging

Even to your old age, I am, even when you turn gray I will carry you; I will carry you and will save you.

—Isaiah 46:4

Spiritual writers Henri Nouwen and Walter Gaffney (1990), in their book *Aging: The Fulfillment of Life*, described the aging process poignantly as a human experience "which overarches the human community as a rainbow of promises" (p. 19). Aging, the authors believe, "can lead us to discover more and more of life's treasures . . . aging is not a reason for despair but a basis for hope, not a slow decaying but a gradual maturing, not a fate to be undergone but a challenge to be embraced" (p. 20). Seymour (1995) also advanced the concept of viewing the aging process in a spiritual light, asserting that as one's physical strength weakens, the spiritual dimension of life may intensify. Supportive of that position is a quotation cited by Seymour from a 150-year-old volume, *Happy Talk towards the End of Life*. "Is your eyesight dimmer? Then the world is seen by you in cathedral light. Is your hearing duller? Then it is just as though you were always where loud voices and footsteps ought not to be heard . . . Yes, for twilight and silence . . . old age makes us like daily dwellers in the house of the Lord" (p. 100). Spiritual issues in later life are "often driven" by such paradoxes, suggest Young and Koopsen (2011) in discussing the "unique spiritual challenges of aging" (p. 315).

Scholars of aging disagree as to whether the older adult becomes more or less involved in both spiritual and religious issues (Bianchi, 1995; Burt, 1992). Admittedly, some of the physical and psychosocial deficits of older age may hinder one's religiosity or religious practice; however, personal spirituality often deepens (Seymour, 1995). If an older person is relatively well, research has shown that religious practice may increase (Ainlay & Smith, 1984; Hunsberger, 1985; Markides, 1983). Membership in a church "is claimed by 73% of women and 63% of men older than 50 years, although fewer attend regularly" (Roen, 1997, p. 356); older adults tend to view the practice of religion as more important than do younger adults (Peterson & Potter, 1997). A church or synagogue may provide social networks for an older adult, as well as delineating a structure within which to live out one's spiritual beliefs. Some church groups may even facilitate health care for the older adult through the support of a parish nurse.

David Moberg (1990) worried, however, that while many religious or faith communities have been concerned about meeting the physical needs of their elders, they may have neglected ministering to spiritual needs (p. 18). Spiritual needs in the older adult are manifestations of the spiritual development associated with the aging process. As Bianchi (1995) pointed out, creatively dealing with the fact of one's mortality is a "major life task" (p. 59), as well as a major faith task. The task can become central to finding meaning in life for an older adult. Boettcher (1985) believed that as an elder's physical and psychosocial world begins to shrink, "an inner expansion of awareness and spirit can develop" (p. 29).

In order to provide spiritual care to an older adult, it is important for the caregiver to have some understanding of the developmental faith tasks of aging (Maltby, 1990). One useful paradigm is that of James Fowler's (1981) stages of faith development. To explain the late adult era, the final two of Fowler's stages are appropriate: conjunctive faith, stage 5, and movement toward stage 6, universalizing faith. Stage 5, or conjunctive faith (midlife and beyond), is a time of attempting to look beyond rational explanations and seeing their limitations. In this stage, the older adult may look back on earlier religious beliefs and traditions, which may have been discarded, and begin to reincorporate them into current attitudes and practice. Fowler (1981) called this a "reclaiming or reworking of one's past" (p. 197). He noted also that this is a time of "opening to the voices of one's deeper self," of one's "social unconscious" (p. 198). Previous prejudices toward people or religions can now be rejected and a new openness created. Despite this movement toward an attitude of justice for all, the individual in stage 5 may remain somewhat torn between preserving his or her own tradition and needs and a "more universal" caring (Koenig, 1994, p. 92).

Fowler's (1981) sixth stage, universalizing faith, occurring in the final years of life, is identified as "exceedingly rare." "The persons best described by it have generated faith compositions . . . inclusive of all being" (p. 200). Persons in the sixth faith stage possess "enlarged visions of universal community," and generally tend to violate "usual criteria for normalcy" (p. 200). These persons are unequivocally committed to a vision involving justice and peace and are willing to sacrifice their lives in the cause (Koenig, 1994, p. 93). This final stage is similar to what has been labeled "mature religious faith," a time when one directs one's concerns away from self and toward the larger society (Koenig, 1994; Maitland, 1991; Payne, 1990).

Promoting spiritual well-being for an older adult may involve such activities as active listening (including presence, touch, and reminiscence) and spiritual support (forgiveness, hope, and prayer) (Gaskamp, Sutter, & Meraviglia, 2006, pp. 9–10); support for an individual's religion and spirituality (McFadden & Kozberg, 2008); and the interventions of spiritual assessment and spiritual care, as well as palliative care if appropriate (MacKinlay, 2008).

▶ Spirituality and Religious Practice in Older Adults

As an outgrowth of and support for one's spiritual development, religious practices may be very important to the quality of life of an older adult. The religious or faith tradition of the elder will direct the nature of specific practices. Studies of religiosity among elders have, however, identified certain practices common to a number of religious denominations. Some of these include prayer and meditation, church membership, participation in religious worship services, study of religious doctrine, and spiritual reading. Halstead (1995) also identified the use of religiously oriented videos, music recordings, and television programs as helpful to elders in practicing their religion (p. 416).

In a study of religious practice among 380 elders, Mull, Cox, and Sullivan (1987) found that 94 percent reported religion to be important in terms of their health and well-being. The well elders highly valued attendance at church or synagogue. For those who had greater physical disability, private religious practices such as prayer and watching religious TV programs became more important (p. 151). Religious practice can be seen as giving life to spiritual beliefs, providing an important spiritual support network for the older adult, and helping an ill elder to transcend physical or emotional suffering by internalizing a transcendent vision in terms of the meaning of life (Hall, 1985).

Religious and/or spiritual practices carried out by older adults have also been found to be associated with positive self-care agency, that is, self-caring activities. A study of 235 seniors concluded that "the older adults who reported routine practice of spiritual growth behaviors also reported having positive self-concepts and took the initiative and responsibility for self-care" (Callaghan, 2006, p. 49). Study implications for nursing included "incorporating spiritual assessments and interventions in caring for older adults" (p. 50). From research such as this, as well as from the extant literature on spirituality, aging, and nursing, a number of issues were identified "for translating evidence into practice" (Hudson, 2008, p. 145). Hudson identified the issues in terms of seven key themes, which include:

1. Spirituality, concept development and models
2. Spirituality and chronic illness
3. Promoting spiritual health and well-being
4. Spirituality and dying
5. Cross-cultural and multifaith issues
6. Spiritual assessment
7. Ethics (Hudson, 2008, pp. 146–148)

Hudson recommended that nurses "carefully consider the place of spirituality within a holistic framework of care for the older person" (p. 149).

As well as general concern for the spirituality and spiritual practice needs of the older adult, it is noted that current "changes from monocultural to multicultural societies challenge nurses to know how to provide culturally and faith appropriate care" (MacKinlay, 2008, p. 151). Like Hudson, MacKinlay also suggests concern about ethical issues: "Ethical perspectives of older people must be carefully addressed in nursing as frail and vulnerable older people struggle with issues of compromised autonomy" (p. 151).

A common religious practice universally identified with most Western and Eastern religions is that of prayer. Despite diminishing physical health, persons of all religious beliefs tend to pray more during their senior years than at any other time in their lives (Finley, 1989). Prayer is a practice with many faces. For a well elder, prayer may involve social interaction when engaged in during group worship services. For an ill or frail elder, private prayer or meditation can help alleviate feelings of loneliness or anxiety. For the confused or cognitively impaired older adult, traditional prayers learned in one's youth can sometimes be remembered and provide comfort. This is reflected in the comments of a chaplain with more than seven years of experience in ministering to nursing home residents. In justifying the inclusion of confused elders in religious rites, the chaplain asserted:

> Even patients who are pretty much out of contact, they are still able to make the sign of the cross; they are still able to say prayers they learned when they were three or four years old. It [religion] is one of the things that goes last, as far as the memory is concerned; well, at least some basic tenets that they hang on to because they were so deeply ingrained. (O'Brien, 1989, p. 144)

Establishing a schedule for times of prayer during the day can be helpful for the newly retired person who may be somewhat "at loose ends"; the person can look forward to this time "not as a duty but as a time of joy and relaxation" (Coupland, 1985, p. 44). Spiritual writer Robert Wicks (1997) suggested that older adults might choose to engage in several types of prayer during the day, including both formal and informal prayers ("conversations with God"), religious reflections, "spiritual letter-writing," and creating of one's own parables (p. 22). Some comforting Psalms that an elder might pray are Psalm 23, "The Lord is my shepherd"; Psalm 25, prayer for guidance; Psalm 34, God as protector; Psalm 62, trust in God; Psalm 71, prayer in old age; and Psalm 121, God's support in trials (Hynes, 1989, p. 49).

▶ Spirituality and Physical Diminishment

Every age has its own beauty. Why be afraid of physical decline when the years bring deeper insight and greater gentleness of action?

—Roger of Taizé, as cited in Finch, 1993, p. 23

When an elder's physical capacities are no longer functional at the level an individual may wish, a sense of inner comfort and peace may still be derived from spiritual beliefs and behaviors. Spiritual and religious practices such as meditation or silent prayer, or having a loving attitude toward others, may be part of a life plan even for the older old person afflicted with a multiplicity of physical deficits. In a study including 31 in-depth interviews with older adults whose health ranged from good to terminal illness, Hungelmann, Kenkel-Rossi, Klassen, and Stollenwerk (1985) found the concept of "harmonious interconnectedness" of relationships to constitute spiritual well-being. The core categories of spiritual well-being identified were "ultimate other," reflecting such concepts as belief and trust in God and religious practice; "other/nature," consisting of expressions of mutual love and forgiveness, and accepting and giving help; and "self," relating to accepting and valuing oneself (p. 150). The investigators reported that, for this population of elders, spiritual well-being represented a "state of peace and harmony . . . linked to past experiences and future hopes and goals" (p. 151).

A nursing diagnosis of alteration in spiritual well-being or spiritual distress in an ill elder may be related to the individual's anger or frustration over an illness or disability. Chaplain Mary Brian Durkin (1992), who ministers to patients on a rehabilitation unit, noted that a disabled patient's suffering was often associated with a negative attitude toward his or her condition. For such a patient the provision of spiritual counseling and support can be a critical element in coping with illness and disability. Sister Mary Byrne (1985) asserted that for some ill elders "spiritual support is their greatest need"; she pointed out that emotional support is not adequate if an older person's problem is of a spiritual nature (pp. 30, 32).

▶ Spirituality and Cognitive Diminishment

Many older adults experience some degree of cognitive impairment as they progress through the aging process. Rice, Beck, and Stevenson (1997) reported cognitive impairment or senile dementia of the Alzheimer type (SDAT) in an "estimated 10.3% of those over 65," and that "the incidence may be as high as 48% in persons over 85 years of age" (p. 29). The authors posited that approximately 75 percent of nursing home residents have some cognitive impairment (p. 29).

The latter statistic was supported during the author's conduct of an exploratory case study of a 230-bed nursing home, labeled "Bethany Manor" (O'Brien, 1989). Because of the large number of Bethany Manor residents manifesting dementia symptoms, an attempt was made, through qualitative interview, to gain at least minimal understanding of their spiritual, physical, and emotional needs. Five dominant themes describing attitude and behavior were derived from data elicited in interviews with a subsample of 24 moderately cognitively impaired residents. These concepts included conformity, related to the residents' desire to please, especially the nursing home staff; privacy, which meant "minding one's own business" and limiting social interactions in the nursing home; activity, relating to activities of daily living in the nursing home, as well as visiting with staff and family; externality, a theme describing the fact that, according to their comments, some residents seemed to "live" in the worlds of family and friends outside of the nursing home; and reminiscence, or telling stories of one's life, even as far back as childhood (O'Brien, 1989, pp. 37–39). Some hints as to a resident's spirituality did emerge in the data, for example, remarks about God, prayer, or attendance at church as a child. One woman commented, "When you look at the handicaps all the people here have, I say God's been good to me" (p. 39); another long-term resident asserted, "I have been brought up as a Christian and my belief is a great support to me now" (p. 47).

As pointed out by Sharon Mooney (2006), "The effect of Alzheimer's disease on spirituality, or on a person's relationship with God, is an area that has not been studied extensively" (p. 9). Thus, Mooney has explored "ways to help dementia patients remember God"; one suggestion was the use of "rituals" associated with a patient's faith tradition. Mooney explained, "For the present generation of older adults with progressive dementia, the importance of rituals as a means of enhancing some degree of orientation to reality, calming emotions and decreasing agitated physical behavior should not be underestimated" by nurses caring for these patients (p. 9).

It is understood that Alzheimer's disease "can create an overwhelming set of circumstances for those diagnosed and for those giving care . . . [and] under such circumstances, many diagnosed individuals and their families cope by drawing on spiritual and religious beliefs and practices" (Stuckey, Post, Ollerton, FallCreek, & Whitehouse, 2002, p. 199). Stuckey et al. assert that "even when persons with dementia are stripped of memory, it is still possible, and perhaps even more likely, to reach them in religious and spiritual pathways" (p. 206). This conclusion is supported by the work of Beuscher and Beck (2008), who conducted a literature review on spirituality and coping with Alzheimer's disease. Their "findings suggest that persons with early-stage Alzheimer's disease draw from their spirituality and faith to find meaning and courage in facing the challenges of cognitive losses" (p. 88). Beuscher and Beck conclude that for nurses, gaining an "understanding of how older persons with Alzheimer's disease cope with their memory loss is critical to the development of evidence-based interventions to minimize the stress of living with the disease" (p. 88).

One of the established nursing interventions for elders with cognitive diminishment is that of reminiscence. The process was studied among a group of 116 older adults with dementia living in long-term care facilities (MacKinlay & Trevitt, 2010). The nurse investigators collected qualitative data, generated prior to and after reminiscence group sessions, to evaluate the success of the project. Study findings revealed that "new relationships were developed among group members that improved life" for the study participants (p. 394). MacKinlay and Trevitt suggested that "spiritual reminiscence offers nursing staff a way of knowing those with dementia in a deeper and more meaningful way" (p. 394).

▶ Spiritual Concerns of the Older Adult

Two key spiritual concerns identified by older adults are loneliness and uncertainty of the future.

Loneliness

Loneliness can be a significant problem for the older adult (Fischer, 1995; Lotito, 1993; Normille, 1992). This is related to the onset of both physical and psychosocial deficits. Such deficits may cause the older person to become distanced from a faith or worship group. Restriction in ambulation can hinder an elder's religious practice in terms of attendance at church or synagogue worship services; impairment in sight and hearing may cause an elder to be sensitive about participating in faith group activities where such a limitation might be noticed. Elders may also retreat from church activities as a result of fatigue or depression associated with the aging process. For the elder not of a religious tradition, loneliness may relate to isolation from former work and friendship or volunteer groups, such as clubs and charitable organizations.

An older adult may take a number of steps to alleviate loneliness, such as making a conscious effort to get out, if able physically. Many churches today have special programs and groups for elders only; these can be social or may involve volunteer activities (Finley, 1989). Also, a number of community programs encourage the participation of the elderly who are mobile. For the homebound elder, church groups and some hospitals have projects such as Senior Connection, through which the ill older person can stay connected by phone to others in the area.

Although loneliness is a phenomenon experienced at some time and to some degree by virtually everyone, the loneliness of the older adult is unique in that it often grows out of loss (Valentine, 1994). An elder's loneliness can be the result of multiple losses: physical (isolation related to disabling health deficit), emotional (deaths of family and friends), social (loss of work-related relationships), financial (inability to travel or participate in social activities due to a fixed income), or spiritual (loss of ability to participate in religious worship services).

Although steps can be taken to alleviate an elder's loneliness, spiritual literature on the concept advises that "aloneness need not be a negative experience": "On the contrary, the emptiness of feeling alone can open one's heart, and make one more perceptive of the presence of God" (Deeken, 1986, p. 41). After a life filled with activity, work, family, and social activities, seniors may find that their aloneness provides a time of peace and quiet joy. For those elders, rather than bringing loneliness, the period of retirement from active work is welcomed as a spiritual journey, a preparation for the transition to eternal life.

Uncertainty of the Future

For the older adult, especially one experiencing illness, uncertainty of the future can be the source of much anxiety. The elder may have already witnessed the lingering illnesses and deaths of relatives or friends, each loss raising anew the specter of one's own mortality. Central concerns for the older adult generally are focused on economics (financial security or lack of security in the later stages of life) and autonomy (being able to care for oneself in illness or having some control over the kind of care received). Associated fears are those related to the possibility of future loneliness and cognitive impairment. The comments of a 77-year-old nursing home resident reflect such uncertainty. "I just don't know about the future. You work hard all your life, but in the end you never know. It's a worry, I'll tell you that for sure."

Some older adults, however, especially those with a spiritual or religious perspective on life, express little fear of the future. An 83-year-old nursing home resident described her present life as satisfactory. "I'm at peace and I hope to die here. I have reached a good age. God has been good to me. The things that could make me wonder about things, worry me, are lost. Death doesn't frighten me" (O'Brien, 1989, p. 45).

▶ Spiritual Needs of the Older Adult

Hammer (1990) identified the spiritual needs of the older adult as relating to the carrying out of religious practices such as grace before meals, Scripture reading, and prayer; for the older or frail elderly, some contact with a former church or faith group is important (pp. 3–4). Forbis (1988) advanced a broader understanding of spiritual need among older adults, identifying such activities as listening to music, reading poetry, and verbalizing fears and anxieties, as well as prayer and spiritual reading (p. 159). Forbis warned that an ill elder who had strong religious beliefs may be fearful of expressing doubts or anxieties to family or friends; such an individual may, however, share these concerns with a nurse who does not have the same expectations as significant others (p. 158).

A key spiritual need of the older adult, regardless of whether the elder identifies with a particular religious tradition, is the ability to find meaning in the aging process (Blazer, 1991). Although this can be the most difficult task of aging in the face of multiple physical, psychological, social, and financial losses, it is also the most challenging dimension of an elder's spiritual journey. Closely linked to this faith task of aging is the need to confront the prospect of death and the dying process. Although those who adhere to a religious tradition generally fear death less than those with no particular religious belief, the prospect of coping with the dying process causes anxiety in most older adults (Berggren-Thomas & Griggs, 1995). In the face of terminal illness, specific spiritual needs for trust, hope, and forgiveness most frequently manifest in an older adult. Related to these needs is the desire for reminiscence, which may help the elder to put present anxieties into the perspective of an entire lifetime.

Trust

Trust, a concept that can be defined as being related to a sense of security in one's future, can be greatly tested during the later stages of the aging process. Fear of the unknown associated not only with death and the dying process but also with the concept of an afterlife poses a great threat to trust in the older adult (Swift & Rench, 1991). The religious elder who has lived according to the tenets of his or her tradition may more easily maintain trust by reflecting on the rewards identified for the faithful. An older adult who does not subscribe to any particular religious belief system will need to draw on personal philosophical beliefs about the meaning of life and one's own contribution to society for support.

Hope

Hope, or the expectation of a positive outcome in the future, is closely linked to trust, especially for the elder from a religious background. Hope is strengthened by an older adult's adherence to strong religious and moral values (Fischer, 1988; Lenarz, 1988; Lotito, 1993). Hope may be more difficult for an ill elder who no longer feels in control of his or her life or future activities. Through a qualitative study to explore the meaning of hope among 12 older adults, Gaskins and Forte (1995) identified hope-related themes related to such factors as health, relationships, material resources, positive emotions, giving service, and reminiscing (p. 19). The most significant and frequently identified theme, however, was that of spirituality. "All of the [study] participants spoke of the important role spirituality played as a source of hope" (p. 19). The authors admitted that all elders in the study identified with a faith tradition, and thus the spirituality theme was often associated with religious practice and belief; hope was, for others, however, described as "having a moral creed for living one's life" (p. 20). And in a study of hope among 94 chronically ill elders residing in a long-term care facility, Beckerman and Northrop (1996) found the most important sources of hope to be faith, relationships, self-esteem, and the ability to give to others. Hope engenders in an elder the spirit to find meaning and joy in life and to maintain a positive sense of self-worth amid diminishing physical and psychological capacities.

Forgiveness

Perhaps the most frequently identified spiritual need for the older adult, especially in the face of serious or terminal illness, is the desire to give and to receive forgiveness. It is rare to find any person, especially one who has lived to elder years, who is not able to acknowledge some attitude or behavior for which he or she would wish forgiveness. The individual from whom the elder desires forgiveness may not be aware of the elder's need; the concern may totally reside in the heart and conscience of the one seeking forgiveness. The other important dimension of the concept relates to an older person's need to extend forgiveness to a person who in the elder's perception has done harm. To give and receive forgiveness are tasks not easily accomplished. Both, noted Fischer (1995), involve "a long and complex process of healing" (p. 127). Much emotional baggage related to old hurts, both given and received, may be deeply ingrained in the elder's persona; they are not easily let go of (Finley, 1989). It is important to remember, also, that desiring to forgive or accept forgiveness does not erase the memories; what forgiveness may accomplish is to "humanize" and incorporate a memory into an elder's current "self-understanding" (Maitland, 1991, p. 160). Healing occurs as the forgiving or forgiven elder reframes his or her self-image and is able to make peace with the past (Bozarth, 1995).

Reminiscence

Another need for the older adult, and one closely linked to giving or receiving forgiveness, is the need for reminiscence. As an individual reviews his or her life story, the need for forgiveness may emerge. There are also many other positive aspects to the act of reminiscence. First, an elder may be strengthened in dealing with present concerns and anxieties by remembering and reidentifying past coping skills used in dealing with stressful experiences. An elder may come to recognize that he or she has "endured beyond [the] ability to endure" (Seymour, 1995, p. 104). This can be a very beneficial memory in terms of facing the unknown future. The process of reviewing past life accomplishments can also serve to suggest what tasks an elder might still undertake, and what legacies can be left (Erikson, 1995, p. 14). In this way, reminiscence may serve as the catalyst for initiating a new career in later life or for helping the older adult to complete some partially finished tasks or activities. Additionally, an elder who reminisces as a social activity with family or friends can offer hard-earned wisdom as a gift to loved ones.

▶ Spiritual Needs in Long-Term Care

Long-term health care for the elderly involves providing "comprehensive, continuous care for older adults in diverse settings" (Collins, Butler, Guelder, & Palmer, 1997, p. 59). These settings include the elder's home or the home of relatives, retirement communities, assisted care facilities, and skilled care nursing homes. The care populations consist of active elders with chronic illness, the homebound elderly, and elders in need of skilled nursing home care. In discussing the need to "revolutionize" long-term care, Patricia Emery (2006), a nursing home director, commented, "Only two populations in this country still face routine and/or permanent institutionalization—convicted felons and the elderly" (p. 16). Some of the positive suggestions for change identified by Emery are "to explore placing control back in their (the elderly) hands" and "allowing them to participate in the decision making processes of life" (p. 22). This can be accomplished, Emery adds, "by providing a home, a sanctuary, a healing environment, where elders experience life and growth" (p. 22).

In a nursing study to explore the relationship between spiritual well-being and positive quality of life, the author conducted both structured and open-ended (conversational) interviews with three populations of older adults: mobile elders living with chronic illness, homebound elders, and nursing home residents (O'Brien, 1997). All study participants were over the age of 65 years. The sample group consisted of 38 mobile elders, 4 older adults who were homebound, and 10 nursing home residents. Data elicited from all three groups reflected a strong association between spiritual well-being, evaluated by a Spiritual Assessment Scale (O'Brien, 1997)—which measures personal faith, religious practice, and spiritual contentment/distress—and quality of life, evaluated in terms of hope (Miller Hope Scale, Miller & Powers, 1988; adapted 1997) and life satisfaction (Life Satisfaction Index-Z, Wood, Wylie, & Sheafor, 1969).

Qualitative data generated through open-ended, conversational interviews (Spirituality and Religiousness Interview Guide, O'Brien, 1997) also demonstrated the presence of hopefulness and life satisfaction among elders with a high degree of personal faith, involvement in religious practice, and lack of spiritual distress, that is, a strong sense of spiritual well-being. Data reflecting spiritual and religious characteristics of chronically ill elders—active elders living with chronic illness, homebound elders, and nursing home residents—are discussed relative to each subcategory.

Active Elders Living with Chronic Illness

Census data for 1989 revealed that 70 percent of men and 77 percent of women over 65 had one or more chronic illness; 81 percent of the men and 90 percent of the women were chronically ill by the age of 80 (Sapp & Bliesmer, 1995, p. 4). In an ethnographic study of spirituality among 12 chronically ill elders ranging in age from 65 to 89 years, Young (1993) identified recurrent themes of "hope, comfort, strength and well-being" as related to spiritual beliefs. The concept of hope was associated with trust in the existence of an afterlife, comfort and strength were derived from an elder's belief in God, and well-being was related to the sense of God's love and care provided both in the present and after death (p. 299). Koenig (1994), who also explored the spiritual needs of physically ill elders, described specific concerns such as the need for meaning and hope, the need for belief in transcendence, the need for spiritual support, the need to carry out religious practices, the need for a feeling of self-worth, the need for love, the need to trust in God, and the need to give to others (pp. 284–291). Ill elders, Koenig asserted, need to be not only prepared for death and the dying process, but also supported "in the life they have remaining" (p. 294).

In the author's study of spiritual well-being and quality of life (O'Brien, 1997) among 38 active (nonhomebound) chronically ill elders, participants ranged in age from 67 to 96 years; 30 were female and 8 were male. Thirty-five persons were white and three were African American. Fifty percent of the group had some college education. Twenty-three of the elders were Roman Catholic, 14 were Protestant, and one was Jewish. Seventy-eight percent of the chronically ill elders attended church at least once a week. Chronic illness conditions included such diagnoses as rheumatoid arthritis, hypertension, cardiomyopathy, asthma, osteoporosis, peptic ulcer, and diabetes mellitus. A number of the study participants also reported multiple diagnoses such as congestive heart failure, arthritis, and hearing loss; hypertension, arthritis, and glaucoma; and hypothyroidism and coronary artery disease.

Although, as noted, the association between spiritual well-being and positive quality of life was strong overall, certain individual scale items revealed interesting findings. Hope, as a concept, was rated high among the group; however, seven of the study participants disagreed with Miller Hope Scale item 4 ("I have energy to do what is important to me"), and over half of the group, 22 (57.8 percent), agreed moderately rather than strongly with the statement. And, although most elders responded negatively to the Life Satisfaction Index-Z item 3 ("This is the dreariest time in my life"), 16 respondents or 42 percent of the group also disagreed with Life Satisfaction Index-Z item 5 ("These are the best years of my life"). One 72-year-old woman penciled in the comment, "These are not the best years of my life, but they're good!" Several respondents commented on item 14 in the Spiritual Assessment Scale ("I am helped to communicate with God by spiritual reading or thinking about religious things"). For example, an 84-year-old woman admitted that because of failing eyesight, reading had become a problem.

The author's analysis of qualitative data elicited in interviews with the 38 chronically ill elders revealed five dominant themes reflecting spiritual well-being among the group: trust, comfort, joy, acceptance, and peace. Trust was associated with the constancy of God's protection, especially during difficult times. Comfort was defined as a sense of well-being received from prayer and spiritual reading, especially the reading of Scripture. Joy was seen as deriving from personal faith beliefs, religious practices, and the support of one's church. Acceptance was related to patience in the face of pain and suffering and faith that God would provide needed support. Peace was achieved in facing death; this was frequently associated with an elder's perception of having lived a "good life," as he or she understood the concept.

Trust

Mrs. Daly, an 88-year-old Roman Catholic diagnosed with congestive heart disease and arthritis, expressed great confidence in God. "I can always count on God to help me in my times of need. My trust in Him affects my whole life; he gives me strength to take part in senior citizen's programs. My belief in God makes me feel great, knowing that He is there watching over me every day, giving me time to spend with my daughter and my grandchildren. I'm healthy and happy. God is very good to me."

Mrs. Kelly, an 81-year-old Catholic who was somewhat more ill with cardiovascular disease, also verbalized trust in God. "I feel as though all my life God has been standing by me. He has always watched over me and helped me get through the pain." Mrs. Kelly added, "But more importantly God showed me how to find love."

Comfort

Mrs. Ann Johnson, an 89-year-old Baptist diagnosed with heart disease and arthritis, described the comfort she received from religion and religious practices. "I pray and am at peace. God and I have a relationship that comforts me. I talk to Him when I am lonely or in need or thankful. My trust in God is part of my everyday life . . . My faith in God got me involved in my church and the people in my church are the bright spot in my life, so I guess God has been a great comfort in my life."

Sixty-five-year-old Miss Smith, a Christian suffering from rheumatoid arthritis, reported comfort from spiritual reading. "I read from a religious book, *My Daily Bread*, which I find very comforting, especially in times of illness or sadness in my life. It keeps me remembering that God will never send me crosses heavier than I can bear."

Joy

Mrs. Davis, a 65-year-old Presbyterian with cardiac disease, described the joy her spirituality and religious practice brought to her life. "I know that I am in God's hands; He is looking out for me and that is a joy. Another thing that brings me a lot of happiness is that I attend Sunday school and church every Sunday. I have been with the same people in Sunday school for almost 29 years. These friends are very dear to me and we help each other in rough times; they are my church support."

Sixty-seven-year-old Mrs. Flaherty, a Catholic suffering from cardiomyopathy, reported, "My joy is from my love of God, which affects my everyday relationships with people. Although I can lose my temper sometimes, I try to be true to my faith and be loving and share the joy with people in my life."

Acceptance

Mr. Anderson, a 70-year-old diagnosed with a brain tumor, spoke about the importance of his Lutheran beliefs and practices in helping him accept his illness. "I know God cares for us in times of sickness. I pray and talk to Him and know that He hears me. He may not always answer the prayers the way I would like Him to do, but He knows what is best for me. I am at peace in my relationship with God. I trust in His Son, Jesus Christ, and know Him as my Lord and Savior. He has given me an inner peace to accept whatever happens, whatever my illness situation may be." Mr. Anderson explained that his church, the Evangelical Lutheran Church of America (ELCA), provided much support. "It gives me strength to deal with my illness. We are a community of believers, and God gives us the assurance that He is with us in time of need, and that He will heal us." Mr. Anderson concluded, "He is a caring and healing God. We are in His hands. Who could ask for anything more?"

Roman Catholic Mrs. Doherty, an 86-year-old suffering from arthritis, observed, "I feel at great peace in my relationship with God. I have been able to accept pain and put difficult times in perspective because I feel that God allows things to happen for a reason. I just trust that God will be watching over me no matter what happens. So in that way I can accept whatever happens."

Peace

Miss Mahoney, a 75-year-old Catholic and a cancer survivor also suffering from congestive heart failure, described the meaning of peace in her life. "I truly am at peace right now. I completely feel at peace in my relationship with God; I always have. There are hard times when you are struggling, but that does not take away your peace, your faith in God. I am at peace about death too; I'm not afraid to die. I know that God will be with me then, as always."

Seventy-eight-year-old Mrs. Pearson, diagnosed with coronary artery disease, explained that as a member of the Baha'i faith, her peace was related to having lived well. "I don't exactly have a relationship with God as in the sense of a 'relationship.' Baha'i's believe that God is all around us. But I do feel at peace with God, because I have led a good life. I honor God every day."

The Homebound Elderly

Chronically ill elders who are homebound or nonmobile and living in assisted care facilities may have significant spiritual needs related to the physical and psychosocial sequelae of their conditions. The physical and emotional pain associated with being homebound requires a depth of faith and spirituality (Burghardt, 1991), as well as spiritual maturity, which Birren (1990) interpreted as the elder's ability to focus on transcendent spiritual values, while still appreciating religious experiences of the past (p. 42).

In studying 26 Protestant, Catholic, and Jewish homebound elders, Brennan (1994) found that personal spirituality was described as giving "meaning and purpose to life" (p. 96). Brennan's study participants understood the difference between the concepts of religion and spirituality, yet perceived them to be interrelated; many described using prayer as a coping mechanism. A specific need expressed by more than half of the study group was the "desire to be able to discuss their spiritual beliefs and feelings with others, especially in times of crisis" (p. 96).

Four homebound elders interviewed for a study of spiritual well-being and quality of life (O'Brien, 1997) ranged from 75 to 91 years of age; all were female and were wheelchair or walker restricted. Three of the women were white and one was African American. Two members of the homebound subgroup were Roman Catholic, one was Mennonite, and the other was a member of the Church of Christ; all were unable to attend worship services because of physical disability. Their illness conditions included rheumatoid arthritis, diabetes and postpolio syndrome, hypertension and cardiovascular disease, and congestive heart failure and hypertension. Quantitative measures for this group revealed a strong relationship between spiritual well-being and positive quality of life.

Qualitative data elicited from the homebound elders reflected one unifying theme that might be described as confident prayer; that is, all four study participants spoke about the depth of their faith and trust in God related to their prayer practices and the prayers of their families and church members. Mrs. Allen, an 83-year-old Mennonite diagnosed with diabetes and postpolio syndrome, described herself as almost totally disabled, yet she displayed a strong faith. "I pray to God daily; He's on my mind all the time. I rely on God and on my church in hard times. God is very accessible. I'm very much at peace in my relationship with God." The remarks of 91-year-old Mrs. McCarthy, a Catholic with multiple diagnoses of congestive heart failure, coronary artery disease, and hypertension, who lives in an assisted care setting, reflected a similar theme. "I believe in God who watches out for me in times of sickness and health. I feel at peace with God; I pray to Him every day and I know He will take me when He is ready." Mrs. McCarthy added, "When I'm sick I also count on the prayers of my family and my church."

Mrs. Clark, an 82-year-old homebound member of the Church of Christ who was diagnosed with diabetes and hypertension, reported that although she could not get out to attend church services, she prayed all the time. "I pray and I know that God is taking care of me in all my trials and tribulations, and I will come out better in the end. I believe that no matter what happens God will be with me. You can trust God all the time." Mrs. Clark also commented on the importance of the prayer support of others. "My family members are all of the same religion and they pray for me, and we pray for each other. Being a Christian has helped keep us together, to keep God in the middle of everything."

Mrs. O'Connell, a 75-year-old Catholic who is wheelchair bound because of arthritis, described the peace she received from prayer. "I do feel at peace when I pray; it affects all the activities of my day. It gives me a positive attitude about things. I pray every day and trust in God and the Blessed Mother to get me through."

Nursing Home Residents

The term *nursing home* is broadly understood as describing a facility that "provides twenty-four hour skilled nursing care at an intermediate [i.e., nonhospital] level" (Simmons & Peters, 1996, p. 7). Data obtained in 1984 identified 19,100 nursing homes with approximately 1.6 million beds; this statistic reflected "a 22% increase over the previous ten years" (Millsap, 1995, p. 99). Presently almost 20 percent of older old adults (over 80) reside in nursing homes, and by the year 2030, the number is expected to triple (Koenig, 1994, p. 353). Mechanisms suggested to enhance the spiritual well-being of elders in institutional settings include "appreciation for the spiritual dimension of life," "spiritual care," "vitality of the spirit" of the setting, "spiritual health of the staff," and "presence of . . . clergy" (Minnix, 2008, pp. 66–67). A study of perception of the meaning and value of spirituality among five residents of a long-term care facility revealed such themes as "meaning," "coping," "positive outlook," "reliance," "comfort and consolation," and "hope for recovery" (Schwartz & Cottrell, 2007, p. 43).

Some characteristics of a contemporary nursing home population include average age in the 80s; most widowed or single; women in 3:1 proportion to men; many having some degree of dementia and/or arthritis or cardiovascular disease; many experiencing impaired vision or hearing, or both; and most requiring assistance with activities of daily living (Holland & McCurren, 1997, p. 97). Data from an urban nursing home with approximately 230 residents revealed a population physical profile heavily laden with such diagnoses as arteriosclerotic heart disease, diabetes mellitus, hip fracture, osteoporosis, arthritis, Parkinson's disease, Alzheimer's disease, and senile dementia (O'Brien, 1989, pp. 22–23).

The multiplicity of health deficits experienced by current nursing home residents requires skill and ingenuity in care planning, including that of spiritual ministry. Malcolm (1987) believed that nurses must work at developing "creative spiritual care" for elderly nursing home residents; she suggested that although usual care plans place symptoms of dementia under a psychosocial need heading, these aspects of an elder's personality may also be "interwoven with the spiritual" (p. 25).

Some religious rituals appropriate for the responsive nursing home resident include Baptism (for one who has never experienced the sacrament earlier in life), Communion (according to the resident's religious tradition), Anointing of the Sick, and celebrations of religious feast days (Simmons & Peters, 1996, pp. 76–83). For the seriously physically or cognitively impaired resident, Simmons and Peters noted that these rituals may be adapted and modified to meet the elder's condition. Many nursing homes are formally affiliated with a particular religious denomination, so the worship services and rites of that tradition may be central to the home's activities; however, arrangements are generally made for religious ministry to residents of different traditions.

The 10 nursing home residents who participated in the author's study of spiritual well-being and quality of life (O'Brien, 1997) ranged in age from 71 to 98 years; 8 were female and 2 were male. Eight of the nursing home residents were African American and two were white; three of the group were married. Group members had been living in the nursing home from 4 months to 5 years; all were wheelchair bound. Five of the nursing home residents were Roman Catholic, two were Baptist, one was Seventh-day Adventist, one was Pentecostal, and one was a Jehovah's Witness. Their collective diagnoses included peripheral vascular disease, bilateral knee replacements, cerebral vascular accident, rheumatoid arthritis, congestive heart disease, diabetes, blindness, right-sided paralysis, and fractured hip.

Quantitative data demonstrated a strong relationship between spiritual well-being and positive quality of life among the group. Interestingly, all of the nursing home residents agreed with the Miller Hope Scale item 4 ("I have energy to do what is important to me"). One might speculate that this group of wheelchair-bound nursing home residents had modified their expectations in terms of those activities for which they perceived energy to be required.

Three dominant themes were derived from qualitative data elicited in interviews with the nursing home group: faith in God and religious beliefs despite illness and disability, and acceptance of nursing home life; devotion, relating especially to private religious practices such as prayer and Scripture reading; and spiritual contentment, or a sense of peace in relation to where the elder is on his or her spiritual journey.

Faith

Mrs. Jackson, an 81-year-old Baptist resident who had experienced bilateral knee replacements, described a powerful faith. "I do believe in God; He gives me strength to do everything I need to do. He has blessed me so in my life; I am able to go on because of Him. Sometimes the road is rough; not everything is smooth. Sometimes it's hard to be in a nursing home. There are some bumps and some knocks but Jesus will be right beside you." Mrs. Jackson added, "I don't ever feel far away from God regardless of what happens. I read the Twenty-third Psalm in the Bible, you know, 'Yea, though I walk through the valley of the shadow of death, I will fear no evil for Thou art with me.' It just makes you forget anything that might have happened."

The remarks of Mrs. Earhardt, a 76-year-old Seventh-day Adventist resident with peripheral vascular disease, also reflected a strong faith. "I have faith in God, a relationship with God, and when I get stressed out or something happens to me, the Lord always makes a way for that to ease over. Then the stress leaves me and the breath of God comes back in me. My faith is everything to me; if the effect of God didn't work in me, I couldn't make it. There is no way that I could make it without the

Lord. I might as well just hang it up and forget it." Mrs. Earhardt concluded, "Faith in God means everything. If you don't have faith in God, you don't have faith in anybody. There is no one I look up to but Jesus. If you believe in His word, He will answer you."

A male nursing home resident, Mr. Martin, an 82-year-old bilateral amputee and member of a pentecostal church, the Church of God in Christ, explained his faith. "Faith is having a personal relationship with Jesus. I believe that to be a child of God, you have to be born again of the Spirit. You can go to Jesus and tell Him anything and He will listen to you. And according to His will, He will grant you what you ask."

Devotion

Mrs. Meehan, an 87-year-old Catholic resident who was recovering from a stroke, described her religious devotion. "I try to stay very close to God through my prayers and church services. Many times I have talked to God; I talk with my God every day, a lot of times a day. I also go to Mass here in the chapel every day and I have a spiritual advisor who I talk to. And I have my rosary too that I say for my family who have gone to God, and for my friends."

An 88-year-old Jehovah's Witness resident, Mrs. Jensen, also recovering from a stroke, spoke especially about the importance of Scripture reading. "I'm at peace with God because I believe deeply in Him through the Bible. I read the Bible every day and I've come through with flying colors. Scripture gives comfort in Jesus. I am a Jehovah's Witness and we believe deeply in Jesus Christ. Jehovah is our great God. I find him in my Bible."

Spiritual Contentment

Seventy-two-year-old Mrs. Annie Smith, a Baptist nursing home resident with hypertension and stroke sequelae, described the contentment brought about by her spiritual and religious beliefs. "I believe in God and in His Son Jesus who care for me in times of trials and tribulations. God is such a consolation to me. And I am content and very confident that I will be taken care of in any matter. I think I've lived according to His commandments and I feel that God directs me in things I have done in my life, so I'm at peace." Mrs. Smith concluded, "I am in constant prayer with God, and I pray day and night or anytime that I feel I need to."

Mrs. Loughlin, a 98-year-old with multiple cardiovascular conditions and a Catholic, also reflected spiritual contentment in her remarks. "I'm at peace at this time in my life. I can't go to church anymore, but I get to the chapel here. I say my rosary in the evening for all my relatives and I pray for the people here. Most of my life God has answered all of my prayers. He is the power and the glory and the strength of my life. And I don't ever feel far away from Him, so I'm very happy here." Mrs. Loughlin concluded, "I thank God for all the lovely privileges I've had in my life; my home, and my family, and some of the beauty of the world. I realize that if it is God's will that I live a little longer then it's OK, but if it is not, then He will take me home to Glory."

Overall findings from the author's study of spirituality and quality of life among three groups of elders—active elders living with a chronic illness, home-bound elders, and nursing home residents—revealed the presence of spiritual values including faith, hope, trust (confidence), joy, acceptance, peace (contentment), and devotion (commitment to prayer for self and others) among the study participants. These study data documenting the spiritual and religious beliefs and practices, as well as the needs, of ill elders are supportive of James Fowler's (1981) final faith stages in which the older adult seeks a deepening of his or her own spiritual life as well as expressing concern over the needs of the larger society.

Continuing Care Retirement Community Residents

In today's world of long-term care, one hears the term *CCRC* (which stands for continuing care retirement community) used even more frequently than *nursing home*, although in fact the modern CCRC generally contains one or several dimensions of the older style nursing home.

The CCRC concept has become popular in the past several decades of long-term care. CCRCs differ significantly in terms of contracts, housing options, services, and costs. Generally, however, a CCRC is expected to be a long-term care facility providing three levels of living options for an older adult: independent living (in a room, apartment, or even a small cottage home); assisted care (single room with meals served in a communal dining room); and skilled nursing care (single- or double-room occupancy). Some CCRCs have separate facilities for dementia patients.

The advantage of the CCRC for many elders is the fact that they can enter the facility on a more independent level and then stay in the same CCRC as physical and/or cognitive needs require more assistance or care. Contracts vary significantly among CCRCs, as do costs. Some facilities provide a life-care contract, guaranteeing that the individual will be cared for until death; for such a contract, the cost of the entrance or admission fee is generally significant. CCRCs also usually require that a potential resident come with Medicare A, B, and D (drug coverage), as well as a health-care supplemental plan such one of those recommended by the Association for Retired Persons (AARP). Some contracts provide services and care for a specified period of time; others include a fee-for-service contract. The latter CCRC usually only requires a minimal entrance fee; however, if assisted or skilled care is later needed, monthly costs will escalate notably.

An important concern for many potential CCRC residents is the presence or lack thereof of spiritual and religious support at the facility. Currently most large CCRCs have a department of "pastoral care" and a chapel to meet the needs of residents from a variety of faith traditions. The sponsorship or the administration of the facility may or may not be associated with a particular religious community or church.

It is only during the past decade that the nursing and health-care literature has begun to address the needs and concerns of the CCRC resident. Generally, the CCRC literatures addresses such issues as home technology, "including the influence of primary care providers" (Courtney, Demiris, Rantz, & Skubic, 2008, p. 195); networking or "social interaction with other people living at the retirement community" or CCRC (Schafer, 2011, p. 795); factors associated with exercise among CCRC residents (Resnick & D'Adamo, 2010); and patient education in a CCRC (Wendel, Durso, Zabel, Loman, & Remsburg, 2003). Interestingly, the concepts of spirituality and religion in the CCRC are seldom addressed. In one paper on the topic of the "therapeutic landscape" and residential transition to a CCRC, Cutchin, Marshall, and Aldrich (2010) did include the fact that symbolism "embedded in the interior and exterior of the buildings on a CCRC campus is typically meant to affirm cultural values of the generation living there as well as provide a sense of who the residents view themselves" to be (p. 120); no examples such as religious symbolism, however, were identified. The authors do present a table comparing pre- and post-move activity of CCRC residents, which includes an item revealing a change in attendance at religious services, but the concept is not explored in depth.

In a qualitative exploration of life in a CCRC entitled "But I Am Not Moving," the investigator conducted interviews with 35 residents primarily focused on the topic of transitions or moving across the three levels of the studied facility's care. Analysis of the data revealed three key themes related to CCRC transitioning that were labeled autonomy, fatalism, and social disengagement (Shippee, 2009, p. 421). The theme of autonomy included such concepts as "being told to move" and "threats to privacy" (pp. 421–422); fatalism included such concepts as "death" and "irreversibility of the move" (p. 423); and social disengagement included the "nature of social interaction" (p. 425). The topics of spirituality and/or religion might only be considered as implicitly addressed in relation to such concepts as fatalism and death.

I spent seven months volunteering in the pastoral care department of a large, 600-bed CCRC. The facility was rich with symbolism in terms of its founders' religious and spiritual orientation. Both the exterior and interior of the buildings were embellished with religious statuary and art reflective of the institutions' spiritual commitment to care for elders. The presence of a department of pastoral care, several chaplains, and three chapels on the campus also reflected the spiritual nature of the CCRC and provided worship opportunities for residents from a variety of faith communities. Daily pastoral care visits were made to all residents and a number of special celebrations were conducted on religious holidays. The pastoral care dimension of caring at this CCRC was described by residents in independent living, assisted living, and the nursing center as being central to their life satisfaction at the facility and also as having been a key factor in their choice of this particular CCRC for their personal retirement.

▶ Spirituality and Quality of Later Life

The quality of life for an older adult depends greatly on the personal spirituality supporting the elder's perception of his or her current life stage. As has been demonstrated in this chapter, some of the physiologic and psychosocial literature presents a rather bleak picture of life and functional ability for an elder; the older a person becomes, the more forbidding the image seems to be. On the other hand, spiritual and religious writing has affirmed the journey of aging as encompassing a time of peace and fulfillment; a "time to be eagerly awaited and warmly embraced" (Sapp, 1987, p. 133). The truth, for most older adults, probably lies somewhere between these two extremes. Certainly there is a greater risk of physical deficit as one ages. Oppenheimer (1991) believed, however, that "realism does not require that we should anticipate all these ills" (p. 43). Some future problems may be prevented by heeding health/illness-related precautions. And, if unexpected health deficits occur, the use of established coping skills, especially those of a spiritual or religious nature, can greatly mediate the negative impact of the condition. As Oppenheimer concluded, some future suffering can be "circumvented"; other suffering needs to be "faced."

In nursing research to explore the meaning of quality of life among residents of a long-term care facility, Aller and Van Ess Coeling (1995) identified three themes descriptive of the concept; these include "ability to communicate with others," "ability to care for self," and "ability to help others" (p. 23). The latter theme also reflects well Fowler's (1981) final stages of faith development, conjunctive faith and universalizing faith, in which an older individual's social conscience takes precedence over the needs of self; the desire to reach out to others becomes primary. As one of Aller and Van Ess Coeling's (1995) elder study respondents commented, "Quality of life, to me, is not only self-betterment, but the betterment of others (p. 23).

A study of 71 elders residing in a nursing home revealed that quality of later life was decidedly subjective. An 88-year-old resident in relatively good physical and mental health admitted that she did not want to do "much of anything" at this point in her life. "I made up my mind I am at the end of my rope. You do sort of get that notion. I have felt I really don't have any incentive to live" (O'Brien, 1989, p. 44). An 83-year-old woman, however, compared her quality of life to that of more seriously disabled residents. "You feel sorry for them. Of course, you say to yourself: 'There but for the Grace of God, go I!' I wake up in the morning and say, 'Thank God, I've got another day.' I mean it" (p. 44).

Contemporary elder adults are living longer and functioning better than ever before. Although obviously some physiologic and psychosocial deficits accompany the aging process, a strong personal faith and participation in religious practices can greatly enhance an elder's quality of life. Chronically ill older adults living in a nursing care facility, as well as those living at home, may enjoy significant spiritual well-being in their later years. The aging adult may take comfort in the wisdom of Brother Roger of Taizé who observed:

> Every age has its own beauty. Why be afraid of physical decline when the years bring deeper insight and greater gentleness of action. (As cited in Finch, 1993, p. 23)

While some older adults are able to maintain a significant degree of physical and psychological health well into their later decades of life—even to the 80th and 90th years—others are struck by illness and disability as aging occurs. For some, the disease processes are diagnosed as progressive and ultimately terminal, thus placing the individual in an end-of-life status—some well before their anticipated time of death.

▶ References

Ainlay, S. C., & Smith, D. R. (1984). Aging and religious participation. *Journal of Gerontology, 39*(3), 357–363.

Aller, L., & Van Ess Coeling, H. (1995). Quality of life: Its meaning to the long-term care resident. *Journal of Gerontological Nursing, 21*(2), 20–25.

Beckerman, A., & Northrop, C. (1996). Hope, chronic illness and the elderly. *Journal of Gerontological Nursing, 22*(5), 19–25.

Berggren-Thomas, P., & Griggs, M. J. (1995). Spirituality in aging: Spiritual needs or spiritual journey. *Journal of Gerontological Nursing, 21*(3), 5–10.

Beuscher, L., & Beck, C. (2008). A literature review of spirituality in coping with early-stage Alzheimer's disease. *Journal of Clinical Nursing, 17*(5), 88–97.

Bianchi, E. C. (1995). *Aging as a spiritual journey*. New York, NY: Crossroad.

Birren, J. E. (1990). Spiritual maturity in psychological development. In J. Seeber (Ed.), *Spiritual maturity in the later years* (pp. 41–53). New York, NY: The Haworth Press.

Blazer, D. (1991). Spirituality and aging well. *Generations, 15*(1), 61–65.

Boettcher, E. (1985). Linking the aged to support systems. *Journal of Gerontological Nursing*, 11(3), 27–33.

Bozarth, A. R. (1995). *Lifelines: Threads of grace through seasons of change*. Kansas City, MO: Sheed & Ward.

Brennan, Sr. M. R. (1994). *Spirituality in the homebound elderly* (Unpublished doctoral dissertation). The Catholic University of America. Ann Arbor, MI.

Burghardt, W. J. (1991). Aging, suffering and dying: A Christian perspective. In L. S. Cahill & D. Mieth (Eds.), *Aging* (pp. 65–71). London, UK: Conciliam.

Burt, D. X. (1992). *But when you are older: Reflections on coming of age*. Collegeville, MN: The Liturgical Press.

Byrne, Sr. M. (1985). A zest for life. *Journal of Gerontological Nursing, 11*(4), 30–33.

Callaghan, D. (2006). The influence of growth on spiritual self-care agency in an older population. *Journal of Gerontological Nursing, 32*(9), 43–51.

Castellaw, L. S., Wicks, M. N., & Martin, J. C. (1999). Spirituality in white older women with arthritis. *Graduate Research Nursing, 1*(1), 1–9.

Collins, C. E., Butler, F. R., Guelder, S. H., & Palmer, M. H. (1997). Models for community-based long-term care for the elderly in a changing health system. *Nursing Outlook, 45*(2), 59–63.

Coupland, S. (1985). *Beginning to pray in old age*. Cambridge, MA: Cowley.

Courtney, K., Demiris, G., Rantz, M., & Skubic, M. (2008). Needing smart home technologies: The perspectives of older adults in continuing care retirement communities. *Informatics in Primary Care, 16*, 195–201.

Cutchin, M., Marshall, V., & Aldrich, R. (2010). Moving to a continuing care retirement community: Occupations in the therapeutic landscape process. *Journal of Cross Cultural Gerontology, 25*, 117–132.

Daly, L., & Fahey-McCarthy, E. (2014). Attending to the spiritual in dementia care. *British Journal of Nursing, 23*(14), 787–791.

Deeken, A. (1986). *Growing old and how to cope with it*. San Francisco, CA: Ignatius Press.

Durkin, M. B. (1992). A community of caring. *Health Progress, 73*(8), 48–53.

Emery, P. (2006). Building a new culture of aging: Revolutionizing long-term care. *Journal of Christian Nursing, 23*(1), 16–24.

Erickson, R. M. (1995). *Late have I loved thee: Stories of religious conversion and commitment in later life*. New York, NY: Paulist Press.

Finch, A. (Ed.). (1993). *Journey to the light: Spirituality as we mature*. New Rochelle, NY: New City Press.

Finley, J. (1989). *The treasured age: Spirituality for seniors*. New York, NY: Alba House.

Fischer, K. (1988). Hope never ends: God's promise to the elderly. *Journal of Christian Nursing, 5*(4), 32–35.

Fischer, K. (1995). *Autumn gospel: Women in the second half of life*. New York, NY: Paulist Press.

Forbis, P. A. (1988). Meeting patients' spiritual needs. *Geriatric Nursing, 9*(3), 158–159.

Fowler, J. W. (1981). *Stages of faith: The psychology of human development and the quest for meaning*. San Francisco, CA: Harper.

Gaskamp, C., Sutter, R., & Meraviglia, M. (2006). Evidence-based guideline: Promoting spirituality in the older adult. *Journal of Gerontological Nursing, 32*(11), 8–13.

Gaskins, S., & Forte, L. (1995). The meaning of hope: Implications for nursing practice and research. *Journal of Gerontological Nursing, 21*(3), 17–24.

Hall, C. M. (1985). Religion and aging. *Journal of Religion and Health, 24*(1), 70–78.

Halstead, H. L. (1995). Spirituality in the elderly. In M. Stanley & P. G. Beare (Eds.), *Gerontological nursing* (pp. 415–425). Philadelphia, PA: F. A. Davis.

Hammer, M. L. (1990). Spiritual needs: A forgotten dimension of care. *Journal of Gerontological Nursing, 16*(12), 3–4.

Haugen, G., Rannestad, T., Hammervold, R., Garasen, H., & Espnes, G. (2013). The relationship between self-transcendence and spiritual well-being in cognitively intact nursing home patients. *International Journal of Older People Nursing, 9*(1), 65–78.

Heriot, C. J. (1995). Developmental tasks and development in the later years of life. In M. Stanley & P. G. Beare (Eds.), *Gerontological nursing* (pp. 349–356). Philadelphia, PA: F. A. Davis.

Hicks, T. J. (1999). Spirituality and the elderly: Nursing implications with nursing home residents. *Geriatric Nursing, 20*(3), 144–146.

Higgens, P. (2013). Meeting the religious needs of residents with dementia. *Nursing Older People, 25*(9), 25–29.

Hogstel, M. O. (1995). Mental health wellness strategies for successful aging. In M. Stanley & P. G. Beare (Eds.), *Gerontological nursing* (pp. 17–27). Philadelphia, PA: F. A. Davis.

Holland, B. E., & McCurren, C. (1997). Aging. In J. M. Black & E. Matassarin-Jacobs (Eds.), *Medical–surgical nursing: Clinical management for continuity of care* (5th ed., pp. 81–104). Philadelphia, PA: W. B. Saunders.

Hudson, R. (2008). Application to practice guidelines. *International Journal of Older People Nursing, 3*, 145–150.

Hungelmann, J., Kenkel-Rossi, E., Klassen, L., & Stollenwerk, R. M. (1985). Spiritual well-being in older adults: Harmonious interconnectedness. *Journal of Religion and Health, 24*(2), 147–153.

Hunsberger, B. (1985). Religion, age, life satisfaction, and perceived sources of religiousness: A study of older persons. *Journal of Gerontology, 40*(5), 615–620.

Hynes, M. (1989). *The ministry to the aging.* Collegeville, MN: The Liturgical Press.

Jolley, D., & Moreland, N. (2011). Dementia care: Spiritual and faith perspectives. *Nursing and Residential Care, 13*(8), 388–391.

Koenig, H. G. (1994). *Aging and God: Spiritual pathways to mental health in midlife and later years.* New York, NY: The Haworth Press.

Lenarz, M. A. (1988). In the dark: A nurse struggles to give hope to the elderly. *Journal of Christian Nursing, 5*(4), 30–32.

Lotito, F. A. (1993). *Wisdom, age and grace: An inspirational guide to staying young at heart.* New York, NY: Paulist Press.

Lueckenotte, A. G. (1997). Older adult. In P. A. Potter & A. G. Perry (Eds.), *Fundamentals of nursing: Concepts, process and practice* (pp. 568–593). St. Louis, MO: C. V. Mosby.

MacKinlay, E. (2008). Practice development in aged care nursing of older people: The perspective of ageing and spiritual care. *International Journal of Older People Nursing, 3*, 151–158.

MacKinlay, E., & Trevitt, C. (2010). Living in aged care: Using spiritual reminiscence to enhance meaning in life for those with dementia. *International Journal of Mental Health Nursing, 19*, 394–401.

Maitland, D. J. (1991). *Aging as counterculture: A vocation for the later years.* New York, NY: The Pilgrim Press.

Malcolm, J. (1987). Creative spiritual care for the elderly. *Journal of Christian Nursing, 4*(1), 24–26.

Maltby, T. (1990). Pastoral care of the aging. In H. Hayes & C. J. van der Poel (Eds.), *Health care ministry: A handbook for chaplains* (pp. 98–104). New York, NY: Paulist Press.

Markides, K. S. (1983). Aging, religiosity, and adjustment: A longitudinal analysis. *Journal of Gerontology, 38*(5), 621–625.

McFadden, S., & Kozberg, C. (2008). Religious and spiritual supports for late-life meaning. *Generations, 32*(2), 6–11.

Miller, J., & Powers, M. (1988). Development of an instrument to measure hope. *Nursing Research, 37*(1), 6–10.

Millsap, P. (1995). Nurses' role with the elderly in the long-term care setting. In M. Stanley & P. G. Beare (Eds.), *Gerontological nursing* (pp. 98–106). Philadelphia, PA: F. A. Davis.

Minnix, L. (2008). Maintaining spirituality in institutional settings. *Generations, 32*(2), 65–67.

Moberg, D. O. (1990). Spiritual maturity and wholeness in later years. In J. Seeber (Ed.), *Spiritual maturity in the later years* (pp. 5–24). New York, NY: The Haworth Press.

Mooney, S. F. (2006). When memory fails: Helping dementia patients remember God. *Journal of Christian Nursing, 23*(1), 6–14.

Morikawa, J. (1974, September). American Baptist news service, Division of communications. *Aging without apology: Living the senior years with integrity and faith.* Valley Forge, PA: Judson Press.

Mull, C. S., Cox, C. L., & Sullivan, J. L. (1987). Religion's role in the health and well-being of well elders. *Public Health Nursing, 4*(3), 151–159.

Normille, P. (1992). *Visiting the sick.* Cincinnati, OH: St. Anthony Messenger Press.

Nouwen, H. J., & Gaffney, W. J. (1990). *Aging: The fulfillment of life.* New York, NY: Doubleday.

O'Brien, M. E. (1989). *Anatomy of a nursing home: A new view of resident life.* Owings Mills, MD: National Health Publishing.

O'Brien, M. E. (1997). *Spiritual well-being and quality of life in chronically ill elders* (Unpublished study funded by Research Grant-in-Aid). The Catholic University of America, Washington, DC.

Odbehr, L., Kvigne, K., Hauge, S., & Danbolt, L. (2015). Spiritual care to persons with dementia in nursing homes: A qualitative study of nurses and care workers' experiences. *BMC Nursing, 14*(70), 1–9.

Oppenheimer, H. (1991). Reflections on the experience of aging. In L. S. Cahill & D. Mieth (Eds.), *Aging* (pp. 39–45). London, UK: Conciliam.

Payne, B. (1990). Spiritual maturity and meaning-filled relationships. In J. Seeber (Ed.), *Spiritual maturity in the later years* (pp. 25–39). New York, NY: The Haworth Press.

Peterson, V., & Potter, P. A. (1997). Spiritual health. In P. A. Potter & A. G. Perry (Eds.), *Fundamentals of nursing: Concepts, process and practice* (pp. 440–455). St. Louis, MO: C. V. Mosby.

Resnick, B., & D'Adamo, C. (2010). Factors associated with exercise among older adults in a continuing care retirement community. *Rehabilitation Nursing, 36*(2), 47–53; 82.

Rice, V. H., Beck, C., & Stevenson, J. S. (1997). Ethical issues relative to autonomy and personal control in independent and cognitively impaired elders. *Nursing Outlook, 45*(1), 27–34.

Roen, O. T. (1997). Senior health. In J. H. Swanson & M. A. Nies (Eds.), *Community health nursing: Promoting the health of aggregates* (2nd ed., pp. 347–386). Philadelphia, PA: W. B. Saunders.

Rykkje, L., & Raholm, M. (2014). Understanding older peoples' experiences of dignity and its significance for caring: A hermeneutical study. *International Journal of Human Caring, 18*(1), 17–26.

Sapp, M., & Bliesmer, M. (1995). A health promotion/protection approach to meeting elders' health care needs. In M. Stanley & P. G. Beare (Eds.), *Gerontological nursing* (pp. 3–12). Philadelphia, PA: F. A. Davis.

Sapp, S. (1987). *Full of years: Aging and the elderly in the Bible and today.* Nashville, TN: Abington Press.

Schafer, M. (2011). Health and network centrality in a continuing care retirement community. *Journal of Gerontology, 66*(6), 795–803.

Schwartz, L., & Cottrell, R. P. (2007). The value of spirituality as perceived by elders in long-term care. *Physical & Occupational Therapy in Geriatrics, 26*(1), 43–62.

Seymour, R. E. (1995). *Aging without apology: Living the senior years with integrity and faith.* Valley Forge, PA: Judson Press.

Shippee, T. (2009). "But I am not moving": Residents' perspectives on transitions within a continuing care retirement community. *The Gerontologist, 49*(3), 418–427.

Simmons, H. C., & Peters, M. A. (1996). *With God's oldest friends: Pastoral visiting in the nursing home.* New York, NY: Paulist Press.

Stagg, F. (1981). *The Bible speaks on aging.* Nashville, TN: Broadman Press.

Stuckey, J., Post, S., Ollerton, S., FallCreek, S., & Whitehouse, P. (2002). Alzheimer's disease, religion and ethics of respect for spirituality: A community dialogue. *Alzheimer's Care Quarterly, 3*(3), 199–207.

Swift, H. C., & Rench, C. E. (1991). *Life, fulfillment and joy in the sunset years.* Huntington, IN: Our Sunday Visitor Publications.

Taylor, C., Lillis, C., & LeMone, P. (1997). *Fundamentals of nursing: The art and science of nursing care* (3rd ed.). Philadelphia, PA: J. B. Lippincott.

Tournier, P. (1983). *Learn to grow old.* Louisville, KY: Westminister/John Knox Press.

Valentine, M. H. (1994). *Aging in the Lord.* New York, NY: Paulist Press.

Wendel, I., Durso, S., Zable, B., Loman, K., & Remsburg, R. (2003). Group diabetes patient education: A model for use in a continuing care retirement community. *Journal of Gerontological Nursing, 29*(2), 37–44.

Wicks, R. J. (1997). *After 50: Spiritually embracing your own wisdom years.* New York, NY: Paulist Press.

Wilkes, L., Cioffi, J., Fleming, A., & LeMiere, J. (2011). Defining pastoral care for older people in residential care. *Contemporary Nurse, 37*(2), 213–221.

Wood, V., Wylie, M., & Sheafor, B. (1969). An analysis of a short self-report measure of life satisfaction: Correlation with later judgments. *Journal of Gerontology, 24*(2), 465–469.

Young, C. (1993). Spirituality and the chronically ill Christian elderly. *Geriatric Nursing, 14*(6), 298–303.

Young, C., & Koopsen, C. (2011). *Spirituality, health, and healing: An integrative approach.* Sudbury, MA: Jones & Bartlett Learning.

CHAPTER 11

Spiritual Well-Being and Quality of Life at the End of Life

Just like the clay in the potter's hand, so are you in my hand.

Jeremiah 18:6

> In the ministry that I have been privileged to be a part of, as far as accompanying those at the end of life, listening is, on any given day, sometimes 95 percent of what I do. I've learned over the years that listening, if passive, really I'm not listening, but an active listening is really hard work. It calls forth from me a disposition or a posture of truly trying to hear at times what is not being said . . . to be sensitive to the fact that pain is often not simply physical, it can be emotional, mental, spiritual. In our present healthcare system, we seem to become so caught up with tasks that we lose sight of really being present. I think when we are present to another person, that is when the greatest active listening takes place.

Caitlin, Nurse Manager of a Palliative Care Unit

For the person at or near the end of life, the words of the Old Testament prophet Jeremiah can be deeply comforting; they express the idea that one is held firmly, yet tenderly, in the hands of the Divine Potter who both created and cares for all His people. In a volume entitled *The Nurse's Calling*, I devoted an entire chapter to interpreting the meaning of Jeremiah's potter's story for practicing nurses (O'Brien, 1991). I believe that, because nurses like to be "in control"—in fact, need to be in control to a degree in caring for our patients—we find the concept of being like "clay" in the hands of a "potter" somewhat difficult to accept.

The same can probably be said for most persons in our contemporary society. We all like to be in control of our lives, our environment, and certainly our health, as much as possible. In regard to our health, many of us spend a great deal of time and energy on such things as exercise programs, shopping for nutritious foods and supplements, and participating in numerous other health promotions or health-enhancing activities.

When, however, a person is faced with a life-threatening, terminal illness, when one accepts the fact of being at or near the end of human life, loss of control becomes a lived and living reality—a living reality that can be both frightening and depressing. But it is precisely at this point in one's life journey that Jeremiah's account of his visit to the "Potter's House" can come alive:

> The word came to Jeremiah from the Lord: Come, go down to the potter's house, and there I will let you hear my words. So I went down to the potter's house, and there he was working at his wheel. The vessel he was making of clay was spoiled in the potter's hand and he reworked it into another vessel, as seemed good to him. Then the word of the Lord came to me: Can I not do with you . . . just as this potter had done? says the Lord. Just like clay in the hands of the potter, so are you in my hand." (Jeremiah 18:16)

A plethora of literature in recent years has documented the relationship between personal faith beliefs, associated with a variety of religious denominations, and positive coping with illness and disability. An ill individual's personal faith, supported by Scripture such as the Jeremiah passage cited previously, can be both consoling and strengthening. This is particularly true in cases of serious or life-threatening illness.

Spiritual care at the end of life has been significantly influenced both early on and today by the teaching of Dame Cicely Saunders, the founder of the hospice movement (Campion, 2011). Compassion for patients at the end of life and their loved ones is an important nursing characteristic of spiritual care (Howard, 2012). Also relevant is the attribute of positive communication, which facilitates "disclosure from patients so that we fully understand their spiritual wishes and concerns" (Nyatanga, 2016, p. 159). Nyatanga advises, "It is important that we do not 'rush' into giving information and advice, as this will stop further disclosure" (p. 159). Treating a person at the end of life with dignity and respect was described as essential by a cadre of 468 nurses (Kisvetrova, Klugar, & Kabelka, 2013, p. 599).

Some barriers to providing spiritual care at the end of life, identified by palliative care nurses, include: "lack of time, skills, privacy and fear of what you may uncover, unresolved symptoms and differences in culture and beliefs" (Keall, Clayton, & Butow, 2014, p. 3197). The perceptions of a group of end-stage heart failure patients revealed several lacunae in their spiritual care that validate certain of the nurses' perceptions; these lacunae were: "having someone to talk to; supportive careers; and staff showing sensitivity/taking care to foster hope" (Ross & Austin, 2013, p. 871). Assessing and fostering hope was also highlighted as an important element of spiritual care at the end of life by Wynne (2013, p. 44).

There is still, however, minimal research documenting the relationship between spiritual well-being or strong faith beliefs and positive quality of life in persons facing the end of life. In an attempt to understand better the spiritual concerns and needs of the terminally ill, three studies were carried out exploring the concepts of spiritual well-being and quality of life at the end of life. Both quantitative and qualitative data reflecting the importance of spiritual well-being in enhancing overall coping and quality of life were collected from persons at or near the end of their lives. The studies included in this chapter are entitled "Spiritual Well-Being at the End of Life: An Experiment in Parish Nursing," "Meeting Spiritual Needs of Elders Near the End of Life," and "The Relationship Between Spiritual Well-Being and Quality of Life in Older Adults at the End of Life."

▶ Spirituality at the End of Life

Your fear of death is but the trembling of the shepherd when he stands before the King whose hand is to be laid upon him in honor.

—Kahlil Gibran, 1980

Myriad definitions of *end of life* may be found, although most authors admit to ambiguity and vagueness in attempting to define the concept. Hamilton (2001) suggests that "end of life care can be defined as medical and other supportive care given to a person during the final six months of life" (p. 74). This statement is immediately followed, however, with the question, "But how do we know which are the final six months?" (p. 74). Other authors have suggested that end of life may be defined as from as long as 2 years prior to death. Ultimately, Hamilton concluded that "Given the difficulty of predicting when and by what process death will come, end-of-life can best be defined . . . as that care which the health care team provides in what they think could be the final days, weeks or months of the patient's life" (p. 74).

The National Institutes of Health (2004) "State of the Science Conference Statement on Improving End-of-Life Care" noted "the evidence does not support a precise definition of the interval referred to as end-of-life or its transitions" (p. 3). The statement added, "There is no exact definition of end of life; however, the evidence supports the following components: (1) the presence of a chronic disease(s) or symptoms or functional impairments that persist but may also fluctuate; and (2) the symptoms or impairments resulting from the underlying irreversible disease require formal (paid, professional) or informal (unpaid) care and can lead to death. Older age and frailty may be surrogates for life-threatening illness and comorbidity; however, there is insufficient evidence for understanding these variables as components of end of life" (p. 3).

A significant amount of contemporary literature suggests the existence of a strongly positive relationship between spirituality (relating to one's relation with the transcendent) and religiousness or religiosity (relating to the practice of one's religious faith) and coping with end of life and the death experience. Harold Koenig (2002), in discussing the role of religion and spirituality at the end of life, observed that "it is often religious faith and support from (a) spiritual community" that gives individuals facing the end of life "greater control over the dying process" (p. 20). Koenig added, "Rather than trying to control everything, faith allows them to give up the need for control and instead to trust that God will control their circumstances based on God's love, wisdom, and unique knowledge about their situations. They say, 'It's all about letting go and letting God, not hanging on and holding tight to that which on this earthly plane is passing away'" (p. 20).

In carrying out a conceptual analysis of spirituality at the end of life, Vachon, Fillion, and Achille (2009) reported the identification of 11 dimensions of the concept: "meaning and purpose in life, self-transcendence, transcendence with a higher being, feelings of communion and mutuality, beliefs and faith, hope, attitude toward death, appreciation of life, reflection on values, developmental nature of spirituality, and conscious aspect" (p. 53). An exploratory study of spiritual care at the end of life concluded that health-care providers view spiritual care as consisting of "fluid interpersonal processes" within "mutually recognized values" instead of "proscribed roles" (Daaleman, Usher, Williams, Rawlings, & Hanson, 2008, p. 406).

In exploring spiritual issues at the end of life, Chaturvedi (2007) notes that "spirituality plays an integral role in the care of the terminally ill" (p. 48). In relation to hospice philosophy and palliative care, the patient's spirituality and spiritual needs are "consistent with these values" (p. 48). "Spirituality," Chaturvedi observes, "includes two main components: faith/religious beliefs and meaning/spiritual well-being" (p. 48). The importance of the concept of "meaning" as a spiritual need at the end of life is supported by McKinnon and Miller (2011), as well as the needs of "hope," "sense of and ultimate spiritual source," "love and acceptance," and "dignity and humanity" (pp. 370–372). A patient and/or family's spiritual perspective, as well as their spiritual values "often sway the decision making process" in relation to end-of-life plans (Keegan & Drick, 2011, p. 159). Keegan and Drick add that "enhancing the spiritual aspect of dying is quite possibly the most challenging as well as one of the most pertinent aspects of care that is long overdue" (p. 160). And while religious beliefs and practices may be significantly different for dying patients, caregivers can in fact come to a "common ground based on basic values, including human dignity, the sacredness of all life, care, nonviolence, selflessness and compassion" in order to begin to develop "method and comportment to provide care" (p. 171).

Spirituality and End-of-Life Care

In a survey of 861 critical care nurses, the purpose of which was to obtain suggestions on ways to improve end-of-life care, spiritual needs did not emerge as a major theme; however, several suggestions were at least indirectly related to the topics of spirituality and religion. These suggestions were the building of a "chapel in the intensive care area for the use of patients' families and hospital staff," creation of a "small walking garden," and the idea that no patient should die alone. "Every patient needs to have someone present with them at the moment of death—to touch them, speak to them, to let them know it's okay to go" (Beckstrand, Callister, & Kirchoff, 2006, p. 41). Under "Miscellaneous findings," the authors also noted a suggestion for "more involvement from ancillary personnel such as pastoral staff" (p. 42).

In describing results of a case study focusing on managing pain at the end of life, clinical nurse specialist Laura Middleton-Green (2008) reported the benefit of using pain assessment tools in order to comprehensively address and manage patient discomfort; and in research exploring interventions providing "consolation" for patients with incurable cancer, it was found that the most successful nursing attitude was marked by such factors as "presence," "understanding," "commitment," "creativity," and "courage" (Langegard & Ahlberg, 2009, p. 99). Comfort care measures appropriate at the end of life identified by nursing home staff included "symptom management," "family care," "interpersonal relationships," and "complementarity between interdisciplinary roles" (Waldrop & Kirkendall, 2009, p. 719). When a multidisciplinary team is involved, "shared decision making" is critical to end-of-life care (Frank, 2009, p. 612). Finally, the concept of staff having "time" was identified as being "essential to the provision of spiritual support" in a hospice setting (Bailey, Moran, & Graham, 2009, p. 42).

The critical care nurses' suggestion for "presence" at the time of death is in fact considered a "spiritual caregiving strategy" by Young and Koopsen and Father Joseph Driscoll. Young and Koopsen (2005) note that "health care providers can provide spiritual care of the dying by dealing with spiritual issues from the individuals' and families' perspectives . . . (one) way is to listen to individuals who have a desire and a need to discuss the experience" (pp. 174–175). Father Driscoll observes, "Spiritual care is so much more than religious care. Spiritual care discovers, reverences, and tends the spirit—that is, the energy, or the place of meaning and values—of another human being" (2001, p. 334).

In describing spirituality and end-of-life care as "a time for listening and a time for caring," Christina Puchalski (2002), MD, cited a survey poll in which end-of-life patients stated that "they wanted warm relationships with their providers, to be listened to, to have someone to share their fears and concerns with, to have someone with them when they are dying, to be able to pray and to have others pray for them" (p. 290). Puchalski concluded, "We need to listen to the dying . . . and be with them, for them. The process of dying can be a meaningful one—one that we can all embrace and celebrate rather than fear and dread" (p. 294).

A lovely symbolic gift, signifying warm relationships for families and patients at the end of life, is described in an article entitled "Compassion in Practice Nursing" (Howard, 2012). In the paper, parish nurse Hilary Howard explains a volunteer project of the making and donating of brightly colored blankets "offered to families as part of end-of-life care" (p. 21). The blankets, Howard reported, "enhance spiritual care to a wide range of individuals . . . the fabrics led to stories being told and listened to about end-of-life experiences and how individuals value compassion" (p. 21).

Palliative care nurse Polly Mazanec asserts that "spirituality can be especially significant in end-of-life care, offering the patient a way to find meaning and purpose in dying as in life" (2003, p. 55). Mazanec also cites the importance of religious rituals for some end-of-life patients. "Spiritual or religious practices (customs) and rituals (more formal ceremonies) often play important roles . . . at a time of transition in one's life. For example, a Roman Catholic ritual known as Anointing of the Sick might be performed for a seriously ill person. Considered 'a sacrament of healing,' it's intended to bring the recipient physical and spiritual strength and to convey God's grace. A Muslim family might request that immediately after death, the patient's body be turned to Mecca, their holiest city" (p. 55).

Milligan (2011) has identified a number of "practical ways in which nurses can identify, support and assist people to meet their spiritual care needs" at the end of life (p. 47). Her examples of spiritual care include "being present," to give patients a sense of "not being abandoned"; "accompanying," to "create a sense of shared humanity"; "harmonizing environment," or providing "spiritual comfort" through a supportive environment"; "encouraging reminiscence and life review," to help the patient "recover a sense of personhood"; "assisting planning," planning for a funeral or memorial service "which requires considerable courage on the part of the dying person and great sensitivity on the part of the nurse"; and "signposting to others," that is, a nurse recognizing when "a patient's need exceeds his/her skills level and to signpost the patient to appropriate specialist help" (pp. 54–55). The latter concept appears to be also supported by Deborah Hayden (2011), who urges nurses to reflect and dialogue about the subject of spirituality and end-of-life care in order to make it more "practically meaningful" (p. 550). Hayden concludes that "'A one size fits all' model for spiritual care is not advocated but there is a need for a clear framework, underpinned by established theory, within which practitioners can locate their own professional work context" (p. 550).

Finally, assessment of spiritual needs and the requirement for spiritual care at the end of life have been addressed by Doka (2011), who suggests that a key in end-of-life assessment may be to "engage both the individual and family in an exploration of their individual and collective spiritual histories" (p. 106). In terms of providing care, Doka points out that "once an assessment of spirituality is made, an individual can be encouraged to connect with their [sic] spiritual strengths" and adds that "often this may involve clergy, chaplains, spiritual mentors or members of their faith community" (p. 106). Doka also notes that other patients' spiritual beliefs and practices can provide comfort and strength; these might include prayer, meditation, and/or religious rituals (pp. 106–107). Rabbi Barry Kinzbrunner (2011) describes a number of end-of-life spiritual assessment models that may be helpful to a nurse, but he admits that "while these structured assessment models have been found useful in many situations, one must be aware that there are still occasions when the spiritual assessment will need to be conducted more informally, using general narrative and/ or life review" (p. 405). "It is up to the spiritual care provider," Kinzbrunner adds, "to determine whether formal or informal methods will be most effective in planning for the care of any individual patient and family" (p. 405).

The following three nursing studies on spiritual well-being at the end of life illustrate well the described themes related to the importance of being present and listening to persons at the end of life; helping them to "let go and let God"; supporting such faith-related practices as reverence, religiousness (religious practice), and devotion; helping patients achieve spiritual peace; and supporting such concepts as "the gift of life" and "the spirituality of community."

▶ Spiritual Well-Being at the End of Life: An Experiment in Parish Nursing

The overall purpose of this study was to explore selected correlates of spiritual well-being and quality of life among a population of persons at or near the end of life, as well as to test the impact of parish nursing intervention on spiritual well-being and quality of life at the end of life. Although initial sample criteria for seriously ill study participants did not include their being at or near the end of life, approximately 75 percent of the study population fit that criteria. Of the 45 participants entered into the study, 31 (69 percent) resided in nursing homes or assisted care facilities, and 39 subjects (87 percent of the group) were over the age of 70 (40 percent were 70 to 79; 29 percent were 80 to 89; and 18 percent were 90 to 96). The conceptual model undergirding the research was the "Middle-Range Theory of Spiritual Well-Being in Illness."

The research method consisted of a quasi-experimental, pretest, posttest design, including a correlational dimension. Methodological triangulation was also employed in data collection; both quantitative and qualitative tools were used to measure key variables in the study.

Sample

Of the 45 cognitively alert adults who agreed to participate in the study, all except one were at or nearing the end of life. The study sample consisted of those individuals who were able and willing to respond to nursing intervention to enhance spiritual well-being, as well as to participate in data collection activities.

Variables/Instruments

Three quantitative tools and one qualitative tool were used to assess the variables of spiritual well-being and quality of life (operationalized in terms of hope and life satisfaction) prior to and following parish nursing intervention.

- The Spiritual Assessment Scale (SAS) (O'Brien, 2003a) is a 21-item Likert-type scale that measures spiritual well-being overall and uses three subscales that assess personal faith, religious practice, and spiritual contentment.
- The Miller Hope Scale is a 15-item tool that measures hope in terms of such issues as meaning of life and attitudes toward the future. This instrument was abbreviated for a more fragile end-of-life population with permission of the author, Dr. Judith Miller (Miller & Powers, 1988).
- The Life Satisfaction Index-Z is a 13-item scale designed to measure satisfaction with life among elder adults (Wood, Wylie, & Sheafor, 1969).
- The qualitative tool is an investigator-developed instrument called the SWBG (O'Brien, 2003a).

The SAS established reliability and validity. Reliability, using Cronbach's alpha, was again established with the study population. All statistics were calculated at time 1 (T1) prior to the parish nursing intervention and at time 2 (T2) following intervention. The SAS total scale measured spiritual well-being as T1: 0.94, T2: 0.92. For subscales, personal faith was T1: 0.95, T2: 0.94; religious practice was T1: 0.86, T2: 0.76; and spiritual contentment was T1: 0.77, T2: 0.87.

The SWBG explores, in narrative responses, the concepts of personal faith, religious practice, and spiritual contentment. Content validity was established by a panel of experts in the area of spiritual well-being and chronic illness.

A demographic data form was used to collect data on the potentially mediating variables of severity of illness (degree of disability), age, gender, religious orientation, religiosity (religious practice) as well as other demographics, including diagnosis, to provide a sample population description.

Nursing Intervention

Following collection of baseline data, a nursing intervention plan was designed and carried out to enhance spiritual well-being and quality of life; each intervention was tailored to the specific spiritual and/or religious needs of the study participant. The experimental parish nursing intervention plan was carried out in context of at least three visits to the study participant, following initial data collection, and prior to postintervention (outcome) data collection. At the time of baseline data collection, the parish nurse assessed the study participant's spiritual needs; a broad intervention plan to be carried out over the next three visits was developed. The interventions differed somewhat based on such variables as a study participant's degree of disability, spiritual beliefs, and/or personal coping style; this, however, represents the norm in contemporary parish nursing intervention. For example, if the study participant was able to read, and had a spiritual history of Bible reading, he or she may have wished to discuss appropriate passages with the parish nurse. If a study participant had impaired vision, the nurse read a relevant Scripture passage to the participant, then initiated discussion of the content.

Some study participants desired the nurse to pray with them; others wished to reminisce about their past lives or speak about the imminence of death and dying with the parish nurse. Several study participants requested that the nurse arrange for specific pastoral care intervention, such as administration of church sacraments, if they had not been receiving such spiritual ministry. In sum, the primary focus of the parish nursing intervention at or near the end of life was to allow the ill person the opportunity to receive whatever spiritual support or comfort he or she needed as death approached.

It should be pointed out that the parish nurse, who visited as a representative of the church and was also a spiritual companion, was also vested with the roles of educator, advocate, referral agent, and counselor. Thus, the nursing intervention visits sometimes included listening to and guiding the study participants in regard to a variety of issues related to their illness or disability. These activities also supported and strengthened the spiritual well-being of the person nearing the end of life.

As was noted in the final report of the study, "Because of the diversity of spiritual needs and concerns among study participants, as well as myriad physical deficits and disabilities, the parish nursing visits varied somewhat in terms of process and content; this was expected for, as with any intervention in the area of spiritual well-being, the nurse cannot plan precisely what will occur as the nurse–patient interaction evolves. Nevertheless, significant findings, both quantitative and qualitative revealed the positive impact of parish nursing intervention on the study participants' spiritual well-being and quality of life" (O'Brien, 2001, p. 11).

Analysis

Quantitative analysis was carried out using appropriate parametric procedures for both correlational and pre–postintervention data such as Pearson's r multiple regression analysis and paired t-test. Although quantitative tools established reliability and validity, reliability scores were again calculated on quantitative tools (overall scale scores and subscales) using Cronbach's alpha procedure. Qualitative data were content analyzed to identify and describe dominant themes that emerged idiosyncratic to the data.

Study Findings

Quantitative data analysis "revealed significant positive increases in study variables following the parish nursing intervention . . . as revealed by evaluation of the paired t-test data. Paired t-tests were computed for all scales. There were statistically significant differences; that is positive increases on all three instruments: The SAS overall (t 0.44 5 5.23, p 0.0005); the three subscales for personal faith (t 0.44 5 3.86, p 0.0005), religious practice (t 0.44 5 3.41, p 0.001), and spiritual contentment (t 0.44 5 4.80, p 0.0005); the Miller Hope Scale (t 0.44 5 2.68, p 0.010); and the Life Satisfaction Inventory-Z (t 0.44 5 2.12, p 0.040). In sum, following the parish nursing intervention, the study participants had a greater sense of spiritual well-being, more hope and a higher degree of life satisfaction than at the initiation of the study" (O'Brien, 2003b, p. 221).

There were also significant positive correlational relationships between the key variables of spiritual well-being and quality of life as measured by hope and life satisfaction.

Following the nursing interventions, qualitative data were also collected and analyzed. From these data, five dominant themes reflecting spiritual well-being emerged including reverence, faithfulness, religiousness, devotion, and contemplation. (Specific details of the study design, analyses, and conclusions may be found in *Parish Nursing: Healthcare Ministry Within the Church* [O'Brien, 2003b, pp. 213–284]).

Significance

This study was of significance to nursing on three fronts: spirituality in nursing, parish nursing, and end of life. Spirituality in nursing is an important dimension of the holistic health-care paradigm that gives attention to body, mind, and spirit. Parish nursing is a newly recognized subfield of nursing. Finally, it addressed nursing's contemporary concern with the quality of life of those who are near or at the end of life.

Data from both clinical nursing practice and nursing research reveal that sick persons who manifest spiritual well-being cope significantly better with illness and disability than those who do not. Even as physical deficits increase, a strong sense of spiritual well-being promotes a perception of hope and comfort for the person nearing the end of life. The Joint Commission mandates, in its regulations, attention to the spiritual needs of those who are being treated in health-care settings. In February 1998, with publication of the *Scope and Standards of Parish Nursing Practice*, the newly created subfield of parish nursing was formally acknowledged by the American Nurses' Association Congress on Nursing Practice. However, minimal research currently documents the impact of parish nurses' interventions on the spiritual well-being of their patients; this is especially true in terms of the parish nurse's intervention with persons at or near the end of life.

▶ Meeting Spiritual Needs of Elders Near the End of Life

Following the parish nursing intervention study just described, an interpretive phe-nomenological study of 15 chronically ill elders (ages 65 to 82 years) near the end of life was carried out. The study sample consisted of five Roman Catholics; four persons who identified themselves broadly as "Christian"; three individuals who were Baptist; and three who were Presbyterian, Episcopalian, and Unitarian, respectively.

The study aim was to identify through open-ended interviews the lived experi-ence of spirituality and/or religious practice, and specifically of spiritual needs, at or near the end of life. Nursing interventions to meet specific spiritual needs were then implemented, as needed, by the parish nurse.

Ultimately, five nursing diagnoses related to spiritual well-being were identified and appropriate nursing interventions initiated; the nursing diagnoses were spiritual alienation, spiritual anxiety, spiritual anger, spiritual loss, and spiritual peace.

Spiritual alienation was evidenced by perceptions of being distanced from God; of feelings of lack of peace in terms of God's care and comfort.

Spiritual anxiety was demonstrated by verbalization of fear of God or lack of trust in God's mercy and forgiveness.

Spiritual anger was reflected in an individual's sense of frustration or outrage at God for real or perceived pain and sufferings in his or her own life or that of a loved one.

Spiritual loss was manifested by feelings of no longer being loved by God, often related to a decrease in former spiritual peace.

Spiritual peace was determined by a study participant's perception of trust, joy, and security in the love, mercy, and compassion of God (O'Brien, 1982, pp. 106–107; O'Brien, 2006, pp. 30–32; details of the study design, analysis, and findings may be found in the article "Parish Nursing: Meeting Spiritual Needs of Elders Near the End of Life" [O'Brien, 2006]).

▶ Spiritual Well-Being and Quality of Life in Older Adults at the End of Life

The overall purpose of this study was to explore the relationship between spiritual well-being and quality of life among a population of ill elders at or near the end of life. A limitation of the earlier referenced study "Spiritual Well-Being at the End of Life: An Experiment in Parish Nursing" related to the religious élan of the private foundation funding the work; that is, it was mandated that all of the study participants belong to one religious denomination, that of the funding institute. As noted, however, statistically significant relationships between spiritual well-being and quality of life were found among the study population, as well as the five dominant themes reflective of spiritual well-being that emerged from content analysis of qualitative data: reverence, faithfulness, religiousness, devotion, and contemplation.

The present study differed from the parish nursing intervention study in four ways.

1. Designation of a correlational rather than an experimental design
2. Broadening of the sample to include persons of all religious faiths and/ or spiritual belief systems
3. Replacement of two previously used measures of quality of life with the McGill Quality of Life Questionnaire (MQOL) developed for end-of-life research
4. Exploration of two additional potentially mediating variables: symptom severity and social support

Two investigator-developed tools were used to measure the latter two variables: the Geriatric Severity of Physical Symptoms Scale (GSPSS) and the Geriatric Social Support Scale (GSSS). Content and construct validity were established on all research instruments.

Aim

The specific study aim was to examine the relationship between spiritual well-being and quality of life in ill elders at or nearing the end of life. Also explored were the effects of potentially mediating variables such as physical symptom severity, social support, and selected demographic variables.

Conceptual Framework

The conceptual model undergirding the research was the "Middle-Range Theory of Spiritual Well-Being in Illness, the core component of which is "the concept of finding spiritual meaning in the illness experience" (O'Brien, 2004, p. 39). Quality of life was understood according to the McGill end-of-life conceptualization, which includes focus on physical, psychological, and existential well-being. Spiritual well-being was described as encompassing an individual's positive attitudes toward his or her personal faith, religious practice, and spiritual contentment.

Method

The research included a correlational design, also employing the concept of methodological triangulation. Both quantitative and qualitative tools were used to measure key variables in the study.

Sample

The sample consisted of 22 ill, yet cognitively alert, elders, 65 years or older, at or nearing the end of life, who were physically able and willing to participate in data collection activities.

Instruments

Four quantitative tools—the Spiritual Assessment Scale (SAS) (O'Brien, 2003a); the McGill Quality of Life Questionnaire (MQOL) (Cohen, 2001); the Geriatric Severity of Physical Symptoms Scale (GSPSS) (O'Brien, 2004); and the Geriatric Social Support Scale (GSSS) (O'Brien, 2004)—were used to assess the variables of spiritual well-being and quality of life, as well as mediating variables of symptom severity and social support. A demographic data form was employed to assess the additional potentially mediating variables of age, gender, religious orientation, marital status, education, and frequency of church attendance.

Following collection of quantitative data, a qualitative tool, the SWBIG (O'Brien, 2003a) was used to explore the study participants' perception of key study variables expressed in narrative form.

Procedure

Study participants were accessed from several urban nursing home/assisted care facilities. After appropriate informed consent procedures had been carried out, quantitative data were collected using the previously noted standardized tools. Following completion of response to the standardized tools, a tape-recorded open-ended interview was conducted with all study participants, employing the identified interview guide to focus the discussion. Because of the fragile nature of the study participant population, i.e., ill elders at or near the end of life, data collection was conducted in two sessions, if needed, in order not to unduly fatigue participants.

Protection of Human Subjects

Study participants, who had signed the informed consent form, were carefully reminded that they could withdraw from the study at any time or refuse to answer any questions without penalty. It was not anticipated that study questions would cause emotional discomfort; however, if a study participant became fatigued or distressed during questioning, the interview was to be immediately terminated and supportive counseling provided. This did not occur. Study participants' confidentiality was assured; data were kept in a locked file and tape recordings destroyed following transcription and analysis.

Data Analysis

Quantitative and qualitative analyses were carried out using appropriate descriptive and interpretive procedures in order to identify patterns of thought and behavior among the study participants.

Significance and Relationship to Future Research

Both previous research and clinical experience have documented relationships between spiritual well-being and positive coping with illness and/or quality of life in chronically ill persons (Koenig, 1999; O'Brien, 2003a). However, little research has been done to explore these relationships among older adults at or near the end of their lives. This study was designed to achieve the following goals:

1. Expand the investigator's previous research in the area
2. Establish reliability of several investigator-developed quantitative tools for use with a population of elders at or near the end of life
3. Explore use of the investigator-developed middle-range conceptual model A Model of Spiritual Well-Being in Illness for use to undergird research with older adults at or near the end of life

Note: It is recognized that there may appear to be some conceptual overlap related to the variables of "symptom severity" and "quality of life" (the McGill Questionnaire contains several items dealing with "recent troubling symptoms"). However, the investigator-developed GSPSS was created to provide a measure of overall (global) and persistent severity of physical symptoms that might significantly mediate the correlational relationship under investigation, as well as interact with the quality-of-life questions relating to immediate physical symptoms (i.e., problems within the last two days prior to the time of interview).

Study Findings
Quantitative Findings

The study participants, as noted earlier, consisted of 22 elders at or near the end of life. Those participating in the research were suffering from a variety of illnesses and disabilities; most individuals identified at least two health problems and a number had as many as five or six. This, of course, was to be expected considering that the study sample consisted of a population of elders at the end of life. Some of the disease conditions and/or disabilities reported included arthritis, diabetes, cardiovascular disease, congestive heart failure, hypertension, chronic obstructive pulmonary disease, lung cancer, prostate cancer, osteoarthritis, esophageal cancer, emphysema, glaucoma, heart arrhythmias, hearing loss, loss of vision (cataracts), memory loss, and depression.

One case example of an end-of-life elder experiencing multiple illnesses and disabilities and being treated with myriad therapeutic remedies was Frances, an 84-year-old widow living in an assisted care facility. Frances's diagnoses included altered cardiac status secondary to hypertension, hypothyroidism, osteoarthritis, left mastectomy secondary to breast cancer, mitral valve prolapse, endocarditis, atrial fibrillation, syncopal episodes resulting in frequent falls, subdural hematoma (evacuated), and gastroesophageal reflux disease (GERD).

Frances's routine medications consisted of Synthroid, 100 mcq qd; Colace, 100 bid; Prilosec, 20 mg qd; Lopressor, 25 mg bid; Fosamax, 70 q wk; calcium, 600 mg 1D qd; Lipitor, 10 mg qhs; Detrol LA, 4 mg qhs; and Extra Strength Tylenol, 2 q 6 hrs PRN.

The study group, which consisted of 18 women and 4 men, reported a variety of religious affiliations including 5 Protestants, 13 Roman Catholics, 1 Jewish person, 1 Quaker, and 2 individuals who did not claim any specific religious affiliation. Ages ranged from 70 to 94 years old including 1 person who was 70 years of age, 2 who were between 71 and 74, 4 who were 76 to 79, 7 persons who were between 80 and 85, 3 who were between 86 and 89, and 5 individuals who were between 90 and 95.

Nine of the study participants had attended high school including 5 who attended for two years and 4 who completed a 4-year program. The other 13 individuals had attended college, including 7 who attended two to four years and 6 who had masters or doctoral degrees in a variety of subjects. Five research participants were single and the other 17 were widowed.

The frequency of being able to attend formal worship services depended on a number of factors such as the physical condition of the study participant, availability of services at the nursing home or assisted care facility (study participants were living in a variety of health-care facilities), and desire. In general, three individuals reported attending some kind of worship service daily, and three attended more than once a week; five attended services once a week; two, once a month; five, several times a year; and three study respondents admitted that they never attended any formal worship services.

Descriptive quantitative findings revealed specific patterns of response on each of the study tools. In responding to the GSPSS, most study participants admitted to pain at least sometimes; this was generally associated with disease conditions such as arthritis or osteoarthritis. Fatigue associated with such diagnoses as congestive heart failure or cancer also was a predominant theme. Difficulty walking was associated with progressive arthritis or age-related vertigo; and difficulties in seeing and hearing were related, respectively, to age-related hearing loss and vision loss from such conditions as glaucoma and cataracts. In some persons, these losses were corrected through the use of glasses and hearing aids. Some age-related memory loss was also admitted to by many study participants.

In responding to the GSSS, a number of end-of-life persons identified little if any social support from family or friends. This was associated with the fact that, for many, their significant others' lives had already been claimed by age-related illness conditions. The study participant was the last member of his or her support system left alive.

Responses to the SAS revealed that most study participants had fairly strong personal faith beliefs and a high degree of spiritual contentment. The lower scale scores elicited by the SAS subscale "Religious Practice (RP)" were associated with lower response on the specific items dealing with belonging to a church and participating in worship services. Many individuals decried the fact that they could no longer drive and thus get out to church on their own. Some of the health-care residential facilities had weekly or biweekly in-house worship services; others were limited in that regard. Another "religious practice" item on which study group members scored lower was the item asking if one had a "spiritual friend or companion." In some cases, it was reported that pastors and/or church members visited frequently; for many, not at all.

On the MQOL, the weakest response from the study group was to the item "I feel that I have control over my life." Obviously, living in a nursing home or assisted care facility greatly decreased an individual's personal sense of control. Despite this response, a large number of study participants responded very positively to the question that asked if "the past two days" had been a "gift." Many reported that, on waking or sometime during the day, they thanked God for "still being here" or "for another day of life." Despite a multiplicity of physical and psychosocial deficits, persons at the end of life frequently wanted to remain alive as long as possible.

These themes are also reflected in the qualitative study data presented later in this chapter.

Finally, there was a strongly positive correlation between the key study variables of spiritual well-being and quality of life. Those study participants who scored higher on the SAS (measuring spiritual well-being), including the subscales that measured personal faith, religious practice, and spiritual contentment, also reported a more positive quality of life as measured by the MQOL. Those persons who perceived a greater degree of social support (GSSS) also scored higher on the SAS and the MQOL. The severity of physical symptoms, as evaluated by the GSPSS did not seem to affect the study participants' spiritual well-being and quality of life significantly.

Qualitative Findings

Six dominant themes related to spiritual well-being emerged from content analysis of open-ended interviews with study participants; these themes included the gift of life; spiritual comfort, which included subcategories companionship of God, faith and prayer, and devotional practices; religious reminiscence; spiritual pain; death awareness; and spirituality of community.

The Gift of Life

The comment that life was a "gift" or "blessing" was a recurring theme related to spiritual well-being elicited from the population of elders at or near the end of life who responded to the Spirituality and Religiousness Interview Guide. Interestingly, although most reported no fear of death and, in fact, suggested that they were simply waiting to be "called by the Lord" or "go to God," study participants still expressed a sense of gratitude for their lives; some reported feeling "blessed to still be here."

Ninety-four-year-old Sarah, who had severe osteoporosis and difficulty walking and seeing, observed, "I am so blessed; life is a gift from God. Oh, I trust in God; others are so much worse off than I."

Seventy-two-year-old Eliza, who was wheelchair bound with a degenerative spinal condition as well as heart disease, commented, "I'm so grateful to have my mind and my hearing. Lord, I'm grateful that I'm part of your little gang down here and I don't have to holler out: 'what's that, again?' Life is a gift and I'm never alone. God will take care of me. Some people just hate being here (nursing home) but I feel privileged that there's a place like this. I can't think of anything more precious in my life than letting God do the controlling. I realized that peace was not going to be what Eliza wanted but what God wanted."

Robert, an 84-year-old with cardiovascular disease, emphasized, "I feel that my life has been a gift and that God's not finished with me yet! The gift I appreciate most is my ability to pray; daily Mass, the Stations, the Rosary, personal prayers; all are increasingly meaningful to me. That is my number one gift in life. That makes my day and alongside it, I still have my wits about me. I can listen to people and make sense of what they are saying. And make some sense in what I am saying. The ability to converse and to share thoughts, to share views and talk about world events." Robert concluded, "They also serve who only stand and wait. I offer each day to God. I'm in a waiting position."

Finally, Anna, a 79-year-old woman suffering from heart failure, arthritis, and osteoporosis, asserted, "Every day is a gift!" She showed the researcher a holy card that stated, "Old age leads to Him and old age will touch me only as He wills." Anna added, "I like the sense of being more available to people than before I retired. I'm more connected to people; there's more sharing."

Spiritual Comfort

A second theme that emerged very strongly in study participant interviews was the spiritual comfort brought about by the individuals' awareness of the companionship of God, their faith beliefs and personal prayer life, and their participation in devotional practices such as attending worship services, reading spiritual books, and/or looking at religious statues and pictures.

Companionship of God

Eighty-seven-year-old Martha, a widow whose husband had long suffered from Alzheimer's disease and who herself had myriad illnesses and disabilities related to vision, hearing, and walking, unhesitatingly stated, "God is my life! I have a beautiful relationship with God. God understands me. I don't say the rosary but I'm never without them, if I was I'd be frantic. I think God would like it because I try to do things for others." Martha added, "I memorize prayers so that I can sit outside on the bench and say them and people won't say: 'Oh, she's praying again': 'Remember O most compassionate Virgin Mary.'"

Ada, a 73-year-old heart disease patient who got around in an electric wheelchair, explained her perception of the constant companionship of God. "I'm never alone. God will always take care of me. His dying on the Cross with open arms. He will forgive everybody. God is just waiting for all of us. The only control I want over my life is what God wants me to be doing every day."

Faith and Prayer

Teresa, a 91-year-old widow suffering from high blood pressure and heart disease and taking multiple medications, asserted emphatically, "I don't know how I could live without my faith in God; that's my anchor. The least little problem I turn to Him. Every night and morning when I get up I kneel down and say the prayer: 'Look down upon me good and gentle Jesus while before thy face I humbly kneel and, with burning soul, pray and beseech thee to fix deep in my heart lively sentiments of faith, hope and charity and true contrition for my sins. Amen.'" Teresa concluded, "I pray every day for my family. Oh, I couldn't live without my faith in God."

Elizabeth, a 79-year-old widow with multiple illnesses including diabetes and heart disease, described her faith and her prayer life. "I pray the rosary. I go to the chapel. I feel so sad for others who don't have faith in God. I don't worry. I talk to God in my own words. God always takes care of me. I know that God loves me; that's my faith."

Rachel, an 86-year-old widow with crippling osteoarthritis, noted, "I pray all the time. I really talk to God. If I'm having a bad day I see people who are so much worse off than I am. I say my rosary and I know how many 'Our Fathers' and 'Hail Marys' it takes to get down the path outside. I trust God but I'm a little afraid of the future." Rachel explained her fear and her prayer, "I pray to God: 'Please God let me die before my mind goes' because I think that's terrible when people are in the last stages of Alzheimer's."

Robert, an 84-year-old single man with arthritis and heart disease, described the importance of his faith and prayer life in the midst of illness. "My sensitivity to pain is modified by my faith. I carry the Cross with Jesus. Without faith my life would be unlivable! God has been very good to me. I've been blessed in more ways than I can express." Robert added, "I feel that I'm making a contribution because I pray for people and I carry crosses."

Finally, 79-year-old Alice described how growing older had changed her prayer life. "Since I have reached the 'golden years,' my morning starts with a 'Thank You' to God for another day of life. When I look back on my life, I realize that I never prayed enough. I pray to God every day to help me accept my pain from arthritis in my knees and in my hips. I pray for my grandchildren who have a rare disease and I pray for my daughter and son-in-law. And, when God takes me, I pray to God that I will go to heaven so that I can see my mother and father."

Devotional Practices

Eighty-seven-year-old Camille, a 30-year insulin-dependent diabetic with congestive heart failure, hypertension, and advanced arthritis, described herself as a "loner." "I don't mingle," she asserted. Camille did, however, report that her devotional faith practices were very important in her life. "I believe God is watching over me. If I feel down I go and sit in the chapel and I feel better. I say my rosary every day. I pray many times during the day. I just look up and say 'Thank you, Lord, for my blessings. Thank you, Lord, that I'm still here.'"

Rita, an 84-year-old widow with multiple illnesses and disabilities including cardiac arrhythmias, hypertension, arthritis, glaucoma in both eyes, and past hip and knee surgeries, spoke about the value of spiritual reading and having religious articles in her room. "I get a little magazine with religious stories and I love it; the stories all end up with God. They all have a spiritual point." Rita also proudly showed off her statue of the Infant Jesus and described the joy of having it in her room to look at.

Another octogenarian, 86-year-old Jeanette, pointed out the crosses hanging on her lampshade that her granddaughters had sent and added, "I have a rosary that my daughter got at the Vatican."

Seventy-seven-year-old Katherine, suffering from emphysema and lung cancer, admitted, "I don't know what I'd do if I didn't believe in God." She explained that watching religious TV programs was very comforting to her. "Watching EWTN [Eternal Word Television Network] gives me support and strength."

Religious Reminiscence

Reminiscence of past life events in general occurred a great deal during open-ended study interviews. Sometimes the "remembering" simply dealt with family occasions or social highlights in an individual's past life. Frequently, however, the reminiscence took on a spiritual tone.

Carolyn, an 87-year-old Quaker suffering from a variety of illnesses including arthritis, bowel dysfunction, and hypothyroidism, reminisced about the joy of her Quaker Meeting experiences. "I wouldn't want to be anything else. We gathered together and waited on the presence of God. I don't like all the 'ups and downs' of the Catholic and Protestant services. I liked a silent meeting with God." Carolyn continued, "We did occasionally sing. I found peace at a 'Gathered Meeting.' We gathered strength from just being together."

Frank, a 67-year-old with chronic lung disease and emphysema who had difficulty breathing, reminisced about the importance of his Church in his life. "It's (emphysema) a constant battle but I lean on God. God put me in this for a reason. I talk to God; I always have and it makes me feel better. I do believe there is a God (repeated several times). Sometimes I like to just sit and meditate in the Chapel; I like the silence. My Church, St. Peter's, was like that; I'm going to be buried in St. Peter's cemetery. That's where my ashes will be. My Church was everything to me so it's important that I have the 'Last Rites' of the Church. That's why I came here (nursing home). It makes me not afraid of the future."

Several other study participants related how they were taught about religion from their parents, especially their mothers. One example was Rebecca, an 87-year-old Jewish widow suffering from angina, arthritis, and diabetes. "My mother taught us a lot about Judaism. We always kept a Kosher household. Her parents raised her in a Kosher household in Russia. She taught us to believe in God and that God will take care of the future. I keep a Star of David from her in my home and it's 41 years old."

Spiritual Pain

A few of the study participants described experiences of spiritual pain, sometimes related to occurrences in their own lives, sometimes to those in the lives of their children or relatives, and occasionally having to do with organized religion.

Rebecca noted sadly that her two daughters had married "outside the faith." "It really shook up me and my husband," but, she added, "I had to accept it if I didn't want to lose my daughters and their husbands are wonderful boys. If there is something special going on in the Synagogue, they will put on yarmulkes and go."

Eighty-seven-year-old Camille reported, "My son was always raised to go to church but he married a girl who was not Catholic and they don't go to church. That makes me very sad and I pray they'll come back to the church."

Eighty-seven-year-old Rita commented, "It hurts me a lot because I have two great-nieces who are not baptized and I worry about that a lot. I pray for them and for the family and that is comforting."

Michael, a 77-year-old widower with prostate cancer and numerous other illnesses, spoke about his disillusionment with his former Church. "I'm not much of any religion now. I only go to church at Christmas. I get depressed and my eyes are not too good. I still have one friend at the church and I get their newsletter but I've become uncertain about the existence of God. Going to church does not impact my life at all." When Michael was asked if he prayed, he responded "No!" He then added, "I'm sorry to upset your statistics!"

Rachel, at 86, noted, "I'm afraid that over the years I've gotten cynical about the church and that hurts. My family doesn't go to church; my husband doesn't go either. I've become disillusioned with the church because my pastor never came to visit me even though I went to his church for over 40 years. My boys were altar boys and I sat right up front every week but he never even came to see me. Now I take a walk outside and talk to God instead of going to church."

Marta, an 82-year-old widow with cardiovascular disease and osteoporosis, spoke about her struggles with joining and quitting a variety of Christian Churches related to weakness in the pastors and congregations. She described leaving one parish community by saying, "Not one member of that church ever consoled me (after her husband's death) so I left. I was so disillusioned with churches and religion." Marta now describes herself as a "secular humanist" and reported that she visited the headquarters of the "American Humanist Society" in Washington, DC, and gets their magazine once a month. Marta added, "It's (humanist society) not a faith group; it's just a way of life."

Death Awareness

Eighty-seven-year-old Rebecca spoke about the imminence of death. "One of my best friends is in the final stages of Alzheimer's and my other best friend has emphysema and can't come to visit me anymore. There is a 90-year-old here who is always talking about death and I say: 'Ruth, God hasn't called you yet, you have to wait your turn.'" She added, "All our turn is coming at this age."

Ninety-year-old Martin, who was experiencing severe hypertension, heart disease, and glaucoma, observed, "After my wife died the day before Christmas, suddenly I didn't know if God was with me or not or if I would die soon. I don't know if there's a hereafter but I imagine she's with God. I talk to her but unfortunately (laughs) she doesn't talk back."

An 82-year-old single woman described a family experience as taking away her fear of death. "I'm not afraid of death. My cousin who was like a sister to me died at 49 of cancer. I knew that if she could do it, I could do it."

An 80-year-old woman with severe diabetes stated calmly, "I ask God sometimes: 'I want to go to be with you.'"

An 86-year-old commented, "I would like to die in my sleep. As long as I'm mentally alert, I'm fine, but I'm afraid of Alzheimer's."

Spirituality of Community

A number of study participants, even though suffering from many personal illnesses and/or disabilities, expressed spiritual satisfaction in reaching out to others less fortunate than themselves. This was possible because the end-of-life study group resided in health-care facilities, either nursing homes or assisted care residences. An example of the spirituality of community in one facility was reflected in an anecdote related by Mary, an 87-year-old widow who had diagnoses of diabetes, congestive heart failure, hypertension, osteoporosis, a past fractured pelvis, glaucoma in both eyes, and who had frequent dizzy spells necessitating her use of a walker. Mary reported that she attended daily Mass because it "makes me feel my life is worthwhile."

Mary gave the following example of the spirituality of community. "I keep to myself mostly but I want to tell you about something that really made me feel good. I was in the chapel one morning when Sister Ann approached me and asked me if I would take Tim to the dining room. He is only about 50 years old but blind and he has to use a cane to go anywhere. I did so and since then we talk to each other often about God. When I am at Mass with him I am very impressed with his gentleness and how he knows all the prayers."

At the conclusion of the open-ended study interviews, many respondents reported that they had truly enjoyed the interview process and the opportunity to reflect on spiritual and religious beliefs as related to the quality of their lives. One study participant, Ruth, called her interviewer three months after their first meeting to request a follow-up visit. Ruth, an 82-year-old widow with cardiovascular disease and osteoporosis, asked for a second visit because, she commented, "Talking . . . gave me comfort." "I've been a worrier all my life," Ruth said and suggested that her anxiety may be related to a kind of spiritual "testing" she was to undergo. She is not sure about the existence of God but admitted that she prays "if there is a God."

▶ Conclusion

This chapter has presented both literature and nursing research supporting a positive relationship between spiritual well-being and quality of life for persons at or near the end of life. The research was undergirded by the author's newly developed middle-range theory of spiritual well-being in illness, which practicing nurses and nurse researchers may use to guide their work with seriously ill patients. The theory evolved from the author's previous research and practice with both chronically and terminally ill persons. The multiple studies, three of which are included in this chapter, well validate the usefulness of the theory of spiritual well-being in illness to guide the assessment of a person's spiritual and/or religious concerns and needs at the end of life.

▶ References

Bailey, M. E., Moran, S., & Graham, M. M. (2009). Creating a spiritual tapestry: Nurses' experiences of delivering spiritual care to patients in an Irish hospice. *International Journal of Palliative Nursing, 15*(1), 42–48.

Beckstrand, R. L., Callister, L. C., & Kirchoff, K. T. (2006). Providing a "good death": Critical care nurses' suggestions for improving end-of-life care. *American Journal of Critical Care, 15*(1), 38–45.

Campion, B. (2011). Spiritual care at the end of life. *Canadian Nursing Home, 22*(1), 16–19.

Chaturvedi, S. (2007). Spiritual issues at the end of life. *Indian Journal of Palliative Care, 13*(2), 48–52.

Cohen, S. R. (2001). *McGill quality of life questionnaire.* Quebec, Canada: Royal Victoria Hospital (personal communication; permission to use tool).

Daaleman, T. P., Usher, B. M., Williams, S. W., Rawlings, J., & Hanson, L. C. (2008). An exploratory study of spiritual care at the end of life. *Annals of Family Medicine, 6*(5), 406–411.

Doka, K. J. (2011). Religion and spirituality: Assessment and intervention. *Journal of Social Work in End-of-Life & Palliative Care, 7*(1), 99–109.

Driscoll, J. (2001). Spirituality and religion in end-of-life care. *Journal of Palliative Care, 4*(3), 333–335.

Frank, R. K. (2009). Shared decision making and its role in end-of-life care. *British Journal of Nursing, 18*(10), 612–618.

Gibran, K. (1980). *The prophet*. New York, NY: Alfred A. Knopf.

Hamilton, J. B. (2001). The ethics of end-of-life care. In B. Poor & G. P. Poirrier (Eds.), *End of life nursing care* (pp. 73–103). Sudbury, MA: Jones & Bartlett Learning.

Hayden, D. (2011). Spirituality in end-of-life care: Attending the person on their journey. *British Journal of Community Nursing, 16*(11), 546–551.

Hermann, C. P. (2007). The degree to which spiritual needs of patients near the end of life are met. *Oncology Nursing Forum, 34*(1), 70–78.

Howard, H. (2012). Compassion in nursing practice. *Primary Health Care, 22*(4), 21–23.

Keall, R., Clayton, J. M., & Butow, P. (2014). How do Australian palliative care nurses address existential and spiritual concerns? Facilitators, barriers and strategies. *Journal of Clinical Nursing, 23*(21/22), 3197–3205.

Keegan, L., & Drick, C. (2011). *End of life: Nursing solutions for death with dignity*. New York, NY: Springer Publishing Company.

Kinzbrunner, B. (2011). Psychosocial and spiritual assessments. In B. Kinzbrunner & J. Policzer (Eds.), *End-of-Life Care: A practical guide* (pp. 393–413). New York, NY: McGraw Hill Medical.

Kisvetrova, H., Klugar, M., & Kabelka, L. (2013). Spiritual support interventions in nursing care for patients suffering death anxiety in the final phase of life. *International Journal of Palliative Nursing, 19*(2), 599–605.

Koenig, H. G. (1999). *The healing power of faith: Science explores medicine's last great frontier*. New York, NY: Simon and Schuster.

Koenig, H. G. (2002). A commentary: The role of religion and spirituality at the end of life. *The Gerontologist, 42*, 20.

Langegard, U., & Ahlberg, K. (2009). Consolation in conjunction with incurable cancer. *Oncology Nursing Forum, 36*(2), 99–106.

Mazanec, P. (2003). Cultural considerations in end-of-life care: How ethnicity, age and spirituality affect decisions when death is imminent. *American Journal of Nursing, 103*(3), 50–58.

McKinnon, S., & Miller, B. (2011). Psychosocial and spiritual concerns at the end of life. In B. Kinzbrunner & J. Policzer (Eds.), *End-of-life care: A practical guide* (pp. 349–377). New York, NY: McGraw Hill Medical.

Middleton-Green, L. (2008). Managing total pain at the end of life: A case study analysis. *Nursing Standard, 23*(6), 41–46.

Miller, J., & Powers, M. (1988). Development of an instrument to measure hope. *Nursing Research, 37*(1), 6–10.

Milligan, S. (2011). Addressing the spiritual care needs of people near the end of life. *Nursing Standard, 26*(4), 47–56.

National Institutes of Health. (2004). *State-of-the-science conference on improving end-of-life care* (December 6–8, 2004). Bethesda, MD: National Institutes of Health.

Nyatanga, B. (2016). Spiritual needs in palliative care and the possibility of being nothing. *British Journal of Community Nursing, 21*(3), 159.

O'Brien, M. E. (1982). The need for spiritual integrity. In H. Yura & M. Walsh (Eds.), *Human needs and the nursing process* (pp. 87–115). Norwalk, CT: Appleton-Century-Crofts.

O'Brien, M. E. (1991). *The nurse's calling: A Christian spirituality of caring for the sick*. Mahwah, NJ: Paulist Press.

O'Brien, M. E. (2001). *The gift of faith in chronic illness*. Washington, DC: The Catholic University of America. Final report submitted to the Our Sunday Visitor Institute, Huntington, IN.

O'Brien, M. E. (2003a). *Spirituality in nursing: Standing on holy ground* (2nd ed.). Sudbury, MA: Jones & Bartlett Learning.

O'Brien, M. E. (2003b). *Parish nursing: Healthcare ministry within the church.* Sudbury, MA: Jones & Bartlett Learning.

O'Brien, M. E. (2004). *A nurse's handbook of spiritual care.* Sudbury, MA: Jones & Bartlett Learning.

O'Brien, M. E. (2006). Parish nursing: Meeting spiritual needs of elders near the end of life. *Journal of Christian Nursing, 23*(1), 28–33.

Puchalski, C. M. (2002). Spirituality and end-of-life care: A time for listening and caring. *Journal of Palliative Medicine, 5*(2), 289–294.

Ross, L., & Austin, J. (2013). Spiritual needs and spiritual support preferences of people with end-stage heart failure and their carers. *Journal of Nursing Management, 23*(1), 87–95.

Vachon, M., Fillion, L., & Achille, M. (2009). A conceptual analysis of spirituality at the end of life. *Journal of Palliative Medicine, 12*(1), 53–59.

Waldrop, D. P., & Kirkendall, A. M. (2009). Comfort measures: A qualitative study of nursing home-based end-of-life care. *Journal of Palliative Medicine, 12*(8), 719–724.

Wood, V., Wylie, M., & Sheafor, B. (1969). An analysis of a short self-report measure of life satisfaction. *Journal of Gerontology, 24*(2), 465–469.

Wynne, L. (2013). Spiritual care at the end of life. *Nursing Standard, 28*(2), 41–45.

Young, C., & Koopsen, C. (2005). *Spirituality, health and healing.* Thorofare, NJ: Slack.

CHAPTER 12

Spiritual Needs in Death and Bereavement

By faith that Abraham obeyed when he was called to set out for a place . . . that was an inheritance given to him, and he set out not knowing where he was going.

Hebrews 11:8

Dying is part of the life cycle. Some of us will be lucky enough to know when we are going to die and be able to do so in a peaceful way surrounded by our friends and families. As far as critically ill and dying patients are concerned, you have to plan. They want spiritual comfort, they want information, they want to trust in having alleviation of pain, they want to die with the best sense of dignity they can, and that is something that I feel that nurses can facilitate.

Joanne, Charge Nurse at a Medical Outpatient Clinic

In this chapter, the spiritual needs of the dying are explored. Also identified are the family's spiritual needs related both to the death and to the bereavement experience. The author obtained empirical data through observation and informal interviews with dying patients and their families, as well as with their professional nursing caregivers.

Recent nursing literature is increasingly paying significant attention to spiritual needs and concerns in death and dying. Discussed are such topics as: "dying care interventions in the intensive care unit" (Kisvetrova, Skoloudik, Joanovic, Koneca, & Miksova, 2016, p. 139); "what constitutes a good or bad death?" (Ko, Kwak, & Nelson-Becker, 2015, p. 422); assisting patients' spiritual path in palliative care (Giske & Cone, 2015); hospice nurses' perspectives and experiences with spiritual care (Tiew, Kwee, Creedy, & Chan, 2013); understanding dying as a transition (Renz, Mao, Bueche, Cerny, & Strasser, 2013); and professionals coping with pediatric death and dying (Forster & Hafiz, 2015).

As an important addition to the concept of theory development in nursing, a middle-range theory of psychological adaptation to death and dying was offered by nurse theorist Marjorie Dobratz (2011). Dobratz's model, which is linked to the adaptation theory of Callistra Roy, includes findings from a number of studies on end-of-life psychological adaptation and provides assumptions and testable hypotheses (p. 370).

Current literature on family bereavement, discussed later in this chapter, also highlights the importance of spiritual and religious beliefs in facilitating long-term adaptation for loved ones (Draper, Holloway, & Adamson, 2013; Black, Santanello, & Rubinstein, 2014).

▶ The Spirituality of Death and Dying

Death is defined physiologically as occurring "when an individual has sustained either (1) irreversible cessation of circulatory and respiratory functions, or (2) irreversible cessation of all functions of the entire brain, including the brain stem" (President's Commission for the Study of Ethical Problems in Medicine, 1981, p. 1). From a theological perspective, death is conceptualized as "the final point of a human person's individual history . . . the decisive act of human freedom in which the person can either accept or reject the mystery of God and thereby put the final seal on his or her personal history and destiny" (Hayes, 1993, pp. 272–273). The spiritual understanding of death is undergirded by an individual's religious belief, that is, faith tradition. In Judaism, attitudes toward death vary both within and among specific traditions: Orthodox, Conservative, Reform, and Reconstructionist. In general, however, Judaism places great value on life as God's gift; there may be uncertainty about the existence of an afterlife (Grollman, 1993; Neuberger, 1994). Christian spirituality views death and dying in terms of the Gospel message of Jesus. Jesus' death provides a model for His followers who accept their sufferings in hope of the eternal reward He promised. For Jesus, death was not an ending but the beginning of eternal life with His Father (Kinast, 1993). Similarly, the Islamic perception of death incorporates the belief that an eternal life is part of God's plan (Esposito, 1990); the death of a loved one is considered only a "temporary separation" (Neuberger, 1994, p. 36).

The study of death and of the dying process teaches us much about the prevailing culture's attitude toward living (Moller, 1990). Historically, a number of theories of death and dying have been advanced; perhaps the best known is Kübler-Ross's (1969), which describes the stages of denial, anger, bargaining, depression, and acceptance. Angelucci and Lawrence (1995) developed a more contemporary nursing schema: "Health Promotion During the Dying Experience." This model includes cognitive-perceptual factors, such as perceived control and perceived benefits of preparing for dying; modifying factors, such as demographics, cultural influences, and social support; and health-promoting behaviors (p. 405). An important dimension of nursing support included in Angelucci and Lawrence's model is concern for meeting the patient's spiritual needs. This is seen as a significant element in promoting quality of life for the dying person (p. 412).

In discussing the "spirituality of dying," Chaplain Sharon Burns (1991) pointed out that to provide holistic care for a terminal patient, medicine and religion must work together. Chaplain Burns views spirituality as the "life principle" of a person's being and asserted that when the body is ill or dying, the spirit must be affected. An important facet of dealing with the spiritual dimension of dying is the introduction of reminiscence and reconciliation, that is, of allowing the patient to review his or her life and to accept the past as well as the present and future (Burns, 1991, p. 50). In this way, the dying person can integrate spiritual beliefs about the meaning and purpose of life with personal experiences and find comfort and consolation in legacies to be left.

In a similar vein, Derrickson (1996) described the spiritual work of the dying process as including the tasks of remembering, reassessing, reconciling, and reuniting. Remembering relates to reminiscence or a life review through which one can recognize the goodness of life, reassessing is the act of redefining personal worth, reconciliation means healing damaged or broken relationships, and reuniting refers to combining the material and spiritual elements of the person and the world (pp. 14–21). As well as engaging in a life review, some other specific tasks that comprise the "work" of dying are conversing with family and friends, which provides the opportunity to say what needs to be said, and giving and receiving forgiveness when needed (Kalina, 1993, pp. 36–38).

Kalina (1993) also identified spiritual signs that death is imminent, such as detachment from material goods; less tolerance for the mundane in conversation and preference for more times of silence; detachment from concern about appearance; and finally, detachment from relationships as the person recognizes that the end is near (pp. 45–46).

How a person dies can reveal a great deal about how he or she lived. So also, the spirituality manifested in death and in the dying process reflects the personal spirituality of the dying person. For a dying individual who adheres to the tenets of a religious denomination that professes belief in an afterlife, the dying process can represent a joyful transition to a better state, a place where the good acts of one's life are rewarded and sins are absolved. For the person who believes that existence of both body and spirit cease with physical death, the dying process may represent a fearful experience, especially if the individual has not fulfilled desired life goals and ambitions. Spiritual care will need to be carefully planned so as to be relevant to the prevailing spiritual and religious beliefs of the dying patient and his or her family. Many deaths occur in the hospital, nursing home, or hospice setting. With changes in the contemporary health-care system, however, more and more terminally ill individuals will die at home. Thus, the provision of spiritual support for patient and family may fall to the home health-care or parish nurse, as well as to hospital, hospice, or nursing home nursing staff.

▶ Spiritual Needs in the Dying Process

The dying process is unique to each person; a multiplicity of demographic, physical, psychosocial, and spiritual values may influence and mediate the experience. Such factors as age, gender, marital status, religious tradition, socioeconomic status, diagnosis, coping skills, social support, and spiritual belief, especially as related to the meaning of life and death, can influence one's management of the dying process. Despite the uniqueness of the individual, however, some universal needs are identified for most dying persons. These include the need for relief from loneliness and isolation, the need to feel useful, the need to express anger, the need for comfort in anxiety and fear, and the need to alleviate depression and find meaning in the experience (Kemp, 1995, pp. 11–16). Kenneth Doka (1993b) posited three broadly circumscribed spiritual goals of the dying person: "(1) to identify the meaning of one's life, (2) to die appropriately, and (3) to find hope that extends beyond the grave" (p. 146). The search for the meaning of life represents an attempt to bring together the dying individual's experiences, activities, and hoped for goals and outcomes; dying appropriately refers to dying in the manner that the individual finds most acceptable; and finding hope that extends beyond the grave relates to the dying person's peace and trust in his or her concept of an afterlife (pp. 146–148). If a dying person is unable to find purpose and meaning in life, he or she may experience guilt from the perception of aspirations unfulfilled (Featherstone, 1997). Other spiritual needs of the dying person identified in the nursing literature include the need for forgiveness and love (Conrad, 1985), for self-acceptance, and for positive relationships with others, including, for some, relationship with God or a deity (Highfield, 1992).

Although the physical and psychosocial needs of the dying may be more readily identified by overt emotional or physical symptoms, spiritual needs can be more difficult to assess. Because one's spiritual and religious beliefs are personal, symptoms of spiritual distress may not be openly displayed and thus may be neglected in the planning of care for a dying patient (Charlton, 1992). Such lack of attention to spiritual needs is not acceptable, however, for nurses attempting to provide holistic care during the dying process (Stepnick & Perry, 1992).

Dealing with spiritual needs of the dying, identified as a central task of caring for the terminally ill, is not easy (Katz & Sidell, 1994). The spiritual needs of a dying person with no formal religious affiliation can be particularly problematic; the individual may "agonize over life and death issues . . . asking 'why me?' questions" (p. 120). However, a religious person facing death may also raise such questions depending on his or her spiritual maturity and experience. Frequently these concerns arise when the dying person is young and has not yet achieved his or her desired life goals. For the nurse caring for such a dying patient, therapeutic intervention may include dealing with the major spiritual issue of anger at God and/or organized religion.

In a study of 40 patients, 20 dying of lung cancer and 20 of heart failure, qualitative interviews elicited data reflecting both spiritual need and spiritual well-being (Murray, Kendall, Boyd, Worth, & Benton, 2004). Some of the spiritual needs identified included "expressions of frustration, fear, hurt, doubt or despair, feeling isolated and unsupported, feeling useless . . . and feeling of losing control" (p. 41). Some signs of spiritual well-being were "having hope, goals and ambitions, social life and place in community retained, feeling valued, coping with and sharing emotions, being able to practice religion and finding meaning" (p. 41). Ultimately the authors concluded that "patients with life-threatening illness, even if still on 'active treatment' need help to cope with the prospect of dying, well before the terminal stage" (p. 44).

Tim, a 37-year-old terminal cancer patient, explained the importance of resolving spiritual issues prior to his impending death. "I guess it's like they say about 'no atheists in foxholes.' Well I'm in more than a foxhole. I need to get things together with myself and God before I go. I'm praying, and a pastor's been coming by to see me. I guess you don't think about all this until it gets near the end, but it's time now; it's definitely time."

▶ Spiritual Support in Death and Dying

Dying patients and their families cope with impending death in a variety of ways, depending on such factors as the age of the patient, the severity of the illness, the patient's religious beliefs, and cultural norms and values. One of the most frequently observed dilemmas is the fluctuation between acceptance and denial of the immediacy of death. Helping dying patients and families to manage the tension between these two attitudes is a key role of the spiritual caregiver (Joesten, 1992). One of the best ways of providing spiritual support in this situation is to allow the patient and family to verbalize their feelings; for a dying person "one of the greatest spiritual gifts" a nurse can give is to listen (Burns, 1991, p. 51).

Nursing literature subscribing to the concept of holistic care points out repeatedly that nurses must include spiritual support as part of the therapeutic regimen for the dying client (Conrad, 1985; Hittle, 1994; Taylor & Amenta, 1994). Some researchers have suggested also that if a nurse is to master the ability to assess and meet the spiritual needs of dying patients, he or she must engage in a personal spiritual journey in the process (MacDonald, Sandmaier, & Fainsinger, 1993; Praill, 1995; Price, Stevens, & LaBarre, 1995). It is impossible for a nurse to undertake the work of therapeutic spiritual support of patients without some understanding and acceptance of his or her own beliefs and attitudes about such issues as spirituality, religion, end-of-life decisions, and the existence or nonexistence of an afterlife. Olson (1997) believes that the "nurse's own spirituality will be reflected in the choice of interventions selected" (p. 132). This may be correct to a degree. The situation can be problematic, however, if nurse and patient have serious divergence in spiritual or religious beliefs and behaviors. The nurse must be comfortable and secure enough in his or her own spirituality and/or religious beliefs to remain open to differing spiritual or religious attitudes and needs on the part of the dying patient.

Some broad areas of spiritual nursing care for dying persons include assisting the patient to find meaning in life, hope, a relationship to God, forgiveness or acceptance, and transcendence (Kemp, 1995, p. 45). Five specific spiritual interventions for dying patients that fall within the purview of the nurse are praying, facilitating the presence of loved ones, allowing the dying person time to share, assisting in the completion of unfinished tasks, and assuring that the dying person has been given "permission" to die (Olson, 1997, p. 133). Nurses caring for dying patients should also attempt to identify the presence of spiritual pain, which may be manifested in terms of "the past (painful memories, regret, failure, guilt); the present (isolation, unfairness, anger); the future (fear, hopelessness)" (Eisdon, 1995, p. 641). Hospice research has documented the fact that spiritual care of dying patients falls within the scope of nursing practice (Hermann, 2001). Assessment of spiritual needs may be complex in end-of-life care (Sheldon, 2000); however, the provision of spiritual care in death and dying has been shown to enhance nurses' personal spirituality (Highfield, Taylor, & Amenta, 2000). A nursing theory recommended to support the provision of spiritual care for the terminally ill is the humanistic theory of Paterson and Zderad (Vassallo, 2001).

Young and Koopsen (2011) point out that dying "is a spiritual event of enormous importance"; "dying," they add, "is a profound process of spiritual transformation" (p. 245). For many, Young and Koopsen comment, dying involves one's attention being turned away "from the outer distractions in the world and turned inward toward a greater peace and comfort in spiritual fulfillment" (p. 245). This contention is supported by the perceptions of 38 hospice patients (Pevey, Jones, & Yarber, 2008), as well as by the research on death attitudes conducted by Dezutter et al. (2009).

Stepnick and Perry (1992) offered a plan to guide nurses in providing effective spiritual care to dying patients, employing a model of the transitional phases of dying. They believe that, although patients may have different beliefs and levels of spiritual maturity, they share some common characteristics and needs as death approaches (p. 18).

Based on Kübler-Ross's (1969) phases of denial, anger, bargaining, depression, and acceptance, some suggested nursing strategies include listening and assuring trust, being nonjudgmental about anger, being sensitive to the pain of the bargaining stage, keeping communication open, and preparing the dying patient for what to expect in terms of the end stages of illness (pp. 19–23).

It is an accepted fact that "nurses regularly encounter death in the care of [their] patients" (Schulling, 2012, p. 55); and death is "not an easy subject as it often feels like failure for family and healthcare professionals" (Rushing, 2012, p. 113). Nurse Arlene Reynolds (2009) thus poses the question, "How can I respond to dying patients?" (p. 197). Reynolds's response involved spiritual care and talking with a patient about his or her spirituality. She concluded that "Sometimes we tend to be overly concerned with the tasks of nursing, and miss moments to make an eternal difference for patients" (p. 197).

In attempting to make such an "eternal difference," however, how do nurses themselves cope with their patients' death and dying? "Where do nurses go for help?" (Peterson et al., 2010, p. 432). After conducting qualitative interviews with 15 nurses, all of whom had cared for dying patients, Peterson et al. concluded that the nurses relied on two sources of support, internal and external: "Internally, nurses found that evaluating the death and relying on professional distance helped them cope. Externally, the nurses looked to peers, religious resources and the patients and families themselves for comfort" (p. 435).

Brian, a master's-prepared psychiatric–mental health nurse, spoke about how he drew on his own spiritual journey in caring for dying patients:

> I hope that I always carry the motto of my former religious community [of nursing brothers], "Christ impels me," to my work with dying patients. Now I haven't done a good job of that every day of my life, I assure you; I'm an "earthen vessel" too. But nursing, for me, is a vocation; and I have always felt very privileged to work with patients in the last chapter of their lives on earth. It's such a rewarding experience. It's a tremendous privilege of being there, of ministering to the dying person.
>
> There was this patient and I was holding one of her hands and her daughter was holding the other, and it was like we were saying: "It's OK, you can let go." And then her daughter asked me to say a prayer, and I just sort of incorporated some ideas, like "you are surrounded by people who love you, and whenever you're ready to go, you can go to God. He's waiting for you." . . .
>
> When the patient dies, you think of what that person has given to you, and how their spirit will live on in you, and that's very special, very gifting.

Maggie, a hospice nurse, spoke about the importance of using touch to calm the anxieties of her patients entering the death experience:

> I will frequently reach out and touch a dying person physically; it's so important when they're scared. I don't think people are afraid to die; they are afraid of the process of dying. It's the loneliness, the isolation, the abandonment, the fear of people not wanting to touch them or care for them . . . What is most fearful is the unknown in the dying process. Are they going to be in pain; are they going to feel loved; is their family going to be there? And then, what happens after? I think we nurses are good about giving physical attention

to dying patients, and even psychosocial, but we're afraid to talk about the spiritual, about the fact that maybe they feel abandoned or forsaken by God. As caregivers, I think we shy away from that. But I've learned that it's really important that people are supported in whatever they feel comes after life, and in their concept of God.

Palliative Care

The World Health Organization (1990) defined palliative care as "the active total care, by a multi professional team, of patients whose disease is not responsive to curative treatment. Control of pain, of other symptoms, and of psychological, social and spiritual problems is paramount. The goal of palliative care is achievement of the best quality of life for patients and their families" (p. 1). Palliation essentially relates to the acts of relieving suffering and restoring peace to those who cannot be cured (Doyle, 1984). Palliative care focuses on immediate quality rather than length of life (Olson, 1997) and integrates physical, psychosocial, and spiritual care in its therapeutic plan (Katz & Sidell, 1994). Palliative care may be carried out in a variety of settings: a hospital, a nursing home, a hospice, or a patient's home. In addition to providing symptom relief and support of positive quality of life, palliative care as an emerging subspecialty of health care also includes promoting the dying person's independence as much as possible, facilitating communication between collaborating care agencies, supporting families and staff during the bereavement period, and influencing care through education and research in the area (James & MacLeod, 1993, p. 6).

Spiritual or religious beliefs may influence both the choice and the practice of palliative care for a dying person (Hamel & Lysaught, 1994). Hamel and Lysaught explained that in palliative care patients' religious beliefs may affect decisions about death and dying by "(a) helping to shape [their] worldviews, (b) giving form to their particular beliefs, (c) giving rise to moral principles and rules, and (d) shaping community character and dispositions" (p. 61). For the dying person whose life history has been consistent with the worldview, beliefs, and moral principles central to his or her religious tradition, a sense of peace and security related to end-of-life decisions will usually be demonstrated; the support of the individual's religious community is also generally evident. In such a case the palliative care interventions should be consistent with the religious tradition of the dying patient. The caregiver should attempt to "build on" the existing beliefs of the patient and support the faith tradition that has provided comfort and sustenance in the past (Murray & Lyall, 1994).

Several authors have addressed the positive relationship between spirituality and quality of life for persons experiencing palliative care (Vivat, 2008; Crang & Muncey, 2008), as well as noting the importance of spiritual support being provided by the health-care practitioner (Narayanasamy, 2007).

Hospice Care

The concept of palliative care was initiated primarily in concert with the hospice movement in Europe and the United States. The first modern nursing hospice of note, St. Christopher's, was founded in Sydenham, England, in 1967, under the direction of Dame Cicely Saunders, MD. The goal of St. Christopher's founder was to provide compassionate and loving care for those who were dying (Saunders, 1981, 1983).

During the medieval period a hospice was considered a place of hospitality for pilgrims on a journey, a stopping off place for travelers. The modern nursing hospice may also be described as a "way station" or "place of transit"; here, however, individuals are helped "to live fully in an atmosphere of loving kindness and grace" as they experience the process of natural death (Stoddard, 1978, p. 10). The goal of providing care and a place for the "weary traveler" to find "rest and safety" has not really changed from medieval times (Cohen, 1979). Most patients are indeed battle scarred and weary by the time they arrive at the hospice seeking relief. The central philosophy of hospice care emphasizes the fact that the outcome will be death, not prolongation of life; thus the care focus is in "comfort not cure" (Kirschling & Pittman, 1989, p. 1).

Hospice care in the United States is generally considered to have begun with the Hospice of New Haven project associated with Yale University, initiated in the mid-1970s. Nurses caring for those with terminal illness, especially nurses whose personal spirituality espoused the Judeo-Christian tradition, eagerly received the hospice message of compassionate care; for those caregivers the hospice concept was a direct reflection of the Scriptural admonitions to provide loving and sensitive care to those who are ill and in need of comfort. In hospice care, the nurse has the opportunity of reflecting a concept that Chaplain Trevor Hoy (1983) believes "lies at the heart" of spiritual care of the dying, and which is expressed in the Twenty-third Psalm: "Yea, though I walk through the valley of the shadow of death, I will fear no evil; for thou art with me" (p. 177). Hoy's position was supported by that of hospice chaplain Ted Harvey (1996) who described the two central concerns of spiritual care for the dying as relating to the patient's emotional well-being and his or her relationship with God (p. 41).

The more modern hospice concept refers to either a facility or a program that supports the dying person's spiritual and religious beliefs and goals (Franco, 1985, p. 80). Related to the complexities of the ever changing health-care system in this country, hospice chaplain Richard Grey (1996) suggested that the hospice mission and identity will continually need clarification. To that end, Grey proposed a psychospiritual care paradigm within which all hospice personnel can situate their particular activities, yet share in the common element of compassionate care. The National Hospice Organization Standards and Accreditation Committee developed a set of hospice service guidelines, which include policies related to admissions and discharge; levels of care; staffing, including a chaplain to provide spiritual care; services; and treatment (The National Hospice Organization, 1996b). A Hospice Code of Ethics has also been created, the first precept being "to remain sensitive to and be appreciative of the ethnic, cultural, religious and life style diversity of clients and their families" (The National Hospice Organization, 1996a, p. 76).

Five palliative care physicians conducted an open-ended qualitative study to assess hospice patients' attitudes toward the discussion of religious and/or spiritual topics with their doctors. From the study data, four dominant themes emerged: "1) treating the whole person, 2) treating with sensitivity, 3) favorable attitudes toward religious or spiritual discussions with doctors, and 4) no preaching" (Hart, Kohlwes, Deyo, Rhodes, & Bowen, 2003, p. 160). The physicians concluded that they were not expected to be "spiritual advisors" for their patients but that many patients did feel positive about speaking about spiritual issues with their doctors (p. 160).

Several nursing studies have explored the prevalence of spiritual care in the hospice setting. Millison and Dudley (1992), in surveying 117 hospice directors in three states, found that many nonclergy hospice personnel were providing spiritual care by listening to patients, teaching meditation or guided imagery, and referring patients to clergy. These authors also found that hospice personnel are a spiritual group, and that those who identified themselves as more spiritual "found greater satisfaction in their hospice work" (p. 63). In a chart review of home visits to 37 hospice care patients, Reese and Brown (1997) discovered that spirituality and death anxiety were the most commonly discussed topics between patients and caregivers.

Laurie, a hospice nurse for five years, spoke about the concepts of death anxiety, spirituality, and caring, as experienced with some of her patients:

> The patients are afraid when they are in the dying process, of what the end will be like; some use their faith to help but even still they can be afraid of the unknown. That's when I think the nurse's caring is so important. Caring is hard to define. I think it's the ability to show compassion, to be able to touch someone. To just sit and listen, especially to their spiritual concerns and feelings and not to be critical or judgmental, to be with the flow of the moment. Time is such a commodity for people who are dying; it's so important to listen to people who are dying. That's spiritual caring I think.

▶ Religious Practices Associated with Death and Dying

For a dying person, religious practices can provide an important dimension of spiritual support and comfort. Even if an individual has become alienated from a religious denomination or church, a terminal illness may be the catalyst for return to the practice of one's faith. This was clearly reflected in the comments of a 47-year-old male patient in the advanced stages of cancer. "I hadn't gone to my church for years; I don't know why. I just stopped going. But lately I've started up again, and I've been reading the Bible. When I die I want to have a church burial and be buried in a Christian cemetery; that's a big thing with my family."

Although the nurse caring for dying patients cannot be knowledgeable about the death-related beliefs and practices of all religious faiths, some familiarity with those of the major Western and Eastern traditions may provide a starting point for the provision of spiritual support. Having some idea of the theological positions and religious practices of different groups may assist the nurse in developing a relationship with a dying person and an empathetic and caring attitude (Head, 1994, p. 310). Anglican priest David Head (1994) believes that such knowledge on the part of a care provider will allow a dying patient to express spiritual or religious concerns more freely, without fear of being misunderstood (pp. 311–312). Ultimately, the best nursing approach to providing spiritual care to a dying person is to request information about religious beliefs and practices directly from the patient or family.

Western Traditions: Judaism, Christianity, and Islam

Judaism

Attitudes toward death for the Jewish patient may vary according to identification with a particular subgroup of Judaism: Orthodox, Conservative, Reform, or Reconstructionist. A Jewish person's approach to the dying process will also be influenced by his or her belief or nonbelief in the existence of an afterlife. Some Jews, especially those of the Orthodox tradition, do not subscribe to the concept of eternal life; they may, however, believe that faithful Jews will be resurrected when the Messiah comes. Some believe that one's good deeds in this life live on in the memories of family and friends. In Judaism, life is highly valued as a gift of God; all efforts to continue a productive life are supported. Thus, facing death may represent an ending of something precious. As Rabbi Julia Neuberger (1994) explained, "It is not so much uncertainty about the afterlife which causes a problem, but the emphasis put on the here and now" (p. 13).

A Jewish person who is dying, especially an Orthodox Jew, will generally receive visits from friends and synagogue members, because the duty to visit the sick is considered a mitzvah or good deed in Judaism. Some contemporary synagogues have established formalized groups called Bikkur Cholim societies, whose express purpose is to visit and minister to those who are ill; Bikkur Cholim members receive training from their synagogues in how to work with the sick. These individuals may also be present at a Jewish person's death and will offer prayers or readings from the Psalms, if desired by the patient or family.

After death occurs, synagogue members from the Jewish Burial Society may come to prepare the body of an Orthodox patient; no action should be taken by hospital or hospice personnel until it is determined whether this will occur. It is also customary that, after death, a Jewish person be buried within 24 hours; an exception may be made for the Sabbath. The formal ritual prayer of mourning, the kaddish, may be recited by a rabbi or family member; cremation and autopsy are avoided. After the burial has taken place, the important task of mourning is initiated. This involves friends and relatives of the deceased visiting at the family's home, or sitting shiva for the next seven days. This mourning period provides the grieving family with the support and care of those close to them and to the deceased person during the time immediately following death. Following shiva, 30 days of mourning, shloshim, continues; during this time the family may resume usual activities but avoids formal entertainment (Grollman, 1993).

Christianity

Three major subgroups within the Christian tradition are the Eastern Orthodox Churches, Roman Catholicism, and Protestantism; in addition, a number of other faith groups are identified as followers of Christ. Virtually all Christian traditions believe in eternal life, as promised in the Gospel message of Jesus. Thus, for the devout Christian, although the dying process can raise anxieties in terms of possible pain and suffering, death itself is viewed as a positive transition to a life with God and to one's eternal reward. Protestantism, which relies on the concept of salvation, trusts that faith will bring the believer into a better world (Klass, 1993). Older adult Christians sometimes express a desire for God to come and "take them home."

As death approaches, the majority of Christian patients and their families welcome a visit from a priest or minister; the pastoral visitor may be from the family's church or can be a hospital or hospice chaplain. These ministers will generally pray and read a Scripture passage with the dying person and their family. Eastern Orthodox Christians, Roman Catholics, and some Episcopalians may request an anointing or the "Sacrament of the Sick" prior to death; they may also wish to make a confession of sins and receive the sacraments of Penance and of Holy Eucharist (Holy Communion).

A priest or family member may cross the arms of the Eastern Orthodox patient after death, situating the fingers to represent a cross.

After death occurs, most Christians will have a period of "viewing" of the body, sometimes called a "wake"; this ritual, which provides the opportunity for friends and family to call, takes place from one to three days after the death, in either the family home or a funeral home. A priest or minister may offer prayers periodically during the viewing. Christian burial services vary according to denomination. Eastern Orthodox, Roman Catholic, and some Episcopalian (Anglo-Catholic) Christians attend a funeral Mass of Requiem for the deceased prior to interment in a church cemetery. Although Mass is still the norm for the Catholic funeral, emphasis is now placed on life rather than death, and the central theme is resurrection; the priest celebrant wears white rather than black vestments. This changed focus, from grieving the death to hope in God's love and trust in the resurrection, indicates "a more healthy biblicism and pastoral practice" (Miller, 1993, p. 42). Other Christians participate in funeral or memorial services of their denominations; some families prefer a private service conducted by a minister in the home. The latter may be desired if cremation is chosen and no formal trip to the cemetery is planned.

Private memorial services are also the norm for the deceased who did not adhere to any conventional religious tradition. As Irion (1993) pointed out, a dying "secularist" also has a spiritual need to find meaning and purpose in life and in death (p. 94). The secular humanist usually places a high value on life and life accomplishments; these may be remembered and honored at a nonreligious memorial service.

Islam

The devout Muslim, like the Christian, views death as representing a spiritual transition to eternal life with Allah (Renard, 1993). Although a terminally ill Muslim may fear the dying process related to possible suffering, the concept of death itself is accepted as the will of Allah. Thus, excessive grieving of death by a Muslim may be considered inappropriate and represent a contradiction of Allah's plan. The death of a loved one should be viewed as only a temporary loss (Neuberger, 1994, p. 36). Islam, like Christianity, holds a belief in "resurrection of the body, final judgement and assignment to heaven or hell" (Kemp, 1995, p. 58).

As death approaches, family members or a Muslim minister, an imam, may read a passage from the Holy Qur'an to comfort the patient and family. The dying Muslim may wish to face Mecca, in the East, and ask forgiveness of Allah for sins. After death occurs, members of the family frequently wish to prepare the body through ritual washing and wrapping in a white cloth. After the body is prepared, the deceased may be laid out in a position facing Mecca.

Burial rites for a Muslim patient can vary, but generally interment takes place in a Muslim cemetery 24 hours after death.

Eastern Traditions: Hinduism, Buddhism, and Confucianism

Hinduism

Hinduism consists of a number of related Indian religious traditions, all of which are centuries old. Although a pantheon of lesser gods is associated with Hinduism, as demonstrated in Indian temples and holy places, most devout Hindus believe in the existence of one supreme being or deity. The many less powerful gods and goddesses are considered to be forms or derivatives of the one deity, with power and interest in specific areas of one's life.

The concept of reincarnation or rebirth influences the dying Hindu's attitude toward death; death itself is viewed as a union with God. How one has lived in this world is influential in how one might return in the next life; this concept is referred to as karma.

Hindu patients often prefer to die at home where they can be more certain of the presence of a priest (Green, 1989a). A Brahmin priest, who performs the death rites, may tie a string or cord around the dying person's neck or wrist, which should not be removed; prayers are also chanted by the priest. Following a Hindu's death, the funeral is usually carried out within 24 hours, and cremation is the traditional ritual.

Buddhism

Buddhism, founded by Gautama Siddhartha, differs from most other major religious traditions in that the Buddhist does not accept the existence of God or of a Supreme Being; Buddhists do, however, acknowledge the presence of a multiplicity of individual gods who are involved and interested in the lives of the Buddhist. Devout Buddhists live according to the "eightfold path" of right belief, right intent, right speech, right conduct, right endeavor, right mindfulness, right effort, and right meditation (Kemp, 1995, p. 60). The ultimate goal of the Buddhist is to reach the interior state of Nirvana or inner peace and happiness; this is achieved after having lived according to the eightfold path.

The Buddhist's attitude toward death is also influenced by belief in the concept of rebirth; death is accepted as a transition and as part of the cycle of life. A Buddhist monk may chant prayers at the death of a devout Buddhist in order to provide peace of mind at the point of death (Green, 1989b). An important dimension of the dying process for a Buddhist is to remain conscious in order to be able to think right and wholesome thoughts (Kemp, 1995). The deceased is generally cremated after death.

Confucianism

Confucianism is the tradition founded by the ancient Chinese scholar and philosopher, Confucius. Confucianism places great emphasis on respecting the memories and the contributions of one's ancestors. Elaborate death and burial rituals allow the bereaved to formally express grief and bring "continuity with the past and with tradition" (Ryan, 1993, p. 85). Ryan (1993) reported that in the Confucian tradition a person is taught to live life in such a way that after death good memories of the deceased may be honored (p. 86). The fate of the deceased in an afterlife depends on the quality of his or her natural life; it is also important that the deceased be properly honored by relatives after death. This relates to a strong belief in a "continuity of life after death" (Neuberger, 1994, p. 48).

The Confucianist's funeral may be an elaborate ritual, its complexity reflecting the status of the deceased. A carefully crafted coffin may be purchased by the family prior to death so that the dying person will know that he or she will be well honored at the burial rites.

▶ Spirituality and the Rite of Burial

The burial rite provides important spiritual support for the family and friends of a deceased person. The planning of one's own funeral or memorial service may provide comfort for the dying person. In contemporary society, as chronically ill persons live longer and are able to anticipate death, they often become involved in the planning of their burial rites. During the early period of the acquired immunodeficiency syndrome (AIDS) epidemic in this country, with many gay men not only anticipating their own approaching deaths but also experiencing the deaths and burial rites of friends, planning the memorial service became a central activity of the dying process. As one 45-year-old man suffering from advanced Kaposi's sarcoma humorously commented, "I've put so much into the plans for my memorial service, it's beginning to resemble the coronation of a king." Despite the humor of the patient's remark, he nevertheless admitted that creating the memorial service plans was very comforting, observing, "This way I don't have to worry about my family having to deal with this when they are grieving my death."

As Rando (1988) pointed out, burial rites help families confront the death of a loved one and begin the grieving process (p. 261). The funeral provides an opportunity for meeting the spiritual, psychological, and social needs of the bereaved (Raether, 1993, p. 214). Some specific therapeutic benefits of the bereavement ritual include confirming the reality of death; acknowledging the loss; providing an opportunity to express feelings; remembering and validating the life of the deceased; accepting the changed relationship with the deceased; supporting family and friends; and, in the case of religiously oriented funerals, placing the meaning of life and death in a religious/philosophical context (Rando, 1988, pp. 266–269).

Burial rites can also be helpful to nurse caregivers who wish to formally terminate relationships with patients who have died. In one clinical research facility, nurses worked extensively with dying children, most of whom returned home to a different geographical location for death and burial; thus, staff requested that the hospital chaplain periodically conduct pediatric memorial services to provide nursing staff the opportunity for formal farewells to the deceased children.

In evaluating the concepts of death, burial, and bereavement, Margaret Holloway (2006) explored the often heard phrase, "Death is the great leveler." Holloway agrees that the thought represents the "acknowledgement that in death our common humanity is affirmed" (p. 834). Holloway goes on, however, to offer the option of a transcultural spirituality of death and bereavement, which means "the challenge . . . is not so much to find a common model . . . as to seek out the means to access the strengths and resources in each other's tradition which affirm our common humanity" (p. 838).

▶ Spirituality and the Bereavement Experience

The body of literature dealing with the postdeath period includes the terms *bereavement*, *grief*, and *mourning*; these are sometimes used interchangeably, all being understood as describing the physical and psychosocial experience of loss following the death of a loved one. Rando (1988) defined *grief* as "the process of experiencing the psychological, social and physical reactions to [one's] perception of loss" (p. 11). *Mourning*, derived from the Greek "to care," is described as "an emotion that results from the universal experience of loss" (Davidson, 1984, p. 6). And Sanders (1989), in her book *Grief: The Mourning After*, distinguishes between the three concepts: bereavement is conceptualized as the overall experience one faces after a loss, grief is viewed as representing the physical and psychosocial reactions an individual experiences while in the state of bereavement, and mourning describes the culturally prescribed behaviors carried out after a death (p. 10).

Historically, the study of the bereavement experience, including the aspects of grief and mourning, began with the work of Eric Lindemann in 1944. His classic study of 101 bereaved survivors of Boston's "Coconut Grove" fire provided the benchmark for our contemporary understanding of the grieving process. Lindemann described the acute reaction to the death of a loved one as including such somatic responses as "a feeling of tightness in the throat; choking with shortness of breath; need for sighing; an empty feeling in the abdomen; lack of muscular power; and an intense subjective distress described as tension or mental pain" (p. 141).

Later scholars of bereavement such as Bowlby (1961) and Parkes (1972) viewed the grief reaction as being of longer duration and consisting of such phases as acute grief, chronic grief, conflicted grief or complicated grief, and prolonged or delayed grief. Writing in 1983, Colin Murray Parkes and Robert Weiss asserted that when grief was uncomplicated, recovery was generally accomplished within one year after the loss; this time period has been extended significantly in recent years, although the one-year anniversary may represent a milestone in the healing process for some mourners.

Extant research also supports the importance of a number of potentially mediating variables related to the bereavement experience: the meaning of the bereavement to the mourner; the relationship between the deceased and the bereaved; the physical, social, material, and psychological resources of the bereaved person; and the spiritual and religious beliefs of the family (Rando, 1988; Sanders, 1989). Sanders's (1989) model, labeled the "Integrative Theory of Bereavement," included the earlier noted variables as well as the external mediator of religious practice. The work of identifying and meeting the spiritual or religious needs of bereaved persons is central to supporting positive coping with grief and loss.

Manifestations of an uncomplicated grief reaction are generally divided into four categories: physical, cognitive, emotional, and behavioral. Some of these as described by Worden (1982) include physical reactions such as stomach emptiness, shortness of breath, tightness in chest and throat, and fatigue; cognitive reactions of disbelief and mental confusion; emotional responses of sadness, guilt, anger, loneliness, numbness, and yearning for the deceased; and behavioral disruptions such as insomnia, loss of appetite, social isolation, crying, and restlessness (pp. 20–23). Worden described the four tasks of mourning during the bereavement experience as accepting "the reality of the loss," experiencing "the pain of the grief," adjusting "to an environment in which the deceased is missing," and reinvesting "emotional energy . . . in another relationship" (pp. 11–15). Rando (1988) suggested specifically that the bereaved person should not isolate himself or herself, accept the support of significant others, obtain information about what to expect in the grieving process, realize that grief may be expressed in a variety of ways, allow himself or herself to cry and to talk about the deceased, and trust that the pain will decrease after a time (pp. 242–248). It is pointed out that "each, person's journey through the grief process is profoundly unique . . . and is experienced spiritually, behaviorally, physically, and cognitively" (Young & Koopsen, 2011, p. 266), and that one's religion and/or spiritual philosophy of life influences his or her attitude toward grief and bereavement (Becker et al., 2007; Lees, 2008; Wortman & Park, 2008).

It is well known that for many dying persons, spirituality and/or religion play(s) an important role in the coping process; the influence of spirituality and religion on bereavement is less well documented. A systematic review of the extant research on spirituality and bereavement revealed that "ninety-four percent show some positive effects of religious/spiritual beliefs on bereavement" (Becker et al., 2007, p. 207). The study authors admit, however, that there was a great "heterogeneity regarding included populations and outcome measurements" (p. 207).

Bereaved persons need and will often accept spiritual support from the family's pastoral care provider, rabbi, minister, priest, or, in some cases, a nurse if he or she is skilled in bereavement counseling and support. Other significant persons who may provide spiritual support for the bereaved are church or faith group members who also understand the grieving person's or family's spiritual and theological perspective on the loss. Whether spiritual care is provided by the pastor, nurse, or church member, intervention should focus on supporting two major tasks of the bereaved individual: letting go of the deceased person and becoming reinvested in current life activities. The spiritual caregiver's challenge in grief and bereavement is to balance the activities of strengthening and disputing; the caregiver must "know when to comfort and support and when to challenge and confront" (Joesten, 1992, p. 144). Joesten observed that an important dimension of spiritual intervention for bereaved persons is the presence of a caring other who is willing to be there and share in the grief and the pain (p. 145); he asserted that the spiritual caregiver assists the bereaved most by being someone who offers hope and honesty amid the darkness of the experience (p. 148).

Finally, it is important to remember, as noted by Young and Koopsen (2005), that for those dealing with loss, "individuals in the early stages of spiritual development may need more external support and communication, while more spiritually developed individuals may use rituals, rites and symbols for comfort" (p. 192).

Death of a Child

There is perhaps no loss so grievous for any person as the loss of a child. Most parents are devastated when one of their children dies, regardless of the age of the child. The common understanding of family, in virtually all societies, is that a child will survive his or her parents. Although family members attempt to find meaning and purpose in the life of the deceased offspring, the task is more difficult in the death of an infant or a very young child. The bereaved parents are often left with great frustration related to unfulfilled dreams and expectations. As Sanders (1989) observed, children represent a parent's legacy for the future; they are to be the bearers of the family tradition (p. 163). A parent may also experience guilt that he or she was somehow not able to protect the child from illness and death.

Sanders (1989) identified some parental responses to bereavement: despair, related to the ability to go on living following a child's death; confusion, related to the parent being unable to accept the reality of the death; guilt that the parent was not able to be responsible for the child's welfare; and anger, associated with the inability to prevent the child's death (pp. 165–169). Death of a child may also affect a marriage if the usual ways of interacting between the spouses are disrupted by the loss (Rando, 1988, p. 170). Many relationships end in separation or divorce as a result of the terminal illness and death of the couple's child.

Parents may find comfort in religious and spiritual beliefs, especially if they were able to integrate these into coping with the child's illness prior to the death experience. A nurse should not, however, attempt to impose such beliefs on a parent or parents with words such as "This must have been God's will," because the bereaved may still need to express feelings of anguish or anger over their loss (Amenta, 1995, p. 206). The nurse can, however, provide the spiritual care of presence by being available to the parents with a loving and listening heart.

A significant amount of research has been done on the impact of the death of a child on surviving parents. One example is exploring parental grief and depression after the death of a child from cancer. In this study, the investigators found that while a "minority" of 58 parents actually met their criteria for parental grief and depression, "almost half of the sample was experiencing significant separation distress associated with persistent longing and yearning for their child" (McCarthy et al., 2010, p. 1321). And in a study of 31 parents whose child had died from cancer it was found that fathers coped by being more "task focused," while mothers were more "child focused" (Alam, Barrera, D'Agostino, Nicholas, & Schneiderman, 2012, p. 1). The researchers concluded that the findings emphasized "the need for tailoring bereavement support services in the family" (p. 2). Finally, a study of the lived experience of six mothers who had experienced the unexpected death of a child revealed a number of helpful coping behaviors employed by the study participants; these included "positive beliefs, faith beliefs, everlasting love, pleasant remembrances, social engagement, and staying connected" (Parker & Dunn, 2011, p. 221). Parker and Dunn observed that "by exploring, through interviews, the lives of mothers who have experienced the loss of a child, healthcare providers may become more aware of the needs of those who grieve" (p. 232).

Death of a Spouse

The death of one's life partner is a traumatic event, regardless of the number of years a couple has been together. The death of a spouse is recognized as emotionally overwhelming and is generally considered one of the most devastating human losses possible (Osterweis, Solomon, & Green, 1984, p. 71). Raphael (1983) posited that conjugal bereavement is one of the most disruptive and potentially stressful experiences that an adult can experience and may affect the essential meaning of the survivor's existence (p. 177). A particular difficulty for the surviving spouse is identity transition; that is, the change in self-image in beginning to view oneself as a single person rather than as one-half of a couple. In the case of a small number of bereaved partners, the inability to identify as a single person has generated feelings of helplessness so severe as to result in suicide (Raphael, 1983).

Some bereaved spouses experience physical symptoms of their grief. Parkes, Benjamin, and Fitzgerald (1969) coined the metaphor of the "broken heart" based on their findings that some widower deaths within six months of bereavement were due to heart disease related to the loss of one's spouse. An important mediator of such mortality and morbidity is the presence of spiritual and social support for the bereaved spouse. Shuchter's (1986) study of 70 bereaved spouses revealed that interaction with significant others helped the bereaved by providing emotional support and caring, and by giving the surviving spouse an opportunity to become involved in the concerns of others (p. 110).

Sanders (1989) found the practice of religion, particularly church attendance, to be a mainstay among bereaved spouses (p. 194). Nurses may have the occasion to provide spiritual care to bereaved spouses who stay in touch after the death of their partner in a hospital setting. If face-to-face interaction is not possible, a written note of condolence from a loved one's nurse can be very meaningful. During the dying process in a health-care facility, staff nurses often become important significant others for the family of the ill person. Any expression of care and concern after the death, such as a letter or a phone call, will convey a deeply appreciated message of spiritual support.

Death of a Parent

The death of a parent frequently represents a loss of security on the part of the bereaved child or children. Although a surviving child may be chronologically an adult at the time of parental death, the loss of love and caring can be great. Even adult children who have undertaken complete support of a frail parent feel keenly the pain of a mother's or a father's death. The nature of the former parent–child relationship is, of course, a mediating variable in the bereavement experience of the offspring. Sanders (1989) believed, however, that even if a parent–child relationship has not been exemplary, a significant bond exists, which is traumatic when broken (p. 202).

The nurse assisting at the death of a parent, even an elderly parent, must be sensitive to the deep spiritual meaning of the parent–child bond. The grief associated with this death experience can be powerful and deep for surviving offspring of any age. Awareness of the significance of this loss will guide the nurse in his or her efforts to provide spiritual support for the grief experience of an adult child as well as that of a bereaved young child or teen.

▶ Spiritual Care in Bereavement: The Healing Process

Clearly, the nurse seeking to provide spiritual care to a bereaved person will need to have some knowledge of the individual's spiritual and/or religious beliefs and practices related to loss and grieving. Respect for the religious attitudes and practices of the bereaved must be clearly communicated by one attempting to provide care and support (Doka, 1993a, p. 191). If a bereaved individual appears to have dysfunctional beliefs related to a particular religious tradition, referral to a clergyperson of the person's denomination or the use of religious books may be helpful (Doka, 1993a). Clinebell (1991) suggested that a caregiver attempting to facilitate the work of the grieving process may want to employ a ministry of caring and presence, responsive listening, counseling as the bereaved attempts to rebuild his or her life, facilitating of spiritual growth, and supporting the bereaved in reaching out to others with similar losses (p. 221). Although the funeral provides an important opportunity for the emotional expression of grief, Clinebell pointed out that it may take many months for the bereaved person to come to terms with a loss, and continued spiritual support is needed during that time. Some postfuneral questions that might encourage the expression of emotions are, "What have you been feeling since the funeral?" "What sort of memories keep coming back?" "How often have you let yourself cry?" "Have you had trouble keeping going?" and "Would you tell me more about the way he/she died?" (p. 224).

In order for healing to be completed, the bereaved person must be able to let go of the deceased. Although this may have appeared to occur at the time of death, when a family member verbally gives a dying person permission to give up, the emotional attachment may remain with the survivor. Many bereaved persons express significant distress at coming to a point at which they have difficulty remembering what the deceased looked like, or even at letting several hours pass without thinking about the deceased. Ruskay (1996) proposed an approach to bereavement care in which the griever is encouraged to incorporate the loss into daily activities and plans; the bereaved person is counseled to incorporate some of the deceased person's interests, for example, gardening, into their lives, thus adding a positive dimension to the grieving process (p. 5).

In discussing bereavement care, Bouton (1996) distinguished between the goals of grief counseling and bereavement care. Grief counseling is envisioned as facilitating the work of grieving to achieve a successful outcome by helping the bereaved person face the reality of the loss; cope with physical, psychological, and spiritual grief reactions; and reinvest himself or herself into life activities. Bereavement care is conceptualized as identifying and resolving the pain and conflict resulting from the loss that may block completion of the grieving process (p. 17).

Additionally, spiritual and religious beliefs are important considerations in the provision of bereavement care. Religious beliefs may be instrumental in defining right or acceptable attitudes and behavior in relation to the bereavement experience (Koenig, 1994, p. 405). Cullinan (1993) conceptualized spiritual care of the bereaved as a "sacred art." While acknowledging the existence of a multiplicity of theories related to the relationships among spirituality, religiosity, and bereavement, Cullinan (1993) viewed spirituality as undergirded and influenced by the individual's faith development, cultural background, and religious or denominational affiliation and practice (p. 197). Such an adaptive type of psychospiritual approach to care, Cullinan argued, will help the bereaved person to cope with the loss in a more positive and healthy way (p. 197).

Personal spirituality and religiosity or religious practice are important mediating variables in coping with death and bereavement. Dying persons' and their families' spiritual and religious beliefs about such concepts as the meaning of life and death, the existence of an afterlife, and the purpose of suffering can influence profoundly how the dying process is experienced. The nurse, sensitive to the spiritual and religious beliefs of a dying patient and his or her family, may be able to provide therapeutic spiritual support and intervention that will mediate the pain associated with the death and bereavement experiences.

▶ References

Alam, R., Barrera, M., D'Agostino, N., Nicholas, D., & Schneiderman, G. (2012). Bereavement experiences of mothers and fathers over time after the death of a child due to cancer. *Death Studies, 36*, 1–22.

Amenta, M. O. (1995). Loss, death and dying. In D. D. Ignatavicus, M. L. Workman, & M. A. Mishler (Eds.), *Medical–surgical nursing: A nursing process approach* (pp. 95–212). Philadelphia, PA: W. B. Saunders.

Angelucci, D., & Lawrence, M. (1995). Death and dying. In M. Stanley & P. G. Beare (Eds.), *Gerontological nursing* (pp. 400–414). Philadelphia, PA: F. A. Davis.

Becker, G., Xander, C. J., Blum, H. E., Lutterbach, J., Momm, F., Gysels, M., . . . Higginson, I. J. (2007). Do religious or spiritual beliefs influence bereavement? A systematic review. *Palliative Medicine, 21*, 207–217.

Black, H. K., Santanello, H. R., & Rubinstein, R. L. (2014). A pragmatic belief system in family meaning-making after death. *Death Studies, 38*(8), 522–530.

Bouton, B. L. (1996). The interdisciplinary bereavement team: Defining and directing appropriate bereavement care. *The Hospice Journal, 11*(4), 15–24.

Bowlby, J. (1961). Processes of mourning. *International Journal of Psychoanalysis, 42*(8), 317–340.

Burns, S. (1991). The spirituality of dying. *Health Progress, 72*(7), 48–52.

Charlton, R. G. (1992). Spiritual need of the dying and bereaved: Views from the United Kingdom and New Zealand. *Journal of Palliative Care, 8*(4), 38–40.

Clinebell, H. (1991). *Basic types of pastoral care and counseling.* Nashville, TN: Abingdon Press.

Cohen, K. P. (1979). *Hospice: Prescription for terminal care.* Germantown, MD: Aspen Systems.

Conrad, N. L. (1985). Spiritual support for the dying. *Nursing Clinics of North America, 20*(2), 415–426.

Cullinan, A. (1993). Bereavement and the sacred art of spiritual care. In K. J. Doka (Ed.), *Death and spirituality* (pp. 195–205). Amityville, NY: Baywood.

Crang, C., & Muncey, T. (2008). Quality of life in palliative care: Being at ease in the here and now. *International Journal of Palliative Nursing, 14*(2), 92–97.

Davidson, G. W. (1984). *Understanding mourning: A guide for those who grieve.* Minneapolis, MN: Augsburg.

Derrickson, B. S. (1996). The spiritual work of the dying: A framework and case studies. *The Hospice Journal, 11*(2), 11–30.

Dezutter, J., Soenens, B., Luyckx, K., Bruyneel, S., Vansteenkiste, M., Duriez, B., & Hutsebaut, D. (2009). The role of religion in death attitudes: Distinguishing between religious belief and style of processing religious contents. *Death Studies, 33*, 73–92.

Dobratz, M. C. (2011). Toward development of a middle-range theory of psychological adaptation in death and dying. *Nursing Science Quarterly, 24*(4), 370–376.

Doka, K. J. (Ed.). (1993a). The spiritual crisis of bereavement. In *Death and spirituality* (pp. 185–194). Amityville, NY: Baywood.

Doka, K. J. (Ed.). (1993b). The spiritual needs of the dying. In *Death and spirituality* (pp. 143–150). Amityville, NY: Baywood.

Doyle, D. (1984). *Palliative care: The management of far-advanced illness.* Philadelphia, PA: The Charles Press.

Draper, P., Holloway, M., & Adamson, S. (2013). A qualitative study of recently bereaved people's beliefs about death: Implications for bereavement care. *Journal of Clinical Nursing, 23*(9/10), 1300–1308.

Eisdon, R. (1995). Spiritual pain in dying people: The nurse's role. *Professional Nurse, 10*(10), 641–643.

Esposito, J. L. (1990). Islam. In J. A. Komonchak, M. Collins, & D. A. Lane (Eds.), *The new dictionary of theology* (pp. 527–529). Collegeville, MN: The Liturgical Press.

Featherstone, S. M. (1997). Coping with loss, death and grieving. In P. A. Potter & A. G. Perry (Eds.), *Foundations of nursing: Concepts, process and practice* (pp. 457–476). St. Louis, MO: C. V. Mosby.

Forster, E., & Hafiz, A. (2015). Paediatric death and dying: Exploring coping strategies of health care professionals and perceptions of support provision. *International Journal of Palliative Nursing, 21*(6), 294–301.

Franco, V. W. (1985). The hospice: Humane care for the dying. *Journal of Religion and Health, 24*(1), 79–89.

Giske, T., & Cone, P. H. (2015). Discerning the health path: How nurses assist patient spirituality in diverse health care settings. *Journal of Clinical Nursing, 24*(19/20), 2926–2935.

Green, J. (1989a). Death with dignity: Hinduism. *Nursing Times, 85*(6), 50–51.

Green, J. (1989b). Death with dignity: Buddhism. *Nursing Times, 85*(9), 40–41.

Grey, R. (1996). The psycho-spiritual care matrix: A new paradigm for hospice caregiving. *American Journal of Hospice and Palliative Care, 13*(4), 19–25.

Grollman, E. A. (1993). Death in Jewish thought. In K. J. Doka (Ed.), *Death and spirituality* (pp. 21–32). Amityville, NY: Baywood.

Hamel, R. P., & Lysaught, M. T. (1994). Choosing palliative care: Do religious beliefs make a difference? *Journal of Palliative Care, 10*(3), 61–66.

Hart, A., Kohlwes, R., Deyo, R., Rhodes, L., & Bowen, D. (2003). Hospice patients' attitudes regarding spiritual discussions with their doctors. *American Journal of Hospice and Palliative Care, 20*(2), 135–139; 160.

Harvey, T. (1996). Who is the chaplain anyway?: Philosophy and integration of hospice chaplaincy. *American Journal of Hospice and Palliative Care, 13*(5), 41–43.

Hayes, Z. (1993). Death. In J. A. Komonchak, M. Collins, & D. A. Lane (Eds.), *The new dictionary of theology*. Collegeville, MN: The Liturgical Press.

Head, D. (1994). Religious approaches to dying. In I. B. Corless, B. B. Germino, & M. Pittman (Eds.), *Dying, death and bereavement: Theoretical perspectives and other ways of knowing*. Sudbury, MA: Jones & Bartlett Learning.

Hermann, C. P. (2001). Spiritual needs of dying patients: A qualitative study. *Oncology Nursing Forum, 28*(1), 67–72.

Highfield, M. F. (1992). Spiritual health of oncology patients: Nurse and patient perspectives. *Cancer Nursing, 15*(1), 1–8.

Highfield, M. E. F., Taylor, E. J., & Amenta, M. O. (2000). Preparation to care: The spiritual care education of oncology and hospice nurses. *Journal of Hospice and Palliative Nursing, 2*(2), 53–63.

Hittle, J. M. (1994). Death and spirituality: A nurse's perspective. *American Journal of Hospice and Palliative Care, 11*(5), 23–24.

Holloway, M. (2006). Death the great leveler? Toward a transcultural spirituality of dying and bereavement. *Journal of Clinical Nursing, 15*(7), 833–839.

Hoy, T. (1983). Hospice chaplaincy in the caregiving team. In C. A. Corr & D. M. Corr (Eds.), *Hospice care: Principles and practice* (pp. 177–196). New York, NY: Faber & Faber.

Irion, P. E. (1993). Spiritual issues in death and dying for those who do not have conventional religious belief. In K. J. Doka (Ed.), *Death and spirituality* (pp. 93–112). Amityville, NY: Baywood.

James, C. R., & MacLeod, R. D. (1993). The problematic nature of education in palliative care. *Journal of Palliative Care, 9*(4), 5–10.

Joesten, L. B. (1992). The voices of the dying and the bereaved: A bridge between loss and growth. In L. E. Holst (Ed.), *Hospital ministry: The role of the chaplain today* (pp. 139–150). New York, NY: Crossroad.

Kalina, K. (1993). *Midwife for souls: Spiritual care for the dying*. Boston, MA: St. Paul Books and Media.

Katz, J., & Sidell, M. (1994). *Easeful death: Caring for dying and bereaved people*. London, UK: Hodder & Stoughton.

Kemp, C. (1995). *Terminal illness: A guide to nursing care*. Philadelphia, PA: J. B. Lippincott.

Kinast, R. L. (1993). Death and dying. In M. Downey (Ed.), *The new dictionary of Catholic spirituality* (pp. 252–256). Collegeville, MN: The Liturgical Press.

Kirschling, J. M., & Pittman, J. F. (1989). Measurement of spiritual well-being: A hospice caregiver sample. *The Hospice Journal, 5*(2), 1–11.

Kisvetrova, H., Skoloudik, D., Joanovic, E., Konecna, J., & Miksova, Z. (2016). Dying care interventions in the intensive care unit. *Journal of Nursing Scholarship, 48*(2), 139–146.

Klass, D. (1993). Spirituality, Protestantism and death. In K. J. Doka (Ed.), *Death and spirituality* (pp. 51–74). Amityville, NY: Baywood.

Ko, E., Kwak, J., & Nelson-Becker, H. (2015). What constitutes a good and bad death? Perspectives of homeless older adults. *Death Studies, 39*(7), 422–432.

Koenig, H. G. (1994). *Aging and God: Spiritual pathways to mental health in midlife and later years.* New York, NY: The Haworth Press.

Kübler-Ross, E. (1969). *On death and dying.* New York, NY: Macmillan.

Lees, J. (2008). A spiritual perspective on loss and bereavement. *International Journal for Human Caring, 12*(2), 90–94.

Lindemann, E. (1944). Symptomatology and management of acute grief. *American Journal of Psychiatry, 101*(1), 141–148.

MacDonald, S. M., Sandmaier, R., & Fainsinger, R. L. (1993). Objective evaluation of spiritual care: A case report. *Journal of Palliative Care, 9*(2), 47–49.

McCarthy, M., Clarke, N., Ting, C., Conroy, R., Anderson, V., & Heath, J. (2010). Prevalence and predictors of parental grief and depression after the death of a child from cancer. *Journal of Palliative Medicine, 13*(11), 1321–1326.

Miller, E. J. (1993). A Roman Catholic view of death. In K. J. Doka (Ed.), *Death and spirituality* (pp. 33–50). Amityville, NY: Baywood.

Millison, M. B., & Dudley, J. R. (1992). Providing spiritual support: A job for all hospice professionals. *The Hospice Journal, 8*(4), 49–66.

Moller, D. W. (1990). *On death without dignity: The human impact of technical dying.* Amityville, NY: Baywood.

Murray, D., & Lyall, D. (1994). Pastoral care. In D. Doyle (Ed.), *Palliative care: The management of far-advanced illness* (pp. 414–427). Philadelphia, PA: The Charles Press.

Murray, S., Kendall, M., Boyd, K., Worth, A., & Benton, T. F. (2004). Exploring the spiritual needs of people dying of lung cancer or heart failure: A prospective qualitative interview study of patients and their carers. *Palliative Medicine, 18*, 39–45.

Narayanasamy, A. (2007). Palliative care and spirituality. *Indian Journal of Palliative Care, 13*(2), 32–41.

The National Hospice Organization. (1996a). Hospice code of ethics. *The Hospice Journal, 11*(2), 75–81.

The National Hospice Organization. (1996b). Hospice services guidelines and definitions. *The Hospice Journal, 11*(2), 65–73.

Neuberger, J. (1994). *Caring for dying people of different faiths* (2nd ed.). St. Louis, MO: C. V. Mosby.

Olson, M. (1997). *Healing the dying.* New York, NY: Delmar.

Osterweis, A., Solomon, F., & Green, M. (1984). *Bereavement reactions: Consequences and care.* Washington, DC: National Academy Press.

Parker, B., & Dunn, K. (2011). The continued lived experience of the unexpected death of a child. *Omega, 63*(3), 221–233.

Parkes, C. (1972). *Bereavement. Studies of grief in adult life.* New York, NY: International University Press.

Parkes, C. M., Benjamin, B., & Fitzgerald, R. (1969). Broken hearts: A statistical study of increased mortality among widowers. *British Medical Journal, 1*(1), 7400–7443.

Parkes, C. M., & Weiss, R. (1983). *Recovery from bereavement.* New York, NY: Basic Books.

Peterson, J., Johnson, M., Halversen, B., Apmann, L., Chang, P. C., Kershek, S., . . . & Pincon, D. (2010). Where do nurses go for help? A qualitative study of coping with death and dying. *International Journal of Palliative Nursing, 16*(9), 432, 434–438.

Pevey, C. F., Jones, T. J., & Yarber, A. (2008). How religion comforts the dying: A qualitative inquiry. *Omega, 58*(1), 41–59.

Praill, D. (1995). Approaches to spiritual care. *Nursing Times, 91*(34), 54–57.

President's Commission for the Study of Ethical Problems in Medicine and Biomedical and Behavioral Research. (1981). *Defining death* (Pub. No. 81-600150). Washington, DC: US Government Printing Office.

Price, J. L., Stevens, H. O., & LaBarre, M. C. (1995). Spiritual caregiving in nursing practice. *Journal of Psychosocial Nursing, 33*(12), 5–9.

Raether, H. C. (1993). Rituals, beliefs and grief. In K. J. Doka (Ed.), *Death and spirituality* (pp. 207–215). Amityville, NY: Baywood.

Rando, T. A. (1988). *Grieving: How to go on living when someone you love dies.* Lexington, MA: Lexington Books.

Raphael, B. C. (1983). *The anatomy of bereavement.* New York, NY: Basic Books.

Reese, D. J., & Brown, D. R. (1997). Psychosocial and spiritual care in hospice: Differences between nursing, social work, and clergy. *The Hospice Journal, 12*(1), 29–41.

Renard, J. (1993). Islamic spirituality. In M. Downey (Ed.), *The new dictionary of Catholic spirituality* (pp. 555–559). Collegeville, MN: The Liturgical Press.

Renz, M., Mao, M. S., Bueche, D., Cerny, T., & Strasser, K. (2013). Dying is a transition. *American Journal of Hospice and Palliative Medicine, 30*(3), 283–290.

Reynolds, A. (2009). How can I respond to dying patients? *Journal of Christian Nursing, 26*(4), 197–198.

Rushing, D. (2012). "Am I going to die, Aunt Deborah?" *Journal of Christian Nursing, 29*(2), 113–116.

Ruskay, S. (1996). Saying hello again: A new approach to bereavement counseling. *The Hospice Journal, 11*(4), 5–14.

Ryan, D. (1993). Death: Eastern perspectives. In K. J. Doka (Ed.), *Death and spirituality* (pp. 75–92). Amityville, NY: Baywood.

Sanders, C. M. (1989). *Grief: The mourning after: Dealing with adult bereavement.* New York, NY: John Wiley & Sons.

Saunders, C. (1981). The founding philosophy. In C. Saunders, D. H. Summers, & N. Teller (Eds.), *Hospice: The living idea* (p. 4). Philadelphia, PA: W. B. Saunders.

Saunders, C. (1983). The last stages of life. In C. A. Corr & D. M. Corr (Eds.), *Hospice care: Principles and practice* (pp. 5–11). New York, NY: Springer.

Schulling, S. (2012). God's dominion over death. *Journal of Christian Nursing, 29*(1), 52–56.

Sheldon, J. E. (2000). Spirituality as a part of nursing. *Journal of Hospice and Palliative Nursing, 2*(3), 101–108.

Shuchter, J. (1986). *Dimensions of grief: Adjusting to the death of a spouse.* San Francisco, CA: Jossey-Bass.

Stepnick, A., & Perry, T. (1992). Preventing spiritual distress in the dying client. *Journal of Psychosocial Nursing, 30*(1), 17–24.

Stoddard, S. (1978). *The hospice movement: A better way of caring for the dying.* Briarcliff Manor, NY: Stein and Day.

Taylor, E. J., & Amenta, M. (1994). Midwifery to the soul while the body dies: Spiritual care among hospice nurses. *American Journal of Hospice and Palliative Care, 11*(6), 28–35.

Tiew, L. H., Kwee, J. H., Creedy, D. K., & Chan, M. F. (2013). Hospice nurses' perspectives of spirituality. *Journal of Clinical Nursing, 22*(19/20), 2923–2933.

Vassallo, B. M. (2001). The spiritual aspects of dying at home. *Holistic Nursing Practice, 15*(2), 17–29.

Vivat, B. (2008). Measures of spiritual issues for palliative care patients: A literature review. *Palliative Medicine, 22,* 859–868.

Worden, J. W. (1982). *Grief counseling and grief therapy: A handbook for the mental health practitioner.* New York, NY: Springer.

World Health Organization. (1990). *Cancer pain relief and palliative care: Technical report series 804.* Geneva, Switzerland: Author.

Wortman, J. H., & Park, C. L. (2008). Religion and spirituality in adjustment following bereavement: An integrative review. *Death Studies, 32,* 703–736.

Young, C., & Koopsen, C. (2005). *Spirituality and health and healing.* Thorofare, NJ: Slack Incorporated.

Young, C., & Koopsen, C. (2011). *Spirituality, health, and healing: An integrative approach.* Sudbury, MA: Jones & Bartlett Learning.

CHAPTER 13

Parish/Faith Community Nursing: Caregiving within the Church Community

The role of parish nurses is basically a reaching out for more whole person ways of ministering to people who are hurting.

Granger Westberg, 1999

The parishioners that I minister to are mostly older and with a lot of health problems physically; some are cognitively impaired as well. But they all love to have the parish nurse come, as a representative of the church, to minister to them. I help them with any health problems or questions. Sometimes I pray with them or read the Bible if they want or sometimes just listen. Older folks love to reminisce about the past. Talking about the good things that happened in the past validates their lives and helps them accept where they are now in the journey of life.

Elizabeth, Parish Nurse

A parish nurse related the following anecdote: At a conference for religious pastors of urban churches, a presentation was given on the topic of parish nursing. Although the parish nurse presenter was described as well prepared and articulate, most of the clergy audience came away admitting that they still "did not know what parish nursing really was." This is a very telling story and reflects the lack of understanding of many contemporary nurses and pastors related to the place of the subfield of parish nursing within the larger profession. This chapter explores the philosophy of parish nursing, including the scope and standards of practice, and the historical background, models, educational preparation, spirituality, parish nursing research, and the present day art and practice of parish nursing. In addition to literature review in the area, empirical examples of parish nursing are presented in data elicited through interviews with contemporary practitioners and recipients of parish nursing.

▶ Parish Nursing/Faith Community Nursing

In the nursing literature on church-related health care, one currently finds both labels: "parish nursing" and "faith community nursing." This is related to the fact that the title changed in some quarters during the past decade.

A Professional Title Change

Before proceeding to discussions of the philosophy, scope and standards of practice, history, and models of parish nursing, it is necessary to address the relatively recent title change for the profession adopted by some—that is, from parish nursing to faith community nursing. Over the past decade, certain practitioners in the field have started informally using the label *faith community nursing*. This title was formally adopted by a number of parish nurses in 2005 with the publication of the American Nurses Association's (ANA) *Faith Community Nursing: Scope and Standards of Practice* (the second edition of this work was published in 2012 by the ANA and the Health Ministries Association [HMA]).

Historically *parish nursing* was the original label adopted for nurses, mostly volunteers, who worked with congregational health issues following the 1970s and 1980s vision of the Reverend Dr. Granger Westberg, the acknowledged founder of the parish nursing concept. This earlier title is reflected in the original publication of the *Scope and Standards of Parish Nursing Practice*. The title formally changed, however, with the publication of the 2005 *Scope and Standards of Practice*: "In the 2005 revision of the ANA *Scope and Standards of Practice*, the term faith community nurse was adopted to be inclusive of the titles of parish nurse, congregational nurse, health ministry nurse, crescent nurse, or health and wellness nurse (ANA and HMA, 2005)" (Gustafson, 2008, p. 1033).

A number of contemporary parish nursing publications use the newer title, highlighting the concept of the faith community rather than the parish. Some examples are: "The Emerging Role of Faith Community Nurses in Prevention and Management of Chronic Diseases" (McGinnis & Zoske, 2008); "State of Research for Faith Community Nursing 2009" (Dyess, Chase, & Newline, 2010); "Services Delivered by Faith-Community Nurses to Individuals with Elevated Blood Pressure" (Monay, Mangione, Sorrell-Thompson, & Baig, 2010); "A Documentation Approach for Faith Community Nursing" (Miller & Carson, 2010); and "Clergy Knowledge and Attitudes Concerning Faith Community Nursing: Toward a Three-Dimensional Scale" (Thompson, 2010).

Some article titles use a combination of the terms *faith community* and *parish*, such as: "Faith Community Nursing/Parish Nursing in a Frontier State" (Peterson, 2011). In a commentary entitled "Nursing in the Church," a master's-prepared nurse with the titles "faith community nurse–health ministry educator" and "parish nurse consultant," admits that currently "parish/faith community nursing is experiencing growing pains" (Hinton, 2012, p. 141).

And, finally, a number of nursing journal articles still employ the earlier classic usage, *parish nursing*, to describe the content, including "Exploring Parish Nurses' Perspective of Parish Nurse Training" (Ziebarth & Miller, 2010); "Parish Nurse-Initiated Interdisciplinary Mobile Health Care Delivery Project" (Mayernik, Resnick, Skomo, & Mandock 2010); and "A Congregation and Parish Nurse Meet an Angel" (Bond, 2011).

Although the more common descriptor found in the contemporary nursing literature seems to be *faith community nursing*, parish nurses Deborah Patterson and Mary Slutz (2011) have argued for retention of the title parish nurse to describe nursing that is based in a Christian congregation. In the article "Faith Community/ Parish Nursing: What's in a Name?" Patterson and Slutz point out that "retaining the language 'parish nurse' promotes a broader understanding of the purpose of this specialty practice, not only as inreach or outreach on behalf of a church or health system, but as a focused and integrated 'parish' ministry" (p. 31). While Patterson and Slutz agree that the title faith community nursing is "appropriate to describe this broad specialty practice across all faiths, the title 'Parish Nurse' should not be abandoned by those working in the context of Christian faith communities" (p. 32). The authors observe that the term *faith community nursing* "does not go far enough to convey the outreach that as Christians [they] are called to ministries of service" (p. 32). Ultimately, Patterson and Slutz concluded that "For a Christian calling, Parish Nurse is an honored title that any registered nurse educated in the specialty and serving a Christian faith community should be honored to hold" (p. 33).

In a recent article entitled "A Renewed Look at Faith Community Nursing," the author reiterates the fact that the terms *parish nursing* and *faith community nursing* continue to be used interchangeably and "have the same meaning" (Schroepfer, 2016, p. 63). The current definition of *faith community nursing*, as identified in 2012 by the American Nurses Association and the Health Ministries Association, is cited by Schroepfer (2016) as: "the specialized practice of professional nursing that focuses on the intentional care of the spirit as part of the process of promoting holistic health and preventing or minimizing illness in the faith community" (p. 63). The greatest strength of faith community nursing is described as "the consistency and trust built between parishioners and the faith community" (p. 65).

Currently the American Nurses Association Credentialing Center (ANCC) offers "Faith Community Nursing" board certification; the offering of certification began in August 2014. Eligibility criteria for the "Faith Community Nursing" certification include: "current active R.N. license; equivalent of 2 years full time practice as a registered nurse; minimum of 1000 practice hours in specialty area of 'Faith Community Nursing' within the last 3 years; a minimum of 30 hours of continuing education in 'Faith Community Nursing' within the last 3 years; and two professional development categories such as academic credits, presentations, publications" and others (Breisch, 2016, p. 13).

Parish or faith community nursing, is presently viewed as a unique resource for the community as "it seeks to support mainstream healthcare providers by encouraging faith groups to employ or appoint part-time registered nurses . . . to help improve public and community health in their local areas" (Wordsworth, Moore, & Woodhouse, 2016, p. 66). The number of parish/faith community nursing programs has increased dramatically since the discipline's formal beginning in 1964; there are now "thousands of FCN nurses serving populations around the world" (Shores, 2014, p. 299). One example in the United States is the parish nurse serving parishioners at St. Bartholomew's Church in Nashville, Tennessee, by providing a variety of health-care programs such as blood pressure screening and nutritional education (Donnelly, 2014). Findings from a study of patients of parish nurses revealed that patient/parishioners, as well as resolving health challenges, reported: "changes in spiritual identity" and "an enhanced understanding of who they were in God/Christ" (Van Dover & Pfeiffer, 2011, p. 1824).

▶ Parish Nursing Defined

The Philosophy of Parish Nursing

Essentially, the philosophy of parish nursing is grounded in the relationship between spirituality or faith beliefs and the conduct of caring for the sick. This might be described best in the following paradigm of "Beatitudes for Parish Nurses," which combines the Scriptural beatitudes identified by Jesus in His Sermon on the Mount (Matthew 5:3–10) with the primary roles identified for contemporary parish nurses: health counselor, health educator (health promoter), health referral agent, health advocate, health visitor, integrator of faith and health, and coordinator of support and volunteer groups.

Beatitudes for Parish Nurses

Blessed are parish nurses who care for the poor, for theirs is

The kingdom of heaven.

Blessed are parish nurses who mourn for parishioners lost, for they will

Be comforted.

Blessed are parish nurses who visit the isolated and the elderly,

For they will inherit the land.

Blessed are parish nurses who advocate for marginalized clients,

For they will be satisfied.

Blessed are parish nurses who minister to those in pain and suffering,

For they will be shown mercy.

Blessed are parish nurses who bring peace to patients who are anxious

And afraid, for they will be called children of God.

Blessed are parish nurses who suffer misunderstanding for the sake of

Their ministry, for they will see God.

Blessed are parish nurses who comfort and care in the Lord's Name, for

Their reward will be great in heaven.

The former director of the International Parish Nurse Resource Center, Ann Solari-Twadell (1999), suggests that the best way to answer the question "What is parish nursing?" is to study the philosophy of the discipline (p. 3). Solari-Twadell notes that in calling the nurse to care for the "whole person," parish nursing includes and, in fact, highlights the individual's "spiritual dimension": "The pastoral dimensions of nursing care are emphasized, with particular attention to the spiritual maturity of the nurse. This begins to distinguish the practice from the traditional community health nurse and to set the parameters for the role" (pp. 3–4). Two key points of Solari-Twadell's identified philosophy are that "parish nursing holds the spiritual dimension to be central to the practice," and "the focus of practice is the faith community and its ministry" (p. 15). The philosophy of parish nursing has been described as the guiding principle to "promote the health of a faith community by working with the pastor and staff to integrate theological, sociological and physiologic perspectives of health and healing into the word, sacrament and service of the congregation" (Lovinus, 1996, p. 7). The parish nurse serves as "a role model for the relationship between one's faith and health" (Solari-Twadell & Westberg, 1991, p. 24).

The parish nurse is considered by most parish nurse educators to be a registered nurse with well-developed clinical and interpersonal skills, a strong personal religious faith, and a desire or felt call to serve the needs of a parish or faith community. A parish nursing philosophy builds on the existing philosophy of caring and commitment already espoused by the nurse as a professional ethic. One parish nurse described her ministry as a vocation. "Nursing in a faith community is a calling, an absolute caring for people and a deep sense of personal faith" (Palmer, 2001, p. 17). Parish nurses are generally noted for their roles as educators and health promoters within a congregation. "They provide information on healthy life styles and ways to prevent illness" (Dunkle, 2000, p. 316); they also, however, tend to patients' "psychosocial and spiritual needs" (p. 316). It is pointed out that parish nurses practice within a specific "cultural community": "in a place of worship where the focus is on meeting spiritual needs; the nurses work with the community leaders as their professional partners" (Trofino et al., 2000, p. 60). As a final point in examining the philosophy of parish nursing, it is important to emphasize that the role or title of parish nurse does not limit one to working with any "particular faith community or religious denomination"; it has, therefore, been suggested by some that the label be changed from parish nursing to "health ministry" or "congregational nursing" ("Parish Nursing," 2000, pp. 8–9).

Scope and Standards of Practice

Between 1996 and 1998, a document identifying the scope and standards of parish nursing practice was developed by the Practice and Education Committee of the HMA. The HMA is a professional organization that represents parish nurses and other health ministers. The scope and standards document was acknowledged by the ANA, Congress of Nursing Practice, in Spring 1998. The introduction to the document states that "Parish nursing promotes health and healing within faith communities" (American Nurses Association, 1998, p. 1). The purpose of the scope and standards document is to "describe the evolving specialty of parish nursing and to provide parish nurses, the nursing profession, and other healthcare providers, employers, insurers, and their clients with the unique scope and competent standards of care and professional performance expected of a parish nurse" (p. 3). The parish nurse scope and standards are based on the ANA's 1991 *Standards of Clinical Nursing Practice* (p. 4). The definition of *parish nurse*, as articulated formally in the scope and standards of practice is, "The most common title given to a registered professional nurse who serves as a member of the ministry staff of a faith community to promote health as wholeness of the faith community, its family and individual members, and the community it serves through the independent practice of nursing as defined by the nurse practice act in the jurisdiction in which he or she practices and the standards of practice set forth in this document" (p. 7).

Some of the parish nurse's roles, as identified in the initial scope and standards of practice, include collecting client health data (health assessment); diagnosing, based on the data; identifying desired health outcomes; health care and promotion planning; implementing interventions; and evaluating client responses (ANA, 1998, pp. 9–14). The nurse also participates in such activities as quality assessment, performance appraisal, education, collegial sharing, ethical decision making, collaboration with the community, research, and resource utilization (pp. 15–22).

As previously mentioned, a second document describing parish nurses' scope and standards of practice was published by the ANA in 2005 under the title *Faith Community Nursing: Scope and Standards of Practice.* Related to the current and ongoing changes in the health-care system, the ANA (2012), in collaboration with the HMA, recently published a second edition of this document. It was reported that "twenty-one practicing RNs who represent the specialty . . . contributed to this edition" (Bennett, 2011, p. 9). The current publication "builds on the 2005 and 1998 editions, as well as *ANA's Nursing: Scope and Standards of Practice,* 2nd Edition" (p. 9).

The second edition of *Faith Community Nursing: Scope and Standards of Practice* "describes the specialty practice of faith community nursing for the nursing profession, faith community nurses, other healthcare providers, spiritual leaders, employers, insurers, health care consumers, families, and members of faith communities" (ANA, 2012, p. 1). In defining faith community nursing, the ANA document points out that the faith community nurse (FCN) "is knowledgeable in two primary areas: professional nursing and spiritual care" (p. 5). The "goals of the FCN are the protection, promotion and optimization of health and abilities; the prevention of illness and injury; and the alleviation of suffering in the context of the values, beliefs and practices of a faith community, such as a church, congregation, parish, synagogue, temple, mosque or faith based community agency" (p. 5).

▶ A Brief History of Parish Nursing

The contemporary concept of parish nursing is usually attributed to Lutheran pastor Granger Westberg, as an outgrowth of his holistic health center project of the mid-1980s. This experimental program of care was supported by the Kellogg Foundation and the University of Illinois College of Medicine (Westberg, 1990). Although Pastor Westberg is appropriately acknowledged as the founder of the current parish nursing movement in the United States, one should also recognize the health-care activities of the early Christian Church, as well as the European models of parish nursing, such as the 19th-century German Christian Deaconesses, the Gemein-deschwestern (Zerson, 1994, p. 20). The earliest deacons and deaconesses of the fledgling Christian community established immediately after the death of Christ considered care of the sick in their homes to be one of the primary ministries of the Church. Following those early centuries and throughout the Middle Ages, men and women felt their calling to minister to the ill and the infirm to be a vocation from God. St. Vincent de Paul, the great minister to the sick in 17th-century France, established "societies of women of the Church who banded themselves together with some simple rules to tend the sick and the poor of the immediate neighborhood. They called themselves the 'servants of the poor'" (Woodgate, 1946, p. 43). These women could surely be considered forebears of contemporary parish nurses.

In the mid-20th century, an article was published in a religious nursing journal entitled "In the Parish" (Cummings, 1960). The nurse author begins the piece by relating the fact that in recent issues of the journal she had read about nurses "in hospitals, in clinics, in schools and in homes" but, she lamented, "Alas, I was not included, for in the parish, is my job" (Cummings, 1960, p. 26). Nurse Cummings describes her role as a parish health counselor in a parish of about 3,500 families and asserts that, at this time, her Church believes that their multidisciplinary health program is "the only one of its kind in the United States" (p. 26). This innovative parish nursing program was focused on such things as care of the chronically ill elders in the parish, education for home care of the ill, referral to community agencies, volunteers service, and home visiting. Nurse Cummings's role as a parish health counselor reads very much like that of the parish nurse of today. Some other parish nursing activities described in the 20th-century nursing literature included a Christian Church–affiliated "volunteer nursing program" to provide care for the ill and infirm in their homes (Martin & Lacoutre, 1953) and an "organized plan for visiting individuals who are ill and lonely" sponsored by a Church Diocesan Council of Nurses ("Council Projects," 1956, p. 42).

In the era of the late 1970s and early 1980s, Pastor Granger Westberg's interest in and support of the concept of holistic health care, including the subfield of parish nursing, began to capture the attention of some members of the larger nursing community. With his support, a parish nursing program was sponsored by Lutheran General Hospital in Park Ridge, Illinois; parish nursing was also initiated at several parishes in the area. As the ministry developed, the International Parish Nurse Resource Center (IPNRC) was created in 1986 under the aegis of Advocate Lutheran General Hospital. Together with a committee of nurse consultants from across the country, the staff of the IPNRC developed a model curriculum for parish nursing education. The IPNRC also began to sponsor annual Westberg Symposiums to provide a forum for parish nurses from across the country to come together to discuss the emerging subfield and its practice. In an October 2001 letter addressed to the "Friends of the International Parish Nurse Resource Center," however, it was announced that the IPNRC would no longer be an agency of Advocate Health Care, the umbrella organization providing support for this parish nursing education effort. It was anticipated that the Westberg Symposiums and some other activities formerly conducted by the IPNRC would continue to be supported in other arenas.

Another previously mentioned parish nursing association, the volunteer membership group called the Health Ministries Association (HMA), was derived from the emerging parish nursing interest of the 1970s and 1980s. The HMA, collaborating author of the *Scope and Standards of Nursing Practice*, is an association for those who serve in health ministry. The group "serves as the professional specialty organization for parish nurses and as such has been accepted by the American Nurses Association for membership in the Nursing Organization Liaison Forum (NOLF)" (FAQ About HMA & Parish Nursing, 2001, p. 1).

As the new millennium dawned, it was estimated that "200 institutions in the United States offered parish nurse education"; no curriculum has been endorsed by the ANA ("The ANA does not endorse curriculum"); "there is no process in place for parish nurses to become certified"; and "parish nursing" has been "designated a specialty practice by ANA," which means that "a parish nurse cannot practice without a license" in his or her state (Story, 2001, p. 3). It was also noted that it will probably take a number of years, and "a minimum of $80,000" before ANA certification exams can be offered (p. 3).

▶ Early Models of Parish Nursing

Four early models of parish nursing have been defined: congregation-based volunteer (CBV), congregation-based paid (CBP), institution-based volunteer (IBV), and institution-based paid (IBP) (Kuhn, 1997, p. 26). The terms *congregational nurse practitioner (CNP)* and *congregational care nurse (CCN)* have also begun to be used to describe the role of the nurse working primarily within a parish or faith community (Souther, 1997). A parish nurse may be employed by a church to work as a member of a ministerial team and provide some nursing services to parishioners; a hospital or other health-care institution may also employ a parish nurse in partnership with a local parish, as a way of bringing health promotion into the community. Wilson (1997) described the parish nurse as "a community health nurse who also becomes God's representative of love, caring and healing on earth" (p. 13). The parish nurse does not compete with the public health nurse, but rather works in concert with other nurses in the community (Schank, Weis, & Matheus, 1996).

Lynda Whitney Miller (1997) developed a contemporary parish nursing model undergirded by the theological perspective of evangelical Christianity. The Miller Model of Parish Nursing contains four major components: "person/parishioner"; "health"; "nurse/parish nurse"; and "community/parish" (p. 18). Miller's goal is to provide Christian nurses with a theoretical base to support the practice of parish nursing (p. 17). A separate parish nursing model called the "Circle of Christian Caring" was created by Dr. Margie Maddox (2001). In her model, Dr. Maddox incorporated a number of activities already in place when she began to serve as parish nurse at a large Presbyterian church. Dr. Maddox noted that as she "worked with the services in which the church was already engaged, the model began to emerge" (p. 11). The Circle of Christian Caring model focuses on the parish nurse roles of health educator, health counselor, referral resource/client advocate, and facilitator of groups and/or processes (pp. 12–13).

Parish Nursing Education

Related to the early emerging models of parish nursing were a variety of educational programs that prepared one for the field of parish nursing. These educational offerings ranged from weekend or weeklong continuing education unit (CEU) programs, which may have awarded from 3 to 6 CEUs, to academic courses in parish nursing, which awarded 3 to 6 credits for the overall program. There were also several post-baccalaureate and graduate programs that focus on the topic of nursing in a faith community. These programs were sponsored primarily by health-care institutions, colleges and universities, seminaries, or other church-related associations. In some instances, community interfaith groups of churches collaboratively put together parish nurse education programs to prepare nurses to serve in their various faith communities. The multiplicity of parish nurse preparation programs were, as noted earlier, conducted in a variety of ways; some of these included "one day to weeklong orientations, continuing education workshops, seminars, distance learning, and ongoing coursework over weeks and months, as well as credit-bearing coursework in BSN, MSN and M.Div. programs offered over the course of a semester or, for some, over several years" (McDermott, Solari-Twadell, & Matheus, 1999, p. 271).

Three examples of early parish nurse programs are:

- A weeklong continuing education program, sponsored by a Christian nursing group, following which the participants were awarded 3 CEUs and were "commissioned" as parish nurses. Requirements for the course included having a state nursing license, some clinical nursing experience, and the desire to work with a faith community.
- A parish nurse preparation program, sponsored by a college and awarding the participants 3 CEUs, which held classes on six alternating Saturdays. This program required that the RNs have at least three years of experience and be partnered with a faith community. The course ended with a "dedication ceremony."
- A university-affiliated program that covered nine days and awarded the participants 5.4 CEUs. As well as including the usual topics described in the following paragraphs, this longer program included participation in several interfaith services and provided student on-site observations and clinical experiences with parish nurses in the community.

Some basic components of most early parish nursing programs included such topics as a theology of health and healing; the nurse's role in spiritual care; history, philosophy, and models of parish nursing; ethical issues in parish nursing; assessment of the individual, the family, and the congregation; documentation and accountability; the functions of the parish nurse, such as health counseling, health education, health referral, coordination of volunteers and support groups, patient advocacy, and integration of faith and health; working with a congregation; health promotion; dealing with grief and loss; and legal considerations in the conduct of parish nursing. Some programs also included classes focusing on such activities as prayer and worship leadership, research, grant writing, service among underprivileged people, and working with a ministerial team.

▶ The Spirituality of Parish Nursing

Although nurses from a variety of religious denominations are currently engaged in parish nursing, it is the nurse's personal spirituality and spiritual vocation to serve the ill that inspire and support the ministry. For Christian nurses, Jesus' blessing, related by the evangelist Matthew "I was ill and you cared for me" (25:36) provides both the catalyst and the reward for their caring for the sick within a faith community. Most parish nurses, many of whom serve on a volunteer basis, carry out their nursing within their own faith communities. This is usually desirable for both nurse and congregation, because the parish nurse is thus familiar with the spiritual and religious beliefs of the congregation and of the pastor. In the future, however, if parish nursing becomes "professionalized" to a greater degree, and if acceptable to a faith community, parish nurses may be hired to work with a church not of their own denomination. This kind of partnering does exist to some degree, in contemporary hospital-based parish nursing programs in which staff parish nurses provide consultation and support to developing church programs from a variety of religious traditions.

Perhaps one of the most critical elements in beginning a parish nursing program with a faith community is to listen to the needs and desires of the pastor and the parishioners. Lloyd and Ludwig-Beymer (1999) in discussing a concept they call VOC or "voice of the customer," note that "parishioners, whom we may think of as clients, patients, or in other terms, must be listened to. Clients are the ones who define quality and set the expectations of performance" (pp. 108–109). A director of a large community-based health ministry program observed that when approached about the initiation of a parish ministry program in their churches, most pastors raise three immediate questions: "How much of my time will this involve?"; "How much money is it going to cost me?"; and "Can I be sued?" The goal is to be able to provide negative answers to all three questions to allay the pastors' anxieties about the burden of establishing a parish nursing program for their congregation.

In this era of continued change within the U.S. health-care system, including such factors as short hospital stays, same-day surgeries, and early discharges, parish nursing, or nursing provided to those in their homes by members of a local faith community, may be critical to a patient's recovery, and perhaps even to his or her survival. No longer are patients, especially older patients or those who live alone, allowed the luxury of remaining in the hospital until they are able to fully function on their own. Health insurance policies rarely cover such extended stays, even if a patient's recovery may be at risk. It is expected that many of the former hospital nursing care services will now be provided by relatives or friends in a home care setting. This makes the role of the contemporary parish nurse vitally important to recovering patients who have no extended family networks and who may depend on their churches for caring support in times of crisis or significant need. It is suggested that individuals of all ages can benefit from the "personal caring and attention offered by a parish nursing model" (Stewart, 2000, p. 116).

The role of the parish nurse, as bridge between the patient and the faith community, incorporates the important activity of discussing spirituality with ill parishioners, a behavior that some clinical nurses admit to finding difficult (Wiebe, 2008). This is a dimension of spiritual care essential to the role of the contemporary parish nurse (Wordsworth, 2007).

One of the first things a parish nurse may find helpful in beginning to work with a faith community, especially a church to which the concept of parish nursing is new, is to do a "needs assessment" of the parish. There are a variety of needs assessment schemas being developed; however, the assessment must take into account certain factors that vary in parishes, such as the mean age of the parishioners, the range of socioeconomic levels in the church, the parish size, and the availability of volunteers to assist with the development of a parish health ministry. Parish nurses report that a critical factor in beginning a new effort with a faith community is the support of the pastor; as noted previously, he or she may have concerns about the time, financial, and/or legal burdens that the establishment of any new program may bring to the church. If, however, the potential parish nurse or health ministry team can predict that the program will be a benefit, rather than a burden, to the church, most pastors will be enthusiastic in their support of the effort.

An example of a professional parish needs assessment is that conducted by the University of Massachusetts, Amherst School of Nursing, at the request of a large urban parish. The school was also asked to assess a newly hired parish nurse. The assessment's aims were to "determine the health status of parishioners; identify their perceived health needs and perceived barriers in meeting those needs; and to assist the church and parish nurse in developing a health program for their faith community" (Swinney, Anson-Wonkka, Maki, & Corneau, 2001, p. 40). The assessment team concluded that the health needs of this faith community were similar to those identified in the goals of "Healthy People 2000," that is, "increased life span in a healthy state, reduced health disparities . . . and access to preventive care" (p. 43). In another study of the health needs and preferences of an individual faith community, in which 67 church members, 6 parish nurses, and the pastor participated, 80 percent of the services desired were educational, including education about such factors as health screening, disease, staying well, spiritual health, and emotional health (Mayhugh & Martens, 2001, p. 15). Some other parish nursing preferences of the faith community studied by Mayhugh and Martens were consultation about health problems, visiting (hospital, home, and nursing home), and coordination and training of volunteers (p. 15).

Although existing church-based parish nursing programs are still new to many faith communities, the number and scope of these ministries is expanding rapidly. In some churches, programs may be limited to such activities as monthly blood-pressure screenings, with occasional health educational programs for the congregation and infrequent home or hospital visiting by members of an "on-call" volunteer team; there may or may not be a parish nurse leading the effort. In other parishes, well-developed parish health ministry programs exist, under the leadership of a paid part-time or full-time parish or congregational nurse.

Depending on the interest and sophistication, in terms of health-care experience, on the part of a pastor and congregation, a church may require that their parish nurse have specific training in parish nursing; be a nurse practitioner; have a number of years of experience in nursing; or simply be a registered nurse who has a commitment and desire to work with a faith community. For example, one church in a moderately sized urban area advertised for a part-time parish nurse who would be a licensed RN in the state with at least three years of experience in nursing; the church also wanted the candidate to have completed a parish nursing preparation course, although the parameters of that course were not specified. It was noted that the nurse's role would include health promotion, disease prevention, education, counseling, advocacy, health screening, and referral. The parish nurse's hours could be "flexible."

Some congregations employing either paid or volunteer parish nurses try to schedule "office hours" at the parish, for example, Wednesdays and Fridays, 9 to noon, so that parishioners can come for private consultation or education. In such a situation, the parish nurse will usually have "on call" hours also. Some of the activities associated with existing parish nursing or health ministry programs, in addition to parish nurse office hours and monthly blood-pressure screening, include exercise classes (especially for seniors), cardiopulmonary resuscitation (CPR) classes, foot care classes, nutritional education classes, diabetes education classes, prenatal classes, bike safety classes for children, self–breast exam classes, substance abuse classes for parents and teens, healthy aging classes, family fitness classes, and classes preparing church volunteers for such ministries as hospital and nursing home visiting, homebound visiting, and respite family care.

The parish nurse may also do some home and hospital visiting as time permits; the nurse's most important role, however, is to serve as the health ministry team leader and coordinator of nonmedical health ministry volunteers. The parish nurse is an advocate for the ill parishioners of a faith community and a source of referral to needed and appropriate community health services.

▶ Parish Nursing Research

In an exploratory study of the parish nursing role, 48 practicing parish nurses identified ways in which they incorporated spiritual care into their activities, including prayer, if acceptable to the client; a caring and compassionate attitude; discussing illness-related spiritual concerns; and conducting or participating in rituals such as healing services and the distribution of Communion (Kuhn, 1997, p. 27). A nursing study of 40 parish nurses, who identified 1,800 client interactions, revealed that although approximately one-half of the nurses' activities dealt with physical problems, the other half related to spiritual–psychosocial issues (Rydholm, 1997). This latter finding is supported by the comments of parish nurse Linda Miles (1997), who asserted that in all of her nursing she included the spiritual dimension of care. "Spiritual nurturing contributes to improved life satisfaction and quality of life, improved health, reduced functional disability, and lower levels of depression" (p. 24).

A number of case study articles describing innovative experiences in parish nursing have been presented in the literature. For example, Dr. Margie Maddox (2003), in "Clinical Experience in Parish Nursing," described a newly created student clinical course in parish nursing; and Gretchen Quenstedt-Moe (2003), in "Parish Nursing and Home Care: A Blended Role?" explored parish nurses adopting a primary role of home visiting that she viewed as helping "fill the gaps left by the fragmented health care system" and that can "help parishioners to find meaningful connections that involve their needs, the parish nurse and God" (p. 30).

In looking at parish nursing as meeting the spiritual needs of elders at or near the end of their lives, a qualitative study of 15 end-of-life older adults revealed the importance of the parish nurse's spiritual care interventions: "1) Sharing of prayer and scripture; 2) Spiritual presence (listening with the heart); and 3) Pastoral counseling (including facilitating participation in religious rituals)" (O'Brien, 2006, p. 30).

The Gift of Faith in Chronic Illness

The author conducted an exploratory pilot study of the impact of parish nursing on persons who were unable to practice their faith because of illness and disability. The aim of the study was to test the effectiveness of a model of parish nursing/health ministry on spiritual well-being, hope, and life satisfaction among persons marginalized from their churches, and to explore the relationship between spiritual well-being and quality of life (measured in terms of hope and life satisfaction) for chronically ill persons. For a study participant distanced from his or her church, or desirous of additional spiritual support, pastoral care intervention was carried out in the hope of increasing spiritual well-being and positive quality of life. Following an initial individual spiritual needs assessment, pastoral care interventions were tailored by the parish nurse for each study participant.

The sample group consisted of six chronically ill individuals: four men and two women whose ages ranged from 45 to 92, with a mean of 74 years. Three patients were married, two were widowed, and one was single. Five individuals were college graduates and one completed high school; one person lived alone, one resided in a nursing home, and four lived with spouses or adult children. Three of the study patients were Protestant (Protestant, Church of God, and United Church of Christ), two were Roman Catholic, and one patient was Jewish. In terms of church attendance, the group reported attending services from once a month (or even daily when possible) to two to three times a year. Church attendance was quite variable depending on illness symptoms and remission and exacerbation of disease conditions. Patients' diagnoses included glaucoma and lupus, cancer, renal failure (dialysis), myasthenia gravis, type II diabetes and hypertension, substance abuse, and stroke. The study group reported degrees of disability as being from minimal to complete; this again varied with exacerbation of illness symptoms.

The initial needs assessment was carried out using three quantitative tools and one qualitative tool: the Spiritual Well-Being Scale (O'Brien, 1999); the Miller Hope Scale (Miller & Powers, 1988; abbreviated with permission of the author); the Life Satisfaction Index-Z (Wood, Wylie, & Sheafor, 1969); and the Spiritual Well-Being Interview Guide (O'Brien, 1999). Following the collection of baseline data, three or more pastoral visits were planned by the parish nurse, with the nursing interventions geared to the health considerations of the study participant. As well as listening to, counseling, and praying with patients, small devotional items such as prayer books, Bibles, religious pictures, or other items requested by a patient were provided to assist in facilitating the practice of his or her faith. At a final pastoral care visit, study participants were again evaluated in terms of spiritual well-being and quality of life.

The sample population was identified through referrals from a local pastor and from a neighborhood parish, neither of whom had staff engaged in parish nursing, and through several informal referrals. All six individuals approached to participate in the study agreed with enthusiasm; appropriate informed consent procedures were carried out prior to initiation of the research.

The initial exploration of the impact of parish nursing on a group of chronically ill persons revealed that all benefited from the pastoral care interventions of the parish nurse. The quantitative measurement tools identified a number of spiritual needs and concerns amenable to pastoral counseling, such as "uncertainty that God might not take care of one's needs"; "getting angry" at God for "letting bad things happen" to oneself or to persons one cares about; frustration about not being able to attend church because of disability; fear of having done some things "for which God might not forgive"; and "uncertainty" about being at peace with God and with God's care. There were, however, a number of positive changes documented in response to these items following the parish nurse's intervention. One example is the case of a 45-year-old man, suffering from several chronic illnesses, who asserted that the parish nurse's visits had helped him a great deal. In his initial assessment, the patient agreed that there were "some things for which [he feared] God may not forgive [him]"; following the parish nursing intervention the study participant disagreed with the item, that is, he no longer was living with the fear that God would not forgive him for perceived transgressions.

The patient's spiritual well-being measures also changed positively on a number of other items following nursing intervention. For example, at baseline interview (Time 1 [T1]), he responded that he was "uncertain" about whether he was at peace with God but at follow up (Time 2 [T2]), he agreed that he was at peace. At T1 he admitted "uncertainty" about three other items: receiving strength and comfort from spiritual beliefs, believing God is interested in activities of his life, and spiritual beliefs supporting a positive image of himself and others as members of God's family, but at T2 the patient responded affirmatively to all three items. At T1, the study participant disagreed that he found "any satisfaction in religiously motivated activities" but at T2 he strongly agreed. At T1, he agreed to having "pain associated with spiritual beliefs," but at T2 he strongly disagreed. Finally, at T1 the study participant admitted to sometimes feeling "far away" from God, but at T2 he disagreed with having any such perception.

It is important to note that this patient also reflected a number of positive changes in terms of hope and life satisfaction following the parish nurse's intervention, including being positive about most aspects of life, being able to set goals, being positive about the future, being valued for who he was, looking forward to doing things he enjoyed, trying to do things important to him, things seeming better, being as happy as when younger, things being as interesting and being as satisfied with life as before his illness, and feeling that he had gotten most of the important things and what he had expected out of life.

In his responses to the qualitative study questions, this study participant also reported a very positive response to the interactions he had had with the parish nurse. The patient had asked for a devotional item that was unfamiliar to the parish nurse and to the study's principal investigator. It was called (he thought) a "prayer box" to help organize his prayers. The patient, who self-identified as Protestant, did not belong to any particular church but did have a strong belief in the existence of God. Through the use of a religious articles catalog, the research team located a small wooden box labeled a "God box"; the box came with a guide for use; it was suggested that the user write out thoughts, concerns, or prayers and place them in the box as one might make entries into a journal. The study participant reported at a follow-up interview that he was delighted with his prayer box. "I use that, I have something in it right now, in the box. The 'God box' I found extremely comforting. I put some real issues that I'm facing and the fact that I was trying to take my will back and get in [God's] way. I wrote it all down on a piece of paper, all my concerns and issues and fears, and then at the end I said 'God I'm putting this in Your hands.' Almost a ceremonial kind of thing. I put it in the box and I prayed over it and then put the box away and walked away."

The patient concluded, "It helped me to be able to put [my concerns and fears] someplace else; to, like, take it out of my head and put it there [in the 'God box']."

Comments of other study participants following the parish nurse's interactions reflected similar positive outcomes, such as "I am at peace with God"; "I don't know how people survive without a trust and faith in God"; "That [practice of faith] is what keeps me going"; "Without your religion, you would be nowhere"; and "God will not let us have more than we can bear without His help; what a peace that gives you."

A participant in a separate study exploring the functions of parish nursing, Angela, a parish nurse for the past five years, described her understanding of the parish nursing role:

> I think being a parish nurse is being a "be-er," rather than a "do-er." We are there to listen, to be a facilitator, to assess and refer. We're not getting into the doctor's or the community health nurse's turf. Here's an example: You see somebody who's had a headache for weeks and they can't sleep and they have been to the doctor. I look at the spiritual dimension. Maybe there's some spiritual problem that is causing the headaches and the not sleeping; something else may be going on. Maybe they need to talk with the pastor. The parish nurse goes into a house and sees that maybe the dishes are not done, or the steps are starting to crack. Maybe there is someone in the church who can help with that. Or you can see that your client is getting confused

and leaving the stove on; maybe you need to do a referral to the VNA. A lot of us work with volunteers also; you can teach them to take blood pressures and vital signs. I do that, as a representative of my church; and arranging for transportation for people who maybe need to go to a doctor or dentist.

Finally, Angela explained how spirituality was incorporated into her parish nursing interventions:

Spirituality is all encompassing. Sometimes, these people, it's all they need. They need somebody to listen and to say "let's talk about this." Then you can assess their needs and minister to them if they need that; counseling or referral or whatever comes up. Sometimes it is just that something is wrecking their spiritual equilibrium; something is attacking their spiritual base. It might be guilt or anxiety about something they feel they did wrong. Sometimes it's easier for a person to talk to a nurse before they go to the pastor . . . I think parish nursing is caring; it is a caring ministry. It's spiritual care, and it's health promotion and it's illness prevention. If we could get people to a healthier life style, a more spiritual life style, then they wouldn't get into trouble and need secondary and tertiary care.

This chapter has explored briefly the basic dimensions of parish nursing, including the discipline's professional title change adopted by some practitioners; philosophy, scope, and standards of practice; the history of parish nursing; early models of parish nursing and parish nursing education; working with a faith community; and parish nursing research. Parish nursing is presently a developing subfield within the larger nursing community, but interest in the area is growing rapidly. New parish nursing education programs continue to be developed by colleges and universities and by church-related organizations. It is hoped that eventually there will be ANA certification for parish nurses. Until this comes about, however, professional nurses who feel called by God to serve within a faith community continue to support and enhance the parish nursing role through their vision and their dedication. The concept of parish nursing is very new and it is also very old; contemporary parish nurses have embraced their ministry with the caring and commitment of the first-century deacons and deaconesses and with the wisdom and understanding of present-day nursing knowledge. Parish nursing, however it develops in the coming decades, is definitely here to stay.

▶ References

American Nurses Association (1998). *Scope and standards of parish nursing practice.* Washington, DC: American Nurses Publishing.

American Nurses Association. (2012). *Faith community nursing: Scope and standards of practice* (2nd ed.). Silver Spring, MD: Author.

Bennett, F. (2011). ANA, HMA to co-publish Faith Community Nursing: Scope and Standards of Practice. *The American Nurse, 43*(6), 9.

Bond, A. (2011). A congregation and parish nurse meet an angel. *Parish Nurse Perspectives, 10*(4), 6–7.

Breisch, A. J. (2016). ANCC offers certification in faith community nursing. *Tar Heel Nurse, 78*(1), 13.

Council projects: Plan for friendly visiting. (1956). *The Catholic Nurse, 5*(1), 42–44.

Cummings, A. L. (1960). In the parish. *The Catholic Nurse, 8*(3), 26–29.

Donnelly, M. E. (2014). Faith community nursing: Health care in the church. *The Tennessee Nurse, 77*(1), 9.

Dunkle, R. E. (2000). Parish nurses help patients, body and soul. In R. Hunt (Ed.), *Readings in community based nursing* (pp. 316–320). Philadelphia, PA: Lippincott.

Dyess, S., Chase, S., & Newlin, K. (2010). State of research for faith community nursing 2009. *Journal of Religion and Health, 49,* 188–199.

FAQ about HMA & parish nursing. (2001). Connections, *The Health Ministries Association Information & Contacts, 1*(2), 1.

Gustafson, C. (2008). The nurse in parish nursing. In M. Stanhope & J. Lancaster (Eds.), *Public Health Nursing* (pp. 1033–1054). St. Louis: Mosby.

Hinton, S. (2012). Nursing in the Church. *Journal of Christian Nursing, 29*(3), 141.

Kuhn, J. (1997). A profile of parish nurses. *Journal of Christian Nursing, 14*(1), 26–28.

Lloyd, R., & Ludwig-Beymer, P. (1999). Listening to faith communities. In P. Solari-Twadell & M. McDermott (Eds.), *Parish nursing: Promoting whole person health within faith communities* (pp. 107–121). Thousand Oaks, CA: Sage Publications.

Lovinus, B. (1996). A healer in the midst of the congregation. *Journal of Christian Healing, 18*(4), 3–18.

Maddox, M. (2001). Circle of Christian caring: A model for parish nursing practice. *Journal of Christian Nursing, 18*(3), 11–13.

Maddox, M. (2003). Clinical experience in parish nursing. *Journal of Christian Nursing, 20*(2), 18–20.

Martin, G., & Lacoutre, C. (1953). Volunteer nursing. *The Catholic Nurse, 2*(2), 13–14.

Mayernik, D., Resnick, L., Skomo, M., & Mandock, K. (2010). Parish nurse-initiated interdisciplinary mobile health care delivery project. *Journal of Obstetric, Gynecologic and Neonatal Nursing, 39*(2), 227–234.

Mayhugh, L. J., & Martens, K. H. (2001). What's a parish nurse to do: Congregational expectations. *Journal of Christian Nursing, 18*(3), 14–16.

McDermott, M., Solari-Twadell, P., & Matheus, R. (1999). Educational preparation. In P. Solari-Twadell & M. McDermott (Eds.), *Parish nursing: Promoting whole person health within faith communities* (pp. 269–276). Thousand Oaks, CA: Sage Publications.

McGinnis, S., & Zoske, F. (2008). The emerging role of faith community nurses in prevention and management of chronic diseases. *Policy Politics Nursing Practice, 9,* 173–180.

Miles, L. (1997). Getting started: Parish nursing in a rural community. *Journal of Christian Nursing, 14*(1), 22–24.

Miller, J., & Powers, M. (1988). Development of an instrument to measure hope. *Nursing Research, 37*(1), 6–10.

Miller, L. W. (1997). Nursing through the lens of faith: A conceptual model. *Journal of Christian Nursing, 14*(1), 17–20.

Miller, S., & Carson, S. (2010). A documentation approach for faith community nursing. *Creative Nursing, 16*(3), 122–131.

Monay, V., Mangione, C., Sorrell-Thompson, A., & Baig, A. (2010). Services delivered by faith-community nurses to individuals with elevated blood pressure. *Public Health Nursing, 26*(6), 537–543.

O'Brien, M. E. (1999). *Spirituality in nursing: Standing on holy ground.* Sudbury, MA: Jones & Bartlett Learning.

O'Brien, M. E. (2001). *The nurse's calling: A Christian spirituality of caring for the sick.* Mahwah, NJ: Paulist Press.

O'Brien, M. E. (2006). Parish nursing: Meeting spiritual needs of elders near the end of life. *Journal of Christian Nursing, 23*(1), 28–33.

Palmer, J. (2001). Parish nursing: Connecting faith and health. *Reflections on Nursing Leadership, 27*(1), 17–19; 45–46.

Parish nursing: Building on the spiritual dimensions of nursing. (2001). *Pennsylvania Nurse, 55*(6), 8–9.

Patterson, D., & Slutz, M. (2011). Faith community/parish nursing: What's in a name? *Journal of Christian Nursing, 28*(1), 31–33.

Peterson, C. (2011). Faith community nursing/parish nursing in a frontier state. *Parish Nursing Perspective, 10*(2), 17.

Quenstedt-Moe, G. (2003). Parish nursing & home care: A blended role? *Journal of Christian Nursing, 20*(3), 26–30.

Rydholm, L. (1997). Patient focused care in parish nursing. *Holistic Nursing Practice, 11*(3), 47–60.

Schank, M. J., Weis, D., & Matheus, R. (1996). Parish nursing: Ministry of healing. *Geriatric Nursing, 17*(1), 11–13.

Schroepfer, E. (2016). A renewed look at faith community nursing. *MEDSURG Nursing, 25*(1), 62–66.

Shores, C. I. (2014). Spiritual interventions and the impact of a faith community nursing program. *Issues in Mental Health Nursing, 35*(4), 299–305.

Solari-Twadell, P. (1999). The emerging practice of parish nursing. In P. Solari-Twadell & M. McDermott (Eds.), *Parish nursing: Promoting whole person health within faith communities* (pp. 3–24). Thousand Oaks, CA: Sage Publications.

Solari-Twadell, P., & Westberg, G. (1991). Body, mind and soul: The parish nurse offers physical, emotional and spiritual care. *Health Progress, 72*(7), 24–28.

Souther, B. (1997). Congregational nurse practitioner: An idea whose time has come. *Journal of Christian Nursing, 14*(1), 32–34.

Stewart, L. E. (2000). Parish nursing: Renewing a long tradition of caring. *Gastroenterology Nursing, 23*(3), 116–120.

Story, C. (2001, April). Carol's corner. *Puget Sound Parish Nurse Ministries, 3,* 1.

Swinney, J., Anson-Wonkka, C., Maki, E., & Corneau, J. (2001). Community assessment: A church community and the parish nurse. *Public Health Nursing, 18*(1), 40–44.

Thompson, P. (2010). Clergy knowledge and attitudes concerning faith community nursing: Toward a three-dimensional scale. *Public Health Nursing, 27*(1), 71–78.

Trofino, J., Hughes, C., O'Brien, B., Mack, J., Marrinan, M., & Hay, K. (2000). Primary care parish nursing: Academic, service and parish partnership. *Nursing Administration Quarterly, 25*(1), 59–74.

Van Dover, L., & Pfeiffer, J. (2011). Patients of parish nurses experience renewed spiritual identity: A grounded theory study. *Journal of Advanced Nursing, 68*(8), 1824–1834.

Westberg, G. (1990). *The parish nurse: Providing a minister of health for your congregation.* Minneapolis, MN: Augsburg.

Westberg, G. (1999). A personal historical perspective on whole person health and the congregation. In P. Solari-Twadell & M. McDermott (Eds.), *Parish nursing: Promoting whole person health within faith communities* (pp. 35–41). Thousand Oaks, CA: Sage Publications.

Wiebe, G. (2008). Why is it so hard to talk about spirituality? *Newsletter of the Parish Nurse Interest Group of the Registered Nurses Association of Ontario, Spring,* 8.

Wilson, R. P. (1997). What does a parish nurse do? *Journal of Christian Nursing, 14*(1), 13–16.

Wood, V., Wylie, M., & Sheafor, B. (1969). An analysis of a short self-report measure of life satisfaction. *Journal of Gerontology, 24*(2), 465–469.

Woodgate, M. V. (1946). *St. Louise de Marillac.* London, England: B. Herdor Book Company.

Wordsworth, H., Moore, R., & Woodhouse, D. (2016). Parish nursing: A unique resource for the community and district nurses. *British Journal of Community Nursing, 21*(2), 66–74.

Wordsworth, H. (2007). Reclaim the spirit. *Nursing Standard, 22*(10), 22.

Zerson, D. (1994). Parish nursing: 20th century fad? *Journal of Christian Nursing, 11*(2), 19–22.

Ziebarth, D., & Miller, C. (2010). Exploring parish nurses' perspectives of parish nurse training. *Nursing 2010, 41*(6), 273–280.

CHAPTER 14

Spiritual Needs in Mass Casualty Disasters

I have not a moment. The whole army is coming into the hospitals. The task will be gigantic. Alas, how will it all end? We are in the hands of God. Pray for us. We have at the moment five thousand sick and wounded. My only comfort is, God sees it, God knows it, God loves us.

Florence Nightingale, December 1854

In trauma, you could be taking care of the person who shot the person in the next bed; or the alcoholic who crashed his car. You do have to focus on, you are taking care of a patient, a person who needs you. You can't narrow it down to just taking care of a body, but you take care of that whole person, including spiritual needs. That person needs you now. It is not your place to judge.

Rosemarie, Head Nurse of a Trauma Unit

This chapter is dedicated to the New York City firefighters and police officers who gave their lives on September 11, 2001; they made the ultimate sacrifice in the hope of helping thousands of their brothers and sisters trapped in a towering inferno. As nurses, they too are anonymous ministers. The firefighters and police officers indeed "stood on holy ground" before God, deeply present in the "burning bush" of the mortally wounded World Trade Center. While the world witnessed, in horror, the absolute evil of the September 11th attack, it also witnessed, in awe, the absolute goodness embodied in the courage and heroism of these ministers of commitment and compassion. They have truly taught us the meaning of spiritual caring in mass casualty disasters. Their fallen comrades now rest in the loving arms of our Father in heaven. They answered His call to serve with the precious gift of their lives; they are, among all persons, most blessed!

The chapter was originally written several months after the September 11, 2001, terrorist attack on America; the attack that resulted in three simultaneous mass casualty disasters situated at the World Trade Center in New York City; the Pentagon, located in a Virginia suburb near Washington, DC; and a rural area southeast of Pittsburgh, Pennsylvania. The chapter content was updated several years ago to include information on the spiritual needs of post-9/11 survivors and witnesses. In this sixth edition of *Spirituality in Nursing*, a further discussion has been added focusing on three recent incidents of international terrorism: the Boston Marathon Bombings, the Paris Terrorist Attacks, and the Brussels Multisite Explosions.

This chapter begins with a brief overview of disaster nursing, including the types and phases of disasters, and selected key disaster service agencies: the Federal Emergency Management Agency (FEMA), the American Red Cross, and the Salvation Army. Following are discussions of the psychosocial impact of mass casualty trauma, spiritual needs in the aftermath of a disaster, and the nurse's role in the spiritual care of disaster victims. The heart of the chapter, however, which includes many examples of spiritual need and spiritual care in a mass casualty disaster, is based on the case example of the terrorist attack on America on 9/11, particularly at the sites of the World Trade Center and the Pentagon. Data were obtained through news reports, writings published after the attack, and the author's personal interviews and experiences with chaplains, firefighters, police officers, and other witnesses of the attack.

▶ Disaster Nursing

Prior to the 9/11 attack in the United States, there was minimal nursing literature addressing the topic of disaster nursing. Most books on the topic of disaster nursing were published in the era of the mid-20th century, the 1950s and 1960s. They included concerns about disasters such as hurricanes, tornados, fires, floods, accidents, and nuclear radiation incidents, such as those caused by an atomic bomb explosion. Although there was some discussion of biologic and chemical warfare, suicidal terrorist attacks, as occurred in the United States on September 11, 2001, were not considered. Some of the early works devoted specifically to disaster nursing include *Disaster Nursing* (Nabbe, 1960); *Disaster Nursing Preparation* (Neal, 1963); *Disaster Handbook for Physicians and Nurses* (American Red Cross, 1966); *Disaster Handbook* (Garb & Eng, 1969); and *Emergency and Disaster Nursing* (Mahoney, 1969). In 1985, Loretta M. Garcia, edited a book entitled *Disaster Nursing: Planning, Assessment and Intervention*. Although these earlier disaster nursing books do include discussions of the psychosocial impact of a disaster, spiritual or religious needs in mass casualty trauma are not included as key topics of discussion. In that era, the assessment of a patient or family member's spiritual or religious need was still considered by many nurses to fall within the role of the pastoral caregiver only; that thinking has changed, and a number of nurses have developed spiritual assessment scales to be used as nursing tools.

Disaster nursing poses multiple challenges in terms of assessment and intervention. As Susan Gardner (1985) notes, "The nurse does not have the luxury of a leisurely assessment; every second counts" (p. 18). Most disaster scenes also include elements of danger and confusion; thus, the "physical and emotional stress factors may be extreme" (Brown, 1985, p. 45). Although disaster nursing is a unique area of nursing, only a modest number of journal articles on the topic are found in the literature; this is probably related to the fact that the majority of nurses have never had disaster nursing experience and never expect to become engaged in such nursing. Publications extant in the nursing literature primarily involve reports of care given in individual disaster situations; these experiences are reflected in such titles as "When the Tornado Hit Worcester: Heroic Nurses Play a Vital Role" (*The Catholic Nurse*, 1953); "Nurses Respond to Hurricane Hugo: Victims' Disaster Stress" (Weinrich,

Hardin, & Johnson, 1990); "In the Wake of Hurricane Andrew: The Development of a Community-Based Primary Care Center" (Horner, Pfeifer, & Clunn, 1994); "Community Health Nursing: Shelter from the Storm" (Christopher & McConnell, 1994); "Disaster Nursing in the Oklahoma City Bombing" (Atkinson, Keylon, Odor, Walker, & Hunt, 1995); "Disaster Relief Efforts After Hurricane Marilyn: A Pediatric Team's Experience in St. Thomas" (Damian, Atkinson, Bouchard, Harrington, & Powers, 1997); "Multiple Accident Victims, All Elderly: Would Our Disaster Plan Be Up to the Challenge?" (Walhout, Tubergen, & Cook, 1998); and "The City of New Orleans Amtrak Train Disaster: One Emergency Department's Experience" (Mickelson, Bruno, & Schario, 1999).

A disaster has been described as "any man-made or natural event that causes destruction and devastation and that cannot be alleviated without assistance" (Hassmiller, 2000, p. 401), and as testing "the adaptive responses of communities or individuals beyond their capabilities and lead[ing] to at least a temporary disruption of function" (Clark, 1999, p. 704). Disasters are generally categorized as falling within two broad categories: natural disasters, such as tornadoes, hurricanes, floods, avalanches, earthquakes, volcanic eruptions, and communicable diseases; and human-generated disasters, including warfare, riots, mass demonstrations, and accidents (Lundy & Butts, 2001, p. 551). A disaster is classified as a "multiple patient incident" if less than 10 casualties have occurred; as a "multiple casualty incident" if there are less than 100 casualties but stress is placed on local health-care facilities; and as a "mass casualty incident or disaster" if the occurrence involves more than 100 casualties and "significantly overtaxes existing health care facilities" (Demi & Miles, 1984, p. 64).

Disaster phases have been identified in various ways, including such stages as predisaster preparation, warning, impact, emergency, and recovery (Taggart, 1985, p. 7); and prevention, preparedness, response, and recovery (Tait & Spradley, 2001, p. 394). Regardless of terminology, the disaster phases are generally considered to include some period of disaster planning or preparation, a time of immediate impact and emergency response, and a recovery period. It is important to remember that nurses involved in responding to a disaster impact may themselves be victims of the disaster, especially if the incident involves an entire community, as in the case of a tornado or flood. Often the nurse will have to put personal or family concerns on a "back burner," to carry out his or her professional responsibilities.

The nurse's role in a disaster response may depend on where the nurse happens to be at the time of impact, such as at home, a hospital, a clinic, or somewhere in the community. If a nurse is in the immediate location of the disaster, he or she may be able to make a direct nursing response through such activities as "assisting in evacuation, rescue, and first aid efforts until the immediate needs of the situation are met" (Taggert, 1985, p. 11). An example is given later in this chapter in the report of a nonnative New York nurse who was visiting the city at the time of the terrorist attack on the World Trade Center. She was able to provide emergency care to rescue workers in need of a variety of kinds of first aid in the initial hours following the collapse of the twin towers.

As noted, there may be a multiplicity of first aid and other emergency care needs at a disaster site that will fall within the purview of the nurse. Some related activities that professional nurses might assist with include providing leadership; maintaining a communication network; organizing the provision of food, warmth, shelter, and social support; and counseling victims who appear to display "panic or hysterical behavior" (Reichsmeier & Miller, 1985, p. 191). Another important role of the nurse responding to a disaster situation is awareness and assessment of the needs of the rescue workers. If the disaster is particularly devastating in terms of multiple injuries or loss of life, "psychological reactions can easily overwhelm relief teams of caregivers unless careful attention is given to meeting basic biological needs, especially the need for rest and sleep" (Reichsmeier & Miller, 1985, p. 199).

Disaster Services

Three agencies are charged with the provision of relief services in mass casualty disasters in the United States: FEMA, the American Red Cross, and the Salvation Army. Each group has specific responsibilities in times of disaster and mass trauma.

Federal Emergency Management Agency (FEMA)

The Federal Emergency Management Agency (FEMA) is an agency of the federal government that is charged with planning for and responding to disasters, both natural and man-made. Since March 2003, it has been a part of the U.S. Department of Homeland Security. The organization "has also been active in the development of nationwide contingency systems for disaster relief" (Switzer, 1985, p. 318). FEMA staff provide leadership in recovery efforts and support to the victims of disasters through both direct and indirect funding of services to provide the necessities of daily life and functioning. FEMA, founded in 1979, has a staff of several thousand full-time workers, supported by reservists who can be activated if needed. FEMA is called in whenever a situation is declared a disaster or in need of emergency services.

The American Red Cross

The American Red Cross, initiated under the direction of nurse Clara Barton in 1881, received its charge from the 58th Congress of the United States to "continue and carry on a system of national and international relief in time of . . . suffering caused by pestilence, famine, fire, floods and other great national calamities" (Nabbe, 1961, p. 10). Thus, the American Red Cross, although not a government agency, has a national mandate to provide relief services in times of great calamity and disaster in our country; the group is also mandated to provide services for the armed forces of the country as needed. The Red Cross is primarily a volunteer organization supported by private contributions and the volunteer work of a number of individuals. A significant role of the American Red Cross is the provision of blood supplies to hospitals in need of supplemental stocks for disaster victims. Other activities carried out by Red Cross nursing staff and volunteers include providing first aid at disaster sites, feeding rescue and recovery workers, providing food and shelter for disaster victims, communicating with families of disaster victims, providing mental health services, and assisting survivors with accessing available resources. The Red Cross suggests that "community health skills and psychological support skills are important assets for a nurse to possess when helping victims after a disaster" (Hanson, Jesz, & Baldwin, 1991, p. 391).

The Salvation Army

The Salvation Army is an international religious organization founded in London in 1865 by William Booth. The "Army" adopted, early on, a military style of organization and dress; this reflects the group's war against evil as well as its witness of the Christian gospel, to which all Army members adhere. Many people think of Salvation Army members primarily as the "bell-ringers," seen on city street corners with their classic red collection buckets. In fact, this activity of collecting money for the poor is only a small part of the Army's ministry. As well as carrying out a number of services for those in need, the Salvation Army embraces the commitment of assisting any community following a disaster incident. Army members can usually be seen at disaster sites involved in such works as feeding survivors and rescue workers, counseling those in need of psychological and social support, providing grief and bereavement counseling, praying with persons desiring spiritual support, and generally assisting victims and their families with whatever needs they present, in attempting to cope with the disaster experience and its aftermath.

▶ Psychosocial Impact of Mass Casualty Trauma

Support provided by the previously identified organizations is critical in managing a mass casualty trauma, because in such situations, the problems, especially the psychosocial problems experienced by both victims and responders, frequently "exceed the medical community's resources to deal with them" (Baker, 1980, p. 149). Two broad categories of disaster victims are identified: primary victims, who "directly experience physical, material and personal losses from the disaster event"; and secondary victims, who "witness the destructiveness of the disaster but do not experience the actual impact" (Bolin, 1985, p. 6). Secondary victims may include both family members and rescue workers involved in a disaster incident. The American Psychiatric Association's DSM-V Classification identifies "bearing witness to a trauma or being confronted by the traumatic experience of a family member or close friend" as a stressor that may have "psychiatric consequences" (Fullerton & Ursano, 1997, p. 59).

It is suggested that "the impact of victimization" may threaten or even "shatter" certain basic assumptions of the survivor: "the belief in personal invulnerability; the perception of the world as meaningful and the perception of oneself as positive [or as being a worthy person]" (Janoff-Bulman, 1985, p. 15). This psychological impact of a disaster has important implications for spiritual need and spiritual care, which are discussed later in this chapter. Obviously some victims of a disaster will be affected by the victimization to a greater degree than others. Some factors that may negatively influence a survivor's ability to cope both physically and psychologically include a history of "previous traumatic life events"; "recent ill health"; the "experience of severe stress and loss"; loss of "social and psychological supports"; and "lack of coping skills" (Cohen & Ahearn, 1980, p. 9). Especially vulnerable, of course, are the elderly, the young, and those with cognitive or mental disabilities (pp. 9–10).

Another group particularly at risk of both physical and psychosocial stress following a mass casualty disaster are the "responders": police officers, firefighters, emergency medical technicians (EMTs) and other medical personnel (physicians and nurses), rescue personnel such as iron or steel workers, and any other individuals who witness the human carnage brought about by a major disaster. In many major disasters, the responding personnel face such traumatic sights as burned, dismembered, or mutilated bodies; these experiences put disaster workers at great risk "for the development of posttraumatic stress" (McCarroll, Ursano, & Fullerton, 1997, p. 37). Thus, it is important for disaster nurses to remember to assess the needs of disaster workers and to provide care for the caregivers as well as the "primary victims" in the days following a major disaster (Newburn, 1993, p. 127).

In one study, a group of firefighters who had been involved in mass casualty disasters were asked what incidents bothered them most in order of significance. They identified as most stressful: (1) "dead or injured children"; (2) "high rise fires with threat to life involved"; (3) "multi-casualty incidents"; (4) "death"; (5) "threat of personal mutilation or death" (Hodgkinson & Stewart, 1998, p. 197). Heroically, the firefighters placed their own potential injury or death at the lowest end of the scale in terms of significance. This fact, in itself, has important implications for the kinds of stressors that surviving firefighters or other rescue personnel might experience in terms of the concept of "survivor guilt." Some rescue workers may question their own survival in the face of massive losses of life at a disaster and even fear a "mission failure" (Hartsough, 1985, p. 27). Emergency workers may also have trouble sleeping or "winding down" after a disaster in which they were exposed to "almost daily horrors of death, destruction and coping with the needs of hurting human beings" (Mitchell, 1986, p. 109). A discussion of the "psychological aftermath" of a disaster for EMT personnel suggests that some negative feelings identified by responders to a mass casualty incident may include "feelings of frustration and powerlessness," "fear," "guilt" ("over real or imagined misjudgments" or "over casual handling of the dead"), and "insecurity" (Butman, 1982, pp. 149–150). Again, the disaster workers' stressors provide important implications for spiritual care in the aftermath of the incident.

For both victims and responders, as well as the planning of long-term care and counseling, "psychological first aid" may be needed at or near the disaster site. This consists of such activities as "instilling confidence," "showing warmth and caring," "providing guidance in stress reduction," and "attempting to assess [the individual's] need for counseling" (Mahoney, 1969, p. 208).

A final group that needs to be considered as having unique and special needs in the wake of a disaster incident is children. Obviously the child's degree of involvement in the disaster, as well as such factors as age, developmental stage, past life experience, and family support, will significantly influence his or her response to a traumatic event. In one nursing study of children who had experienced Hurricane Andrew in 1992, it was reported that children ages 5 to 12 described life as "weird" after the storm; the children's families and schools, however, served as primary resources in helping them cope with the life changes necessitated by the disaster (Coffman, 1994, p. 363). There are a number of books that might help parents or disaster nurses working with children who survive a mass casualty incident in which loved ones were lost; one example is *Your Grieving Child* (Dodds, 2001).

A great deal has been written about posttraumatic stress disorder (PTSD) following a disaster; the physical and psychological signs and symptoms vary widely among victims and responders. Dr. Michele Davidson (2001), pointed out that because Americans were exposed to incredible "images of death and destruction at the hands of the terrorists" in the September 11th attack, some may continue to experience some degree of PTSD "for months or even years to come" (p. 10). Some common symptoms of PTSD include fatigue, irritability, restlessness, fear, anxiety and depression, nightmares, difficulty sleeping, lack of appetite, difficulty concentrating, headaches, GI upsets, and a multiplicity of other physical complaints. After the World Trade Center disaster, some New Yorkers reported anxiety at hearing loud noises, especially if they involved an aircraft passing overhead. A variety of therapeutic interventions may be employed to ameliorate these symptoms and help the sufferer on the road to recovery; some basic steps in therapy include "initial exploration of the stress event," "establishing the therapeutic alliance," and "working through thoughts and feelings" about the event (Marmar & Horowitz, 1988, pp. 93–97).

The "critical incident stress syndrome (CISS)" is a fairly recent concept identifying a stress reaction of disaster workers appropriate for psychological intervention. This may occur in EMTs, physicians, nurses, police, firefighters, and other rescue workers after a traumatic incident causes interference with their ability to function, or later results in a strong emotional reaction (Kennedy & Charles, 2001, p. 391). The CISS is defined as "responding to a scene and becoming overwhelmed by what one sees, hears, touches, or smells; and experiencing normal reactions of an abnormal event" (Kennedy & Charles, 2001, p. 391) such as can occur at the site of a mass casualty trauma. A therapy recommended to counter the stress of emergency workers in a disaster is the psychological debriefing process labeled the "Critical Incident Stress Debriefing (CISD)" (Mitchell, 1986, p. 109). In this process, the emergency workers are allowed to vent their emotions after a disaster through a peer support group led by a mental health professional. CISD is reported to assist "emergency personnel in understanding their reactions" and reassuring them "that what they are experiencing is normal and common to most of those who were involved in the incident" (Mitchell, 1986, p. 109).

▶ Spiritual Needs in the Aftermath of a Disaster

While mass casualty disasters may pose seemingly overwhelming physical and/or psychosocial challenges, many people find strength and comfort in their spiritual beliefs. Some individuals can accept that a disaster may be beyond human understanding but accept the event as a "test of faith in God's plan; prayer, meditative practices and faith communities can provide strength and support" (Walsh, 2007, p. 213). It is admitted, however, that "meeting the religious and spiritual needs of a trauma patient is an important, yet often overlooked" dimension of nursing care (Killough, 2005, p. 183).

The topic of spiritual needs immediately after, and in the long term following, a mass casualty disaster is vast. A disaster victim's or a responder's spiritual needs may involve a desire for personal prayer or prayer with a clergy person; a loving hug or words of support from a relative, friend, or caregiver; formal religious rituals in cases of death or critical wounding of loved ones; and myriad other kinds of spiritual or religious support. Much will have to do with the nature of the disaster, the role of the individual in the disaster, and the personal spiritual or religious orientation of the victim or responder. Examples of need and kind of spiritual/religious care provided are best presented in context of a specific disaster incident. Thus, much of the pastoral care literature addressing disaster response is described in such a context. The same is true of this chapter, which, as noted earlier, focuses on the spiritual need and spiritual care involved in the September 11th attack on America. Prior to discussion of the spiritual needs of Pentagon and World Trade Center victims and responders, however, an overview of the extant literature on spiritual care in earlier mass casualty disasters is presented.

In 1966, a tornado devastated a large area near Topeka, Kansas, taking 17 lives and destroying over 800 homes; thousands were left homeless. A chaplain from the Menninger Foundation summarized the reports of the spiritual care provided by local pastors as primarily involving counseling survivors in terms of their everyday needs. The pastors' interventions represented loving, caring church support, and it was noted that "no one reported . . . a discussion on God's will or providence" (Klink, 1966, p. 200). Another widely explored early disaster was that of the 1972 Buffalo Creek experience, in which a local coal mine waste heap collapsed, killing 125 people and leaving hundreds homeless. Shortly after the disaster, local chaplains responded to the scene to provide whatever emergency pastoral care the victims desired; a plan for long-term care was also initiated to focus on "intense unresolved grief; disaster syndrome; and loss of community" (Jordan, 1976, p. 160). A 1974 tornado in Louisville, Kentucky, killed 40 people and left over 900 homeless. Some of the pastoral care strategies reported after this disaster included assisting victims to verbalize the "trauma" (i.e., getting the person to talk), helping victims deal with the stress of "uprootedness" and "loss of possessions," and dealing with problems of "isolation and disillusionment" (Reed, 1977, pp. 98–106). Also in 1974, another Kentucky tornado left 77 people dead and more than 1,000 injured. Some of the key spiritual ministries provided by local pastors included visiting victims in hospitals, attending a mass funeral service, helping rebuild homes, giving last rites and conducting individual funeral services, and collecting money for victims (Chinnici, 1985, p. 248).

Following a 1980 tornado in Grand Island, Nebraska, in which more than 1,000 homes were destroyed, a pastor found that his congregation particularly needed to deal with the meaning of the event. His sermons thus dealt with such topics as the stages of loss, empathy for the victims, and the challenge to help those in need (Allen, 1982, p. 464). Hurricane Andrew devastated areas of Florida in August 1992, leaving many injured and homeless; there were a number of stress-related deaths following the storm. Florida pastors reported that stress was reduced with the help of two spiritual orientations: humility, or the ability to admit that one was not "in charge" in a disaster, and the sharing of disaster experiences with a "community that understood and empathized" (Dudley & Schoonover, 1993, pp. 588–589). Sometimes, the pastors note, these communities were made up of "Christian congregations, but just as often . . . of old friends, neighbors or strangers" (p. 589). Two other disasters described in the pastoral care literature are those of the 1992 impact of Hurricane Iniki, west of Honolulu, and the 1997 Red River flood that devastated Grand Forks, North Dakota. Spiritual care following these disasters included pastors' encouraging victims to take care of each other "reinforcing a living community that became a living reminder of God's love and care" (Moody & Carr, 1996, p. 27), and encouraging citizens to become a community of Christ "by planned and random acts of kindness" (Hulden, 1997, p. 31).

The descriptions of spiritual care and spiritual need included in the reports described here focus primarily on the actual ministries of pastors and congregations in meeting the early needs of disaster victims and their families. Several pastors, however, admit that the question of "why" begins to be articulated as initial stressors fade and long-term coping begins. A victim's or survivor's request for an answer to the "why" of evil or suffering is perhaps the most difficult issue for a spiritual caregiver to address, quite simply because there is no clear answer. The question of why becomes even more sensitive when a disaster or trauma affects the very young. Following a 1989 school disaster in the Hudson Valley, New York, in which 10 children died and many others were injured, questions were reported such as "They were so innocent: how could God allow this?" (Cullinan, 1993, p. 227). It is generally believed that "religion can play a role in assigning meaning" to disasters (Kroll-Smith & Couch, 1987, p. 26); yet, an individual, even a religious person, may be left questioning his or her "trust in God's benevolence" following a devastating disaster (Pedraja, 1997, p. 7).

In discussing the theology and "theodicy or Divine Justice" (Kropf, 1988, p. 57) of disasters, theologians note the difficulty of reconciling three propositions generally held by most religious people: "God is loving and perfectly good"; "God is omnipotent"; and "There is evil and suffering in the world" (Chester, 1998, p. 488). This is the problem presented in the Old Testament book of Job, which, in fact, concludes without giving the reader a satisfying answer as to why Job, ostensibly a good man, had to suffer; the focus of the book is on Job's faith in the midst of suffering. It is suggested, however, that although Job's God may be "inscrutable . . . he speaks and he cares" (Cohn, 1986, p. 276). As movingly put by author David Toole (1999) in an essay on the theology of natural disasters, "But what must we ask of the suffering of the innocents . . . we mourn the deaths and cheer only the possibility that somewhere amidst disaster God is at work judging and saving the world" (p. 561).

In his best-selling book *When Bad Things Happen to Good People*, Rabbi Harold Kushner (1981) took a similar position. "God does not cause our misfortunes," he notes. "Some are caused by bad luck, some are caused by bad people, and some are simply an inevitable consequence of our being human and being mortal, living in a world of inflexible natural laws" (p. 134). Rabbi Kushner adds that because a tragedy that befalls us is "not God's will . . . We can turn to Him for help in overcoming it, precisely because we can tell ourselves that God is as outraged by it as we are" (p. 134). Rabbi Kushner's position is strikingly reminiscent of a mother's comment at the time of her son's dying. "Even when I was screaming at God, because, you know, why and why and why? Even when I was angry with him, I knew that God was crying with me" (O'Brien, 1992, p. 67).

A nursing study of older adult survivors of the 2005 Gulf Coast Hurricane Katrina was carried out to explore the needs of elder populations following major trauma. Of the 224 study participants, almost half added open-ended comments to a standardized questionnaire. One important topic mentioned was spirituality. The investigators reported that "some participants wrote strong expressions of faith, belief in God and spirituality. Many gave blessings to the volunteers and the military who came to their aid" (Langan & Palmer, 2012). Examples of other study participants' spirituality-related comments reported by the researchers were: "'Everything we have belongs to our heavenly Father,' 'He will take care of his children,' and 'Pray'" (p. 131).

▶ The Disaster Nurse's Role in Spiritual Care

Perhaps the most important thing that a nurse caring for a disaster victim can do, in terms of spiritual care, is to reinforce the fact that the trauma a patient has experienced was not caused by God, or brought about by any behavior on the victim's part. This can free a victim from possible feelings of guilt, help restore his or her faith in God, and allow the individual to, as Rabbi Kushner suggests, "turn to God for help" in overcoming the suffering caused by the disaster. Before attempting to provide more specific spiritual care such as praying with a patient or clergy referral, a nurse can do an on-the-spot spiritual assessment by asking a few simple questions related to a disaster victim's spiritual or religious tradition, such as finding out what kind of pastoral care or prayer life they have been used to and what might support them both immediately and in future coping with the disaster. Family members, if available, can provide much of this information. Also, a variety of volunteer clergy members are usually present at disaster sites; their intervention may be very helpful in assisting the nurse with both assessment and planning for a patient's future, especially if the victim is to be hospitalized.

Not all nurses will or need to feel comfortable in providing such spiritual care as praying with a patient; they may, however, feel at ease giving a supportive hug. Nurses in disaster situations should, however, be prepared to assess a patient's spiritual needs, especially if the victim is seriously or mortally wounded. For example, a critically injured Roman Catholic victim would be greatly comforted to receive an anointing or "the Sacrament of the Sick"; this could be done on the spot, if a priest is available. It is doubtful that any priest would come to a disaster site without bringing the holy oil needed for the sacrament. If the patient should die either at the disaster site or in transport to a hospital, the fact that the "last rites" of the Church had been administered prior to his or her death would be very meaningful to a Catholic family.

It can also be helpful for a disaster nurse to provide clergy referral to less seriously injured victims for future spiritual care and counseling. It is very important to refer patients to pastors who are willing and able to listen to the sometimes graphic and gruesome reports of a disaster scene "in a nonjudgmental and practical way but with a sensitivity to the theological implications for the victim" (Williams, 1998, p. 330). Because of the "trust many people have in ministers" they often become natural crisis counselors (Clinebell, 1991, p. 183). Nurses also are "natural crisis counselors" and natural providers of spiritual care, because they are often the people most closely involved with a victim immediately after a disaster. Guidelines suggested for pastoral caregivers working with trauma victims can also be useful for disaster nurses regarding the provision of spiritual support and spiritual care; some of these include "non-judgmental acceptance of the survivor," a posture of " support and advocacy," an understanding of "posttraumatic distress," "willingness to be exposed to the survivor's recounting of the traumatic experience," and recognition that grieving may be a lifelong process (Foy, Drescher, Fitz, & Kennedy, 1993, p. 631). The authors also note that the spiritual caregiver should provide for "pastoral self-care" (p. 631). Pastoral or spiritual self-care is a given for any nurse attempting to provide spiritual care for victims of a mass casualty disaster.

During trauma care, such as that associated with mass casualty occurrences, "healthcare providers face a variety of challenges to addressing the spiritual needs of a patient" (Killough, 2005, p. 183). Some trauma victims may have to deal with personal issues such as "despair, hope, sin, eternity, love, guilt, shame, fear . . . medical care providers may be unable to address all of these issues in an effective manner. But by acknowledging and respecting the real dynamics of victims' faith and belief systems," nurses may begin to meet the needs of patients and families (p. 185). It is noted that "many healthcare practitioners turn to their own spirituality to manage stress and find answers" (Urden, 2012, p. 5). One neonatal intensive care unit (NICU) nurse reported that during the storm Katrina, she "took on the role of spiritual director in the nursery" (Danna & Cordray, 2010, p. 120). The nurse added: "I was a confidante . . . I was always supportive, mostly because of my own belief" (p. 120).

Two other anecdotal reports of nursing roles in spiritual care are those of Snyder, Terzioglu, and Keeling (2011), who describe church-related health-care services they provided to Haitian refugees after the 2011 earthquake there; and the experiences of a young nurse who worked with patients following the 2011 tornado in Joplin, Missouri (Ericksen, Ericksen, & Painter, 2012).

▶ The September 11, 2001, Terrorist Attack on America: Spiritual Needs and Spiritual Care

The Attack

Although explorations of spiritual needs and spiritual care at the Pentagon and the World Trade Center disaster sites are addressed separately, an overview of the terrorist attack on America, including that of the Pennsylvania plane crash, is initially presented; this is to set the tone for that day of tragedy for the citizens of the United States.

In the early hours of September 11, 2001, four large passenger jet aircraft were hijacked by terrorists intent on causing death and destruction in key areas of the United States. At approximately 8:45 a.m., a hijacked American Airlines jetliner, Flight 11 out of Boston, bound for Los Angeles and carrying 20,000 gallons of fuel, crashed into the 110-story north tower (Tower 1) of New York City's World Trade Center at a level between floors 90 and 100. The building immediately burst into flames. At 9:03 a.m., a hijacked United Airlines jet, Flight 175 from Boston, bound for Los Angeles and also fully loaded with fuel, crashed into the south tower (Tower 2) of the World Trade Center between floors 78 and 87 and exploded. Both buildings were now on fire. At 9:45 a.m., American Airlines Flight 77 from Washington, DC, bound for Los Angeles and fully fueled, crashed into the western side of the Pentagon, exploding into flames; a huge section of the building soon collapsed. At 10:10 a.m., United Airlines Flight 93 from Newark, New Jersey, and bound for San Francisco crashed into a field in rural Somerset County, Pennsylvania. It is hypothesized that this fourth hijacked plane may have been headed for the United States Capitol or the White House. It is believed that only the actions of some courageous passengers—who, according to reported cell phone conversations, overpowered the hijackers and took control of Flight 93—prevented a fourth major mass casualty disaster from happening on September 11. At 10:05 a.m., the 110-story south tower of the World Trade Center collapsed in on itself from the heat of the fire melting its steel structure; at 10:28 a.m., the north tower of the World Trade Center also collapsed from the top down. Hundreds of people raced through the streets of Manhattan, fleeing the deluge of debris raining down on the city from the collapsing towers. Some trapped World Trade Center employees leapt to their deaths, perhaps in hope of a miraculous escape from the flames engulfing their offices. Later that afternoon, World Trade Center Building 7, a 47-story structure, also collapsed from the fire.

The country's initial reaction to the first jet crash into the north tower of the World Trade Center was one of shock over a terrible accident. Eighteen minutes later, after the second tower was hit, it was clear that this disaster was not accidental, and all nonmilitary planes in U.S. airspace were immediately grounded. The Port Authority of New York closed all tunnels and bridges into the city and many buildings near the World Trade Center were evacuated. There was a recall of all New York City firefighters to respond to the World Trade Center disaster site. Forty minutes after the second tower was hit, and the Pentagon had been attacked, the country knew that an "act of war" had occurred. President Bush was temporarily evacuated aboard Air Force One; many government office buildings in Washington, DC, were also evacuated. Fighter jets were deployed from military air bases across the country, and all inbound trans-atlantic flights were diverted to Canada. The Pentagon announced that five warships and two aircraft carriers had been deployed from a Virginia naval station to protect the east coast from further attack. The president informed the country that a national emergency had been declared, and U.S. military worldwide were placed on high alert. The number of casualties was unknown in the immediate aftermath of the attacks, but the estimates were staggering; the entire country was in shock. The president begged for prayers for the thousands of victims and their families.

Some months after the attack on America, the numbers of missing, dead, and wounded were still changing, but it had generally been determined that 266 people, including the hijackers, lost their lives in the four plane crashes; 189 people were killed in the Pentagon attack; and close to 3,000 became victims of the World Trade Center disaster. Of the World Trade Center lives lost, 343 represented fallen members of the New York City Fire Department, 75 were New York Port Authority officers and staff members, and 23 were New York City police officers. The City of New York was overwhelmed with funerals and memorial services and with bereaved and grieving families. All of America, and indeed the world, grieved for so many innocent lives lost in this unbelievably painful mass casualty disaster that struck the country with such force and such surprise. Everyone had a story to tell: where they were when the attack occurred; who they knew in New York or Washington that they had worried about; how they expressed their pain, their grief, and their sympathy for the suffering victims. Some of these anecdotes, as well as the author's own experiences and insights in gathering data for this chapter, are woven throughout the following pages describing spiritual needs and spiritual care following the attack on America.

The Pentagon

On September 11, the famous Pentagon, an East Coast hub of U.S. military operations, located only a few miles from the nation's capital, was grievously damaged by the terrorist attack. The disaster resulted in the loss of 189 lives and numerous injuries. American Airlines Flight 77 slammed into the western side of the Pentagon between corridors 4 and 5: "The plane blasted through rings E, D, and C, and parts of it were found between rings C and B" (Cannon, 2001, p. 31). Newscasters across the country noted, with awe, that only the fact that the plane happened to hit a portion of the Pentagon that had recently been renovated, saved hundreds, if not thousands, of lives. The newly reinforced side wall kept the floors from collapsing for about half an hour, thus allowing many Pentagon staffers to escape before that portion of the building came down.

I live and work at The Catholic University of America in Washington, DC, about four miles from the Pentagon. And I, like everyone else in the area, worried and grieved and prayed with and for the victims of September 11. The Pentagon attack seemed like a lesser disaster, compared to the carnage at the World Trade Center, but the impact was in no way minor to the victims, their families, and the brave responders to the disaster site. My university held a moving candlelight memorial service the week of September 11 for those who died at the Pentagon and also those who died in Pennsylvania and New York; we desperately needed to do something, and turning to God in prayer seemed the most important step in coping with what had befallen our country.

Washington, DC, as New York, never got the huge number of mass casualties initially expected; nursing students and faculty at Catholic University were ready to help but the call never came; sadly, there were not enough survivors at either site to overwhelm the existing health-care systems. To view the Pentagon disaster site in the early days was shocking; to see the gaping hole left in this so familiar building, the distinguished center of military operations. To view the grieving families, waiting at the perimeter of the Pentagon disaster site in the hope that a missing loved one might be found alive, was heartbreaking. The wife of one missing soldier asserted, "I'm not going home without him."

The Chaplains

It's not the collar, it's the color.

—**Washington, DC**, Fire Department Chaplain

One of the first people I spoke with about the spiritual needs of Pentagon disaster victims was Reverend "Smith" (all names used in reporting interview data are pseudonyms), a Washington, DC, police and fire chaplain. He had been paged with the DC Fire Department immediately after the attack and had been at the site, ministering to the wounded, to their families, and to the rescue workers each day for weeks. Chaplain Smith reported that there had been a spiritual presence at the Pentagon disaster site 24/7 since the attack. When I asked whether the religious denomination of a person providing spiritual care to disaster survivors mattered to the victims and rescue workers, he replied, "No, it's not the collar; it's the color!" Rev. Smith explained that what was important, especially to rescue workers, was the "color" of his badges, representing the police and fire departments of Washington, DC; he was "their chaplain" and, thus, the chaplain for the survivors and families following a disaster. Rev. Smith explained that "working with people of diverse religious backgrounds is one of the challenges of disaster response chaplaincy. "My role is to coordinate with chaplains of other faiths, ministering to victims and rescue workers; being there and dispensing hugs and thank you's." Rev. Smith also added that a primary ministry, in his role as fire and police chaplain, is for the emergency responders. "You are there for them."

Rev. Smith described his "church" at the Pentagon disaster site as a "tent" that had been set up for the chaplains to provide spiritual care; this was also a place where a stressed-out rescue worker could come for a massage or just to "talk." The chaplains' tent was a "safe place where people could come for refuge." The chaplain explained that "Spiritual care is critical in such a setting; a situation that was that traumatic." He noted, "It was three days before a secure perimeter was established. The fire burned from 9 am on Tuesday to 6 am on Wednesday; lots of people were there waiting for survivors, praying for them." An additional witness of the importance of spiritual need and spiritual care at a disaster site was reflected in FEMA's designating a room for "Meditation and Prayer" (a "Quiet Room") for any staff members seeking a place apart.

Chaplain Smith reported that the spiritual care staff were assisted by staff members from the Red Cross and the Salvation Army who also prayed with and counseled victims and disaster workers at the site. He observed that spiritual counseling after a disaster may also bring out a victim's other life problems, such as with their marriage or relationship with God. Rev. Smith reported that volunteer chiropractors were also a "real asset for those lifting and carrying," especially steel workers and plumbers. This kind of human caring seemed relevant to the topic of spiritual care in the postdisaster situation; the roles of steel workers and plumbers were critical in attempting to rescue survivors who might be trapped in the rubble.

Chaplain Smith admitted that some people he spoke with did "ask why?" "There's nothing wrong with that," he asserted. "I don't have the answers. Some people may be angry with God but that's where faith and prayer come in. My job is to be," he added, "being present." A great deal of his ministry involved "listening, praying and saying 'thank you' to the rescue workers."

When I asked Chaplain Smith how he coped with his own stress in the face of ministering at the Pentagon disaster site, he commented, "My anxiety was that I could not rush to New York to assist my brother chaplains there, but here they said to me 'Who will care for us if you go to New York?'" Rev. Smith added that his faith, his family, and his friendships with other chaplains who were close friends provided his personal spiritual support. Finally, Rev. Smith suggested three pamphlets helpful in responding to spiritual need and providing spiritual care in mass casualty disasters: *Bringing God's Peace to Disaster* (Church World Service, 2001a); *Bringing God's Presence to Survivors* (Church World Service, 2001b); and *Cooperative Faith-Based Disaster Recovery in Your Community* (Church World Service, 2001c).

The Firefighters

It's more like eagerness, not really fear; you can't wait to get in there. Like we were itching to get in there. It's like: "Let's go; let's go; let's go! Let's get in there! We gotta get in there. C'mon; c'mon!"

—**Washington, DC** firefighter on arrival
at the Pentagon site on September 11

I was truly hesitant to ask to speak with any firefighters because of the incredible trauma they had recently experienced in witnessing the human carnage at the September 11th disaster sites, as well as because of the great losses they had suffered within their ranks in the City of New York. Nevertheless, my desire to try and understand, even a little, the heroism and spiritual caring of these men and women who rush to enter those places others rush to leave overcame my shyness. Through informal networking, I met a DC firefighter who graciously agreed to speak with me. Michael was a young firefighter, but seasoned through a number of years of volunteer experience and also through a number of years of "only wanting to be a firefighter," before actually beginning his firefighting career.

Michael belongs to one of the DC engine companies that was off-duty on September 11 when they were called in to respond to the Pentagon alarm. I'll let Michael take up the story from here:

> I drove to the firehouse as fast as I could. We keep our gear at the firehouse; I changed into my uniform, got my stuff. They had called in everybody off-duty and put us into groups; what we were supposed to do. They had additional engines and ladder trucks to operate throughout the city; about 130 firefighters were sent to the Pentagon. We served as relief to the companies that were at the initial alarm. There was still a good amount of fire throughout the building. The companies that were there were saying it was "pretty bad" inside; just bodies and people charred pretty bad. So, I was expecting it to be pretty bad. One of the guys I came with, we were talking about it and pretty much expecting the worst so we tried to be prepared for it.

Mike paused, "Something like this; you pretty much couldn't believe what had happened. It's like the whole world's changed after this. It's still hard to take in, even now." He continued:

By the time we went in we really weren't expecting to find people alive but we had hope that we'd find somebody; I had hope. Not right around the exact impact of the plane because it was pretty much uninhabitable; it looked like a big fireball had gone through that entire ring of the building and you knew that pretty much everybody in that area, it looked like they had died. But areas around there where the plane didn't exactly hit, it looked like they might have been habitable by people so we started doing searches, and hoping. Mostly around the impact area we found bodies, badly charred; sometimes it was really difficult to tell where the bodies were or if we were really seeing bodies.

But if you know that somebody's in there; if you have the slightest inclination that somebody might be alive in there, you go above and beyond. You're pushing it as far as you can go to try and save whoever might be in there. I had some hope that somebody might be in there; alive still! I was talking with one of the guys and we said: "somebody's got to be in there; we're going to find somebody. We gotta keep going!" And I remember being so exhausted; just so exhausted. The heat; the concrete in that building was just containing the heat. I mean I've been in worse fire conditions but we were looking for fire in the walls, hot spots, you don't have a lot of visibility and we wear about 40 pounds of gear; we also have an air bottle and carry some kind of tool like an axe to have the ability to cut through something if you need to. And the guy I was with, we kept encouraging each other. We were just like: "Let's go; let's go."

At this point in our meeting, I asked Michael if he had been afraid on arriving at the Pentagon disaster site and preparing to enter the burning building. His response, as cited previously, bears repeating, because it reflects so beautifully the spiritual caring of the firefighter:

It's more like eagerness; not really fear. You want to get in there. Like we were really itching to get in there. It's like: "Let's go, Let's go, Let's go! Let's get in there! We gotta get in there! C'mon, c'mon!"

At the point of arrival at a fire, or to use Mike's expression, "when we roll up on a fire," the firefighter employs all of his training to put aside fear and direct his energies to the task of rescue at hand; the lives of the victims always come before the firefighter's own safety.

A final question that I had for Michael was about his personal faith; how it supported his ministry as a firefighter and whether experiences such as that of the Pentagon disaster response were something that firefighters in general wanted or needed to talk to a spiritual counselor about. Mike replied, "Well, most guys don't really talk about the stuff that bothers them too much. What I've noticed is guys kind of joke after something like this just kind of to get your mind off it; try to not think about the bodies or whatever. I talked a little bit to a guy I was with; he's pretty spiritual so I felt kind of comfortable talking with him; he's kind of on the spiritual level." Mike continued:

And I pray a lot. There was one thing that was kind of burned into my head at the Pentagon. There was this one man; you could tell that when the place was hit he wasn't killed right away, like the other people. It looked like he had been trying to make it to a doorway and he had his ID out and I thought "Oh, man. I think he was trying to keep his ID out so somebody could identify him." And I said that to my friend; it was like I wanted to say that to somebody. I wanted to say something about it. And then, that was it. I didn't tell anybody else or say anything more. But, seeing that guy trying to get out of the Pentagon, that'll probably stay with me forever. And he was going the right way, too. Oh, man, this guy was heading the right way!

Michael completed his response to my question about his own faith life, "I do pray. I pray every morning before I go to work. I pray every night. I always pray the night before I go to work. When I pray I just ask God to be with me, for Jesus to be with me, to just guide me and help me; that's all. And I know a couple of other guys who pray a lot; I think a lot of others do too but they might not want anybody to know that."

Mike summarized his experience, "Like I tell [family] all the time, I'm glad I was able to be part of it [the Pentagon response]; to do something because it would have crushed me if I couldn't do anything. And every time I see the World Trade Center, I think, 'Oh, I wish I could have been there; to do something.'" He concluded, "I mean I wanted to be part of the Pentagon [response] but at the same time I wish I could have been part of the World Trade Center too. It's just frustrating! I mean I wish I could have done something!"

As a postscript to my meeting with Michael, he told me after our interview that he had recently been to New York to attend the funeral of one of his firefighter friends whose life was lost in the World Trade Center response.

A Prayer for Firefighters

Dear Father in Heaven, guide and protect your beloved firefighters—who daily risk their lives in ministry to brothers and sisters in need.

Grant them courage in the face of danger, strength in times of challenge, and compassion in the midst of suffering.

Guard all firefighters with the power of your loving care, Dear Lord—for they are truly Your own. Bless these heroic men and women who bravely rush to enter the places others rush to leave.

Amen.

There were many post–September 11th stories, in both the local and national news, describing the heroic efforts of firefighters, police, military personnel, and civilians who assisted others to escape during the early minutes of the attack on the Pentagon. As well as the chaplains, these heroic rescuers provided spiritual care in responding to both the physical and psychological needs of disaster victims at the site. Most survivors interviewed by the media attributed their escape from the disaster to God and to his "ministers" who had led them out of the fiery building.

The World Trade Center

It is difficult to know how to begin to describe the myriad kinds of spiritual needs and spiritual care manifested at the site of the overwhelming mass casualty disaster that occurred at the World Trade Center on September 11. As soon as the impact of the first plane on the World Trade Center's north tower was witnessed in New York, chaplains began to head to the scene. One of the first to arrive was the now-famous Franciscan New York Fire Department chaplain, Father Mychal Judge. According to accounts, Father Mike, as he was known by the firefighting community, immediately rushed into the burning north tower to begin ministering to the injured. As he knelt to give the last rites, the anointing of the sick, to a fallen firefighter, he removed his helmet in reverent prayer; he was struck in the head by falling debris and killed instantly while engaged in the ministry he loved. A group of firefighters picked up Father Mike's body, carried it to a nearby church, and laid him down before the altar; a fitting place for Father Mychal to begin his eternal rest.

I was told by a New Yorker friend that another New York priest quickly made his way to the disaster site and began blessing and giving absolution to firefighters, en masse, as they rushed into the burning building to search for survivors. This is a very consoling thought, spiritually, for the families of those who lost their lives in the effort to save others. A young firefighter, being transported to the World Trade Center with 50 other firefighters, is quoted as saying, "There was this chaplain on the bus and he was giving absolution to everyone" (Sullivan, 2001, p. 5). Father Benedict Groeschel (2001a), also a New York Franciscan, wrote, "I am sure that the first priests on hand, like Father Mychal Judge, the fire chaplain who lost his life ministering to the dying, gave general absolution as soon as they arrived on the scene. It may have been the biggest general absolution in history" (p. 242).

The Recoveries

Medical personnel poured into New York City with plans to set up triaging facilities near the disaster site, and also to help staff local hospitals. The volunteers were initially welcomed but, after a few hours, it became clear that, as in the Pentagon attack in Washington, DC, there would not be an overwhelming number of live casualties; the mortality would be much higher than the morbidity following the disaster. Those who did not get out of the towers quickly would not be getting out at all. The most critically important spiritual care, at that point, aside from that needed by rescue workers and family members, was the need for religious rituals to accompany the recovery of victims' bodies. To that end, a temporary morgue site, staffed by an interdenominational group of chaplains, was set up at the nearby Chelsea Piers.

Heart-wrenchingly tender scenes began to be replayed over and over on TV screens across the country, as news cameras at "Ground Zero" recorded the finding of bodies in the days following the September 11th attack. When the body of a uniformed police officer or a firefighter was identified, the deceased was draped in an American flag, and rescue workers stopped their digging to form two long lines of honor guards before which the heroic victim's remains were carried. One journalist reported that some of the men prayed as a fallen brother's remains passed by; others sang hymns. "Some of the men have beautiful voices," she wrote, "and sing the ancient chants; I heard one softly singing the Dies Irae" (Vitullo-Martin, 2001, p. 8). Many staid police officers', firefighters', steel and construction workers', and EMTs' eyes were moist with tears during these impromptu memorials carried out at the World Trade Center disaster site.

The disaster victims' remains were immediately taken from the site to the makeshift morgue set up at Chelsea Piers. There, volunteer chaplains waited to receive the recovered bodies with a prayerful ritual of remembrance. One chaplain reported, "We were about a block away from 'Ground Zero.' All around us were huge piles of rubble, and a tremendous amount of work was going on with diggers and power shovels" (Groeschel, 2001b, p. 23). He continued, "Our task was to conduct a short service each time the remains of a victim's body were brought into the morgue. In the course of . . . six hours we held a service eight times" (pp. 23–24). Another clergyman who had ministered at the Chelsea Piers morgue, Father Philip Murnion (2001a), described the ritual. "Most of the time is spent in waiting . . . Then when a rescue worker arrives with remains, we all jump to our feet and a chapel-silence fills the air . . . all wait as one or two of the clergy step forward and call all to prayer; all the other workers want to make sure this is done. We pray briefly, using our own words and the words of our ritual for the deceased, committing the person to God's love, and perhaps praying for the family . . . all remain quiet for a few seconds" (p. 1). Father added, "The respect, actually reverence, shown to each remain, however small, is extraordinary. It is as if the very fact that full bodies are only rarely retrieved has made the least part of a body all that much more important. The sacred character of each life is so fully honored" (p. 2). Father Murnion concluded his reflections from the World Trade Center morgue site by poignantly expressing a spiritual response to the disaster. "The magnitude of the tragedy and the complexity of forces involved in the attack make almost any response seem inadequate. The hymn lines that occurred to me are from the Stabat Mater: 'Is there one who would not weep, whelmed in misery so deep?' Yet the powerful exertion of compassion-seeking-understanding evident at the site looks to faith and church for grounding, bonding, and action worthy of us as a people" (p. 2).

Manhattan churches of all denominations opened their doors to those in need: to exhausted rescue workers and to family members searching desperately for a loved one missing in the disaster. Quickly, victims' families began to establish personal prayer sites "mounting photos of their loved ones in nearby parks, at the receiving hospitals, at the medical examiner's office . . . and at the armory that served as a clearing house for the names of those missing" (Murnion, 2001b, p. 2). When some asked, "Where was God on September 11th?" clergymen answered with such responses as, "God was there in the seat with every person who went down in the fiery inferno . . . He was in the fireman's suit and behind the police badge. God was there in the elevators and the stairwells of the World Trade Center" (Stover, 2001, p. 79).

For many survivors and families, the Internet became a spiritual "lifeline" to access information, search for survivors, and share personal stories of pain, suffering, hope, and survival in the aftermath of the attack (Terrell & Perry, 2001, p. 67). Spiritual and religiously affiliated organizations and churches providing services to victims and families of the World Trade Center disaster were listed on the Internet; they included such groups as The Salvation Army, Catholic Charities, Healing Works, the Southern Baptist Convention, Church of God Ministries, Christian Reformed Church, United Jewish Appeal Federation, United Methodist Committee on Relief, Evangelical Lutheran Church of America, National Presbyterian Church, Episcopal Church Center of N.Y., YMCA, World Vision, Association of Gospel Missions, World Relief, the Society of St. Vincent de Paul, and many others. Services offered on websites by these organizations included prayer and counseling (crisis and grief counseling), financial support, pastoral counseling (spiritual ministry), emergency services for survivors (food, clothing, shelter), school outreach to children, help with burial costs, emergency day care, legal counseling, job counseling, mental and physical health care, and general assistance for rescue and recovery workers. Approximately three months after the disaster, there were 7,450 websites listed under the heading World Trade Center disaster and spiritual need. Especially in the aftermath of mass casualty disasters, churches and other religiously affiliated groups include provision for physical and mental health needs, as well as materials needed to sustain daily life, as part of their spiritual ministry to victims and survivors.

As noted, another source of spiritual support provided by the Internet was the opportunity for survivors, especially those who had escaped from the World Trade Center, or nearby areas, to tell their stories. Many disaster victims posted lengthy accounts of their experiences, their fears, their horror at the devastation, and their narrow, for some, escapes. Sharing experiences on websites, sometimes anonymously, gave the survivors a chance to vent painful emotions, to say thank you to sometimes unknown rescuers, and to express gratitude, often to God, for simply being alive. Some of the Internet writers ended their narratives with an expression of gratitude for the website and the opportunity it provided to share their experiences. It was interesting to discover that although the majority of stories, especially the most emotional anecdotes, were authored by New Yorkers who were intimately involved with the disaster, a number of people from as far away as California and Washington State felt the need to express their thoughts and feelings. One writer from Kirkland, Washington, ended a narrative with the words, "Thank you for this website!"

Many people from both New York and elsewhere visited the disaster site, "Ground Zero," in the days after the attack. There were mixed feelings about this both on the part of victims' families and rescue workers. No one wanted this sacred place, where so many suffered and died, to become a "tourist attraction"; most visitors, however, came out of a desire to grieve, to pray, and to pay homage to the victims, especially to those who gave their lives so heroically in a mission of rescue. It was admitted shortly after the attack, by psychologist and spiritual writer Eugene Kennedy (2001), that "We cannot deal with this event. We can only respond to it and that requires that we enter into the mystery of loss" (p. 17). Kennedy points out the importance of people expressing their grief over such a massive loss of life. "Nothing is more human," he asserts, "than our need to do that work of mourning that nobody can do for us" (p. 17).

The Chaplains

Aside from the stories of absolution given to rescue workers, and rituals provided at the morgue site, there are a number of accounts of other ministries provided by chaplains at the disaster site on the day(s) of and weeks after September 11. Father James Martin (2001a), a New York Jesuit, described his arrival at the disaster site when he came to provide spiritual support two days after the attack. He reported that he was attempting to minister to a soldier at the site but could hardly tear his eyes away from the overwhelming scene before him. "I make an effort to ask after the soldier's welfare. But instead he ministers to me. 'That's OK, Father,' he says, 'Everybody stares when they see it. It's hard to see, isn't it?' He hands me a face mask" (p. 8). As he went about the disaster site listening and supporting and caring for the rescue and recovery workers, some of whom had lost friends and coworkers in the attack, Father Martin reported, "Suddenly I realize that I am standing beside grace. Here are men and women, some of whom tell me 'I lost a buddy in there,' who are going about their business; the business that includes the possibility of dying. 'Greater love has no person,' said Jesus, 'than the one who lays down his life for another.' And that is what this looks like. Here it is" (Martin, 2001a, p. 9).

Five days after the attack, Father Martin (2001b) and several fellow priests went back to the disaster site to say Mass for the rescue workers in a makeshift chapel at the World Trade Center "Ground Zero" ruins. "In a dusty plaza, we discover a cast off table, which we cover with a sheet. Borrowed chalices and patens from a nearby Jesuit church sit next to a Poland Springs water bottle, a hardhat and a gas mask . . . we assemble . . .

with our gas masks. In a few minutes a small group of people gathers around the table—all visibly tired, all covered with sweat, all blanketed in ash" (p. 29). Father Martin (2001b) noted that the gospel reading for the day was "heart-breakingly appropriate": "the shepherd who rescues his lost sheep . . . we speak of searching, rescuing, hoping and loving . . . many come to receive communion" (p. 29). After Mass, one of Father Martin's companions came to him and said, "Have you seen the sign?" Large poster boards had been placed around the disaster site with spray-painted messages to indicate services or activities: "'Morgue', says one sign. 'Eye Wash Station,' says another" (p. 29). And, a sign written by someone unknown to us, Father Martin reported, had been placed "a few feet from our little altar. It reads: 'Body of Christ'" (p. 29).

There was so much written and replayed on national news reports about the hundreds of funerals in New York that attempting to describe even a few would take up a chapter in itself: the haunting bagpipe melody of "Amazing Grace," which accompanied the fire engine–borne caskets of so many of New York's bravest; the tears of the widows, the children, the parents, the coworkers, the ministers; the moving sermons on pain and suffering and hope in eternal life. An excerpt from a homily offered by Edward Cardinal Egan at a Memorial Mass for rescue workers at St. Patrick's Cathedral reflects the spirituality of those who gave their lives in attempting to save others:

> All of us have our fears. These heroes of ours had theirs too. But they conquered them. Millions of tons of stone and steel were falling all around them. Hurricanes of dirt, dust and debris were engulfing them. There was no light with which to see. There was no air with which to breathe. All the same, they did what they always do. They guided, they protected, they defended, they shielded, they rescued. And in so doing they handed over their lives for the safety and well-being of others. If this is not triumph, I do not know what triumph might be. Triumph over fear. Triumph over caring only for oneself. Triumph over all that makes us less than the Lord would have us be. Triumph that defines heroes; wondrous, glorious heroes. (Egan, 2001, p. 133; cited with permission of Edward Cardinal Egan)

The account of one Catholic parish in Staten Island gave some idea of the enormity of the loss for individual communities and of the need for spiritual rituals in the aftermath of the attack on America. St. Clare's parish lost 30 parishioners in the disaster; 11 were firefighters. It was reported that "Some of the most heartrending funerals and memorial Masses have been in St. Clare's red-brick church, like the one for Louis J. Modaferi, the Captain of Staten Island's Rescue Company 5 . . . Rescue Company 5 was wiped out on September 11" (Golway, 2001, p. 6).

Several weeks after the disaster, I had the opportunity to interview a New York City chaplain who had been working with the New York Fire Department since the attack. One of the first things Chaplain Kelly commented on was the fact that so many victims of the World Trade Center disaster were young; that was especially true among the ranks of the police and firefighters, of whom a great number were in their forties, thirties, and even twenties. Another particularly heart-wrenching aspect of the losses among the 343 firefighters was the fact that some were from the same families, for example, a father and son. It was incredibly difficult for families that so many World Trade Center victims' bodies were never recovered.

At the initial alarm, Father Kelly commented, "No one thought the buildings would collapse. One small engine company, with only seven men, was assigned to the 40th floor of Tower 2. The elevator, with all seven firefighters, went up and the building came down. They have never been heard from since. Another trauma was the terrorist nature of the disaster: the homicide, the mutilated bodies, and the loss of public safety personnel; people think 'if policemen and firemen are killed, who will protect us?'"

Father Kelly related the difficulty of ministry at the morgue. Although he had not done the work himself, several clergy he knew were involved and he noted that when they came back from a six-hour tour at the morgue, they said it "felt like 6 months": "It was very hard; they had to wear masks and gowns, they saw the mutilated bodies . . . we saw the indignity of death."

Father Kelly, whose role was to provide information, in conjunction with the fire department, on CISD and available counseling services, commented on the firefighters' culture. "You know, firemen don't have a choice. You don't stand by and watch the World Trade Center burn down; you go in and fight the fire. Also, if a firefighter is down [if he is dead or injured] he is never left alone. If a firefighter is injured in the line of duty, there will be an intense search for that person and the firefighters reserve the right and honor and privilege of retrieving and removing the body. They do it with a sense of ritual and dignity. They never canceled their presence at the site even for the Thanksgiving and Christmas holidays."

Father Kelly described the experience of "numbing" after the World Trade Center disaster:

> People saw terrible trauma; people jumping out windows, that will be replaying over and over but you selectively process; you can't take it all in. Some people at the site saw the WTC come down but said they didn't hear anything. The site of the WTC disaster looks like one of those movies where you see the world after an atomic bomb had dropped and you say "this cannot be real." You say to yourself "this cannot be the World Trade Center; where I'm standing, right now!" You just can't take it in. Everyone is in shock about the situation. I met a widow outside a firehouse and she just said: "I'm not going home until my husband comes home."

People needed to tell their personal stories over and over again, Father Kelly noted. And the question of "Where was God?" came up. He added:

> Some people can fall back on their faith, for others that doesn't work. There were so many memorial services with similar messages being preached. Some may say: "It's not enough." It was especially hard on the firefighters' widows because they all go to each other's husband's services to be supportive and then have to live their own pain all over again. Some people are angry with God and questioning God. They know we don't have the answers but what they want is for us to be with them in the questioning: to give them the freedom, the permission to question.

Another very difficult dimension of this tragedy, in terms of the grieving process, Father Kelly pointed out, was the absence of remains for so many victims' families.

> Physical remains give us a sense of how someone died. In the initial weeks there were a number of people living in hope; they were sustained by a belief that "my loved one is trapped in a void. There are a lot of cafeterias, so he's in a cafeteria and has food and water; he's safe." But at the end of two weeks, the operation seemed to move from rescue to recovery and there was little hope of survivors. There was some controversy over it but finally the city

decided to issue death certificates for those who were missing; some families didn't want to come and pick them up because it was the end of hope.

Finally, Father Kelly observed that to be a compassionate minister in a disaster such as that of the World Trade Center attack, "you have to walk a fine line; to be able to grieve with those you serve yet not break down completely. You must exercise some boundaries or compassion fatigue can creep up. Some of the survivors will tell you that they just don't know if they can cope. I tell them if you can just borrow some of my strength, I know you can make it. I have faith in you. I have no doubt you will survive with time."

Father Kelly concluded his sharing with an assessment of the firefighters' spiritual mission. "Firefighters are physically very strong, very fit but their gift is compassion. They have selected a profession where the primary and most important skill is to save people, and they fight fires too. But the most important concern of any fireman fighting a fire is are there any people trapped inside. They are there to save lives; there is great sensitivity. They have a compassion orientation."

The Firefighters

On that fateful day, life changed for everyone in America; but for none more than for the citizens of New York City; and surely for none more than the renowned FDNY, the Fire Department of New York City. The entire country cried and grieved and prayed with the victims and their families. As a colleague from the Midwest said in a phone call on the afternoon of September 11, "Today we are all New Yorkers!" On September 11, the world witnessed, in horror, the absolute, unmitigated evil of the terrorist destruction of the World Trade Center; on September 11, the world also witnessed, in awe, the absolute, unmitigated goodness of the hundreds of New York City firefighters and police officers who rushed into the towering inferno in the hope of saving at least some of the thousands of men and women trapped in the burning building. A *Newsweek* report described the scene immediately after the attack. "Scores of firemen were pouring in [to the Trade Center] . . . the men were climbing the stairs under staggering loads of state of the art gear . . . helmets . . . turnout coats . . . boots . . . compressed air cylinders for breathing . . . radios . . . and assorted axes and hand tools [that] weighed between 80 and 100 pounds per man" (Thomas, 2001/2002, p. 54).

Initially, those at the site hoped that the buildings would remain standing. When the towers collapsed, they took with them not only thousands of World Trade Center workers but also hundreds of firefighters who were so bravely climbing the stairs in search of survivors. Many deaths, especially those of the uniformed officers of the New York City Police Department and the New York City Port Authority, occurred in the midst of great courage and caring. The details of a multitude of brave rescues and rescue attempts, carried out by both police officers and civilians, have been documented; many others remain known only to God, who has now welcomed these courageous men and women into His loving arms. By far, however, the greatest loss of life among uniformed rescuers occurred within the heroic ranks of the Fire Department of the City of New York. In that one rescue effort, 343 firefighters were lost, including 21 fire station captains; 19 battalion chiefs; 46 lieutenants; 251 firefighters; the fire department chaplain, Father Judge; a fire marshal; a deputy commissioner; 2 assistant chiefs; and the chief of the FDNY, Chief Peter J. Ganci. New York Mayor Rudolph Giuliani (2001a) described the spiritual commitment of his firefighters. "When firefighters run into a burning building, they don't stop to wonder whether the people inside are rich or poor, what race they are, or what religion they practice. Their thoughts are focused solely on the individuals inside that need to be saved." The mayor concluded poignantly, "Their actions represent the purest example of love for humanity" (p. 8).

Many bodies of these caring and compassionate men were entombed in the smoldering ruins of the disaster site. In the days and weeks following the disaster incident, New York City firefighters worked tirelessly, alongside police officers, EMTs, iron workers, construction engineers, and a variety of other rescue workers, to attempt to retrieve the bodies of their fallen brothers. This was risky and dangerous work because the remaining World Trade Center skeletal structure was unstable and the air was toxic with dust and fumes from the fallen concrete and the fires that smoldered for more than 100 days after the attack. The task was critically important to the New York City firefighters, however, because the firefighter's code is to never leave a fallen brother. The World Trade Center site was never without the presence of New York City firefighters during the weeks and months in which the rescue and recovery efforts were carried out. Twenty-four hours a day, seven days a week, FDNY members kept vigil over the place, the "sacred ground," where the bodies of so many of their brother firefighters, "New York's bravest," rested beneath the enormous pile of rock and rubble. The need to find a spiritual dimension to the horror of the disaster, especially for those involved in the recovery efforts, was evident from the beginning of the work. One powerful spiritual symbol embodied in the ruins was a 20-foot cross, which had evolved naturally out of the intersection of two fallen beams, part of the wounded World Trade Center steel structure. "This cross," it was noted, became "a startling witness to faith for hundreds of thousands of people who were deeply grieved by the terrorist attack" (Groeschel, 2001b, p. 13). A chaplain offered a blessing of the cross and prayed with the workers at its foot.

It was reported that FDNY's engine 54 "sent fifteen men to the first call for help; none returned. The forty-five firefighters left behind worked 24-hour shifts and returned to the attack site on their own time to search for their comrades" (McBride, 2001, p. 15). In reflecting on the behavior of his firefighters after September 11, Mayor Rudolph Giuliani (2001b) explained the firefighters' spiritual philosophy and mission. "It is human instinct to run away from a fire. Firefighters train themselves to run toward fire, determined to save . . . lives" (p. xvi); and Fire Commissioner Thomas Von Essen (2001) described the FDNY as a family: ". . . a family of men and women linked by a unique bond and a noble calling: to save lives at whatever cost" (p. xix). It is important to remember that, as well as the professional and human commitment to save lives and fight fires, the "legal responsibility for the command of a disaster scene usually rests with the Fire Chief and his officers" (Brown, 1985, p. 51). At the World Trade Center disaster, one of the first firefighters lost was the courageous and respected FDNY Chief, Peter J. Ganci, who was reportedly in the center of the disaster scene providing leadership and support for his men when the first building collapsed.

So many brave firefighters were lost . . . so many stories warrant telling. One exquisitely beautiful and yet heartbreaking account of the disaster's impact on the FDNY is reflected in the book *Brotherhood* (Hendra, 2001). Included in *Brotherhood* are pictures of all of the New York City firehouses that lost members at the World Trade Center site. The fronts of many fire stations were turned into religious shrines by neighbors who left flowers, candles, prayer cards, pictures, and statues to honor the dead and the missing. The firefighters' personal spirituality is reflected over and over in the messages they, themselves, posted over fire station doors. Some examples include Rescue 4, Engine 292: "Pray for Our Brothers" (nine names of missing firefighters are listed); Squad 18 FDNY: "We Pray and Hope for Our Brothers" (the names of seven firefighters follow); Engine 290, Ladder 103: "God Bless Our Heroes; Gone But Not Forgotten" (nine firefighters' names are identified); Engine 165, Ladder 85: "To All Our Lost Brothers; Forever Rest in Peace. God Bless You"; FDNY Engine 23: "We Are Missing the Following Members (six firefighters' names listed)—Please Keep Them in Your Prayers"; Engine 230: "Please Say a Prayer for Our 6 Missing Brothers"; and Engine 37, Ladder 4: "God Bless Our FDNY Brothers." Many of the signs thanked the neighbors for their care, their support, and their prayers. The firefighters at Engine 37, Ladder 4, added a touching comment; after thanking the community for their support, the sign concluded with the words: "We Are Still Here for You!" (Hendra, 2001).

The Police Officers

NYPD, the New York City Police Department, proudly referred to as "New York's Finest," lost 23 of its members in the World Trade Center disaster. While overshadowed in numbers by the FDNY mortality, the loss of that many officers in one incident was a grievous assault to the NYPD; and, of course, to the loved ones they left behind. One New York police officer interviewed several months after the attack commented, "I pray more now but I don't ask for anything; I just say 'thank you' for being alive!"

I was able to speak with an NYPD officer who, although not at the World Trade Center site on September 11, had worked with victims and families in Manhattan immediately after the attack and later at the Staten Island recovery landfill. Officer Kevin O'Connor, who also has a brother in the NYPD, was off-duty at the time of the attack; as with the firefighters, he immediately reported to duty. Officer O'Connor's role in the first days following the disaster was to assist several local hospitals to help with family notification as patients were coming in, and to work with family members in taking missing person reports. Officer O'Connor admitted that, although he knew the work he was doing was important for the victims' families, it was difficult not to be down at the site. "You want to be down there helping out. I mean, there could be people trapped that you want to help but with the police department, you don't know what else is going to happen so you have to do other things too." Officer O'Connor noted that an NYPD buddy also shared a similar desire. "We both were going through the same thing; like you want to be down there helping out; we should be down there digging. You want to be in the heart of it."

A site had been set up for family members to come and report missing loved ones, and Officer O'Connor commented that having a social worker there to work with the families was helpful; he added, "I've been doing this for 18 years and you just try to be as consoling as you can."

A part of Officer O'Connor's investigation did take him to the World Trade Center site in the early days and he described his initial reaction. "I remember the first time I went down there, it was nighttime with the lights all lit up; it looked like a movie set. I mean, it was so huge, and to see all those guys working, it was like 'Holy Smokes,' this is unbelievable!" I suggested to Officer O'Connor that he must see a lot as an officer with the NYPD; his response was simply, "This tops anything I've seen before!" He also commented on the gratitude of New Yorkers for the police, firefighters, and other rescue workers. "You see people cheering along the road for all the workers. It was a travesty but I tell you, you saw New York coming together. We got donations at the police stations, the firehouses; there was stuff coming in to go down to the site, because the cops were doing 12 hour tours, 7 days a week. You really didn't have time to go home, so people were sending in all kinds of stuff: food, toothbrushes, toothpaste, change of clothes, shampoo. Soup to nuts, you name it. What we needed, we got it. There were just tables full of stuff."

After Officer O'Connor acknowledged the support of the New York citizens, I commented that the entire country had, in effect, laid a mantle of heroism on the NYPD and FDNY for their response to the World Trade Center attacks; I suggested that they probably did not, however, walk around feeling like "heroes." Officer O'Connor just gently replied, "Nah!"

In the later weeks after the terrorist attack, Officer O'Connor's role was to work with sometimes as many as 500 other NYPD officers at the Staten Island landfill where the debris from the World Trade Center site was taken for processing and investigation. The officers were still looking for body parts and/or crime scene objects such as the black box from the hijacked aircraft. Officer O'Connor did not complain about the mission but when I asked if the work was difficult, he did admit that "As dreary as the site is, the landfill is just as dreary a place. It's a dreary place to be. You do 12 hour shifts; you go and leave in the dark." He added, "The first couple of weeks it was set up with army tents; you would have thought it was Desert Storm." Officer O'Connor observed that the presence of the Salvation Army was helpful because they cooked for the recovery teams; he also said he had met several chaplains who were providing a spiritual presence at the landfill.

I asked Officer O'Connor if personal spirituality was helpful to him and his family coping with the World Trade Center disaster; he replied:

> Oh, sure. We're Roman Catholic and we go to church every Sunday. My [8-year-old] daughter goes to Catholic school and I know some kids in her school lost parents. The religion helps when we talk to her and the school helped. She's very smart and the day it happened she knew about it and she knows that her daddy is a police officer but she said: 'Oh my daddy is [on vacation].' She knew I wasn't there. But it is a concern of hers; she's brought it up a couple times, and not that we don't want her to know about it [the attack] but we try to make it that it is not something she has to be worried about; that's for us as parents to worry about and we wouldn't let anything happen to her.

A last question I had for Officer O'Connor was whether counseling or debriefing groups, such as CISD, would be helpful to him. He replied that "talking to people that are going through the same emotions that you are is helpful; it helps to hear that somebody else has the same things going through their mind that you do. The buddy that I traveled with that day [September 11], we were going through the same things; we wanted to be down there to help."

In summary, I believe that Officer Kevin O'Connor's response to the World Trade Center disaster modeled that of many other officers and firefighters in primarily wanting to "be there" to help others; yet, also, of being willing to "carry on" with whatever tasks were assigned, as part of the overall commitment of service reflected in the commonly used descriptor of the NYPD as "New York's Finest."

A Prayer for Police Officers

Dear Father in heaven, guide and protect Your beloved police officers
who daily risk their lives in the service of those in need. Grant them

strength in conflict, courage in danger, and compassion for those who suffer. Hold all police officers in Your loving arms, Dear Lord, for they are truly Your own. Bless these brave men and women whose call to serve preserves the peace and justice of our world. Amen.

The Nurses

Because the number of living casualties was, sadly, not great, much of the nursing of survivors was carried out by regular hospital staff nurses, especially those working in burn and surgical intensive care units, both in New York and Washington, DC. One trauma nurse from St. Vincent's Hospital in New York commented that the unit was much less busy than she expected, "the victims just didn't have a chance to get out" (Ostrowski, 2001, p. 36). Overall, "St. Vincent's treated 264 patients in the first hours after the attack; 51 were in critical condition" (Ostrowski, 2001, p. 36). Some volunteer nurses and EMTs were involved in caregiving at both disaster sites. Pamela Charles (2001), a pediatric oncology nurse visiting New York on September 11, provided basic first aid at the World Trade Center site, especially the washing of rescue workers' eyes and treating cuts and burns in the hours immediately after the attack. One young firefighter broke into tears and told her that he had just lost his whole unit; she reported, "All I could do was hug him" (p. 44). Charles (2001) admitted that at first she wondered why a FEMA director had requested three nurses as well as three doctors to come to the site, when he could have had all surgeons. At the end of her tour, she concluded that the FEMA official "understood what traumatized, weary rescue workers needed was caring. And that," she noted, "is what nursing is all about" (p. 44).

Nurses at St. Vincent's opened a Family Support Center the day following the disaster, to provide a place where victims' loved ones could come to try to locate survivors. The center also gathered a group of volunteer mental health professionals to help "people cope with a range of experiences related to the tragedy, from losing a family member to being displaced" ("The Road Back," 2001, p. 94).

Much of the spiritual care provided by nurses immediately after the attack on America will remain known only to those individuals involved in the nurse–patient interactions and to God. Spiritual caring on the part of nurses will continue for these disaster victims and their families for years, however, as the long-term stress reactions influence the lives and functioning of many of their patients.

Now, as we have passed the 10th anniversary of the devastating 9/11 attack on America, the case study articles by nurses involved in caring for survivors have dwindled. More contemporary disaster nursing literature has begun to focus on the tremendous medical and nursing caregiving needs engendered by Hurricane Katrina, which devastated the city of New Orleans and several other Gulf Coast regions in the fall of 2005. Joyce Martin (2006), a family nurse practitioner working in a 120-bed hospital in "the oldest part of New Orleans," documented her experience in an article entitled "Riding out Hurricane Katrina." Martin admitted at one point, "I cried, feeling hopeless and abandoned. 'Where is God?' I asked" (p. 37). In the end, however, her personal spirituality and biblical faith in Psalm 107 supported her. "Then they cried unto the Lord in their trouble and he delivered them out of their distresses. And he led them forth by the right way, that they might go to a city of habitation." Listening to those words, Martin observed, she knew that "God had not abandoned us" (p. 37).

▸ Spiritual Needs of Post–9/11 Survivors and Witnesses

It has taken some time and some distance from the 9/11 attacks on America for psychologists and health-care providers to study and publish findings related to spiritual needs and the impact of spirituality and/or religion on survivors of and witnesses to the trauma. Ai, Evans-Campbell, Aisenberg, and Cascio (2006) explored how styles of spiritual or religious coping affected the reaction to 9/11 among 457 college students. These researchers reported that "students sought meaning and answers to existential questions via religious/spiritual means even though many were not active participants in formalized religious practices" (p. 34). This finding, the authors assert, "can point to particular treatment modalities which may support an individual's coping with trauma" (p. 34). At the other end of the life-span age spectrum, Monahan and Lurie (2007) employed focus groups to study the reactions of 24 senior citizens to the 9/11 trauma; the seniors ranged from 65 to 87 years of age. In their discussions the group members "raised the issue of spirituality and how (for some) traumatic events questioned their belief systems while others turned to their beliefs for strength" (p. 36).

A national survey of 890 individuals was undertaken to explore the relationship between spirituality and religiosity and physical and mental health after the 9/11 attacks (McIntosh, Poulin, Silver, & Holman, 2011). It was reported that after three years, and employing "numerous controls, religiosity and spirituality were independently and differentially related to mental and physical health. Both predicted positive affect, and neither predicted cardiovascular ailments. Religiosity alone predicted fewer mental health ailments . . . spirituality alone predicted fewer infectious ailments" (p. 505). And, in a study of firefighters who participated in the post–9/11 recovery process, it was found that there was a significant spiritual need associated with the task of finding bodies (Kelly, 2011). The study author considers this need to find the bodies of friends and loved ones "in light of the gospel accounts of the disciples' contact with the resurrected body of Jesus" (p. 516) and describes "the need for sensory contact with the loved body . . . as a crucial element in the process of grief" (p. 516).

Owens, Schieffler, and Kahn (2011) reflected on healing and hope related to the impact of Hurricane Katrina, considering the 9/11 trauma as a backdrop. The authors accept that "healing is not immediate; it takes time and is a process," however, they also observe that "religion has provided rituals and ceremonies to assist in the healing process for millennia" (p. 477). In a religious context, it is noted, "the goal of healing is to assist the individual and community to come to terms with traumatic events and to experience the closure that is needed to continue beyond traumatic events" (p. 477).

Finally, it is important to remember that individuals bereaved due to a traumatic death often have unique spiritual and/or religious needs. Chapple, Swift, and Ziebland (2011) conducted interviews with 40 people bereaved through violent or traumatic incidents that happened to loved ones. The qualitative interviews revealed that while some people "said that after the death they felt angry or cynical about religion . . . many people turned to spirituality or religion for help" (p. 1). Those who turned to religion reported that "through spirituality or religion they found practical support, comfort, help in making sense of what had happened, belief in continued existence beyond death, a way of ensuring 'continuing bonds' and healing" (p. 1).

▶ Spirituality and International Terrorism

During recent decades, acts of international terrorism "have become an unfortunate reality worldwide" (Tuchner, Meiner, Parush, & Hartman-Maier, 2010, p. 29); devastatingly, "bombs aimed at civilian populations are the most common weapons used by terrorists throughout the world" (Alfici, Ashkenazi, & Kessel, 2006, p. 1155). The resultant disasters involve "emergent and unpredictable situations" (Doubler, 2014, p. 6), which can "disrupt a society by provoking intense fear and shattering all sense of personal and community safety" (Murphy, 2010, p. 46). These terrorist-induced disasters may cause loss of life, destruction of property and often interruption in health-care services (Nash, 2015, p. 425). Throughout the world "it is commonly acknowledged that nurses play an integral part" in any disaster response (Veenema et al., 2016, p. 188). Nevertheless, not a great deal is known about nurses' spiritual and ethical preparation for dealing with the health-care emergencies that follow a mass casualty disaster (Johnstone & Turale, 2014), nor about the spiritual concerns and needs of the survivors and their families.

In our contemporary society the threat of such international terrorism is a persistent concern resulting, for some, in continuous or at least intermittent feelings of stress and anxiety. In this 21st-century élan of fear and insecurity many people turn to spirituality and/or religion for consolation and comfort. While traumatic events, such as those experienced in a terrorist-induced disaster, can challenge an individual's faith, they can also strengthen religious beliefs and "lead to an increase in religious activity" (Hussain, Weisaeth, & Heir, 2011, p. 1027). It has been noted that after such devastating occurrences "religious beliefs can develop . . . religion and spiritual beliefs (which) can be helpful in psychological recovery" (Hussain et al., p. 1027).

In one study of disaster survivors it was found that "religious comfort, i.e., maintaining a positive relationship with God, was associated with positive adjustment and even buffered the impact of resource loss" (Cook, Aten, Moore, Hook, & Davis, 2013, p. 360). In one research effort with post-9/11 survivors, religiosity and spirituality were shown to reduce both mental health deficits and physiological ailments (McIntosh, Poulin, Silver, & Holman, 2011, p. 505). Two other studies of the impact of the 9/11 attacks revealed that: survivors displayed "positive mental health and positive spiritual outcomes when embracing spiritual coping attitudes, prayer and attending religious services" (Meisenhelder & Cassem, 2009, p. 218); and, further, that a lessening of anxiety and sense of calm were remarkably related to "the use of positive spiritual coping strategies" (Meisenhelder & Marcum, 2009, p. 46).

As noted earlier in this chapter, the definitions of disaster vary; a recently proposed theory indicates that it is "a threatening or occurring event of such destructive magnitude as to dislocate people, separate families, destroy property and injure or kill people" (Sterling, 2014, p. 60). The two primary kinds of disasters identified are those which are natural and those which are human initiated. Human-initiated disasters "refer to disasters related to human error or human action that cause significant damage to the environment, people or property" (Baack & Alfred, 2013, p. 281). A number of recent human-induced disasters have fallen into the category of terrorist acts.

While there are also a variety of definitions of the term *terrorism*, it is generally understood to consist of a philosophy and resultant behavior in which violence or threatened violence is employed to achieve a particular end. The concept of "international terrorism" is described by the Federal Bureau of Investigation (FBI) in the

United States as consisting of three characteristics: acts dangerous to human life that violate federal or state law, intimidation of a civilian population or government, and transcending of national boundaries by perpetrators (FBI Definitions of Terrorism in the U.S. Code, 2016). The present discussion of spirituality and international terrorism will focus on three contemporary instances of such terrorism: the Boston Marathon Bombings, the Paris Terrorist Attacks, and the Brussel's Multisite Explosions.

The Boston Marathon Bombings

April 15, 2013, was the scheduled day for the famous Boston Marathon to take place in that city. As well as providing an opportunity for runners with myriad abilities to test their skills, the marathon welcomed a variety of onlookers, among them families with young children, retirees, and visitors to the area. Security was in place but a police presence was not unduly visible and the early part of the marathon went off without incident. After the winner and some of the fastest runners had completed the race, however, two bombs were detonated in immediate proximity to the finish line where crowds of observers had gathered to cheer on the participants. The explosions killed 3 civilians and injured over 200 others; over a dozen of the victims required traumatic amputations. Two Boston hospitals needed to call in emergency personnel to care for the wounded on that Patriot's Day: Massachusetts General Hospital (Hemingway & Ferguson, 2014) and Beth Israel Deaconess Medical Center (Knudson, 2014).

Spiritual and religious attitudes and activities related to the bombings were documented in local and national media reports. Churches of various denominations, in Boston and throughout the country, held worship services to pray for those who had perished as well as for the survivors and their loved ones. Victims of the bombings spoke of the courage of first responders, many of whom were themselves marathon runners or visitors. The spiritual caring reflected in the compassion of individual fellow citizens was frequently applauded by the injured. A universal response manifested by survivors was a strengthening of their faith beliefs even in the midst of suffering. There was also a positive coming together of members of different faith traditions in support of the victims and their families expressed through these various interdenominational prayer and memorial services. Media reporting in the weeks and months after the bombing continued to acknowledge the importance of spiritual and religious beliefs in helping individual survivors, especially amputees, achieve long-term adaptation to the trauma of the experience.

The Paris Terrorist Attacks

For some time the city of Paris had been on a degree of alert to the possibility of another terrorist attack following the January 7, 2015, armed invasion of the *Charlie Hebdo* magazine headquarters as well as a local supermarket. During those attacks 17 people were killed and more than 20 individuals were seriously wounded. As the days after the *Charlie Hebdo* incident passed, a fragile sense of calm seemed to descend on the city. This peace, however, was to be short-lived for on November 13, 2015, a multiplicity of terrorist attacks was leveled on the citizens of Paris.

In the November terrorist attacks, 130 individuals were killed and 368 wounded, some critically (BBC World, 2015). The deaths and injuries were the results of suicide bombers' explosions and armed gunmen shooting randomly at patrons of restaurants, cafés, and a music venue. The most devastating and lethal of the Paris attacks consisted in the armed terrorists entering a crowded social club, blocking the exits, and randomly shooting guests who had come to enjoy an evening of music. During this one terrorist attack, close to 100 Parisians were killed and many more were seriously wounded. The post–attack scene at the music club was described as one of absolute horror and devastation with bodies of the dead and wounded scattered everywhere.

As the entire world watched in anguish, prayer services were immediately initiated at churches of many denominations. Large crowds of people filled the pews of local parishes and congregations to demonstrate their solidarity and sympathy with the citizens of Paris, as well as with all French people and their government. While citizens of the United States, as well as those of many countries, could not be present geographically to comfort the Parisian victims and their families, spiritual support was manifested through attendance at religious services and visits to memorial sites at French embassies across the globe. One U.S. national news anchor noted, in a commentary on the Paris terrorist attacks, that on November 13, 2015, all of us were "French" in heart and in spirit.

The Brussels Multisite Explosions

As a consequence of the 2015 vicious terrorist attacks on the ordinary citizens of Paris, Belgians, especially residents of the capital, Brussels, had been experiencing some anxious days. Many wondered if one of the Belgian cities might be next. Sadly, the feared possibility occurred with two major attacks on Brussels a little over four months later, on March 22, 2016. In these terrorist attacks, 32 Belgian citizens were killed and over 300 injured; two explosions occurred, one at the Brussels airport at Zaventem; the second at the central Brussels Maalbeek metro station (BBC World, 2016).

While the multisite Brussels explosions resulted in fewer victims being directly affected compared to the numbers killed and wounded in Paris, the psychological and spiritual impact on the small country and its citizens was no less devastating. The country had for some time feared the possibility of such terrorism on its own soil and now it had happened. Was there more to come?

As with the Paris attacks, the international community, especially religious organizations represented by a variety of faith traditions, offered prayers of support and sent messages of sympathy for the victims and their families. All services at the Brussels airport were initially shut down following the destruction and death caused by the terrorist explosion. On April 5, however, only a few weeks after the attack, one of the first flights of a Belgian aircraft from Brussels arrived in the United States at Dulles International Airport. To demonstrate the solidarity and care of the American people, the plane was welcomed with a ceremonial water canon salute and a cadre of airport employees lined up on the tarmac waving Belgian flags. One of the Belgian passengers, interviewed by the media, asserted that the warmth of the U.S. reception was both spiritually supportive and greatly appreciated. As with those impacted by the Boston and Paris attacks, Brussels survivors demonstrated amazing spiritual courage in professing their determination to continue to live each day as fully as possible.

Although the innocent citizens touched by the three international terrorist attacks described previously were of different cultures and countries, and held a variety of religious faith beliefs, there were common spiritual needs and spiritual responses to the incidents. For many, physical security was shaken, yet, in the midst of suffering, victims repeatedly expressed gratitude for their caregivers and for the support of many members of the human family who had expressed solidarity and sympathy. Survivors also frequently verbalized their continued religious faith and trust in the goodness of God and of life; this was reflected in multiple national and international media reports.

After a terrorist disaster the immediate response from the health-care community is to care for the wounded and save lives. However, "it is well documented that the real work comes during the period of disaster recovery, helping the individuals affected cope with the psychological consequences and preventing or minimizing complications associated with physical health comorbidities" (Giarratano, Savage, Barcelona-Demendoza, & Harville, 2014, p. 259). In the discussion following a recent study on trauma, faith, and service delivery to victims of international terrorism, the research team noted the importance of spiritual support in helping victims and their families achieve healthy adaptation following a traumatic disaster event. The researchers pointed out that "faith based assessment and helping interventions can serve as vehicles to express God's love, which is important since some victims may (be experiencing) . . . feelings of helplessness, diminished personal control and doubt about their relationships, environment and cultural and belief systems" (Furman et al., 2016, p. 75). In light of this finding, the authors suggested 21 generic, spiritually based, strategies for potential intervention following a terrorist incident. Some of these included: advising victims on the use of spiritual books or writings, praying with and for survivors, encouraging survivors' participation in a spiritual support system or organized religious activity, facilitating attendance at spiritual rituals, suggesting the use of self-reflective journaling, discussing beliefs about what happens after death and making referral to a clergy member or other spiritual advisor if welcomed by the survivor (Furman et al., pp. 87–88).

Many of the identified interventions can be appropriately carried out by nurses caring for post-terrorist attack victims. Not all nurses may or must feel comfortable in providing direct spiritual intervention themselves. It is pointed out, nevertheless, that a nursing assessment of patients' spiritual needs is a professional responsibility. Thus, if appropriate and acceptable to a survivor, a nurse may always make a referral to a trained pastoral care provider of the person's faith if the practitioner identifies a spiritual need and is not comfortable with intervening him- or herself.

This chapter was challenging to write, because the topic of spiritual need in mass casualty disasters is vast and variable. Spiritual needs in the immediate and long-term periods following a disaster are very much related to the particular disaster incident and to the overall needs of the victims and their families. The heart of the chapter is, as noted earlier, focused on the spiritual needs of those involved in the September 11th attack on America. In this updated edition of *Spirituality in Nursing: Standing on Holy Ground* an additional discussion of spirituality and international terrorism has been included centering on three recent events: the Boston Marathon Bombings, the Paris Terrorist Attacks, and the Brussels Multisite Explosions. That topic is also vast and we are only beginning to study the impact of these disasters on those more directly involved as victims, family members, and rescue workers. It is believed, however, that this initial exploration of spiritual need and spiritual care following international terrorist attacks will help nurses caring for all victims of trauma, especially those involved in mass casualty incidents.

▶ References

Ai, A., Evans-Campbell, T., Aisenberg, G., & Cascio, T. (2006). Diverse sociopolitical reactions to the 9/11 attacks and associations with religious coping. *Journal of Religion and Spirituality in Social Work, 25*(2), 19–42.

Alfici, R., Ashkenazi, I., & Kessel, B. (2006). Management of victims in a mass casualty incident caused by a terrorist bombing: Treatment algorithms for stable, unstable, and in extremis victims. *Military Medicine, 171*(12), 1155–1162.

Allen, R. J. (1982). How we respond to natural disaster. *Theology Today, 38*(1), 458–464.

American Red Cross. (1966). *Disaster handbook for physicians and nurses.* Washington, DC: Author.

Atkinson, P., Keylon, K., Odor, P. S., Walker, G., & Hunt, L. (1995). Disaster nursing in the Oklahoma City bombing. *Insight, 20*(3), 30–31.

Baack, S., & Alfred, D. (2013). Nurses' preparedness and perceived competence in managing disasters. *Image, the Journal of Nursing Scholarship, 45*(3), 281–287.

Baker, F. J. (1980). The management of mass casualty disasters. In H. W. Meislin (Ed.), *Priorities in multiple trauma* (pp. 149–157). Germantown, MD: Aspen Systems.

BBC World. (2015, December 9). Retrieved from http://www.bbc.com/news/world/europe-34818994

BBC World. (2016, March 23). Retrieved from http://www.bbc.com/news/world/europe-35

Bolin, R. (1985). Disaster characteristics and psychosocial impacts. In B. J. Sowder (Ed.), *Disasters and mental health: Selected contemporary perspectives* (pp. 3–28). Rockville, MD: National Institutes of Mental Health.

Brown, R. L. (1985). Management and triage at the disaster site. In L. M. Garcia (Ed.), *Disaster nursing: Planning, assessment and intervention* (pp. 45–70). Rockville, MD: Aspen Systems.

Butman, A. M. (1982). *Responding to the mass casualty incident: A guide for EMS personnel.* Akron, OH: Emergency Training.

Cannon, A. (2001). The other tragedy: The attack on the Pentagon left heroes, victims, survivors. *U.S. News & World Report, 131*(24), 20–32.

Chapple, A., Swift, C., & Ziebland, S. (2011). The role of spirituality and religion for those bereaved due to traumatic death. *Mortality, 16*(1), 1–19.

Charles, P. (2001). What I learned at ground zero. *RN, 64*(12), 42–44.

Chester, D. K. (1998). The theodicy of natural disasters. *Scottish Journal of Theology, 51*(4), 485–505.

Chinnici, R. (1985). Pastoral care following a natural disaster. *Pastoral Psychology, 33*(2), 245–254.

Christopher, M. A., & McConnell, K. (1994). Community health nursing: Shelter from the storm. *Caring, 13*(1), 37–39.

Church World Service. (2001a). *Bringing God's peace to disaster.* New York, NY: Author.

Church World Service. (2001b). *Bringing God's presence to survivors.* New York, NY: Author.

Church World Service. (2001c). *Cooperative faith-based disaster recovery in New York.* New York, NY: Author.

Clark, M. J. (1999). *Nursing in the community.* Stamford, CT: Appleton & Lange.

Clinebell, H. (1991). *Basic types of pastoral care and counseling.* Nashville, TN: Abingdon Press.

Coffman, S. (1994). Children describe life after Hurricane Andrew. *Pediatric Nursing, 20*(4), 363–368; 375.

Cohen, R. E., & Ahearn, F. L. (1980). *Handbook for mental health care of disaster victims.* Baltimore, MD: The Johns Hopkins University Press.

Cohn, R. L. (1986). Biblical response to catastrophe. *Judaism, 35*(3), 263–276.

Cook, S. W., Aten, J. D., Moore, M., Hook, J. N., & Davis, D. E. (2013). Resource, loss, religiousness, health and posttraumatic growth following Hurricane Katrina. *Mental Health, Religion and Culture, 16*(4), 352–366.

Cullinan, A. (1993). Spiritual care of the traumatized: A necessary component. In K. J. Doka & J. D. Morgan (Eds.), *Death and spirituality* (pp. 227–242). Amityville, NY: Baywood Publishing Company.

Damian, F., Atkinson, C., Bouchard, A., Harrington, S., & Powers, T. (1997). Disaster relief efforts after Hurricane Marilyn: A pediatric team's experience in St. Thomas. *Journal of Emergency Nursing, 23*(6), 545–549.

Danna, D., & Cordray, S. (2010). *Nursing in the storm: Voices from Hurricane Katrina.* New York, NY: Springer Publishing Company.

Davidson, M. (2001). Not-so-frightening facts about posttraumatic stress disorder. *Nursing Spectrum, 11*(24), 10–11.

Demi, A., & Miles, M. S. (1984). An examination of nursing leadership following a disaster. *Topics in Clinical Nursing, 6*(1), 63–78.

Dodds, B. (2001). *Your grieving child.* Huntington, IN: Our Sunday Visitor Publications.

Doubler, A. (2014). Exploring the laws and ethics with disaster nursing. *Ohio Nurses Review, 89*(2), 6–7.

Dudley, C. S., & Schoonover, M. E. (1993). After the hurricane: Pastoral lessons from Andrew. *Christian Century, 110*(6), 588–590.

Egan, E. C. (2001). Homily at the Mass for deceased police officers, firefighters, healthcare and emergency service workers. In B. J. Groeschel (Ed.), *The cross at ground zero* (pp. 129–135). Huntington, IN: Our Sunday Visitor.

Ericksen, C., Ericksen, M., & Painter, S. (2012). No time to fear: New nurse assists patients following Joplin tornado. *Journal of Christian Nursing, 29*(1), 38–39.

FBI definitions of terrorism in the U.S. Code. (2016). Retrieved from http://www.fbi.gov/about-us /investigate/terrorism/terrorisn-definition

Foy, D. A., Drescher, K. D., Fitz, A. G., & Kennedy, K. R. (1993). Posttraumatic stress disorder. In R. J. Wicks & R. D. Parsons (Eds.), *Clinical handbook of pastoral counseling* (Vol. 2, pp. 621–637). Mahwah, NJ: Paulist Press.

Fullerton, C. S., & Ursano, R. J. (Eds.). (1997). Posttraumatic responses in spouse/significant others of disaster workers. In *Posttraumatic stress disorder: Acute and long-term responses to trauma and disaster* (pp. 59–75). Washington, DC: American Psychiatric Press.

Furman, L. D., Benson, P. W., Moss, B., Danbolt, T., Vetvik, E., & Canda, E. (2016). Reflections on collective trauma, faith, service delivery to victims of terrorism and natural disaster: Insights from six national studies. *Social Work and Christianity, 43*(1), 74–94.

Garb, S., & Eng, E. (1969). *Disaster handbook* (2nd ed.). New York, NY: Springer Publishing Company.

Garcia, L. M. (Ed.). (1985). *Disaster nursing: Planning, assessment and intervention.* Rockville, MD: Aspen Systems.

Gardner, S. S. (1985). Skills in rapid field assessment. In L. M. Garcia (Ed.), *Disaster nursing: Planning, assessment and intervention* (pp. 17–43). Rockville, MD: Aspen Systems.

Giarratano, G., Savage, J., Barcelona-deMendoza, V., & Harville, E. (2014). Disaster research: A nursing opportunity, *21*(3), 259–268.

Giuliani, R. W. (2001a). Introduction. In R. Sullivan (Ed.), *In the land of the free: September 11 and after* (pp. 6–10). New York, NY: Life.

Giuliani, R. W. (2001b). Prologue. In T. Hedra (Ed.), *Brotherhood* (pp. xv–xvi). New York, NY: American Express Publishing Corporation.

Golway, T. (2001). An advent of mourning. *America, 185*(18), 6.

Groeschel, B. J. (2001a). Divine mercy at ground zero. In J. Farina (Ed.), *Beauty for ashes: Spiritual reflections on the attack on America* (pp. 242–250). New York, NY: Crossroad.

Groeschel, B. J. (2001b). *The cross at ground zero.* Huntington, IN: Our Sunday Visitor.

Hanson, C., Jesz, B. L., & Baldwin, S. S. (1991). The American Red Cross: A nursing oriented overview of services. *Journal of Emergency Nursing, 17*(6), 390–394.

Hartsough, D. M. (1985). Effects of stress on disaster workers. In D. M. Hartsough & D. G. Myers (Eds.), *Disaster work and mental health: Prevention and control of stress among workers* (pp. 27–34). Rockville, MD: National Institutes of Mental Health.

Hassmiller, S. B. (2000). Disaster management. In M. Stanhope & J. Lancaster (Eds.), *Community and public health nursing* (pp. 400–415). St. Louis, MO: Mosby.

Hemingway, M., & Ferguson, J. (2014). Boston bombings: Response to disaster. *AORN Journal, 99*(2), 277–288.

Hendra, T. (2001). *Brotherhood*. New York, NY: American Express Publishing Corporation.

Hodgkinson, P. E., & Stewart, M. (1998). *Coping with catastrophe, a handbook of post-disaster psychological aftercare* (2nd ed.). London, England: Routledge.

Horner, D., Pfeifer, D., & Clunn, P. (1994). In the wake of Hurricane Andrew: The development of a community-based primary care center. *Nursing and Health Care, 15*(2), 61–63.

Hulden, J. (1997). The Red River rises. *Sojourners, 26*(4), 31.

Hussain, A., Weisaeth, L., & Heir, T. (2011). Changes in religious beliefs and the relation of religiosity to posttraumatic stress and life satisfaction after a natural disaster. *Social Psychiatry and Psychiatric Epidemiology, 46*(10), 1027–1032.

Janoff-Bulman, R. (1985). The aftermath of victimization: Rebuilding shattered assumptions. In

C. R. Figley (Ed.), *Trauma and its wake* (pp. 15–35). New York, NY: Brunner/Mazel Publishers.

Johnstone, M., & Turale, S. (2014). Nurses' experiences of ethical preparedness for public health emergencies and healthcare disasters: A systematic review of qualitative evidence. *Nursing and Health Sciences, 16*(1), 67–77.

Jordan, C. (1976). Pastoral care and chronic disaster victims: The Buffalo Creek experience. *The Journal of Pastoral Care, 30*(3), 159–171.

Kelly, K. (2011). Bereavement, doubt and the loved body: A 9/11 meditation. *Journal of Religion and Health, 50*(1), 516–520.

Kennedy, E. (2001). Ancient rituals of grief must not be hurried. *National Catholic Reporter, 38*(5), 17.

Kennedy, E., & Charles, S. C. (2001). *On becoming a counselor*. New York, NY: Crossroad.

Killough, W. B. (2005). Acknowledging spiritual dynamics during trauma care. *Topics in Emergency Medicine, 27*(3), 183–185.

Klink, T. W. (1966). Pastoral work in a disaster: Debriefing with comments. *The Journal of Pastoral Care, 20*(2), 194–200.

Knudson, L. (2014). Hospital preparedness for a mass casualty event. *AORN Connections, 100*(3), 1–10.

Kroll-Smith, J. S., & Couch, S. R. (1987). A chronic technical disaster and the irrelevance of religious meaning: The case of Centralia, Pennsylvania. *Journal for the Scientific Study of Religion, 26*(1), 25–37.

Kropf, R. W. (1988). National disaster or "act of God"? The search for the missing link in theodicy. *Dialogue & Alliance, 2*(1), 57–65.

Kushner, H. S. (1981). *When bad things happen to good people*. New York, NY: Avon Books.

Langan, J., & Palmer, J. (2012). Listening to and learning from older adult Hurricane Katrina survivors. *Public Health Nursing, 29*(2), 126–135.

Lundy, K. S., & Butts, J. B. (2001). The role of the community health nurse in disasters. In K. S. Lundy & S. Janes (Eds.), *Community health nursing: Caring for the public's health* (pp. 546–573). Sudbury, MA: Jones & Bartlett Learning.

Mahoney, R. F. (1969). *Emergency and disaster nursing* (2nd ed.). Ontario, Canada: Macmillan.

Marmar, C. R., & Horowitz, M. J. (1988). Diagnosis and phase-oriented treatment of post-traumatic stress disorder. In J. P. Wilson, Z. Harel, & B. Kahana (Eds.), *Human adaptation to extreme stress* (pp. 81–103). New York, NY: Plenum Press.

Martin, J. (2001a). The laying down of life (at the World Trade Center). *America, 185*(9), 7–9.

Martin, J. (2001b). World Trade Center Journal. *America, 185*(10), 28–29.

Martin, J. (2006). Riding out Hurricane Katrina. *Journal of Christian Nursing, 23*(2), 34–37.

McBride, J. (2001). Kindness at ground zero. In J. Waldman (Ed.), *America September 11th: The courage to give* (pp. 9–15). Berkeley, CA: Conari Press.

McCarroll, J. E., Ursano, R. J., & Fullerton, C. S. (1997). Exposure to traumatic death in disaster and war. In C. S. Fullerton & J. R. Ursano (Eds.), *Posttraumatic stress disorder: Acute and long-term responses to trauma and disaster* (pp. 37–58). Washington, DC: American Psychiatric Press.

McIntosh, D., Poulin, M., Silver, R., & Holman, E. (2011). The distinct roles of spirituality and religiosity in physical and mental health after collective trauma: A national longitudinal study of responses to the 9/11 attacks. *Journal of Behavioral Medicine, 34*, 497–507.

Meisenhelder, J. B., & Marcum, J. P. (2009). Terrorism, posttraumatic stress, coping strategies and spiritual outcomes. *Journal of Religion and Health, 48*(1), 46–57.

Mickelson, A. S., Bruno, L., & Schario, M. E. (1999). The City of New Orleans Amtrak train disaster: One emergency department's experience. *Journal of Emergency Nursing, 25*(5), 367–372.

Mitchell, J. T. (1986). Healing the helper. In Center for Mental Health Studies of Emergencies (Ed.), *Role stressors and supports for emergency workers* (pp. 105–118). Rockville, MD: National Institutes of Mental Health.

Monahan, K., & Lurie, A. (2007). Reactions of senior citizens to 9/11: Exploration and practice guidelines for social workers. *Social Work in Health Care, 45*(1), 33–47.

Moody, J., & Carr, C. (1996). After the hurricane. *The Christian Ministry, 27*(1), 25–27.

Murnion, P. J. (2001a). Bleecker & Elizabeth. *Church, 17*(4), 2.

Murnion, P. J. (2001b). *Reflections from WTC morgue site*, 15 October, 2001 (Unpublished report cited with permission of the author).

Murphy, S. A. (2010). Women's and children's exposure to mass disaster and terrorist attacks. *Issues in Mental Health Nursing, 31*(1), 45–53.

Nabbe, F. C. (1961). *Disaster nursing*. Paterson, NJ: Littlefield, Adams & Company.

Nash, T. J. (2015). Unveiling the truth about nurses' personal preparedness for disaster response: A pilot study. *MEDSURG Nursing, 24*(6), 425–431.

Neal, M. V. (1963). *Disaster nursing preparation*. New York, NY: National League for Nursing.

Newburn, T. (1993). *Disaster and after*. London, England: Jessica Kingsley Publishers.

Nightingale, F. (1854). To Caroline Fleidner, December 1854. Cited in B. M. Dossey (2000). *Florence Nightingale: Mystic, visionary, healer*. Springhouse, PA: Springhouse Corporation.

O'Brien, M. E. (1992). *Living with HIV: Experiment in courage*. Westport, CT: Auburn House.

Ostrowski, M. (2001). Terrorism at home: A nurse's view from ground zero. *RN, 64*(11), 35–37.

Owens, D., Schieffler, D., & Kahn, M. (2011). Healing and hope in the midst of devastation: Reflections on Katrina in the aftermath of September 11. *Journal of Religion and Health, 50*, 477–480.

Pedraja, L. G. (1997). In harm's way: Theological reflections on disasters. *Quarterly Review, 17*(1), 5–24.

Reed, J. P. (1977). The pastoral care of victims of major disaster. *The Journal of Pastoral Care, 31*(2), 97–108.

Reichsmeier, J. L., & Miller, J. K. (1985). Psychological aspects of disaster situations. In L. M. Garcia (Ed.), *Disaster nursing: Planning, assessment and intervention* (pp. 185–202). Rockville, MD: Aspen Systems.

The road back: A new center in New York's Greenwich Village helps people to cope with the World Trade Center attack. (2001). *American Journal of Nursing, 101*(11), 94.

Snyder, A., Terzioglu, F., & Keeling, A. (2011). Striving for the "new normal": The aftermath of international disasters. In B. Wall & A. Keeling (Eds.) *Nurses on the front line: When disaster strikes* (pp. 253–264). New York, NY: Springer.

Sterling, Y. M. (2014). Nursing caring during catastrophic events: Theoretical, research and clinical insights. *International Journal of Human Caring, 18*(1), 60–65.

Stover, S. (2001). God was there. In *In the line of duty, a tribute to New York's finest and bravest* (p. 79). New York, NY: Regan Books.

Sullivan, R. (Ed.). (2001). In the land of the free: September 11 and after. Special issue. *Life: A commemorative, 1*(8), 1–128.

Switzer, K. H. (1985). Disaster planning: Assessing and using community resources. In L. M. Garcia (Ed.), *Disaster nursing: Planning, assessment and intervention* (pp. 307–344). Rockville, MD: Aspen Systems.

Taggert, S. B. (1985). Background and historical perspective. In L. M. Garcia (Ed.), *Disaster nursing: Planning, assessment and intervention* (pp. 1–16). Rockville, MD: Aspen Systems.

Tait, C., & Spradley, B. (2001). Communities in crisis: Disasters, group violence and terrorism. In J. A. Allender & B. W. Spradley (Eds.), *Community health nursing: Concepts and practice* (pp. 391–407). Philadelphia, PA: Lippincott.

Terrell, K., & Perry, J. (2001). The day the web was a lifeline. *U.S. News & World Report, 131*(15), 67.

Thomas, E. (2001/2002). The day that changed America. Special issue. *Newsweek* (December 31, 2001–January 7, 2002), 40–71.

Toole, D. C. (1999). Divine ecology and the apocalypse: A theological description of natural disasters and the environmental crisis. *Theology Today, 55*(1), 547–561.

Tuchner, M., Meiner, Z., Parush, S., & Hartman-Maeir, A. (2010). Relationships between sequelae of injury, participation and quality of life in survivors of terrorist attacks. *OTJR: Occupation, Participation and Health, 30*(1), 29–38.

Urden, L. (2012). Caring for the critically ill patient. In L. Urden, K. Stacy, & M. Lough (Eds.), *Priorities in critical care nursing* (pp. 1–7). St. Louis: Mosby.

Vitullo-Martin, J. (2001). Firefighters and cops: What provoked the shuffle? *Commonweal, 128*(20), 8.

Veenema, T., Griffin, A., Gable, A., Macintyre, L., Simons, N., Couig, M., Walsh, J., Lavin, R., Dobalian, A., & Larson, E. (2016). Nurses as leaders in disaster preparedness and response-A call to action. *Image, the Journal of Nursing Scholarship, 48*(2), 187–200.

Von Essen, T. (2001). Foreword. In T. Hedra (Ed.), *Brotherhood* (p. xix). New York, NY: American Express Publishing Corporation.

Walhout, M. F., Tubergen, C. R., & Cook, K. J. (1998). Multiple accident victims, all elderly: Would our disaster plan be up to the challenge? *Nursing, 28*(11), 56–60.

Walsh, F. (2007). Traumatic loss and major disasters: Strengthening family and community resilience. *Family Process, 46*(2), 207–225.

Weinrich, S., Hardin, S. B., & Johnson, M. (1990). Nurses respond to Hurricane Hugo: Victims' disaster stress. *Archives of Psychiatric Nursing, 4*(3), 195–205.

When the tornado hit Worcester: Heroic nurses play vital role. (1953). *The Catholic Nurse, 2*(1), 43–45.

Williams, T. (1998). Diagnosis and treatment of survivor guilt. In J. P. Wilson, Z. Harel, & B. Kahana (Eds.), *Human adaptation to extreme stress* (pp. 319–336). New York, NY: Plenum Press.

CHAPTER 15

The Spirituality of Servant Leadership in Nursing

The greatest among you must become like the youngest and the leader like the one who serves.

Luke 22:26–27

> Several of the nurses that I work with said that they saw servant leadership and nursing as synonymous.
>
> Caitlin, Nurse Manager of a Palliative Care Department*

> In a nursing vocation, a calling to serve, sometimes you have to extend yourself to do the right thing and be caring and compassionate in that calling. . We had a patient who was dying in the critical care unit, and one of the evening staff was hesitant to let the family members stay because it was past visiting hours. But, as the critical care unit (CCU) supervisor, I said they could stay because it was important; the patient was aware of what was happening. I think you have to cross over and put yourself in the place of the patient and family.
>
> Anne, Supervisor of a Critical Care Unit

---

*Major sections of this chapter have been taken from the following chapters: Chapter 1, "Called to Serve: The Nurse's Vocation of Caring"; Chapter 4, "Nursing's Call to Servant Leadership"; Chapter 5, "A Model of Servant Leadership for Nursing"; and Chapter 8, "The Spirituality of Servant Leadership in Nursing." O'Brien, M. E. (2010). Servant leadership in nursing: Spirituality and practice in contemporary healthcare. Sudbury, MA: Jones & Bartlett Learning. Used with permission of the publisher.

The concept of servant leadership in nursing is both old and new, both ancient and modern. From the beginning of time individuals have been called forth from their societies to serve the needs of the ill and the injured. Nursing's tradition of service is well documented through historical accounts of the lives of nursing leaders from the advent of the pre-Christian and Christian communities, through the Middle Ages and into the post-Reformation era.

In this chapter, the 21st-century concept of servant leadership is examined in terms of its philosophy and behavioral characteristics both generally and in regard to servant leadership's specific relevance for nursing. First, the seminal work of Robert Greenleaf, who popularized the term in 1977, is described. Also included are findings from an extensive examination of current servant leadership literature published by Greenleaf disciples and other students of the subject. The writings of contemporary nursing scholars of servant leadership are reviewed as well. Following this introduction, a nursing research study, identifying and describing the attitudes and behaviors of a cadre of contemporary nurse servant leaders, is described. From the narrative data obtained through open-ended interviews with the nursing leaders, a model of servant leadership for nursing was created.

Since Greenleaf first proposed the notion that a true leader, in any venue, must be a servant of those he or she leads, the concept has been embraced by a number of business and industrial organizations, as well as educational communities. It is only more recently, however, that the practice of servant leadership has captured the attention of health-care institutions, and more specifically of nurses practicing in those facilities. Recent nursing servant leadership articles do, however, strongly support the adoption of servant leadership as the most appropriate leadership philosophy and practice for nursing and health care.

Both nursing history, reflecting the profession's tradition of service, and the attitudes and activities of 21st-century nurses, reveal powerfully the spirituality of servant leadership already existing in the nursing community. Poignant stories of caring and compassion, from the earliest understandings of the needs of the sick to the conceptualization of modern medicine, present an elegant mosaic of servant leadership in nursing. In the following pages, this mosaic is displayed in a rainbow of brilliant hues reflecting the myriad ministries carried out by servant leaders in nursing.

Recently the philosophy of servant leadership has received "growing interest in academia and among clinical healthcare leaders . . . nursing studies in the U.S. show that servant leadership is related to job satisfaction and better performance" among staff (Gunnarsdottir, 2014, p. 53). There is currently a "rising interest in the interrelationship between leadership and spirituality, and unprecedented religious and spiritual diversity are creating new challenges and opportunities for the field of nursing management" (Reimer-Kirkham, Pesut, Swatzky, Cochrane, & Redmond, 2012, p. 1037). It is suggested that when nurse managers embrace principles of servant leadership they can obtain better staff productivity and patient outcomes (Waterman, 2011, p. 24). In essence, servant leadership in nursing is described as: "about being of service to others horizontally, the colleagues you work with every day to help them become the best they can be. It is about developing others, supporting them for success by offering yourself freely as a resource and committed to being there for them when they need you" (Mahon, 2011, p. 5).

▶ Servant Leadership: A Sacred Calling

The contemporary concept of servant leadership was first conceived by Robert K. Greenleaf; his classic book on servant leadership initially having been published in 1977. In posing the question, "Who is the servant-leader?" Greenleaf (1977) answered: "The servant-leader is servant first. . . . It begins with the natural feeling that one wants to serve, to serve first . . . That person is sharply different from one who is leader first . . . The difference manifests itself in the care taken by the servant-first to make sure that other people's highest priority needs are being served" (p. 27). The "best test" of this, Greenleaf asserts, is to pose the questions: "Do those served grow as persons? Do they, while being served, become healthier, wiser, freer, more autonomous, more likely themselves to become servants?" (p. 27). Greenleaf adds: "The natural servant, the person who is servant-first, is more likely to persevere and refine a particular hypothesis on what serves another's highest priority needs than is the person who is leader-first and who later serves out of promptings of conscience or in conformity to normative expectations" (p. 28). Ultimately Robert Greenleaf's position was that a good leader in any organization must, in fact, be a servant first; that is, in his conceptualization, a servant leader.

As noted earlier, over the past several decades, Robert Greenleaf's servant leadership concept has been embraced and operationalized by a number of business and educational institutions and organizations, including some health-care facilities, in the conduct of their corporate management. Numerous books and articles by Greenleaf disciples have been and continue to be published addressing the various aspects of the servant leadership spirit and spirituality (Agosto, 2005; Blanchard & Hodges, 2003, 2005; Hunter, 2004). Distinguished among these scholarly writings are those of Larry C. Spears (2003, 2004a, 2004b). Of significant importance in understanding the concept of servant leadership is Spears's identification of the "Ten Characteristics of the Servant-Leader." In 2003, Spears (2003) reported, "After some years of carefully considering Greenleaf's original writings, I have identified a set of ten characteristics of the servant-leader that I view as being of critical importance to the development of servant-leaders" (p. 16). These characteristics include "listening, empathy, healing, awareness, persuasion, conceptualization, foresight, stewardship, commitment to the growth of people, and building community" (pp. 16–19).

In an article entitled "A Review of Servant Leadership Attributes: Developing a Practical Model" authors Robert F. Russell and A. Gregory Stone (2002) presented an overview of the servant leadership literature with the goal of developing a broad servant leadership model. Larry Spears's 10 characteristics of the servant leader were noted; however, Russell and Stone suggested, based on their literature review, that a group of 20 servant leader attributes might be identified. These included nine functional attributes: "vision, honesty, integrity, trust, service, modeling, pioneering, appreciation of others," and "empowerment" (p. 146). Also included were 11 "accompanying attributes of servant leadership": "communication, credibility, competence, stewardship, visibility, influence, persuasion, listening, encouragement, teaching," and "delegation" (pp. 146–147). Russell and Stone noted that three of Spears's characteristics: listening, persuasion, and stewardship, are included in their list and that others are "incorporated under broader categories" (p. 146).

A number of research studies have been conducted during the past decade exploring such servant leadership topics, including the examination of leadership practices and principles identified by servant leaders (Taylor, Martin, Hutchinson, & Jinks, 2007), which explored 12 categories of leadership: "integrity," " humility," " servanthood," "caring for others," "empowering others," "developing others," "visioning," "goal setting," "leading," "modeling," "team-building," and "shared decision making" (p. 408); a comparison of transformational leadership versus servant leadership (Stone, Russell, & Patterson, 2004); two explorations of the role of values in servant leadership (Russell, 2001; Washington, Sutton, & Field, 2006); construction of two instruments to measure servant leadership characteristics: a servant leadership assessment tool (Dennis & Bocarnea, 2005) and development of a servant leadership scale (Barbuto & Wheeler, 2006); a correlational study of servant leadership, leader trust, and organizational trust (Joseph & Winston, 2005); and a case study of servant leadership at a religiously affiliated educational institution (Winston, 2004).

A research study exploring the role of nurse–midwives as servant-leader care providers for Amish women was conducted by nurse–midwife Victoria L. Wickwire (2006). Employing the framework of servant leader characteristics identified by Larry Spears, Dr. Wickwire developed a "Concept of Care Model" that included the following concepts: "listening (affirmation, engagement); empathy (understanding, acceptance); healing (wholeness and health); awareness (encouragement, interaction); persuasion (building consensus and trust); conceptualization (helping others through change, commitment); foresight (intuitiveness, incorporating lessons of the past); stewardship (decreased misunderstanding, servant caring); commitment to the growth of people (helping ministries, humility in caring); and building community (instilling love, compassion)" (p. 145).

While the concept of servant leadership as originally conceived by Robert Greenleaf is not inherently spiritual or religious in nature, one can indeed locate a human "sacredness" in its underlying philosophy. Servant leadership "begins with the natural feeling that one wants to serve, to serve first" and "the care taken by the servant leader [is] to make sure that other people's highest priority needs are being served" (Greenleaf, 1977, p. 27). Servant leaders are to place others' needs before their own and to serve those over whom they assume leadership. Surely these characteristics of the servant leader bring to mind the scriptural model: "The Son of Man came not to be served but to serve and to give his life as a ransom for many" (Mark 10:45). This conceptualization is validated in writings such as those of servant leadership scholars Ken Blanchard and Phil Hodges (2005) who authored the book *Lead Like Jesus: Lessons from the Greatest Leadership Role Model of All Time*. Blanchard and Hodges (2005) assert that "Jesus modeled the heart of a true servant leader by investing most of his ministry time training and equipping the disciples for leadership" (p. 46). They point out that at the end of his ministry, Jesus told his disciples, "I no longer call you servants . . . I call you friends," because he wanted them to grow into greatness in their discipleship after he went to the Father (p. 46).

Echoing a similar theme is the 2008 book *Black Belt Leader, Peaceful Leader: An Introduction to Catholic Servant Leadership* by counselor and Aikido martial arts sensei Tim Warneka, who presents a global image of servant leadership for the world community. Warneka observed poignantly that "today's world cries out for people who can lead with a global perspective. We need leaders who lead from the heart as well as the mind . . . leaders who can act ethically, intentionally, and with respect . . . Most of all we need leaders who understand that the primary function of a leader is to serve, not to be served" (p. xi).

The 10 principles of servant leadership identified by Tim Warneka (2008) include "(1) Love, (2) Humanity, (3) Right Use of Power, (4) Leadership as Spiritual Practice, (5) Leadership as a Journey of Faith, (6) Building an Embodied Peaceful Presence, (7) Valuing Community, (8) Seeking Personal Transformation, (9) Understanding the Universal, and (10) Lifelong Learning" (p. 32). And, in a recent book on leadership in health care, nursing leaders Tim Porter-O'Grady and Kathy Malloch (2011) speak about the concept of "spiritual intelligence" in leadership; central among the authors' "Ten Spiritual Rules of the Road" is "Prayer as a tool of leadership" (p. 484). "Prayer," the authors explain, "harnesses the spiritual forces within and without to help create the stamina to carry on" (p. 486). Thus it seems that prayer should also be included in the criteria for a committed servant leader of today whose role is to "carry on" in the service of those he or she leads.

When looking at the description of servant leadership as described by Greenleaf; Spears, Russell, and Stone; Blanchard and Hodges; Warneka, and others, one is struck by the relevance that the theory has for professional nursing. The identified characteristics, attributes, and principles of servant leadership seem to read like a list of ideal behavioral characteristics of the contemporary nursing leader. And indeed they are representative of many nursing servant leaders' practice as is clearly demonstrated in the research findings discussed in later sections of this chapter.

▶ Servant Leadership in Nursing

During the past few decades, nurses have written extensively about the various understandings of leadership and leadership theory; nurse authors have written significantly little, however, about the concept of servant leadership. Leadership is defined in a 2008 edition of the book *Nursing in Today's World* as "the ability to guide, motivate and inspire, and to instill vision and purpose" (Ellis & Hartley, p. 471). In order to provide leadership, the authors add, one must "be able to influence the beliefs, opinions and behaviors of others and to persuade others to follow (one's) direction" (p. 471). Leadership is also defined as a "process of influence"; a leader "influences others to move in the direction of achieving goals" (Carroll, 2006, p. 3). Leadership, it is pointed out, is "not limited to people in traditional positions of authority" (p. 3).

In a chapter entitled "Leadership and Followership," nurses Theresa Valiga and Sheila Grossman (2007) identify six leadership competencies that they note are derived from a presentation given by Warren Bennis, an influential scholar of leadership. The competencies, which are not incompatible with the theory of servant leadership, include the following: "Leaders must foster a clear vision with an endowed purpose that is owned by the people involved with the leader . . . Leaders must keep reminding people of what is important . . . Leaders must be optimistic and see possibilities . . . Leaders must create a culture of candor . . . Leaders must mentor others and acknowledge their ideas and accomplishments . . . Good leaders must be in tune to getting results" (p. 9).

In describing leadership as a "peak and perk of professional development" for nurses, Mary Schira (2007) observed that "although a leader may be seen as someone who takes charge during a time of crisis or difficulty, most leaders are individuals who work every day among a group of people to encourage high levels of performance and quality" (p. 290). Schira lists the "characteristics and attributes we value in leaders" as "communication, openness, motivation, vision, passion, risk-taking, environment control," and "shares rewards" (pp. 291–293).

Nursing authors suggest that there is "more than one way" of leading (King & Cunningham, 1995, p. 3); that "leadership behavior impacts staff nurse empowerment, job tension, and work effectiveness" (Laschinger, Wong, McMahon, & Kaufmann, 1999, p. 28); and that leadership is the "key to quality outcomes" in nursing (Perra, 2001, p. 68).

A type of leadership style, somewhat akin to that of servant leadership, which is generally included in the nursing leadership literature, is that of transformational leadership. Transformational leadership theory describes leadership behavior in which "both leaders and followers act on one another to raise their motivation and performance to higher levels" (Carroll, 2006, p. 9). It is pointed out that transformational leadership "depends on the concept of empowerment, in which all parties are allowed to work together, to the best of their ability, to achieve a collective goal. The process transforms both the leader and the follower . . . (and allows for) innovation and change" (p. 9). Some attributes of transformation are identified as "self-knowledge," "authenticity," "expertise," "vision," "flexibility," "shared leadership," "charisma," and "ability to inspire others" (Dossey, 2005, pp. 6–14). In a study of transformational leadership in two different kinds of nursing units, it was found that leaders in "nursing developmental units" demonstrated more transformational leadership behaviors than those in "conventional clinical settings" (Bowles & Bowles, 2000, p. 76). It was concluded that the leaders in nursing developmental units may have been more skilled and have more environmental support for transformational behaviors than those in conventional settings (p. 76).

In discussing the "evolution of leadership in nursing," British nurse manager Nadeem Moiden (2002) observed that as new nursing leadership theories emerge, they are compared with older theories and a "more achieved style of nursing leadership may emerge" (p. 25). Staff nurse Claire Welford (2002) points out that nursing leadership needs to ensure that the workplace will become a place where all participants are positively motivated and "led through change" (p. 11). In order for change to occur, however, nursing leaders will need to "move away from traditional leadership practices and behaviors" (Fedoruk & Pincombe, 2000, p. 20). A theory that could undergird the establishment of a supportive and growth-producing nursing environment is that of servant leadership.

Although the concept of servant leadership described earlier seems most appropriate to explain the desired spirit and practice of leaders in the professional nursing community, there is, as noted, a paucity of nursing literature exploring and/or identifying the concept within professional nursing. In a recent computer search of the extant nursing and allied health literature, only 22 articles were found addressing the practice of servant leadership in nursing; several of these were brief and did not demonstrate how servant leadership might be practiced in the nursing community.

In a one-page commentary on servant leadership in *Professional Nurse*, Stephen Prosser (2002) described the concept of servant leadership generally and identified Spears's 10 characteristics of servant leadership, but did not discuss the relevance of the concept to nursing (p. 238). In another commentary in *Reflections*, the journal of Sigma Theta Tau, president Fay L. Bower (1994), also described Greenleaf's conceptualization of servant leadership and related his leadership style to her understanding of leadership in the honor society of nursing (pp. 4–5). In an article in a 2004 issue of *Patient Care Staffing Report*, entitled "Shared Governance and Servant Leadership Are Drawing Nurses to New Hospital," the chief nursing officer at a newly opened facility is described as expressing her vision of leadership, mentioning that "servant leadership" would be a "watchword" at the hospital; how the concept would be incorporated was not elaborated (Weber, 2004, p. 3).

Related to the report of employing servant leadership in a hospital setting, four other articles were found that also supported the initiation of servant leadership in health-care facilities. In the journal *Health Progress*, it was noted that two hospitals belonging to the Catholic Health Association (CHA) "have developed programs to better integrate servant leadership into their culture" (Yanofchick, 2007, p. 7). A newsletter of a rural medical center highlighted the positive value of implementing a "culture of servant leadership" (Englert, 2007, p. 1). The importance of servant leadership in the long-term care setting was described as "an alternative to the traditional power-based approach" as "it encourages collaboration and valuation of all workers" (Downs, 2007, p. 39). Also, Sarah Mullally, chief nursing officer for England, challenged British nurses to adopt patient-focused leadership styles, one of which was servant leadership. Mullally (2001) observed, "Servant leaders . . . inspire, create collaboration, coach, are consistent, are confirming, promote continuous development and improvement. Servant leaders create matrix organizations and promote reconciliation and have a genuine concern for others. They recognize the possibility of human failure and see discipline as part of the developmental process" (p. 27)

The servant leadership concept applied to organizational health in general was described by Larry Spears (2004b) in an article in *Reflections on Nursing Leadership*, including explanations of his 10 characteristics of the servant leader. Spears noted that "servant leadership truly offers hope and guidance for a new era in human development and a prescription for creating healthy organizations" (p. 26); and the British journal *Nursing Management* published a paper entitled "The Servant Leader," which provided some examples from the National Health Service (Howatson-Jones, 2004).

Two nurse-authored articles found in the *Nurse Leader* and the *Health Care Manager*, respectively, addressed selected characteristics of servant leadership as applied to nursing. In the *Nurse Leader*, Patricia Campbell and Pamela Rudisill (2005) identified and described how 6 of Larry Spears's 10 characteristics of servant leadership might be applied in the role of the nursing leader. "Listening" was described as important for nursing leaders who may not consider all variables "within and outside of our control" (p. 27). "Awareness," it was suggested "permits the nurse leader to plan and implement strategies to address needs in a proactive manner" (p. 7). "Persuasion," the authors noted, reflected a leader perceived by staff as "a consistent, fair and reasonable individual . . . who can exhibit a strong and persuasive influence" (p. 27). "Foresight," was viewed as essential for nurse leaders "who must be visionary leaders with a road map in place for followers" (p. 27). "Stewardship" was described as "the responsibility and accountability for managing resources in an appropriate manner" (p. 28). And finally, "Commitment to the growth of individuals," the authors assert, permits "the involvement of nursing staff in the decision-making process" and "results in positive outcomes" (p. 28).

And, in an article published in *Health Care Manager* entitled "Nursing Leadership: Serving Those Who Serve Others," authors Sandra Swearingen and Aaron Liberman (2004) describe the history, philosophy, and application of the servant leadership concept; the latter discussion focusing on the meaning of Spears's 10 characteristics of servant leadership for the nursing community. In discussing "listening," the authors not only suggest that the nurse leader must listen to his or her "own inner voice" but add, "Truly listening to what nurses are saying about their profession is the first step of solving many of its problems" (p. 102). "Empathy" was noted as important to the "distinct generations working in the profession" (p. 102). "Healing" was seen as "desperately needed to heal relationships among those that heal others" (p. 103). "Awareness" was related to the current need for nurse leaders to be "aware of the influences on their industry and the resulting problems that stem from the state of health care today" (p. 103). "Persuasion" was related to "avoidance of top-down leadership," which is "oppressing the nursing profession" and the fact that "consensus building in nursing leadership is an area that needs development" (p. 104). "Conceptualization" included the "vision to create healthy, healing, work cultures" (p. 104). "Foresight" was associated with the fact that "leadership must take lessons from the past, incorporate them with the present and foresee the consequences of the decisions on the future" (p. 104). "Stewardship," was viewed as "first and foremost a commitment to serving the needs of others" (p. 104). "Commitment to the growth of people," was related to the idea that "nurses . . . need and want mentorship. There is always something new to learn" (p. 105). And finally, in describing the importance of "building community," the authors point out, "most healthcare workers spend more waking hours at work than they do in their own homes . . . there is a need to build communities to meet the needs of all stakeholders in the organization" (p. 105).

A 2004 fundamentals of nursing text contains a chapter on leadership, delegation, and collaboration that includes a subsection entitled "servant leadership." In the discussion it is pointed out that "a number of authors believe that the servant leadership approach is valuable in healthcare applications" (Friedman & Mullens, p. 485). In a 2006 nursing text on leadership and management, the author applauds servant leadership as a new and innovative kind of leadership strategy for nurses: "When applied to health care, servant leadership is an attractive alternative to the traditional bureaucratic environment experienced by nurses" (Huber, p. 22). Huber further describes servant leadership as a model that "enhances the personal growth of nurses, improves the quality of care, values teamwork and promotes personal involvement and caring behavior" (p. 22).

The understanding of servant leadership for nursing articulated by Diane Huber is also supported by Mark Neill and Nena Saunders (2008) in their paper "Servant Leadership: Enhancing Quality of Care and Staff Satisfaction". Neill and Saunders observed that "servant leadership encompasses a powerful skill set that is particularly effective in implementing a team approach to the delivery of nursing practice" (p. 395). They add that the "model not only encourages the professional growth of nurses" but also "simultaneously promotes the improved delivery of healthcare services through a combination of interdisciplinary teamwork, shared decision making and ethical behavior" (p. 395).

The value of the philosophy and practice of servant leadership has been identified as supporting nursing research (Jackson, 2007); as supporting nursing education (Neill, Hayward, & Petersons, 2007; Robinson, 2009); as facilitating healing (Ramer, 2008); and as supporting and transforming health-care organizations (Deckard, 2009; Schwartz & Tumblin, 2002).

A 1999 commentary published in the journal *Clinical Systems Management* observed that while the concept of servant leadership has received attention in the press, "little empirical research exists to support the theory or the anecdotal evidence used in the popular press material" (Farling, Stone, & Winston, p. 19). The authors add, "The concept of servant leadership lacks support by well-designed and published empirical research" (p. 19). Both the paucity of literature exploring the concept of servant leadership in the professional nursing community and the commentary in

Clinical Systems Management asserting the need for empirical research on servant leadership, provided impetus, support, and encouragement for the nursing study discussed in the later sections of this chapter.

▶ Research on Servant Leadership in Nursing

Several nursing leaders conducted a study to explore the "attitudes towards collaboration and servant leadership among nurses, physicians and residents" (Garber, Madigan, Click, & Fitzpatrick, 2009, p. 331). Servant leadership was measured using the Barbuto-Wheeler Servant Leadership Questionnaire. In this study, nurses scored higher than physicians for both collaboration and servant leadership characteristics: "The servant leadership findings indicate that RNs have a more positive self-perception of themselves as servant leaders than do physicians" (p. 337). One explanation the investigators offer is the fact that "for servant leadership, the role of the nurse has traditional roots that value taking care of others while physicians are more likely to view their role as the leader or authority in caring for the patient" (p. 338).

In evaluating ethnographic data from a community health agency, nurse educator Bonnie Sturm (2009) identified three key categories or themes that reflect servant leadership among community health nurse leaders; these include "respect and valuing of one as a unique individual," "affirmation of professional judgment and fair treatment regarding workload," and "collaboration with supervisors and administrators in a spirit of willingness" (p. 82). Sturn concluded that "a servant-leadership model can support personal and professional growth, empowering nurses to play a leadership role and thereby increasing nurse collaboration, satisfaction and retention" (p. 82).

Kate Mahon, president of the Canadian Association of Critical Care Nurses, wrote "in praise of servant leadership," describing it as "horizontal service to others" (2011). Mahon noted her personal experience with nurse servant leaders that provided "great satisfaction" and a positive feeling about her work. She asserted: "The result of this type of servant leadership is a workforce that rises together to meet the challenges . . . high morale and strong collegial relationships exist" (p. 5). Mahon's views are supported by Harold Waterman (2011), who asserts that "leaders can obtain the most from their staff and deliver better services by embracing a more egalitarian model of management" (p. 24). Waterman summarizes: "The principles of servant leadership can help leaders frame their decisions with service and community in mind, and focus on client care and the quality of services offered. Servant leadership emphasizes the importance of providing high quality services by releasing leaders from quality checklists . . . [which] [e]nsures that clients and their relevant others are treated with respect and compassion" (p. 26).

The importance of a servant-leader orientation for nurse managers was explored in a large multihospital setting. The study explored "the impact of nurse managers' servant leadership orientation on nurse job satisfaction" (Jenkins & Stewart, 2010, p. 46). Findings of the study supported the belief that "behaviors and attitudes of the nurse manager do impact employee job satisfaction. Departments where staff perceived that managers had higher servant leadership orientation demonstrated significant positive impact on individual employee satisfaction" (p. 46). The investigators reached the natural conclusion that a "health care environment might be enhanced by a more servant-oriented management approach" (p. 46.)

To date the literature on servant leadership in general, as well as servant leadership in nursing, has focused primarily on the leadership of an individual whose role is that of work supervisor; one whose position places him or her in charge of other employees in an organization. This is certainly relevant for many nursing leaders. Nurses in the hospital setting are administrators, supervisors, head nurses, charge nurses, team leaders, or may hold a variety of other positions that place them in charge of other staff members. The same is true in the educational setting, where nursing faculty members may be deans, associate deans, area chairs, program managers, research team leaders, and so forth.

It is important to remember, however, that essentially all nurses are leaders in relation to their roles in caring for patients, family members, study participants, and students. Thus, nurses ministering at the bedside, or in such settings as a clinic, the operating room, or the emergency department, are also servant leaders for those patients and, in some cases family members, committed to their care. Research nurses are servant leaders for their study participants during a patient's participation in a protocol. And in the educational setting, individual faculty members are charged with the responsibility of being servant leaders for their students. Nurses' lived experiences of carrying out the servant leadership role in these various nursing settings were explored in the following phenomenological study of the lived experience of servant leadership in nursing practice.

▶ The Study: Servant Leadership in Nursing

In order to explore the current vocational identity of nursing, the author first initiated a study among 35 professional nurse leaders, employing the phenomenological method of Max van Manen (O'Brien, 2011). The primary aim of the study's Phase 1, entitled "Called to Serve: The Lived Experience of the Nursing Vocation," was to explore and describe the lived experience of nursing as a spiritual calling to serve, as understood by contemporary practicing nurse leaders. The term *spiritual* could be understood by the nurses in a religious and/or a humanitarian sense.

An overarching concept that emerged from analysis of the data, elicited in the Phase 1 interviews, was that of "service." The attributes of service—or servanthood—as described in the published characteristics of servant leadership, were frequently reflected in the documented perceptions and experiences of the nurse leader study participants.

Building on initial analysis of the comments shared by the 35 Phase 1 nurse leader study participants, a second group of 40 nursing leaders was added to the project sample; this effort was labeled study Phase 2. The purpose of the study's second phase was to validate the nursing leaders' perceptions of the lived experience of servant leadership as a concept, as identified in the literature by such scholars of servant leadership as Greenleaf (1977), Spears (2004a), and Russell and Stone (2002). Focused interviews were directed to an exploration of how individual nurse leaders understand and demonstrate characteristics of servant leadership in their day-to-day practice of nursing. The purposive nursing sample included in study phases 1 and 2 was drawn from the population of nursing leaders who consider nursing to be a spiritual calling as well as a profession.

The ultimate goal of the project was to use the data elicited in practicing nurse leaders' interviews to support development of a "Model of Servant Leadership in Nursing." This model may be incorporated in the curricula of schools of nursing, as well as in continuing education programs in medical care centers such as hospitals, clinics, nursing homes, hospices, home health agencies, and churches (where parish or congregational nursing programs exist).

Study Methodology

The nursing servant leadership study design was that of hermeneutic phenomenological inquiry employing the method of exploration and analysis as articulated by Max van Manen (1984, 1990). Overall, van Manen understands hermeneutic phenomenological research as encompassing the following six significant activities:

> (1) Turning to a phenomenon which seriously interests us and commits us to the world; (2) Investigating experience as we live it rather than as we conceptualize it; (3) reflecting on the essential themes which characterize the phenomenon; (4) describing the phenomenon through the art of writing and re-writing; (5) manipulating a strong and oriented pedagogical relation to the phenomenon; and (6) balancing the research context by considering parts and whole. (van Manen, 1990, pp. 30–31)

Study Sample Overview

The purposive sample for the overall study (phases 1 and 2) consisted of a total of 75 professional nursing leaders who admitted to perceiving nursing as a calling to care for the sick. As noted, 35 nurses participated in the first of the two study phases described earlier; 40 nurse leaders were added to study Phase 2. All study participants were registered nurses, with leadership experience, currently employed in a variety of settings including nursing administration, management, education, research, and practice. Nurses engaged in practice represented myriad settings such as the hospital, clinic, rehabilitation center, long-term care, and home care. Nurse participants practiced in differing specialty areas such as medical–surgical nursing, critical care, pediatrics, psych–mental health care, obstetrics and gynecology, community health, school health, and rehabilitation nursing. Nurse respondents had the following credentials: diploma registered nurse (RN), associate degree in nursing (ADN), baccalaureate degree in nursing (BSN), master's degree in nursing (MSN), doctorate in nursing science (DNSc) or doctor of philosophy in nursing (PhD, RN) and reflected a variety of religious faith traditions.

Nursing leader project participants were both male and female. No age criteria were specified; however, study respondents must have practiced nursing for at least one year prior to interview; most, being nursing leaders, had practiced for much longer periods of time. An attempt was made to include nurses from a variety of age categories and representing varied lengths of time in nursing.

Data Collection

Prior to conducting study interviews, the investigator's biases and presuppositions were identified and bracketed as appropriate to van Manen's (1990) requirement that hermeneutic phenomenological research be "presuppositionless" (p. 29). van Manen describes "bracketing" as "the act of suspending one's various beliefs in the reality of the natural world in order to study the essential structures of the world" (p. 175).

For the presently described study Phase 1, two instruments were used to guide data collection. First, study participants were asked to complete a demographic data form from which a demographic study subject profile of nursing leaders was created. Demographic items included the study participant's age, gender, nursing education, religion, nursing leadership role, nursing area of specialization, work setting, and length of time in nursing.

Next, an investigator developed a focused interview guide, exploring the lived experience of nursing as a vocation or spiritual call to care for the sick, was employed to direct questioning. The Nursing Vocation Interview Guide (NVIG) contained one broad phenomenological question addressing the meaning of nursing as a vocation or calling to care for the sick, followed by a number of probes that explored such topics as the meaning of a nurse's personal spiritual call to serve the sick; how one's call to care for the sick attracted the person to nursing; how the vocation is lived out in one's nursing practice; whether one's perception of nursing as a vocation had changed over time; and whether any specific patient care interactions could be cited that were supported by the nurse's perception of his or her vocation to care for the sick.

The NVIG was submitted to a panel of experts in the area of nursing leadership in order to obtain content validity of the instrument (phenomenological question and probe items); construct validity was obtained through review of the nursing vocation and servant leadership literature.

Study Phase 2 consisted of an exploration and validation of the nursing servant leadership themes that had been identified in the secondary analysis of data obtained in study Phase 1. This was done through repetition of the broad phenomenological question about the meaning of one's vocation to serve the sick and a number of probing questions related to the Phase 1 that identified nursing servant leadership themes and subthemes.

Phase 2 study participants also completed the demographic data form used in study Phase 1.

Procedure

Nurse leader study participants were initially accessed through the investigator's contacts within the nursing administration, management, education, research, and practice communities; purposive "snowball" sampling was also employed in order to obtain referrals for additional project respondents. After appropriate informed consent procedures were carried out, qualitative study interviews of approximately one hour were conducted; all interviews were tape-recorded in order to preserve the purity of the data. For confidentiality, audiotapes were destroyed following transcription.

Protection of Human Subjects

Study participants who had read and signed the "informed consent" form were reminded that they might refuse to answer or discuss any question, and that they could withdraw from the study at any time. It was not anticipated, nor did it happen, that the study question or probes would cause (caused) emotional discomfort; however, should this have occurred, an interview would have been terminated and appropriate supportive intervention provided by the investigator. The principal investigator and interviewers involved in phases 1 and 2 of the project completed the NIH "Human Participant Protection for Research Education Tutorial."

Data Analysis

Audiotaped interviews were transcribed verbatim. Qualitative data analysis was carried out according to the guidelines for phenomenological–hermeneutical analysis as articulated by Max van Manen. The analytic stages of the van Manen method included phenomenological reflection (reading and rereading the interview texts); thematic analysis (aimed at identifying underlying themes in the life-world descriptions); composing thematic statements (descriptions of key themes that emerge in data analysis); and phenomenological writing (summarizing study findings related to the phenomena of interest) (Speziale & Carpenter, 2003, p. 59).

Initially, as observed earlier, one overarching concept, that of service, was identified as undergirding the practice of professional nursing among the sample population of nursing leaders. This led initially to development of five nursing vocation attitudinal themes and one subtheme describing nurse leaders' perceptions of nursing as a spiritual calling to serve the sick. In secondary analysis of Phase 1 data and analysis of Phase 2 study data, nine nursing servant leadership themes and 16 subthemes were identified and validated.

Study Sample Details

Study Sample—Phase 1

The 35 nurse leader study participants interviewed for Phase 1 of the Called to Serve research ranged in age from 26 to 69 years; the largest number, 14 (40 percent) were in the 51–60 years age group. The next largest group was from 41–50 years with 10 nurses or 29 percent of the sample population. Only 1 nurse was in the youngest (21–30 years) age range; this was probably because nurse leaders were specifically sought for the purposive sample.

Of the total sample, 15 (43 percent) were master's-prepared nurses; 11 had achieved a BSN degree and only 2 nurses were diploma graduates. Of the total sample, 22 (63 percent) of the nurses were Roman Catholic, 12 were Protestant, and 1 nurse was a member of the Jewish faith. Twenty nurse leaders practiced in a hospital setting; 10 in schools or universities and 4 in clinics. Of the sample group, 27 (77 percent) had been in nursing for 11–40 years, with 5 having practiced between 41 and 50 years.

The most frequently identified area of specialization was medical–surgical nursing (13, or 37 percent); pediatrics was next, capturing 7 nurses. Four nurses specialized in the critical care areas, 2 in maternal–child, 2 in oncology–research, and 1 each in the areas of emergency nursing, public health, OB/GYN, recovery room, quality management, preoperative nursing, and perinatology.

Leadership roles among the Phase 1 study sample of 35 nurse leaders included the following categories: administrator—2; manager—3; supervisor—1; head nurse—8; charge nurse—9; team leader—4; nurse practitioner—1; nurse educator—5; and nurse researcher—2. None of the Phase 1 study group identified themselves as clinical specialists. Specific nursing leadership roles within these categories included:

- Administrator (vice president of nursing in a hospital or administrator of critical care areas)
- Manager (manager of a high-risk pregnancy unit, quality management compliance officer, or public health case manager)
- Supervisor (supervisor of an outpatient diabetic clinic)
- Head nurse (head nurse of a medical–surgical unit, head nurse of a medical–surgical clinic, or head nurse of a critical care unit)
- Charge nurse (charge nurse of one of the following: medical–surgical unit, pediatric clinic, OB/GYN unit, recovery room, or emergency room)
- Team leader (team leader on a medical–surgical unit, pediatric/family-centered care unit, or psychiatric/mental health unit)
- Nurse practitioner (adult health nurse practitioner)
- Educator (nursing educator in pediatrics, critical care, or medical–surgical nursing)
- Researcher (oncology research nurse)

(The demographic profile of Phase 2 study participants is presented in the following section.)

Study Sample—Phase 2

The 40 nurse leader study participants interviewed for Phase 2 of the research ranged in age from 23 to 69 years; the age ranges were fairly evenly distributed, with 11 (27.5 percent) of the nurses in the 31–40 age group; 9 (22.5 percent) in the 41–50 age group; and 11 (27.5 percent) in the 51–60 age group. Six nurses were under 30 years of age and only 3 were older than 60. As with study Phase 1, the nurses tended to be older as nursing leaders were solicited for participation in study Phase 2.

Of the sample, 12 (30 percent) of the sample were master's-prepared nurses; 17 (42 percent) had achieved a BSN degree; and only 3 nurses were diploma graduates. Six nurse leaders had doctoral degrees; 5 nurses had earned the PhD and 1 a DNSc degree.

Of the Phase 2 sample, 22 (55 percent) of the nurses were Roman Catholic, 15 were Protestant, 1 nurse was a member of the Jewish faith, and 1 nurse was Muslim. Two other study participant nurses identified themselves, one each, with the labels "spiritual" and "agnostic," respectively; one nurse stated "none" (no religion) in regard to the demographic category of religion, and one nurse responded "NA" (not applicable) on the religion classification category.

Of the sample, 27 (67.5 percent) nurse leaders practiced in a hospital setting, 5 in schools or universities, 5 in clinics, and 3 nurses worked in private medical or legal offices. Of the group, 14 (35 percent) had been in nursing for 1 to 10 years; 10 nurses had practiced for 11 to 20 years, and 9 from 21 to 30 years. Six members of the group had been in nursing for 31 to 40 years, and 1 nurse had practiced for over 40 years.

The most frequently identified areas of specialization were medical–surgical nursing (13, or 32.5 percent), and critical care nursing (12, or 30 percent). Three nurses were involved in trauma nursing and/or postanesthesia-care nursing, and 2 were psych–mental health nurses. Other categories of nursing specialization identified by study group participants included: home health care, maternal–child and family nursing, occupational health, palliative care, renal nursing, health policy, perioperative nursing, pain management, emergency department nursing, women's health, oncology, and community health.

Leadership roles among the Phase 2 study sample of 40 nurse leaders included the following categories: administrator—5; manager—6; supervisor—3; head nurse—2; charge nurse—9; team leader—6; nurse practitioner—5; and nurse educator—4. Specific nursing leadership roles within these categories included:

- Administrator (vice president of nursing in a hospital, administrator of critical care areas, administrator/director of occupational health, assistant department head of medical–surgical nursing, or director of palliative care)
- Manager (nurse manager of a critical care area, nurse manager of surgical services, nurse manager of a renal department, nurse manager of health policy law, division officer of ambulatory care, or division officer of medical–surgical nursing)
- Supervisor (supervisor of home health care, supervisor of intermediate care and postanesthesia care, or supervisor of perioperative care)
- Head nurse (head nurse of a medical–surgical unit or senior certified registered nurse anesthetist [CRNA] in a trauma unit)
- Charge nurse (charge nurse of medical–surgical unit, maternal–child unit, critical care unit, trauma unit, or chemotherapy treatment unit)
- Team leader (team leader on a critical care unit, medical–surgical unit, trauma unit, or oncology unit)
- Nurse practitioner (nurse practitioner, adult health nurse practitioner, family nurse practitioner, community health nurse practitioner, or psychiatric–mental health nurse practitioner)
- Educator (university-based nursing educators, medical–surgical nursing; psych–mental health nursing, or nursing theory and research; or nurse educator in a hospital emergency department)

Summary Demographic Profile of All 75 Nurse Leader Study Participants

The combined sample group of 75 nurse leaders who participated in Phase 1 and Phase 2 of the Called to Serve study were, in the main, between the ages of 30 and 60 years; baccalaureate, master's, or doctorally prepared; predominantly Christian; practiced nursing in hospitals, clinics, or universities; and represented a wide variety of nursing specialty areas, with medical–surgical nursing and critical care as the leading categories. The total sample of 75 nursing leaders included 7 administrators, 9 managers, 4 supervisors, 10 head nurses, 18 charge nurses, 10 team leaders, 6 nurse practitioners, 9 nurse educators, and 2 nurse researchers.

Study Findings

Phase 1: Nursing Vocation Attitudinal Themes

The five attitudinal themes reflecting nursing leaders' perceptions of the meaning of a nursing vocation or nursing's call to serve included the following:

- A blessed calling (subtheme—a Christian mandate)
- Passionate caring
- Ingrained in the spirit
- The extra mile
- A privilege

All of the attitudinal themes were labeled using the exact wording of one or more of the nurse leader study participants. Other nurse study participants were identified with possessing a particular vocational attitude or perception if his or her comments reflected the theme either directly or with related thoughts. For example, for the theme "a blessed calling," while a number of nurses used the words *blessed calling*, some described nursing itself as a blessing, a blessed vocation, or stated that they felt blessed to be a nurse, as the sample responses reflect. The five nursing vocation attitudinal themes provided the basis for the perceptual dimension of the nursing servant leadership model. Examples of data from which the attitudinal themes were derived include the following:

- A blessed calling—"Nursing is a blessed calling; a spiritual calling to serve the sick" (64, DNSc, educator, community health)
- A Christian mandate—"My faith tells me that I should go out and heal the sick; that is what the Bible says. I believe that since I am a Christian" (65, PhD, RN, educator, adult health)
- Passionate caring—"Nursing is about serving another human being . . . you have to be passionate about caring for others" (59, PhD, RN, educator, pediatrics)
- Ingrained in the spirit: "Nursing is something that has been ingrained in the spirit; you just know that you are called to do it" (43, BSN, charge nurse, critical care)
- The extra mile—"Viewing nursing as a vocation helps me go the extra mile. I think if I did not see nursing as a calling . . . I probably wouldn't go the extra mile" (32, BSN, team leader, medical–surgical)
- A privilege—"It was pretty awesome . . . I realized during my nursing education that my being able to serve was a privilege. Nursing is a privilege . . . I am doing what I was called to do" (52, MSN, rehabilitation unit head nurse)

Finally, as noted, many of the Phase 1 study participants described nursing as a "service," for example, in the words of a 40-year-old case manager in public health: "I see nursing as a call to serve, to serve others, especially those who are not as fortunate as I am."

Combined Findings from Phase 1 and Phase 2

In the following discussion the servant leadership findings from the secondary analysis of the Called to Serve Phase 1 study data, elicited from 35 nurse leaders, and from analysis of the Phase 2 study data, generated in interviews with 40 additional nursing leaders, are combined. Empirical examples of the 75 nursing leader perceptions and experiences, reflecting 9 key nursing servant leader behavioral themes and 16 subthemes emerging from the Phase 1 and Phase 2 analyses, are identified and described. Finally, an overall conceptualization of the lived experience of servant leadership in nursing is presented in both textual and diagrammatic forms. As well as a written description of the Model of Servant Leadership for Nursing, a symbolic representation of what the conceptualization presents, in graphic form, the pathways between and among the nursing vocation attitudinal themes (presented in the preceding section) and the nurse servant leadership themes and subthemes, displaying the overall concept of servant leadership in nursing.

Nursing Servant Leader Behavioral Themes

Whoever serves, let it be with the strength that God supplies, so that God may be glorified in all things.

—**1 Peter** 4:11

Analysis of interview data from the overall study sample population of 75 nursing leaders revealed the following 9 key nursing servant leadership behavioral themes and 16 related concepts or subthemes:

- Listening with the heart (the sounds of silence, the mystery behind the visit)
- Giving of yourself (crossing over, compassionate care)
- Doing ministry (making connections, the wounded healer, a sacred trust)
- Assessing needs (being grounded, taking time out)
- Becoming an advocate (to protect and defend)
- Discerning decisions (staying focused)
- Making a difference (doing your best, generating excitement, a nurturing environment)
- Being there to serve (beyond the ordinary)
- Embracing a higher purpose (a caring vocation)
  Data examples reflecting these key themes include:
- Listening with the heart—"I learned as a nurse that just listening to patients, really listening with the heart, was one of the greatest healers for many kinds of suffering . . . not just listening for the words (patients) are saying but listening with your heart because you really care and the patient knows that you care" (69, PhD, RN, educator, adult health)
- Giving of yourself—"Nursing is much more than just going to work and having a job. You really are giving yourself, giving of yourself to help other people. My job is a vocation . . . that I give of myself every day" (36, BSN, team leader, pediatrics)
- Doing ministry—"When I do nursing, when I care for someone who is sick, I have a real feeling that I am ministering to that person; that I am doing ministry . . . Nursing is definitely a ministry and when you do nursing you have a sense of doing ministry" (64, DNSc, nurse practitioner, community health)
- Assessing needs—"I have to be supportive and be aware of what the patients' needs are. I feel like that is my job . . . that is my first priority" (33, BSN, team leader, medical–surgical)
- Becoming an advocate—"(In nursing) You really have to become an advocate more than anything" (45, MSN, team leader, medical–surgical/critical care)
- Discerning decisions—"When it comes to decision making in nursing, I think discernment is the most important quality that you can have . . . the patient's life can depend on a nurse discerning the right decision" (69, PhD, RN, educator, adult health)
- Making a difference—"It's important knowing that I make a difference . . . my knowledge, my skills, my touch, just being there makes a difference" (52, PhD, RN, educator, critical care)
- Being there to serve—"My real role is to be the patients' advocate; to be there to serve them" (52, BSN, charge nurse, perioperative)
- Embracing a higher purpose—"I think nursing is a higher calling . . . The higher purpose is ordained. It is something that you are called to do and you know it when you are there; you embrace that higher purpose" (43, BSN, head nurse, school health)

Finally, a charge nurse in a medical–surgical unit spoke very movingly of the meaning of servant leadership in her practice:

> I think of service in its entirety, as a leader; service is the foundation of my role as a nursing leader. Because if I didn't place myself to be available and to serve others then I would not consider myself a good leader. I think of the many times when I have been in charge. It is always about serving the group and what can I do to help you make your day a better day. In that respect I am pretty much putting myself in the hands of others. What is it that I can do to serve you so that you can have a better day; so that we can work together as a team? And you are not putting yourself just in the service of your coworkers, but you are putting yourself in the service of other staff, of patients, and families. I think especially in nursing, it is a profession that is based on helping others in service. That is what it means to be a good nurse servant leader. I think that service is the foundation of leadership in nursing.

▶ A Model of Servant Leadership in Nursing

Following analyses of the Phase 1 and Phase 2 Called to Serve study data, a model of servant leadership for nursing was created. From initial analysis of the Phase 1 study data, five attitudinal themes emerged representing the nursing leaders' perceptions of and experiences in the lived experience of a nursing vocation of caring for the sick. These themes are "a blessed calling," which describes the nurse leaders' understanding of their vocation as a spiritual calling to serve; "passionate caring," a theme identifying the depth of feeling that nurse leaders possessed for their ministry to the sick; "ingrained in the spirit," which demonstrated the nurse leaders' innate self-identification with professional nursing; "the extra mile," an expression used by the study group of nurse leaders to describe their perceived degree of commitment to their vocation; and "a privilege," which was a theme representative of the nurse leaders' appreciation of and gratitude for their vocation as nurses.

A subtheme that emerged from data analysis related to a blessed calling was that of "a Christian mandate." As the majority of nurse leader study participants were Christian, many described their calling as related to Christ's mandate to care for the sick; some nurses quoted Scripture, especially Matthew 25:36, as the guiding principle for their nursing practice (details of the themes and subthemes are presented in the previous sections).

The five key nursing vocation attitudinal themes are related because they describe five major facets of a professional nurse's practice: the nurse's calling or attraction to the work (a blessed calling); the nurse's emotional investment in the ministry of caregiving (passionate caring); the nurse's personal sense of appropriateness of his or her vocational choice (ingrained in the spirit); the nurse's depth of commitment to the work (the extra mile); and the nurse's gratitude for the vocation of nursing (a privilege).

To summarize: During the initial data analysis, from which the described themes emerged, it was recognized that the nurse leaders almost universally, at some point during an interview, spoke of nursing as being a "service," a role in which the goal was "to serve" others and to embrace the concept of "servanthood." This emphasis on service directed the investigation to an exploration of the concept of "servant leadership" in nursing, the living out of which might, of course, be mediated by the nurse leaders' specific leadership role in an institution and by his or her length of time in nursing.

In order to describe the "lived experience" of servant leadership in nursing, a secondary analysis of the Phase 1 study data and analysis of the Phase 2 study data were carried out. The 9 key nursing servant leadership themes and 16 subthemes that emerged from the secondary analysis were found to be supported by contemporary servant leadership literature as discussed earlier in this chapter.

The 9 themes and 16 subthemes related to servant leadership identified from content analysis of data elicited from the study group of 75 nursing leaders included:

- Listening with the heart (the sounds of silence, the mystery behind the visit)
- Giving of yourself (crossing over, compassionate care)
- Doing ministry (making connections, the wounded healer, a sacred trust)
- Assessing needs (being grounded, taking time out)
- Becoming an advocate (to protect and defend)
- Discerning decisions (staying focused)
- Making a difference (doing your best, generating excitement, a nurturing environment)
- Being there to serve (beyond the ordinary)
- Embracing a higher purpose (a caring vocation)

As with the five nursing vocation attitudinal themes, the nursing servant leadership themes and subthemes are related in that considered together they reflect a beautiful tapestry of nursing practice as carried out by one who is a true servant leader in the profession. Nurse servant leaders listen with their hearts both to the words and to the silence of those for whom they care; attempt to cross over to truly understand the problems and concerns of their staff, patients, family members, or students; give of themselves consistently in their compassionate caring for those they serve; work to remain grounded so that they can continually assess the needs of those for whom they care; advocate for all those under their care; perceive nursing as having a higher purpose and conceptualize how best that can be achieved in day-to-day practice; remain alert to discern right decisions for those they serve; accept the responsibility of serving those entrusted to their care; continually strive to make a difference and to achieve positive outcomes for those under their care; and attempt to use their leadership positions to nurture the environment wherein they practice.

As **FIGURE 15-1** demonstrates, a description of servant leadership in nursing involves a vocational perception of the profession as encompassing a strongly positive attitude toward one's calling, a passion for the ministry, a feeling of belonging in nursing, a desire to do more than required, and a deep gratitude for nursing as a personal life vocation. These attitudes direct the nurse to become a servant leader, a ministry that might, of course, be somewhat mediated by the nurse's leadership role and length of time in nursing. And, flowing from the attitudinal perception of nursing as a calling to serve, are the servant leadership characteristics, operationalized for nurses in terms of the 9 nurse servant leadership themes and 16 subthemes reflecting heartfelt caring, understanding of others' problems and needs, giving of oneself in nursing ministry, accepting responsibility for the good of those under one's care, being a servant of others, and doing one's best to achieve a positive outcome for all of those for whom the nurse servant leader is responsible.

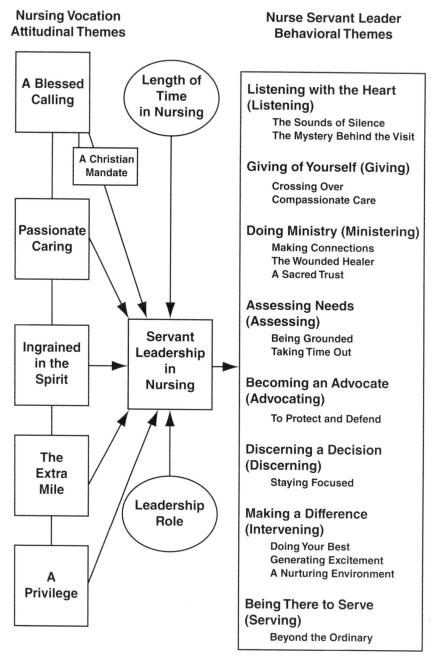

**Nursing Vocation
Attitudinal Themes**

**Nurse Servant Leader
Behavioral Themes**

A Blessed Calling

Length of Time in Nursing

A Christian Mandate

Passionate Caring

Ingrained in the Spirit

Servant Leadership in Nursing

The Extra Mile

Leadership Role

A Privilege

Listening with the Heart (Listening)
  The Sounds of Silence
  The Mystery Behind the Visit

Giving of Yourself (Giving)
  Crossing Over
  Compassionate Care

Doing Ministry (Ministering)
  Making Connections
  The Wounded Healer
  A Sacred Trust

Assessing Needs (Assessing)
  Being Grounded
  Taking Time Out

Becoming an Advocate (Advocating)
  To Protect and Defend

Discerning a Decision (Discerning)
  Staying Focused

Making a Difference (Intervening)
  Doing Your Best
  Generating Excitement
  A Nurturing Environment

Being There to Serve (Serving)
  Beyond the Ordinary

FIGURE 15-1   A model of servant leadership in nursing.

The Spirituality of Servant Leadership

You are my servant whom I have chosen.

—**Isaiah** 43:10

If I did not have that spiritual deep grounding, that persistence of faith that tends to support you in your nursing career, I am afraid I would be relying on other alternatives to make me happy. I really believe that spirituality is very healing not only for the patient but also for the nurse who is a servant leader. It is a reflection of who you are as a person . . . You have to have some kind of belief in yourself and in a higher being in a meaningful, purposeful way of what it is to be not only yourself but as a nurse too. You have to have the spiritual aspect in your nursing life in order to survive.

Agnes, Supervisor, Medical Outpatient Clinic

I think having a spiritual commitment to your profession, to your calling, is an aspect of being a good nurse; an aspect of the role of a nurse servant leader. You are going beyond the usual expectations. Nursing is obviously not just a job; you do what you do at work or institution but also away from there. If somebody was to know you away from the hospital, they would know that you show the same characteristics away from your normal nursing environment. That is what the role of a nursing servant leader is. You are showing leadership because that is your way of life, helping others. Caring for others is your vocation as a leader. Viewing nursing as a calling adds a definite spiritual dimension to the profession.

Linda, Charge Nurse, Medical–Surgical Unit

Although the philosophy of servant leadership, as originally described by Robert Greenleaf in 1977, did not have an overtly religious undergirding, the concept can, by its very nature, be considered spiritual in the broadest sense of the word. Greenleaf asserted that "the servant-leader is servant first . . . [servant leadership] begins with the natural feeling that one wants to serve, to serve first" (p. 27). By describing a servant leader as an individual whose first interest is that of serving others, Robert Greenleaf distinguished the servant leader from the person for whom leadership is first; one who seeks a leadership role "perhaps because of the need to assuage an unusual power drive or to acquire material possessions" (p. 27).

Greenleaf's philosophy describes not a self-serving leader but a self-giving leader; one who puts the needs and concerns of those he or she serves before personal interests. This can lead to an interpretation of servant leadership as spiritual; that is, as deeply humanitarian for some, and as deeply religious for others.

A nonreligious understanding of servant leadership presents a humanistic philosophy of caring that places the good of others in the human family, especially others for whose leadership one is responsible, as a central concern of the leader; the leader sees servant leadership as moral and good for the functioning of an organization and for all of its members.

A religious understanding of the concept reflects a model of servanthood as presented in spiritual teachings such as those of the Judeo-Christian tradition. In both

Old and New Testament writings the concepts of service and servanthood are taught as the ideal attributes for one who wishes to live a holy and religiously attuned life. In the Torah or Old Testament passages the concept of service is particularly related to service of the God of Israel: "The Lord, your God, shall you fear; him you shall serve, and by his name alone you shall swear" (Deuteronomy 6:13). New Testament passages reflect Jesus as role model of the servant leader in mandates such as, "Whoever wishes to become great among you must be your servant, and whoever wishes to be first among you must be slave of all. For the Son of Man came not to be served but to serve, and to give his life as a ransom for many" (Mark 10:42–45).

Thus, there can be found both a spiritual and a religious significance to the philosophy of servant leadership as identified and described by Robert Greenleaf as well as by others who have followed his lead in exploring the concept. Greenleaf's philosophy of servant leadership supports the firmly held belief of many spiritual and religious people that it is in fact "better to give than to receive."

As Greenleaf (1977), a devout Quaker, observed, "Servant-leaders are healers in the sense of making whole by helping others to a larger and nobler vision and purpose than they would be likely to obtain for themselves" (p. 240). This spirituality is reflected in Ken Blanchard and Phil Hodges's (2005) book *Lead Like Jesus: Lessons from the Greatest Leadership Role Model of All Time*, in which the authors observe, "Self-serving leaders think they should lead and others should follow. Servant leaders, on the other hand, seek to respect the wishes of those who have entrusted them with a season of influence and responsibility" (p. 47).

The majority of nurses are, by the very essence of their calling and their profession of caring for the sick, natural servant leaders. They choose to undertake the vocation of nursing, with all of its challenges and difficulties, because they are men and women who embrace the spirituality of giving to others; they recognize, in the words of Francis of Assisi, that it is truly in giving that one receives. Nurses are servant leaders in body, mind, and spirit.

Frequently nurses are stretched almost to the limit of their physical abilities in working long hours, with heavy patient loads or overwhelming staffing responsibilities; they may go home physically exhausted, especially after the 12-hour nursing shifts initiated in some contemporary hospitals. Nurses must constantly pursue continuing education, keeping their minds alert and becoming educated to new medical knowledge and new technologies upon which a patient's very life may depend. And nurses give constantly of their spirits, listening with a caring and empathetic heart, to the worries and concerns of their staff, their patients, and their patients' families. Nursing servant leaders often expend a great deal of energy agonizing over the problems and concerns of those they lead; this is the vocation of nursing. This is the vocation of servant leadership. This is the spirituality of servant leadership in nursing.

▶ References

Agosto, E. (2005). *Servant leadership: Jesus and Paul*. St. Louis, MO: Chalice Press. Barbuto, J. E., & Wheeler, D. W. (2006). Scale development and construct clarification of servant leadership. *Group & Organizational Management, 31*(3), 300–326.

Blanchard, K., & Hodges, P. (2003). *The servant leader: Transforming your heart, head, hands and habits*. Nashville, TN: Countryman.

Blanchard, K., & Hodges, P. (2005). *Lead like Jesus: Lessons from the greatest leader of all time*. Nashville, TN: Thomas Nelson.

Bower, F. L. (1994). Servant leadership . . . president's message. *Reflections, 20*(4), 4–5.

Bowles, A., & Bowles, N. B. (2000). A comparative study of transformational leadership in nursing development units and conventional clinical settings. *Journal of Nursing Management, 8*(2), 69–76.

Campbell, P. T., & Rudisill, P. T. (2005). Servant leadership: A critical component for nurse leaders. *Nurse Leader, 3*(3), 27–29.

Carroll, P. (2006). *Nursing leadership and management: A practical guide*. Clifton Park, NY: Thomson Delmar Learning.

Deckard, G. J. (2009). Contemporary leadership theories. In N. Borkowski (Ed.), *Organizational behavior, theory and design in health care* (pp. 203–222). Sudbury, MA: Jones & Bartlett Learning.

Dennis, R. S., & Bocarnea, M. (2005). Development of the servant leadership assessment instrument. *Leadership and Organization Development Journal, 26*(8), 600–615.

Dossey, B. M. (2005). Florence Nightingale's tenets: Healing, leadership, global action. In B. M. Dossey, L. C. Selanders, D. Beck, & A. Attewell (Eds.), *Florence Nightingale: Healing, leadership, global action* (pp. 9–15). Silver Spring, MD: American Nurses Association.

Downs, F. C. (2007). The servant leadership worldview in long-term care nursing. *Annals of Long-Term Care, 15*(8), 36–39.

Ellis, J. R., & Hartley, C. L. (2008). *Nursing in today's world: Trends, issues and management*. Philadelphia, PA: Lippincott, Williams, and Wilkins.

Englert, J. (2007, February 1). Rural facility received Baldrige for 2006: Culture of servant leadership at core of success. *HealthCare Benchmarks and Quality Improvement* (newsletter), 1–2.

Farling, M. L., Stone, A. G., & Winston, B. E. (1999). Servant leadership: Setting the stage for empirical research (abstract). *Clinical Systems Management, 7*(5–6), 19.

Fedoruk, M., & Pincombe, J. (2000). The nurse executive: Challenges for the 21st century. *Journal of Nursing Management, 8*(1), 13–20.

Friedman, L. H., & Mullens, L. A. (2004). Leadership, delegation and collaboration. In R. Daniels (Ed.), *Nursing fundamentals: Caring and clinical decision making* (pp. 477–489). Clifton Park, NY: Delmar Learning.

Garber, J., Madigan, E., Click, E., & Fitzpatrick, J. (2009). Attitudes towards collaboration and servant leadership among nurses, physicians and residents. *Journal of Interprofessional Care, 23*(4), 331–340.

Greenleaf, R. K. (1977). *Servant leadership: A journey into the nature of legitimate power and greatness*. New York, NY: Paulist Press.

Gunnarsdottir, S. (2014). Is servant leadership useful for sustainable Nordic health care? *Nordic Journal of Nursing Research and Clinical Studies, 34*(2), 53–55.

Howatson-Jones, I. (2004). The servant leader. *Nursing Management, 11*(3), 2–24.

Huber, D. L. (Ed.). (2006). Leadership principles. In *Leadership and nursing care management* (pp. 1–32). Philadelphia, PA: Saunders Elsevier.

Hunter, J. C. (2004). *The world's most powerful leadership principle: How to become a servant leader*. New York, NY: Waterbook Press.

Jackson, D. (2007). Servant leadership in nursing: A framework for developing sustainable research capacity in nursing. *Collegian: Journal of the Royal College of Nursing Australia, 15*(1), 27–33.

Jenkins, M., & Stewart, A. (2010). The importance of a servant leader orientation. *Health Care Management Review, 35*(1), 46–54.

Joseph, E. E., & Winston, B. E. (2005). A correlation of servant leadership, leader trust and organizational trust. *Leadership and Organization Development Journal, 26*(1), 6–22.

King, K., & Cunningham, G. (1995). Leadership in nursing: More than one way. *Nursing Standard, 10*(12–14), 3–14.

Laschinger, H. K. S., Wong, C., McMahon, L., & Kaufmann, C. (1999). Leader behavior impact on staff nurse empowerment, job tension and work effectiveness. *Journal of Nursing Administration, 29*(5), 28–39.

Mahon, K. (2011). In praise of servant leadership: Horizontal service to others. *Canadian Association of Critical Care Nurses, 22*(4), 5–6.

Moiden, N. (2002). Evolution of leadership in nursing. *Nursing Management, 9*(7), 20–25.

Mullally, S. (2001). Leadership and politics. *Nursing Management, 8*(4), 21–27.

Neill, M. W., Hayward, K. S., & Peterson, T. (2007). Students perceptions of the interprofessional team in practice through application of servant leadership principles. *Journal of Interprofessional Care, 21*(4), 425–432.

Neill, M. W., & Saunders, N. S. (2008). Servant leadership: Enhancing quality of care and staff satisfaction. *The Journal of Nursing Administration, 38*(9), 395–400.

O'Brien, M. E. (2011). *Servant leadership in nursing: Spirituality and practice in contemporary health care.* Sudbury, MA: Jones & Bartlett Learning.

Perra, B. M. (2001). Leadership: The key to quality outcomes. *Journal of Nursing Care Quality, 15*(2), 68–73.

Porter-O'Grady, T., & Malloch, K. (2011). *Quantum Leadership* (3rd ed.). Sudbury, MA: Jones & Bartlett Learning.

Prosser, S. (2002). Servant leadership. *Professional Nurse, 18*(4), 238.

Ramer, L. M. (2008). Using servant leadership to facilitate healing after a drug diversion experience. *AORN Journal, 88*(2), 253–258.

Reimer-Kirkham, S., Pesut, B., Swatzky, R., Cochrane, M., & Redmond, A. (2012). Discourses of spirituality and leadership in nursing: A mixed method analysis. *Journal of Nursing Management, 20*(8), 1029–1038.

Robinson, F. P. (2009). Servant teaching: The power and promise for nursing education. *International Journal of Nursing Education Scholarship, 6*(1), 1–15.

Russell, R. F. (2001). The role of values in servant leadership. *Leadership and Organization Development Journal, 22*(2), 76–83.

Russell, R. F., & Stone, A. G. (2002). A review of servant leadership attributes: Developing a practical model. *Leadership and Organization Development Journal, 23*(3), 145–157.

Schira, M. (2007). Leadership: A peak and perk of professional development. *Nephrology Nursing Journal, 34*(3), 289–294.

Schwartz, R. W., & Tumblin, T. F. (2002). The power of servant leadership to transform health care organizations for the 21st-century economy. *Archives of Surgery, 137*(12), 1419–1427.

Spears, L. C. (2003). Introduction: Understanding the growing impact of servant-leadership. In R. K. Greenleaf (author); H. Beazley, J. Beggs, & L. C. Spears (Eds.), *The servant-leader within: A transformative path* (pp. 13–27). New York, NY: Paulist Press.

Spears, L. C. (2004a). Practicing servant-leadership. *Leader to Leader, 34,* 7–11.

Spears, L. C. (2004b). Prescription for organizational health. *Reflections on Nursing Leadership, 30*(4), 24–26.

Speziale, H. J., & Carpenter, D. R. (2003). *Qualitative research in nursing: Advancing the human perspective.* Philadelphia, PA: Lippincott, Williams, and Wilkins.

Stone, A. G., Russell, R. F., & Patterson, K. (2004). Transformational versus servant leadership: A difference in leader focus. *Leadership and Organization Development Journal, 25*(4), 349–361.

Sturm, B. (2009). Principles of servant-leadership in community health nursing. *Home Health Care Management & Practices, 21*(2), 82–89.

Swearingen, S., & Liberman, A. (2004). Nursing leadership: Serving those who serve others. *Health Care Manager, 23*(2), 100–109.

Taylor, T., Martin, B. N., Hutchinson, S., & Jinks, M. (2007). Examination of leadership practices of principals identified as servant leaders. *International Journal of Leadership in Education, 10*(4), 401–419.

Valiga, T. M., & Grossman, S. (2007). Leadership and followership. In R. A. Patronis Jones (Ed.), *Nursing leadership and management* (pp. 3–12). Philadelphia, PA: F. A. Davis.

van Manen, M. (1984). Practicing phenomenological writing. *Phenomenology and Pedagogy, 2*(1), 36–69.

van Manen, M. (1990). *Researching lived experience: Human science for an action sensitive pedagogy.* New York, NY: The State University of New York Press.

Warneka, T. H. (2008). *Black belt leader, peaceful leader: An introduction to Catholic servant leadership.* Cleveland, OH: Asogomi Publishing International.

Washington, R. R., Sutton, C. D., & Field, H. S. (2006). Individual differences in servant leadership: The roles of values and personality. *Leadership and Organization Development Journal, 27*(8), 700–716.

Waterman, H. (2011). Principles of servant leadership and how they can enhance practice. *Nursing Management, 17*(9), 24–26.

Weber, D. (2004). Shared governance and servant leadership are drawing nurses to new hospital. *Patient Care Staffing Report, 4*(7), 1–3.

Welford, C. (2002). Matching theory to practice. *Nursing Management, 9*(4), 7–11.

Wickwire, V. L (2006). *Amish childbearing beliefs and practices and the implications for nurse-midwives as servant-leader care providers* (Unpublished doctoral dissertation). Andrews University, Berrin Springs, Michigan.

Winston, B. E. (2004). Servant leadership at Heritage Bible College: A single-case study. *Leadership and Organization Development Journal, 25*(7), 600–617.

Yanofchick, B. (2007). Servant leadership: Bring it home. *Health Progress, 88*(5), 6–7.

CHAPTER 16

Prayer in Nursing: The Spirituality of Contemplative Caregiving

When you call me, when you go to pray to me, I will listen to you.

Jeremiah 29:12

I pray about my nursing every day; I couldn't do nursing without prayer. I wouldn't have become a nurse without prayer. Nursing is a very active profession but it's a prayerful vocation also; that's the spiritual part of our caregiving.

Elizabeth, Charge Nurse, Medical–Surgical Unit

In a small but powerful book on prayer, Benedictine Mary Clare Vincent (1982) observed "a life without prayer doesn't work" (p. 1). I would add that nursing without prayer doesn't work. For contemporary nurses, prayer is, I believe, more necessary to support their caring for the sick than in any preceding era. Complex moral and ethical issues, related both directly and tangentially to our practice, abound in the current world of health care. Therapeutic procedures involving a variety of extraordinary measures to prolong human life (some of which are admittedly positive) become more sophisticated each year, and medical research on such frightening issues as the cloning of human beings hovers on the fringe of acceptable medical discourse in certain quarters.

If, in fact, we subscribe to the spiritual vision of our profession's founder, how can we not believe in the importance and value of prayer for a nurse? For it was Florence Nightingale (1859) who reminded us, in the late 19th century, that "God's precious gift of life is often placed literally in [the nurse's] hands" (pp. 70–71).

What a sacred commission Nightingale issued to her followers—to hold in our hands "God's precious gift of life." How can we be faithful to such a blessed ministry without the grace of prayer? And yet, in this era of health-care reform, of managed care and—restructured nursing roles, what does prayer mean for the contemporary nurse?

How can time for prayer be found in a caregiving system in which all activities must be cost effective, as mandated by the institutions where we carry out our nursing activities? The purpose of this chapter is to address these and related questions and concerns for present-day nurses; the ultimate goal is to explore the practice of prayerful, contemplative caregiving in the world of 21st-century nursing.

Nurse authors Aru Narayanasamy and Mani Narayanasamy (2008) have identified some guidelines for prayer in clinical nursing. These include the following: "Prayer should not be forced on patients or staff forced to pray for patients"; "Prayer should be part of nursing care if spiritual needs are identified"; "If nurses are willing to pray they should be encouraged if patients need it" (p. 397).

Nurse educator Carrie Demeron (2012) has observed that some nurses may "associate prayer as an intervention in providing spiritual care, yet prayer is elemental to our professional development" (p. 10). "While striving to permeate our personal lives with prayer," Demeron adds, "we can infuse unceasing prayer into our nursing practice" (p. 10). It may, admittedly, be difficult for contemporary practicing nurses to find the time to incorporate personal prayer into their busy workdays; the topic of finding time for prayer is discussed later in this chapter.

One spiritual writer has taken up the topic of prayer associated not only with the time-related intensity of today's world but also with the technology-related intensity of most of our lives. In his book, *Prayer in the Digital Age*, Matt Swaim (2011) points out that for many people today times of "silence," so necessary for a prayerful life, are something to be avoided. "Silence," he asserts, "is the great fear of the modern age" (p. 3).

I believe that we nurses often long for periods of silence; however, we remain continually attached to such mobile devices as netbooks, smartphones, electronic readers, MP3 players, and any other equipment that we believe can keep us "connected" to family and friends. However, these devices also keep us *away* from God, to whom we are connected in prayer. As Swaim (2011) observed: "We can accuse God of silence all we want, but an honest assessment of ourselves will most likely reveal that our antennae are not usually pointing in the proper direction to pick up the signal we claim we want to receive" (p. 28).

Our nursing pioneers did not have the sophisticated technology of the 21st century; perhaps that is why, as is demonstrated in nursing's history, so many early nurses turned to prayer for support and inspiration for their ministry of caring for the sick. From the time of our founder, Florence Nightingale, prayer has been an integral part of the armament that guides and guards nurses in the caring profession.

Today the topics of prayer and meditation at the bedside are identified as appropriate spiritual care activities for nurses if acceptable and welcomed by the patient. Nurses Beth Hubbartt and Donald Kautz (2012) published an article to assist nurses in "providing prayer for patients of all faith traditions" (p. 42). The authors present "guidelines for conducting an assessment to determine the patient's prayer preferences, strategies for overcoming barriers to prayer, resources for finding suitable prayers for healing and some short, practical prayers for nurses and patients" (p. 42). Hubbartt and Kautz (2012) point out that "prayer can help achieve peace and promote feelings of calm, relief, rest and well-being" for one who is ill (p. 43).

Meditation, "as a bedside spiritual intervention," is advocated by nurse educator Roxane Chan (2014, p. 84). Chan asserts that "meditation as a healthcare intervention may promote well-being of the body, mind and spirit uniquely through measurable and lasting physiological changes" (p. 84). Meditation, she adds "whether secular or spiritual," allows the patient to focus on "a single thought or sensation which conveys a sense of comfort" (p. 86). Prayer and attendance at religious services can also provide comfort to dementia patients, especially those nearing the end of their lives (Higgins, 2013, p. 25).

▶ Reclaiming Our Spiritual Heritage: A History of Prayer in Nursing

From its inception, nursing the sick has been considered a vocation or calling; in the early days, especially, nursing was viewed as a ministry of God and of His Church and was guided and strengthened by the prayer of the caregiver. Our nursing forebears, on whose strong shoulders we contemporary nurses stand, understood this calling; they responded by including prayer as a central and critical component of their nursing ministries. Tales of nursing prefigures from the early deacons and deaconesses of the first century, through the medieval monastics such as Saint Catherine of Siena, up to members of the post-Reformation religious orders, are replete with anecdotes indicating the prayerfulness with which nursing ministries were undertaken. For these men and women, committed to a religious vocation of caring for the sick, God's call, heard in prayer, not only was the incentive for undertaking the ministry but also was the very fiber from which a daily tapestry of nursing activities was woven.

As early as the mid-19th century, Florence Nightingale's life and writings modeled a variety of prayers. In a letter to her aunt Hannah, written in 1846, Nightingale described her prayer of petition: "I never pray for anything temporal . . . but when each morning comes, I kneel down before the Rising Sun and only say: 'Behold the handmaid of the Lord, give me this day my work to do, no, not my work, but Thine'" (Dossey, 2000, p. 33). A Nightingale diary entry acknowledges the author's listening to the Lord in prayer: "God called me in the morning and asked me: 'Would I do good for Him, for Him alone without reputation [self-interest]'" (p. 65). Nightingale's mystical bent and her gift for contemplation are reflected in a famous quote from *Notes for Devotional Authors*: "Where shall I find God? In myself. That is the true mystical doctrine. But then I myself must be in a state for Him to come and dwell in me" (Macrae, 1995, p. 10).

In a letter to a cherished mentor and friend, Dr. Benjamin Jowett, Nightingale articulated a beautiful prayer of acceptance of God's will for her life:

> Behold the handmaid of the Lord; be it unto me according as Thou will. What a wonderful favor to be chosen as many thousands before, to be the handmaid of the Lord. What return does God expect from me; with what purity of heart and intentions should I make an offering of myself to Him? And when that offering is made, what a life ought I to lead? I give myself up entirely to Him that He may do with me whatever it pleases Him. (Dossey, 2000, p. 334)

Nightingale displayed the great value she placed on the prayers of others in a letter written to a friend, after learning of the Crimean soldiers' desire to pray for her: "Now I had rather have the men's prayers than a vote of thanks from the House of Commons. And I think there can be no more precious acknowledgement of service done for them" (Vicinus & Nergaard, 1990, p. 205). She went on to say, however, that the War Office should not order the men to pray for her but they should be "left to pray willingly," observing: "This is my feeling . . . not because I do not value the prayers of the men but because I value them so much" (p. 205). Finally, Nightingale shared both her Trinitarian theology of prayer and her concept of God's response to prayer in a commentary on the spiritual life:

> God does not refuse to answer the longing, devoted spirit which says: 'Speak Lord, for thy loving child heareth.' He hears as the Father; he answers as the Son, and as the Holy Spirit. I could not understand God if He were to speak to me. But the Holy Spirit, the Divine in me, tells me what I am to do . . . this voice is ever beyond and above me, calling me to more and more good. (Calabria & Macrae, 1994, p. 127)

Nursing publications in the United States began to proliferate in the early 20th century; following Nightingale's lead, a number of articles of the era dealt with the importance of prayer in the life of a nurse. One example is an article published in *The Public Health Nurse* in June 1923, in which the author asserted that "all who embrace nursing as a life profession must have as a secret source of their ministering contacts a prayerful relationship with God" (White, 1923, p. 283); and in a 1926 commentary in *The Trained Nurse and Hospital Review*, another author suggested that nurses approach a bedside from a posture of prayer and added, poetically, that thus, "They meet the waning hopes of the poor bedridden soul with the radiant beams of a morning glimpse of God" (Lumpkin, 1926, p. 628).

The author of a 1937 textbook, *The Art and Science of Nursing*, advised that the nurse may offer a patient a form of "spiritual therapy" such as "reading from the Bible or saying a prayer" (Rothweiler, 1937, p. 332). In her 1945 classic, *The Nurse: Handmaid of the Divine Physician*, Mary Berenice Beck (1945) authored a nurse's prayer that read, in part, "I am thine own, great Healer, help Thou me, to serve Thy sick in humble charity" (p. xvii). A "Night Nurse's Prayer," published in *The Catholic Nurse* in 1954, included the concept of seeing Christ in all of one's patients: "I looked at my patient there in his bed, but I felt I was seeing the thorn-crowned head" (Maher, 1954, p. 30). And in a 1956 book on moral issues in nursing, an entire chapter is devoted to "The Nurse: A Woman of Prayer." The authors assert, "Because the nurse's vocation is so singularly Christlike, it is imperative that she work though Him, and in Him and with Him. The nurse will find the solution to most of her difficulties, will see her vocation in a new light, through personal contact with Christ. Prayer is that personal contact" (Hayes, Hayes, & Kelly, 1956, p. 134).

As to contemporary publications in nursing, many "fundamentals" texts include some reference to prayer as a dimension of the nurse's practice. A literature search for journal articles focused on the relationship between nursing and prayer revealed 102 publications extant from 1989 to 2012; a search for prayer as a key concept in nursing journal articles under such headings as spiritual care, nursing care, spirituality, nurse–patient relations, and ethics identified over 21,319 items.

▶ Prayer and Contemporary Nursing: Why Should We Pray?

One Saturday morning, at an early service on The Catholic University campus, the Dominican priest celebrant chose as the topic for his homily the question, "Why should we pray?" Although I was, admittedly, still a bit drowsy from a late night of writing, my ears immediately perked up. I really need to "get" this, I thought. At the preacher's first comment, however, my heart sank, for he began to quote the great scholar and doctor of the Church, Thomas Aquinas. Aquinas, the celebrant explained, taught that we should pray because of the principle of "secondary causality." "Oh, oh," I lamented to myself, much as I respect and honor the sainted Aquinas, "it's much too early for a philosophical discourse on prayer."

However, and there's usually a "however" in anecdotes such as this, our wise and sensitive homilist was understanding of both the hour and the spiritual needs of the small congregation gathered for worship. He immediately acknowledged that the phrase *secondary causality* sounded pretty intimidating, and he explained that what Aquinas really meant was that God, in His abundant love, allows us, in prayer, to participate as cocreators in his work in the universe. As an example, the preacher cited the concept of rain; because God who created the world knows that the earth needs rain, why should we pray for rain? Not, surely, to attempt to twist God's arm, but rather to cooperate with him in seeking the response to a need.

With this thought in mind, my nurse's imagination was quickly borne away to a past clinical experience. I remembered standing with a mother at the bedside of a 14-year-old who had just been diagnosed with a highly malignant anaplastic astrocytoma and making comments like, "I'll be praying for Michael," and "You are both in my heart and my prayers." God certainly knew that Michael was desperately ill. He knew that Michael and his mother needed His comfort and support, and He knew that I, as a nurse, needed His strength and His tenderness to minister to this family. So, why pray for these things?

Suddenly Aquinas's teaching made sense. Yes, God our Father, in His omnipotence, knows our needs, our desires, and our hopes. But in His great wisdom, He also knows that we desire to participate with Him in the fulfillment of these needs, these desires, and these hopes; when we perceive problems, we long to be part of the solutions. Of course outcomes may not always be as we wish; that's why we must pray as Jesus prayed: "Father . . . not my will but yours be done" (Luke 22:42). But when we pray about the things that are important to us, we recognize the importance of God for us. Whenever we have a personal encounter that involves great joy, great sorrow, or even a profound insight, the first thing most of us do is run to the phone (or perhaps to email in this age of communication technology) to share the experience with someone we love. Should it not be the same with the One we love most deeply and who loves us with an everlasting love, the One who is the source of our strength and the center of our lives? Why should we pray? How can we not pray?

▶ The Use of Scripture for Prayer in Nursing

Spiritual writer Peter Kreeft (2000) advises that "praying by reading the gospels prayerfully and 'listeningly' is one of the very best ways to pray" (p. 34). Although it might seem a given that listening to or meditatively reading the word of God is helpful to prayer, the topic bears some exploring.

How does one begin the exercise of praying with Scripture? I remember one of the supervising ministers in my hospital chaplaincy program warning us that although we should surely encourage Scripture reading among our patients, we should not advise a neophyte to begin studying Scripture without any guidance. There is a multiplicity of spiritual books to assist in the exercise of praying with Scripture, such as *Pray the Bible* by Page Zyromski (2000), and many relevant chapters in books on prayer. Some examples are "Listening at Prayer with the Written Word" (Groeschel, 1997), "Pondering the Word" (Casey, 1996), and "Contemplating Scripture" (Barry, 1987). There are also Bible dictionaries and commentaries that help explain the meaning of more obscure Scripture passages, as well as providing the history of the holy word; one simple and useful example is the *Collegeville Series on Books of the Bible* (1987).

For some of us, it may be easier to begin with the New Testament—with Scriptures familiar from our worship services: the four gospels; the Acts of the Apostles; and the letters of Jesus' disciples: Paul, James, Peter, John, and Jude. Or we may wish to pick an Old Testament passage with which we also have some familiarity, such as the story of Jeremiah and the Potter's Wheel (Jeremiah 18:1–6), or the prophet Isaiah's promise that those who hope in the Lord will "soar as with eagle's wings" (Isaiah 40:31). The Psalms are also a wonderful guide to prayer as they are the prayers that Jesus prayed. Each psalm has a unique theme that might be relevant to a particular prayer concern such as praise, thanksgiving, and trust; prayer in time of illness; prayer in distress; confidence in God; prayer for help against unjust enemies; prayer for protection; and prayer for faithfulness.

Two excellent commentaries on the Psalms that may be helpful to nurses are *Psalms: A Spiritual Commentary* by the late Trappist Father Basil Pennington (2008), and *Seven Sacred Pauses: Living Mindfully through the Hours of the Day* by Benedictine spiritual writer Sister Macrina Wiederkehr (2008). In the latter book, Sister Macrina provides poetic commentary on the Psalms contained in the sevenfold "Liturgy of the Hours," sometimes referred to as the "Divine Office." In earlier times, the praying of the Liturgy of the Hours was generally considered a practice reserved for priests or nuns living in monasteries. Today, however, many laypeople of different faith traditions find great comfort in praying the Liturgy of the Hours. Some pray the Hours alone in their homes; others join communities of religious men or women in order to pray together as members of a worshipping community.

In terms of the history of our own profession, it has been well documented that Florence Nightingale was an avid reader of the Bible; she wrote many annotations on the Scriptures in which she personally identified with the struggles and experiences of biblical figures (Dossey, 2000, p. 338). This kind of personal acknowledgment of God's word is a wonderful way to integrate Scripture into our prayer lives. Finally, a helpful guide to the overall value of Scripture for our profession is the book *The Nurse with an Alabaster Jar: A Biblical Approach to Nursing* (O'Brien, 2006).

▶ Finding Time for Prayer in Nursing

Brother Lawrence of the Resurrection (1973), sometimes described as the "saint of the pots and pans" for his kitchen ministry, asserted, "It is not necessary for being with God to be always at church. We may make an oratory of our heart wherein to retire from time to time to converse with him" (p. 48). Jean-Pierre De Caussade (1975), the master of abandonment to Divine Providence, taught that "the duties of each moment are shadows which hide the action of the Divine will" (p. 23). And, soldier saint Ignatius Loyola believed that for those who "want to love and serve God in all things" love should be manifest "more by deeds than by words" (Barry, 1987, p. 119).

Other scholars of prayer suggest that we may incorporate prayer into our busy days through such activities as thinking of God as we are walking about or working at some manual task; praying the "Jesus Prayer," using a brief formula such as "Come Lord Jesus"; or simply repeating the name of Jesus and meditating on the holiness of ordinary tasks, especially those involving the care of a brother or sister in need. Nursing practice, in its many and varied dimensions, surely lends itself to the latter kind of prayerful meditation.

The authors and editors of a number of contemporary clinical nursing journal articles identify prayer as a dimension of the nurse's role. The cover design for a spring 2000 issue of *The Clinical Journal of Oncology Nursing* promoted an article on spiritual care, highlighting the concepts of healing, medicine, faith, and prayer. Prayer has been identified as part of the role of holistic nurses (Lewis, 1996, pp. 308–315); intensive care unit (ICU) nurses (Holt-Ashley, 2000, pp. 60–67); oncology, hospice, and parish nurses (Sellers & Haag, 1998, pp. 338–354); and as a general nursing intervention in a variety of other nursing areas (Mason, 1995). It is, thus, a given that most nurses, or at least many nurses, consider prayer to be an important dimension of their practice. But then we must return to the topic of finding time for prayer, or for creating an "oratory of the heart," in the midst of our busy schedules.

Spiritual writer Pierre Wolff takes up the topic boldly by entitling a chapter on prayer "How Can I Pray When I Am Too Busy?" Wolff responds by describing the married relationship of two friends; it is a "love story," he says, "as prayer is." In the anecdote, Wolff explains how his friends, although busy with work, children, and community activities, find time to nurture their love for each other. They may have just a minute to say "I love you," or a longer time to spend being together, but constantly sharing their care for each other has become a way of life (Wolff, 1995).

Another strategy that helps me to remember to "pray always," or to try, as Wolff suggests, to pray even when I am too busy, is to decorate my living and work spaces with spiritual/religious pictures and thoughts. I have a beautifully carved wooden crucifix on my office wall, given to me many years ago when I entered religious life, and a print of Domenico Fetti's 1622 oil painting entitled *The Veil of Veronica*, which one of my students brought me from the National Gallery of Art. Above my computer is a special favorite, a framed print of Jean-Francois Millet's magnificently prayerful painting *The Angelus*. The mid-19th-century scene depicts two young farmers, standing heads bent in prayer, in a potato field, as the sun sets in the background. In the distance one can perceive the faint outline of a village church steeple, its bells tolling the evening Angelus to call the community to prayer. Looking at this print always makes me want to stop for a moment and pray, wishing that I might be united with these young peasant farmers who interrupted their field work to pay homage to their Lord.

The attraction to particular religious symbols or religious art will be different, of course, for each of us. But being surrounded by things that touch the heart and lift the spirit can be very helpful in supporting an ongoing prayer life. There will, in the trajectory of one's developing spiritual life, always be times of distraction and dryness. Nevertheless, using natural God-given gifts such as religious art or uplifting spiritual meditations may strengthen one's commitment to prayer and inspire perseverance in attempting the seemingly impossible gospel mandate to "pray always."

A number of contemporary books on prayer both encourage and support the practice of leading a prayerful life in the midst of myriad professional and social responsibilities; some of these include: *Contemplation in Action* (Rohr, 2006), *The World Is Our Cloister* (Kavanaugh, 2007), *How to Be a Monastic and Not Leave Your*

Day Job (Tvedten, 2008), *The World Is My Cloister: Living from the Heart Within"* (Talbot, 2010), *Jean Vanier, Essential Writings* (Whitney-Brown, 2010), *The Universal Monk* (Talbot, 2011), and *Sanctuary of the Soul* (Foster, 2011).

▶ Prayer and Nursing Practice: A Nurse's Sabbath

There are many ways to approach a discussion of prayer and nursing practice, because our workplaces are so varied in the current profession. We are hospital nurses, clinic nurses, nurse practitioners in offices, home care nurses, long-term care nurses, parish nurses, military nurses, and nurses employed in other disciplines and settings too numerous to list here. Within these arenas, we are nurse clinicians, nurse administrators, nurse managers, nurse educators, and nurse researchers. We are told in the gospel of Jesus that when we care for the sick, we care for Him, that, in fact, our nursing becomes our prayer. But are all of our nursing tasks of equal value? Do they all constitute living the gospel message of Jesus?

A tale from the desert fathers reminds us that a great variety of good works are blessed by the Lord: "For scripture says that Abraham was hospitable and God was with him. And David was humble and God was with him. And Elias loved solitary prayer and God was with him. So, do whatever you see your soul desires according to God." (Vincent, 1982, p. 44). I love that desert fathers story, because it reminds me that there are many options for serving the Lord for us as nurses; there are many prayerful ministries of caring for the sick that reflect the gospel message, "I was ill and you visited me."

Contemporary literature demonstrates health-care providers' interest in prayer related to such clinical topics as holistic care (DiJoseph & Cavendish, 2005), serious illness (Hanson et al., 2008), severe head injury (Vannemreddy, Bryan, & Nanda, 2009), open heart surgery (Ai, Tice, Huang, Rodgers, & Bolling, 2008), chemotherapy for recurrent ovarian cancer (Johnson et al., 2009), chronic pain (Wachholtz & Pearce, 2009; Andersson, 2008), and mental health issues (Lewis, Breslin, & Dein, 2008).

In order, however, to be sensitive to prayer, to the need for prayer in the nursing workplace, nurses also long to have some private time, some "Sabbath time," to be alone to talk with and to listen to the Lord.

The Sabbath is an important day for many major religious traditions; it is a time of rest and relaxation from the workweek, but most importantly, it is a time of prayer, both individual prayer and community prayer. Most Christian denominations hold communal worship services each Sunday (or Saturday, for some). For Roman Catholics, Sunday or Saturday evening Mass is a mandate of the Church, and for many Jewish communities, Sabbath temple worship is expected each week. Because of the importance of the concept, theologian Abraham Heschel (1979) wrote a book, now a classic, entitled *The Sabbath, Its Meaning for Modern Man*. In it, Heschel wrote: "Six days a week we wrestle with the world, wringing profit from the earth; on the Sabbath we especially care for the seed of eternity planted in the soul. The world has our hands, but our soul belongs to Someone Else" (p. 13).

The problem, of course, is that nurses often do not have a "Sabbath" in terms of a particular day of the week. Our Sabbath may consist of 8 to 12 hours staffing an ICU or an emergency room; we may be out in the community doing home care visits for those unable to travel because of illness or disability; or we might even be physically at our respective churches, yet involved in such activities as blood-pressure screening or health counseling in the role of parish or faith community nurse. It's true that such nursing ministries can themselves constitute prayerful efforts, yet we truly do need some time and place of Sabbath, apart, for our personal communion with the Lord. How can this be accomplished?

The Sabbath spirituality of Abraham Heschel holds that on the Sabbath we must attempt to avoid the tyranny of things and "try to become attuned to holiness in time" (p. 13). I suggest that because we nurses may not always have one full Sabbath day during a week, although when possible that would surely be desirable, we may, instead, try to create several small Sabbath experiences within the seven-day period. During those mini-Sabbath times, we can embrace Heschel's concept of becoming "attuned to holiness." Our Sabbath experiences might take place on a quiet Sunday evening, a free Wednesday morning, or a Friday afternoon, before a family dinner or weekend activities take over our lives. Communal worship services may need to be worked around our nursing schedules, but finding the time is always possible. Nurses are consummate improvisers; one thing I am certain of is that if a nurse sets out to make something work, it will work.

What I am suggesting is surely not new; it's the way a number of nurses have created their Sabbath times for many years. In the early days of nursing education, or "training" as we called it back then, students, and sometimes graduate nurses, had only one free afternoon a week and that rarely fell on a Saturday or a Sunday. And yet, as our history documents, nurses throughout the centuries have included a prayerful spirituality as a significant dimension of their nursing practice. The challenge for us, as contemporary nurses, is to continue in the footsteps of those who have gone before us and to continue our commitment to a prayerful and sacred covenant of caring as we carry out our nurse–patient interactions in the sophisticated health-care milieu of the 21st century.

▶ The Ethics of Praying with Patients

It is not the purpose, and it is beyond the scope, of this text to undertake an in-depth ethical discussion of the topic of nurses praying with patients. It is important to note, however, that the ethics of nurses' prayerful interventions has been and continues to be raised in the contemporary nursing literature. A nurse educator and a staff nurse take on the issue directly in their article "To Pray or Not to Pray: A Question of Ethics" (French & Narayanasamy, 2011). These authors discuss such ethical concerns as informed consent, intention, and authority; they point out that "despite the religious beliefs of the nurse, intentions to proselytize must be avoided to protect patient autonomy and to avoid abuse of the nurse's authority" (p. 1198). French and Narayanasamy advise that in the clinical setting nurses should "only offer prayer if they have received consent, provided local policies and protocols are in place to support prayer as a therapeutic intervention" (p. 1203).

In a paper entitled "Examining the Ethics of Praying with Patients," Winslow and Winslow (2003) offer five guidelines to help nurses make appropriate ethical decisions about praying with patients; these include: provision of "spiritually respectful care" (p. 172), following "patients' expressed wishes regarding prayer" (p. 173), "absence of any pressure [on] patients to relinquish their spiritual beliefs" (p. 174), nurses' understanding of "their own spirituality" (p. 175), and prayer with patients being "consonant with the nurse's integrity" (p. 176). Winslow and Winslow conclude that prayer may be a helpful part of the care nurses provide; it must, nevertheless, "be guided by ethical reflection" (p. 176).

Finally, a team of physicians and ethicists provided ethical guidelines for prayer in hospitals quite similar to those identified by nurse authors. These included: "respect (for) patients and their religious beliefs," acting "in the patient's best interests," and "maintaining personal integrity" (Lo et al., 2003, p. 414).

Historically, as noted earlier in this chapter, nurse authors have suggested that nurses praying with patients is an appropriate nursing intervention. Writing in the 1970s, Granger Westberg (2009), the identified founder of parish nursing, advised that a nurse should offer a prayer for a patient if asked, but he warned that "no nurse ought to force prayer upon a patient" (p. 7). Nurse educator Mary Sweat (2009) commented that praying with patients is a "privilege and a responsibility" (p. 181). She also provided ethical guidelines for nurses, however, and pointed out that "prayer isn't magic" (p. 181). Prayer was identified as an important resource for nurses as it "frequently sustains coping and brings comfort" (Taylor, 2003, p. 179); and while admitting that "teaching nursing students to pray with their clients is a basic nursing intervention" (Lantz, 2007, p. 35), professor of nursing Cheryl Lantz also cited important ethical principles to consider including respect, (patient) autonomy, and client advocacy (p. 36).

Finally, the literature reveals that while many studies have demonstrated "positive associations between prayer and wellbeing" in hospitalized patients (Hollywell & Walker, 2008, p. 637), it is strongly advised that "ethical boundaries must be respected" in praying with patients. "It is essential that doctors and nurses acknowledge the disparities of power and information that operate in the health care setting" (Cohen et al., 2000, p. 45).

In conclusion, many older and current nursing articles support the appropriateness and importance of nurses praying with their patients. A number of these articles include a caveat related to ethics and/or ethical guidelines for prayer as a nursing intervention. For those nurse authors who do not specifically address the ethics of praying with patients, it may be assumed that such activities would be guided, as is all nursing care, by the general ethical principal of beneficence; that is, of doing no harm to the patient.

▶ References

Ai, A. L., Tice, T., Huang, B., Rodgers, W., & Bolling, S. (2008). Types of prayer, optimism and well-being of middle-aged and older patients undergoing open-heart surgery. *Mental Health, Religion and Culture, 11*(1), 131–150.

Andersson, G. (2008). Chronic pain and praying to a higher power: Useful or useless? *Journal of Religion & Health, 47*(2), 176–187.

Barry, W. A. (1987). *God and you: Prayer as a personal relationship.* New York, NY: Paulist Press.

Beck, M. B. (1945). *The nurse: Handmaid of the divine physician.* Philadelphia, PA: J.B. Lippincott.

Calabria, M. D., & Macrae, J. (1994). *Suggestions for thought by Florence Nightingale.* Philadelphia, PA: University of Pennsylvania Press.

Casey, M. (1996). *Toward God: The ancient wisdom of western prayer.* Liguori, MO: Liguori Press.

Chan, R. R. (2014). Mantra meditation as a bedside spiritual intervention. *MEDSURG Nursing, 23*(2), 84–100.

Cohen, C., Wheeler, S., Scott, D., Edwards, B., Lusk, P., & The Anglican Working Group on Bioethics. (2000). Prayer as therapy: A challenge to both religious belief and professional ethics. *Hasting Center Report, 30*(3), 40–47.

Collegeville Series on Books of the Bible (1987). Collegeville, MN: The Liturgical Press.

De Caussade, J. P. (1975). *Abandonment to divine providence.* New York, NY: Image Books.

Demeron, C. (2012). Influence your practice: Pray! *Journal of Christian Nursing, 29*(1), 10.

DiJoseph, J., & Cavendish, R. (2005). Expanding the dialogue on prayer relevant to holistic care. *Holistic Nursing Practice, 19*(4), 147–154.

Dossey, B. M. (2000). *Florence Nightingale: Mystic, visionary, healer.* Springhouse, PA: Springhouse Corporation.

Foster, R. J. (2011). *Sanctuary of the soul: Journey into meditative prayer.* Downers Grove, IL: InterVarsity Press.

French, C., & Narayanasamy, A. (2011). To pray or not to pray: A question of ethics. *British Journal of Nursing, 20*(18), 1198–1204.

Groeschel, B. (1997). Introduction. In B. Groeschel & J. Monti (Eds.), *In the presence of our Lord* (p. 15). Huntington, IN: Our Sunday Visitor Publishing Division.

Hanson, L., Dobbs, D., Usher, B., Williams, S., Rawlings, J., & Daaleman, T. (2008). Providers and types of spiritual care during serious illness. *Journal of Palliative Medicine, 11*(6), 907–914.

Hayes, E. J., Hayes, P. J., & Kelly, D. E. (1956). *Moral handbook of nursing.* New York, NY: The Macmillan Company.

Heschel, A. (1979). *The Sabbath: Its meaning for modern man.* New York, NY: Farrar, Straus and Giroux.

Higgins, P. (2013). Meeting the religious needs of residents with dementia. *Nursing Older People, 25*(9), 26–29.

Hollywell, C., & Walker, J. (2008). Private prayer as a suitable intervention for hospitalized patients: A critical review of the literature. *Journal of Clinical Nursing, 18*(1), 637–651.

Holt-Ashley, M. (2000). Nurses pray: Use of prayer and spirituality as a complementary therapy in the intensive care setting. *AACN Clinical Issues: Advanced Practice in Acute and Critical Care, 11*(1), 60–67.

Hubbartt, B., & Kautz, D. D. (2012). Prayer at the bedside. *International Journal for Human Caring, 16*(1), 42–47.

Johnson, M., Dose, A., Pipe, T., Peterson, W., Huschka, M., Gallenberg, M., . . . Frost, M. (2009). Centering prayer for women receiving chemotherapy for recurrent ovarian cancer. *Oncology Nursing Forum, 36*(4), 421–428.

Kavanaugh, J. (2007). *The world is our cloister.* Winchester, UK: O Books.

Kreeft, P. (2000). *Prayer for beginners.* San Francisco, CA: Ignatius Press.

Lantz, C. M. (2007). Teaching spiritual care in a public institution: Legal implications, standards of practice and ethical obligations. *Journal of Nursing Education, 46*(1), 33–38.

Lawrence of the Resurrection. (1973). *The practice of the presence of God.* Mount Vernon, NY: Peter Pauper Press.

Lewis, C. A., Breslin, M. J., & Dein, S. (2008). Prayer and mental health: An introduction. *Mental Health, Religion & Culture, 11*(1), 1–7.

Lewis, P. J. (1996). A review of prayer within the role of the holistic nurse. *Journal of Holistic Nursing, 14*(4), 308–315.

Lo, B., Kates, L., Ruston, D., Arnold, R., Cohen, C., Pulchaski, C., . . . Tulsky, J. (2003). Responding to requests regarding prayer and religious ceremonies by patients near the end of life and their families. *Journal of Palliative Medicine, 6*(3), 409–415.

Lumpkin, G. T. (1926). The Christ spirit which makes the hospital great. *The Trained Nurse and Hospital Review, 77*(6), 628.

Macrae, J. (1995). Nightingale's spiritual philosophy and its significance for modern nursing. *Image, 27*(1), 10.

Maher, A. (1954). A night nurse's prayer. *The Catholic Nurse, 2*(4), 30.

Mason, C. H. (1995). Prayer as a nursing intervention. *Journal of Christian Nursing, 12*(1), 4–8.

Narayanasamy, A., & Narayanasamy, M. (2008). The healing power of prayer and its implications for nursing. *British Journal of Nursing, 17*(6), 394–398.

Nightingale, F. (1859). *Notes on nursing: What it is and what it is not.* London, England: Harrison, Bookseller to the Queen.

O'Brien, M. E. (2006). *The nurse with an alabaster jar: A Biblical approach to nursing.* Madison, WI: NCF Press.

Pennington, B. (2008). *Psalms: A spiritual commentary.* Woodstock, VT: SkyLight Publications.

Rohr, R. (2006). *Contemplation in action.* New York, NY: Crossroad.

Rothweiler, E. L. (1937). *The art and science of nursing.* Philadelphia, PA: F.A. Davis.

Sellers, S. C., & Haag, B. A. (1998). Spiritual nursing interventions. *Journal of Holistic Nursing, 16*(3), 338–354.

Swaim, M. (2011). *Prayer in the digital age.* Liguori, MO: Liguori Publications.

Sweat, M. T. (2009). OK to pray? *Journal of Christian Nursing, 26*(3), 180–181.

Talbot, J. M. (2010). *The world is my cloister: Living from the heart within.* Maryknoll, NY: Orbis Books.

Talbot, J. M. (2011). *The universal monk: The way of the new monastery.* Collegeville, MN: Liturgical Press.

Taylor, E. J. (2003). Prayer's clinical issues and implications. *Holistic Nursing Practice, 17*(4), 179–188.

Tvedten, B. (2008). *How to be a monastic and not leave your day job.* Brewster, MA: Paraclete Press.

Vannemreddy, P., Bryan, K., & Nanda, A. (2009). Influence of prayer and prayer habits on outcome in patients with severe head injury. *American Journal of Hospice and Palliative Medicine, 26,* 264–269.

Vicinus, M., & Nergaard, B. (1990). *Ever yours, Florence Nightingale: Selected letters.* Cambridge, MA: Harvard University Press.

Vincent, M. C. (1982). *The life of prayer and the way to God.* Petersham, MA: Saint Bede's Publications.

Wachholtz, A. B., & Pearce, J. (2009). Does spirituality as a coping mechanism help or hinder coping with chronic pain? *Current Pain and Headache Reports, 13,* 127–132.

Westberg, G. (2009). Granger Westberg on nursing and prayer. *Parish Nurse Perspectives, 8*(3), 7.

White, F. S. (1923). At the gate of the temple. *The Public Health Nurse, 15*(6), 283–285.

Whitney-Brown, C. (Ed.). (2010). *Jean Vanier, essential writings.* Maryknoll, NY: Orbis Books.

Wiederkehr, M. (2008). *Seven sacred pauses: Living mindfully through the hours of the day.* Notre Dame, IN: Sorin Books.

Winslow, G. R., & Winslow, B.W. (2003). Examining the ethics of praying with patients. *Holistic Nursing Practice, 17*(4), 170–177.

Wolff, P. (1995). *The hungry heart.* Liguori, MO: Triumph Books.

Zyromski, P. (2000). *Pray the Bible.* Cincinnati, OH: St. Anthony Messenger Press.

CHAPTER 17

The Spirituality of Caring: A Sacred Covenant Model for Nursing Practice

I have made a covenant with my chosen one.

Psalm 89:3

> There is a sacredness in the caring that we do as nurses. We touch our patients spiritually and they touch us; that's the heart of what it means to be a nurse. The nurse–patient relationship is something beyond other relationships. It's a holy kind of relationship. It's about reverencing those we care for, respecting the sacredness of their lives no matter how ill or how disabled they might be. We are truly blessed in this relationship of caring.

Mary, Nurse Educator in Clinical Nursing

The purpose of this chapter is to introduce a new caring model, a "Sacred Covenant Model of Caring for Nursing Practice," as well as to present an overview, including history and contemporary understanding, of the spirituality of "caring," which has been described as an essential element of nursing practice. In the process of exploring the concept of nurses' caring in the world of 21st-century health care, a newly created "covenant-oriented" model of caring is identified and described; this model is based on empirical data from two recent studies of caring behaviors reported by practicing nurses from a variety of clinical settings. The concept of a covenant-oriented model of caring is also supported in the nursing literature.

New understandings of the concept of "caring," as central to the practice of professional nursing, are continually being offered in the literature. As noted, "nursing is a caring profession and caring is perceived to be vital in promoting successful patient outcomes" (Desmond, Horn, Keith, Kelby, Ryan, & Smith, 2014, p. 35). Key attributes of nurses' caring include: treating patients with courtesy and respect" and "listening carefully to patients" and their concerns (p. 35). Additional characteristics of nurses' caring are: "respect for patients' autonomy" (Taylor, Park, & Pfeiffer, 2014, p. 2612); compassion and treading "gently and softly" in approaching spiritual caring (Pfeiffer, Gober, & Taylor, 2014, p. 2886); listening to the "voices" of nursing staff in "caring theory based practice" (Dyess, Boykin, & Bulfin, 2013, p. 167); "connectedness with inner space" (Rykkje, Eriksson, & Raholm, 2011, p. 40) and "sensitivity" especially in caring for the elderly (Ranheim, Karner, & Bertero, 2011, p. 1).

A simultaneous concept analysis of caring theory and nursing practice included nine interrelated concepts that mediated care; these included "caritas," "sense-making as a movement of embodied reflection," "gaining meaningfulness," "caring in distress," "becoming aware," "embodied moments of presence," "confirmations and abstractions," "marginalization of caring," and "intention of caring" (Ranheim, Karner, & Bertero, 2012, p. 80). And, a positive relationship between a nurse's spiritual health and his or her professional commitment and caring was found in a recent study of 619 clinical nurses evaluated using several spiritual care attitude and behavior scales (Chiang, Lee, Chu, Han, & Hsiao, 2016). In a chapter entitled "A Theory of Caring," nurse ethicist Sara Fry (1991) explored three traditional models of caring: the cultural model of caring, the feminist model of caring, and the humanistic model of caring (pp. 162–165). Under the heading of "moral foundations for a pluralistic model of caring," however, Fry also described a "covenant-oriented" model of caring. In explaining this model, Fry stated: "Authentic nurse caring is based on . . . the maintenance of fidelity in the relationship with the patient; hence, it is a covenant model of care" (p. 166). She added: "A focus on covenant suggests that . . . fidelity is the basis for nurses' caring . . . it includes the elements of compassion and doing for others . . . it also includes respect for persons and the protection of human dignity which are elements fundamental to the nurse-patient relationship" (p. 166). Fry presented a linear representation of a "Covenant Model of Caring," which included five concepts: compassion, doing for others, respect for persons, protection of human dignity, and fidelity (p. 167).

The Sacred Covenant Model of Caring offered here supports Sara Fry's early suggestion and addresses lacunae on the concept of covenant-oriented caring in the nursing literature. The model builds on the author's earlier study findings related to the concept of nurses' caring, which revealed both the sacredness and the covenantal nature of the caring relationship. These include: "A Sacred Covenant" in *The Nurse's Calling: A Christian Spirituality of Caring for the Sick* (M. E. O'Brien, 2001), "A Sacred Covenant: Prayer and the Nurse-Patient Relationship" in *Prayer in Nursing: The Spirituality of Compassionate Caregiving"* (M. E. O'Brien, 2003), "The Bible and the Nurse Patient Covenant" in *The Nurse with an Alabaster Jar: A Biblical Approach to Nursing* (M. E. O'Brien, 2006), and "The Sacred Covenant of Caring" in *A Sacred Covenant: The Spiritual Ministry of Nursing* (M. E. O'Brien, 2008). The present model is also grounded in new qualitative data derived from the two earlier referenced studies of contemporary practicing nurses; this research is discussed later in the chapter.

▶ The Spirituality of Caring in Nursing

The spirituality of caring in nursing may be envisioned as comprised of three concepts: (1) a calling of service, (2) a blessed trust, and (3) a commitment to reverence. The term *spirituality* is generally understood as referring to one's personal relationship with transcendence or a transcendent being, God. Theologian Joann Conn (1990) suggested that for Christians spirituality "means one's entire life as understood, felt, imagined and decided upon in relationship to God, in Christ Jesus, empowered by the Spirit" (p. 972). Dominican Richard Woods (1993) pointed out that Christian spirituality "arose within the Jewish spiritual tradition of," among other things, "God's abiding presence" and "faithful covenant love" (p. 938). Nurse author Kathleen Krebs (2001) observed that the "spiritual aspect of caring" has become "an integral part of health and healing" (p. 55); she asserted also that predictions of the greatest advances in our society "will not come from technology but from our deeper understanding of what it means to be a human, spiritual being" (p. 55). And theorist Carol Montgomery (1992) noted that the "spiritual nature" of nurses' caring "serves as an important resource from which the caregiver can derive meanings that sustain him or her through loss or other stressors associated with caring" (p. 50).

Philip Burnard (1997), in a chapter discussing "ethical and spiritual issues in caring in nursing," addressed the sometimes raised question: considering the "unavoidable inequality of cared for and carer, 'Why bother to care?'" (p. 32). Ultimately, Burnard concluded his discussion with the observation that "caring is so much a part of nursing that if nurses do not care, then they are not fully practicing nursing" (p. 32). Burnard's conclusion is clearly supported by the caring data elicited from practicing nurses who have participated in the author's research. And, although not specifically addressing the spirituality of caring, one of the early nursing theorists of caring, Kathryn Gardner, identified three conditions critical to caring that reflect a spiritual stance toward the concept: "1. Awareness and knowledge of the care receiver's need for care, 2. An intention of the caregiver to act and actions based on that knowledge and 3. A positive change in the recipient of care as a result of caring solely on the basis of the welfare of others" (Gardner, 1992, p. 242). Surely there is a spiritual motive undergirding caring that is perceptive of another's need and based "solely on the welfare of others."

In discussing the "emotional cost of caring," Verena Tschudin (1997) points out that caring can at times be so emotionally draining as to leave one "spiritually bankrupt"; thus, in caring theory there should exist "a deliberate and wise concern for the mental and spiritual nature of the carer" (p. 155). Montgomery (1993), who also discusses the emotional demands of caring, asserts that in order to cope with the stresses that may be associated with caregiving, one of the best resources is a "spiritual understanding," which allows carers to deal with the sufferings of those they care for (pp. 112–113). Often nurses incorporate spiritual actions or activities in their caregiving. Nurse Charlotte Barry (1994) relates a tender experience of caring for a dying patient. One of the tasks she included in her physical care of the semiconscious patient was to tape a rosary, which she found lying in the bed, to her patient's hand. After the patient's death, one of the nurse's caring acts, for which the family expressed special gratitude, was "the taping of the rosary beads to [the patient's] hands so they would be with her always" (pp. 73–74).

A Calling of Service

In discussing the ethics of serving others, Constance Milton (2005) quotes the American Nurses Association's *Code of Ethics for Nurses*, which speaks of the nurse's commitment to the patient and family. Milton asserts: "Nursing exists to serve others" (p. 21). The concept of "being there to serve" and its subconcept of "going beyond the ordinary" in caring for the sick were key themes in a study of servant leadership among contemporary practicing nurses (M. E. O'Brien, 2011, pp. 192–199). Nurse respondents were pleased to discuss their professional roles in terms of a call to serve others: "The idea of servanthood, of being of service to the sick, was not in any way perceived as placing the nurse in a lower position. It was in fact considered a privilege to serve the sick. For a number of nurses . . . the positive attribution placed on the concept of service was derived from the Christian scripture; that is from the example of Jesus, who as 'the Son of Man came not to be served but to serve' (Matthew 10:45)" (M. E. O'Brien, 2008, p. 193).

In early 20th-century nursing, most U.S. hospitals had nursing support offices with labels such as "The Department of Nursing Service" or "The Nursing Service Office." Over the past few decades, however, most large urban hospitals have changed their nursing office titles to "Office of Nursing Administration" or similar language. In certain quarters, nurses refrain from using terms such as *calling*, *vocation*, and/or *service* to describe nursing. These words seem, to some few, to indicate a less than professional description for the conduct of nursing the sick. Interestingly, however, in talking with senior nursing practitioners, and often with younger nurses, there is generally a sense of pride and gratitude for the "calling" or "vocation" of service to those in need. Nurses are proud to be nurses, to have been blessed (in their words) to a "calling of service."

What does it mean to be called to a "calling of service"? The term *calling*, or more properly *vocation*, has many definitions. In the language of spirituality, a calling or vocation generally is understood as a call from God, or "a divine call to undertake a particular activity" (Holland, 1990, p. 1087). A nurse's calling, viewed in the spiritual sense, may indeed be described as a holy calling and a calling of service: "Nursing is not only a respected profession, it is a beautiful and holy vocation. Caring for the sick is not only a job, it is a ministry, a ministry to the weakest, the neediest, the most fragile of our brothers and sisters in the human family" (M. E. O'Brien, 2008, p. 3); "we as nurses are called to care, called to love in a special way, those who are ill in their bodies, in their minds or in their spirits" (M. E. O'Brien, 2001, p. 2).

Theologian Mikael Lundmark (2007) analyzed the writings of two nursing theorists of caring in regard to their understanding of the concept of "vocation as a motivational factor for nursing" (p. 767). Ultimately Lundmark concluded that the caring models of both Ann Bradshaw and Katie Eriksson "advocate a vocational understanding of nursing as being essential to nursing theory" (p. 778). The theorists' perceptions are supported by the article "Why Spirituality Is Essential for Nurses," in which authors Stephen Wright and Julia Neuberger (2012) argue that "engaged spirituality is the key to improving nurses' ability to . . . remain compassionate toward patients" (p. 19). And in their book *Being Called to Care*, nurse theorists Mary Lashley, Maggie Neal, Emily Slunt, Louise Berman, and Francine Hultgren (1994) share multiple chapters documenting the importance and centrality of the nurse's call to caring for the ill and the infirm; some topics include: "What Does It Mean to Be Called to Care?" "Ways of Responding to the Call," "Living the Call Authentically," "Vulnerability: The Call to Woundedness," and "Keeping the Call Alive".

Over the past several decades there have been a number of published studies of the nurse's calling in the extant literature. Three examples of these include: (1) "Nursing Care as a Calling" in which quantitative data from 179 practicing nurses revealed that those nurses who perceived their profession as a "calling" were "excellent in supporting both the individual patient and his or her family" (Raatikainen, 1997, p. 1111); (2) "Re-calling the Spirit of Nursing," a phenomenological study in which 9 registered nurses were asked to reflect on their calling as nurses; the result was that "feeing like a nurse creates possibilities for authentic caring" (Spence & Smythe, 2008, p. 243); and (3) "Why Did I Become a Nurse?", a study of 12 registered nurses and 11 nursing students in which two dominant themes describing study participants' reasons for entering nursing were "Opportunity for Caring" and "My Vocation in Life" (Eley, Eley, Bertello, & Rogers-Clark, 2012, p. 1546).

A Blessed Trust

It seems that one cannot begin a discussion of the dimension of nursing's spirituality of caring labeled "a blessed trust" without calling to mind one of Florence Nightingale's best loved quotes: "And remember every nurse should be one who is to be depended upon . . . she must have a respect for her own calling because God's precious gift of life is often literally placed in [the nurse's] hands" (Nightingale, 1859, p. 71). What a blessed trust nurses have been assigned by Nightingale, a trust essential to a ministry that may at times truly place "God's precious gift of life" in the nurses' hands.

Trust is generally understood to "denote a confidence or a sense of security in the reliability of someone else . . . the term is a relational one, describing the quality of the relationship among two or more persons" (Schreiter, 1993, p. 982). The concept of trust may also be linked to fidelity. A spiritual example of that relationship suggests that "whatever faithfulness, whatever trust we have in God, finds it's assurance in God's own fidelity to us . . . in the covenants God made with Noah and Abraham" (Baynham, 1993, p. 406). What does this concept of trust, this concept of a blessed trust, actually mean for the nurse's role of covenantal caring? Many nursing authors respond to this question in their descriptions of the primacy of trust in the nurse–patient relationship.

Catherine Snelson (1992) discussed trust as a "caring construct with the critically ill: Trust as a care construct is embedded in the nurse-client relationship in critical care" (p. 157). Snelson explains: "In the context of such a short and intense relationship frequently experienced in critical care, it is imperative that critical care nurses quickly understand the patient's perspective of trust in order to implement professional nursing care" (p. 157). Clinical nurse specialist Anne Katz (2011) pointed out that for the past decade nursing has been identified in Gallup polls as "the most trusted profession" (p. 101). Andrea Gregg (2011), a past president of the Florida Nurses Association, notes that "trust in care providers is an essential element in re-establishing well-being lost due to illness" (p. 5). "Thus," Gregg adds, "trustworthiness is one—perhaps the most important—moral virtue among professions, like ours, that help people during times of vulnerability" (p. 5).

In a qualitative exploration of the understanding and experience of trust among seven new graduate nurses, findings suggested that the nurse must first establish rapport with a patient before he or she can "achieve a trusting relationship" (Belcher, 2009, p. 142). After examining the concept of trust in mental health care, researchers Piippo and Aaltonen (2008) reported that trust is "closely connected to autonomy and power; patients feel that trust increases as their experience of autonomy increases" (p. 2867). Finally, a concept analysis of nurse–patient trust was undertaken to clarify the meaning of the term and to determine its relevance to nursing practice (Bell & Duffy, 2009). The authors of this study concluded that the defining attributes of trust in the nurse–patient relationship are: "expectation of competence, goodwill of others, fragility and vulnerability and element of risk" (p. 50). Ultimately a definition of trust in the nurse–patient relationship was identified as "the optimistic acceptance of a vulnerable situation, following careful assessment, in which the truster believes that the trustee has his best interests at heart" (p. 50).

But, what does it mean to label this concept a *blessed* trust? In theological and spiritual dictionaries very few entries are listed under "blessed"; those found usually describe a religious ritual carried out for a specific purpose. Two definitions found in general dictionaries, however, do seem to reflect the understanding of nurses who use the adjective to describe their caring, that is: "to make or pronounce holy" (*Webster's Third New International Dictionary*, 2002, p. 233) and "divinely or supremely favored" (*The Random House Dictionary of the English Language*, 1966, p. 158). Some examples of nurses' comments incorporating the adjective blessed are: "Nursing is a blessed calling; a spiritual calling to serve the sick"; I am truly blessed [to be a nurse]. It's a blessed calling. I am blessed to love my job so much," and "If I didn't think nursing was a blessed calling or ministry and felt like it was just a job, I would not be here presently as a nurse" (M. E. O'Brien, 2011, p. 102). The interpretation, in reviewing those nurses' expanded comments on nursing as a blessed calling, is that nurses truly see their caring in terms of spirituality, or a holiness of purpose, and they feel that this makes the nurse's caring attitudes and behaviors unique.

A Commitment to Reverence

A third characteristic of nursing's spirituality of caring is that of the nurse's commitment to reverence. This attribute of a nurse's spirituality is critical to the caring displayed by professional nurses. Nurses often have to undertake difficult and/or unpleasant tasks, both physical and emotional, in caring for their patients. While such nursing activities are necessary to enhance healing and promote health, they may be uncomfortable, embarrassing, and sometimes painful for both patient and nurse. Thus, a posture of spiritual gentleness, a posture of reverence, in undertaking such nursing actions is essential to promoting and achieving a philosophy of committed caring on the part of the nurse.

Nurse theorist Rosemarie Parse (2009) defined reverence as "a virtue, a quality that is primordially grounded in unconditional love" (p. 1). Nurse Kathy Okland (2002) advises nurses to "remember reverence" as "that feeling of profound respect and awe . . . for nursing and everything it entails" (p. 18). A theological definition of reverence includes the concepts of both justice and charity toward those for whom one cares (T. C. O'Brien, 1979, p. 3040). From the time of Florence Nightingale, nurses and nursing activities have been imbued with a reverence for the sacredness of human life. Another of Nightingale's well-loved quotes describes such reverence in poignant words: "Nursing is an art, and if it is to be made an art, it requires as exclusive a devotion, as hard a preparation, as any painter's or sculptor's work. For what is having to do with dead canvas or cold marble compared with having to do with the living body, the temple of God's spirit" (as cited in Baly, 1991, p. 68). Inherent in Nightingale's request for devotion and preparation among her followers was a mandate for commitment to reverence in the newly founded profession of nursing.

Writing in 1962, Madeleine Vaillot published an entire book on commitment to nursing, in which she suggested that the committed nurse "asks to be judged in terms of the values to which she subscribes . . . as a nurse" (p. 13). Nurse and spiritual writer Verna Benner Carson (1989) observed that "commitment requires that nurses make themselves available to others as long as those clients need support" (p. 168). Carson added:

"A committed nurse shares in the loneliness, anxiety and suffering experienced by a client and does not pull out of the relationship when it becomes uncomfortable" (p. 168). Nurse Julia Barcott (2006) explained her understanding of the meaning of commitment by describing an intense clinical situation of caring; she concluded that in that and similar situations: "The basic ability to try and bring respect, compassion and dignity to patients and their families had brought out the true nature of nursing" (p. 11). In these writings, nursing authors support the assertion that commitment and reverence go hand in hand for the contemporary practicing nurse.

▶ Nurses' Caring as a Sacred Covenant

A critical and constant dimension of the nurse–patient relationship is, as noted earlier, the degree of trust engendered between the interacting parties. The element of trust is lived out in nurse–patient partnerships in terms of a covenant relationship. Although not always formally articulated as such, the presence of an understood covenant between a patient and nurse not only supports the concept of trust between the partners, but it also sets up parameters for appropriate behaviors and attitudes. This covenant can be viewed as sacred given the nature of the intimacy, indeed the holiness, of the nurse–patient relationship. Examining the term *covenant* from a spiritual/theological perspective supports an understanding of the concept of nursing practice as involving a sacred covenant.

Caring as a Covenant

The word *covenant* is derived "from the Hebrew word *berith*, which means 'a binding agreement or pact'" (Senior, 1993, p. 237). The concept of covenant is "one of the Bible's most important and pervasive means of describing the relationship between God and the community of faith" (p. 237). Examples of covenant abound in the Scriptures, beginning with God's covenant with Abraham in the Old Testament (Genesis 12:1–3). In the Old Testament theology, Yahweh's covenant with Israel "established bonds of loyalty and responsibility between God and humanity" (Boadt, 1984, p. 547). The New Testament covenant relates to Jesus Christ as the "Son of David and fulfillment of the Messianic prophecies," as depicted in Luke 22:20 (Nowell, 1990, p. 243). Irene Nowell observes that "covenants may be between equals or superior and inferior (p. 243). In the case of God's covenant with Abraham, Nowell points out, "The covenant binds God; Abraham is the free recipient . . . since the covenant with Abraham binds only God, it is unconditional. It cannot be broken" (pp. 243–244).

The concepts of contract and covenant are differentiated by spiritual writer Henri Nouwen. A contract is viewed as an agreement that may cease if one partner fails to keep the commitment. Nouwen (2003) comments that "the Lord did not establish a contract with the people but a covenant" (p. 63) and cites the supporting Scripture: "'The Lord God says: Does a woman forget a baby at her breast or fail to cherish the son of her womb? Yes, even if these forget, I will not forget you' (Isaiah 49:15)" "And," Nouwen continues, "the one who understands this covenant responds: 'If my father and mother desert me, the Lord will care for me still'" (p. 63). In contrast, a covenant, as envisioned by Nouwen (2003), underlies the spiritual care relationship. He asserts, "In the covenant there is no condition put on faithfulness. It is the unconditional commitment to be of service" (p. 63). Ultimately Nouwen points out that in a covenantal relationship the caregiver cannot "expect a return for good services" (p. 63); he advises, "God did not offer us a contract but a covenant and challenges those of us who want to make this covenant visible in the world to never make human success a criterion of their love for others" (pp. 64–65).

Many of the covenant-related concepts found in the theological and pastoral care literature have relevance for the nurse–patient relationship:

Bonds of loyalty and responsibility—The nurse's commitment to employ all of his or her knowledge and skill to provide the best possible care for the patient, and, in turn, the patient's responsibility to comply, to the best of his or her ability, with the prescribed treatment regimen.

No conditions put on faithfulness—The nurse will not cease to care lovingly for the patient, regardless of attitudes such as apathy, anger, or even outright noncompliance on the part of a patient.

An unconditional commitment to be of service—Regardless of potentially mediating issues such as fatigue or personal stress, a nurse will unfailingly try to be available to serve the needs of the patients under his or her care.

No expectation of a return for good services—The degree of the nurse's care and compassion cannot be predicated on the patient's, or family's, gratitude; for physical or emotional reasons, or perhaps both, such thanks may not always be demonstrated.

The Isaiah Scripture (49:15) cited earlier provides a moving example of God's covenantal constancy. Thus, for the nurse called to a ministry of service, whether in nursing practice, nursing education, nursing administration, or nursing research, the theological concept of covenant serves to teach, to guide, to strengthen, and to inspire. The concept of the personal covenantal relationship of God to His people provides a powerful model for the caring and supportive nurse–patient relationships that reflect the art as well as the science of nursing.

As well as the theological literature, the concept of covenant-oriented nurse–patient caring has been explored in the medical and nursing literature. The relationship of trust between patient and caregiver, in the ministry of health care, is identified by Bruhn (2005) as: "the lost art of the covenant" (p. 311). In exploring this lost art of covenant in the nursing community, theorist Ann Bradshaw (1999) cites the Nightingale era of altruism in her article, "The Virtue of Nursing: The Covenant of Care". Bradshaw notes that traditionally, "To become a nurse was not just to enter into a contractual obligation dependent on reward, it was to enter into a covenant that was regardless of reciprocation" (p. 478). Bradshaw concludes that, "The moral reasons to submit oneself to the service of people who are strangers and who may seem at times unappreciative, unattractive, difficult . . . still apply as they did in the Nightingale day" (p. 479).

Nurse Mary Cooper (1988), in examining covenantal relationships as grounding for a nursing ethic, asserted that, "The nurse's duty of fidelity to the patient is dictated by his or her previous choice to become a nurse and thereby to embrace the professional and moral responsibility inherent in such a choice" (p. 57). Cooper's understanding is supported by nurse authors Neville Strumpf and Kristie Asimos in a chapter discussing the covenant between patient and nurse practitioner. Strumpf and Asimos (1996) believe that, "The covenant between nurse practitioner and patient is rooted in the profession's moral and ethical foundations and its abiding commitment to people in need" (p. 176).

The Sacredness of Caring

To adequately describe the sacredness of caring would take many more definitions and examples than can be included in this chapter. However, the term *sacred* is found in the nursing literature less frequently than one might expect. In considering the nurse–patient covenant, it has been stated that "the sacredness of the nurse's caring relationship with a patient derives directly from the sacredness of the nurse's vocation, of his or her call to care for the most vulnerable members of our society, the ill and the infirm" (M. E. O'Brien, 2008, p. 11). In attempting to define the term *sacred*, one is often referred to other terms such as *holiness*, *spirituality*, or the *relationship to God*. Thus, "recognizing someone or something as sacred can make us step back, somewhat in awe of the meaning and power embedded in the adjective. And so it should with our precious vocation of ministering to the sick, our covenant to care for God's fragile ones" (p. 12).

Perhaps one of the best ways to illustrate the meaning of the term *sacred*, or *sacredness*, in caring is through the words of a practicing nurse: "In describing the spiritual rewards of caregiving, Andrew who had worked extensively with the terminally ill, described his patient interactions as 'holy places we share when we have time together.' Andrew explained: 'There is a sweetness in being with these persons even when they are very ill and death is imminent; it gives one the incredible sense of holding a sacredness'" (M. E. O'Brien, 2001, p. 89). A community health nurse describes her nursing as a "sacred path," relating a caregiving anecdote of a time when she did not understand how important her caring was to a fragile patient until she received a beautiful note of thanks. The nurse concluded: "Now, years later, I'm more convinced than ever that nursing is a divine way to connect with others" (Gerber, 2007, p. 43). A clinical nurse specialist described her ministry in a poem as "The Sacred Place of Nursing," identifying caring as a central concept (Davidson, 2009, p. 14). In further support, nursing practice was conceptualized as "a sacred healing dance" by nursing leaders Fran Biley and Nancy Chiocchi (2007).

Two nursing studies exploring the sacredness of nursing practice are: "Sacred Journeys of Nurse Healers" (Hemsley & Glass, 2006) and "Effects of Sacred Space Environment on Surgical Patient Outcomes: A Pilot Study" (Schmock, Breckenridge, & Benedict, 2009). In the first research effort, a phenomenological study of the "sacred journeys" of 11 nurse healers, data revealed five essential themes, which included "belonging and connecting, opening to spirit, summoning, wounding and healing journey" (Hemsley & Glass, 2006, p. 256). In the second study, Schmock, Breckinridge, and Benedict reported that when a "sacred space" was created for surgical patients there were significant findings in terms of the patients' perceptions of nurse caring (p. 49). The latter study of sacred space brings to mind a hospital chaplaincy experience of working with critically ill children. On the medical center unit where the children were housed, each child's room was considered a safe place and, except in emergencies, no painful treatments were carried out in that space.

Concept Analysis of the Sacred Covenant

There are a number of nursing journal articles reporting the findings of concept analyses of caring. Examples of these include: "An Analysis of Caring" (Sourial,

1997), "An Evolutionary Concept Analysis of Caring" (Brilowski & Wendler, 2005), "Concept Analysis: The Moral Construct of Caring in Nursing as Communicative Action" (Sumner, 2006), "Emotional Labour Underlying Caring: An Evolutionary Concept Analysis" (Huynh, Alderson, & Thompson, 2008), and "Nursing Care: A Concept Analysis" (DalPezzo, 2009).

For the present analysis of the concept of a sacred covenant of caring, the procedure identified by Lorraine Walker and Kay Avant (2011) has been employed. The Walker and Avant process steps for the analysis include, after selection of the concept, determination of the "aims of the analysis," identification of "uses of the concept," determination of "defining attributes," identification of a "model case," identification of "antecedents and consequences" of the concept, and definition of "empirical referents" (p. 160).

The concept to be analyzed as a type of covenantal caring is that of a sacred covenant. The aim of the analysis is to clarify the meaning of the sacred covenant as a caring method in clinical nursing practice. The term *sacred covenant* is a key concept in a newly developed model of caring for nursing. The model can be used to guide nurse–patient interactions in clinical practice. The defining attributes of the concept of the sacred covenant are derived from the literature cited earlier. These include a calling of service, a blessed trust, and a commitment to reverence.

A model case of sacred covenant–oriented nursing care is that of Nurse Katie and her geriatric patient, Marie.

Marie was 94 years old, and "ready to meet her Maker," she liked to tell her nurses at the long-term care facility where she had resided for the past 5 years. Most of Marie's friends had already gone home to the Lord, and there really never had been any blood relatives to speak of; Marie created "family", she said, "wherever" she "lived and worked." She had created a "family" at the nursing home and Katie, a young nurse, was one of her favorite "children."

Not too many young nurses go into geriatric nursing; it does not seem quite as exciting or challenging as the ICU [intensive care unit] or the emergency room. But Katie was an exception, a very special exception. She had just graduated from a distinguished baccalaureate program in nursing and decided she wanted to work with elders; Katie reasoned: "they could be my own grandmother or grandfather some day!"

Marie and Katie hit it off right from the beginning; they were both Irish, both loved to tease, and neither cared much for "whiners"; they discovered lots of areas of mutual agreement. As Marie grew more fragile, and Katie more acclimated to being a geriatric nurse, their friendship deepened. Some days, after her shift was over, Katie would stay on and just sit at Marie's bedside, so Marie "would feel like she really did have family at the nursing home," Katie explained.

As a damp and dreary fall rapidly turned to winter for the nursing home residents, Marie's health began to fail dramatically. She seemed to be constantly coughing from a chronic bronchitis that the medications just could not seem to get a hold of; then, one day Marie spiked a vicious temp, and her lungs began to fill with fluid. The house physician proposed hospitalization, but Marie would have none of it; this was her home, she said, and she wanted to "die at home."

I loved to watch Marie and Katie holding hands during those final days; the tiny, frail elder, with her snow white hair and parchment-like skin; the beautiful, dark-haired nurse, exuding life and energy from every pore of her strong, young body. Katie did so much for her "adopted" grandmother. It wasn't just the "things" she gave her. Oh, of course, Katie often brought in small gifts like a special lotion or cream to soothe Marie's tender skin, or a small container of ice cream to tempt her waning appetite. But what touched my heart most was the tender and gentle way Katie had of nursing her precious patient: her unfailing kindness, and her consistent patience, her continual loving care.

Katie knew that Marie was going to die and admitted that she, Katie, was much more afraid than her friend; she really wanted to be with Marie, but she had never seen a patient die before. Katie wasn't sure if she could do it, that is, until the time actually came. And then, there she was, once anxious Katie, tearfully and tenderly cradling Marie in her arms, while the Chaplain said a final blessing. Katie truly became a nurse that day; she exemplified a beautiful sacred covenant of caring as she midwifed her beloved patient into eternal life with the Lord. (M. E. O'Brien, 2003, pp. 83–84)

Some antecedents of the sacred covenant of caring are bonds of loyalty and responsibility on the part of both nurse and patient, no conditions put on the nurse's faithfulness, an unconditional commitment by the nurse to be of service, and no expectation by the nurse for a return for good services. Potential consequences of the sacred covenant of caring are a sense of sacredness in caring on the part of the nurse and patient, a spiritual bonding for both nurse and patient, and the creation of a sacred space leading to spiritual openness in nurse–patient interactions. The nursing behaviors expected when caring is guided by the sacred covenant model of care are respecting life, being present (and listening with the heart), comforting with compassion, creating meaningful bonds, and becoming a patient advocate. Finally, empirical referents of a sacred covenant model of caring are case studies of clinical nursing nurse–patient interactions such as that of Katie and her geriatric patient Marie described here.

▶ The Spiritual History of Covenantal Caring in Nursing

In a chapter entitled "The Historical Tradition of Care," nurse theorist and historian Dr. Ann Bradshaw described the importance of the "moral dimension of care." Bradshaw (1997) noted, "the attitude of the carer, the way he or she expresses care and responds to the person who needs care, that unquantifiable quality of genuine compassion, kindness, gentleness and understanding alongside skill, knowledge and competence, are the very essence of good health care." (p. 12). "To care," Bradshaw added, "is to protect and to honour" (p. 13). "Nightingale," Bradshaw pointed out, "is the great exemplar of nursing" and "personified the traditional nursing ethic of care. Nightingale's vision of nursing grew out of a profound faith in God which rooted and grounded her life" (p. 16).

Many of our preprofessional "nurses" practiced just such a "covenantal" kind of caring, from Veronica of Jerusalem, who risked the wrath of Roman soldiers to wipe the face of Jesus on his painful journey to the cavalry, to the early Christian deacons and deaconesses who opened their homes to the ill and infirm. Following these courageous and caring men and women came the monastic nurses, who welcomed lepers to their monasteries, and the first military nurses, the Crusader Knights, who rescued fallen comrades in the midst of armed conflicts and tended their wounds.

Perhaps the most well-known early role model of covenant-oriented caring during the Middle Ages was Catherine of Siena who, in the 14th century, risked her own life and health to unselfishly minister to victims of the Black Plague, which had devastated Europe. Many now revere Catherine as the patroness of contemporary nursing.

At the time of the Reformation and afterward, a number of Catholic and Protestant religious orders were founded for care of the sick. Notable among these were the Daughters of Charity and the Kaiserswerth Deaconesses. With the advent of the Nightingale era, and the initiation of professional nursing, women called to minister formally to the sick indeed undertook a covenant-oriented commitment to caring. Anecdotes abound in the literature describing the devotion and dedication expected of and practiced by these early nurses. One example is an article published in 1914 in the fledgling *American Journal of Nursing* entitled "The Place of Religion in the Life of the Nurse." The author asserts: "We need cultured nurses, we need educated nurses, we need spiritual nurses . . . nurses who feel it is their duty to leave a better patient than they met, who feel their sphere is confined only by heaven itself" (Emerson, 1914, p. 863). Writing in 1923, in *The Public Health Nurse,* another author advised that, "All who embrace nursing as a life profession must have as a secret source of their ministering the ability . . . to give their help in the name of God" (White, 1923, p. 283). In a 1926 paper published in *The Trained Nurse and Hospital Review*, registered nurse Mary McDermott commented that "nurses' lives must include the pursuit of truth and goodness" and central to that activity, she added, was study of the Bible (p. 501).

A poignant reflection of the covenant-oriented care of the time is demonstrated in the epic poem "Mary's Nurse," published in 1929 in *The American Journal of Nursing.* The anonymously authored poetic meditation described a "visiting nurse" of the era attending to a young mother-to-be on Christmas Eve; the nurse suggested that on this night they should think of another young mother-to-be, Mary, awaiting the birth of her child in a stable in Bethlehem. The nurse observed that Joseph, Mary's husband, had probably sought out a local woman to assist with the birth; as the two made their way to the stable, the meditation continued, "Mary's 'nurse' began to sing of Israel's Messiah and thought to herself 'How glorious 'twould be to nurse into the world the Little Lord . . . some day perhaps a woman such as I will have that blessing and that happiness but I can only bring some comfort now to a poor young girl in a wretched cattle stall'" ("Mary's Nurse," 1929, p. 1445). The meditation concludes with the visiting nurse imagining Joseph's expression of amazement at the care and generosity of "Mary's nurse" who stayed with the Holy Family throughout the night; when Joseph tried to express his gratitude, the woman replied simply: "It is not hard to nurse the sick for those whose lives are given so. To tend the maimed, the ill, that is a joyous life, a life complete" (p. 1445).

The kind of caring provided by the visiting maternity nurse, meditating on "Mary's Nurse," was the "gold standard" for nursing of the day. In her 1922 classic *Textbook of the Principles and Practice of Nursing,* educator Bertha Harmer asserted: "Nursing is rooted in the needs of humanity and is founded on the ideal of service. Its object is not only to cure the sick and heal the wounded but . . . to minister to all those who are helpless or handicapped . . . the final test in the last day . . . is . . . did ye visit the sick, the hungry? Nursing includes all of this" (p. 3). A 1929 textbook, *Ethics and Art of Conduct for Nurses,* contained a chapter, "The Nurse's Devotion," which identified the characteristics of a nurse as "love for the sick, tenderness, generosity, self-forgetfulness and appreciation for the nobility of the calling" (Garesche, 1929, p. 259). Such devotional caring was also advised in a 1940 article entitled "Vocational Guidance and the Nurse," which identified the Lord's Gospel message as the impetus for the nurse's calling (Miriam, 1940, p. 448).

From the 1940s through the 1960s, most nurses received their "training" at religiously affiliated hospital schools of nursing. Thus, the philosophy of a covenant-oriented kind of caring continued to support the practice of the profession. Books such as Mary Berenice Beck's *The Nurse: Handmaid of the Divine Physician*, written in 1945; Hayes, Hayes, and Kelly's *Moral Handbook of Nursing*, published in 1956; and numerous journal articles, although not using the term *covenant*, described the nurse's role as one of spiritually inspired caring for the sick.

An article entitled "Sanctity and Nursing" asserted: "The vocation of nursing is a royal road to sanctity. It has ever been so, from ancient times, in medieval towers, in centuries of the first nursing orders of religious . . . among the laity who as professional nurses or as untrained good neighbors have reached out their hands to comfort and cure the sick and attend the dying" ("Sanctity and Nursing," 1952, p. 39). The anonymous author concluded that in the future the Lord will say, "'Come in, I was hungry and you fed me . . . sick and you nursed me . . .' In that gathering of the blessed, nurses will stand, surrounded by those they helped physically and spiritually, those who, in turn, helped their nurses ascend that hill that leads to eternal bliss" (p. 39). In another 1952 article, the nurse author observed that, "From the time a girl decides that she wants to be a nurse, in her own mind and heart she feels almost a vocation—a real God given desire to help others. This deeply spiritual glow is produced by thoughts of genuine and unlimited help and service that she might offer to her fellow-man" (Stark, 1952, p. 48.). "Basically," Stark concluded, "the principle behind nursing is service—service to God through service to humanity" (p. 48). The concept of nursing as a vocation of service is also addressed in a 1953 paper that points out that "for every nurse it is very important to have a right and clear idea of vocation. Only in finding and doing what God wills can anyone be happy" ("A Mission Nurse," 1953, p. 15). The author adds that nurses "exercise a unique apostolate," which ultimately will "merit to hear from the lips of our Lord those joyful words, 'Come, ye blessed of my Father and possess the Kingdom prepared for you from the foundation of the world for I was sick and you visited me'" (p. 17).

Two 1954 nursing journal articles addressed a covenantal kind of caring, one identifying the nurse as a "modern Veronica" derived from the author's witness of nursing "Veronicas" "figuratively wipe the bleeding face of the Mystical Body of Christ in dying cancer patients" (Miller, 1954, p. 20). In the second paper, nursing is described as "a privilege and a responsibility" (Sulzbach, 1954, p. 57) flowing from the inspiration of Florence Nightingale "for all who dedicate themselves to the care of the sick" (p. 58). A 1955 article identifies the nursing vocation as a "call to greatness" in a life "devoted to service of the sick and suffering" (Stemler, 1955, p. 27). Writing in 1962, Wright described nursing as "one of those healing arts which has about it all the clear marks of a divine vocation" (p. 35). The author added: "I think that there is no single pledge or vow pronounced by anyone, by religious, by public officials, by soldier, that is more sublime than the solemn pledge that the nurse makes" (p. 37).

And finally, in describing a self-identified "creed for nurses," nurse author Esther Mathewson (1963) suggested such characteristics for the nurse as humility or the "challenge to live . . . in the realization that we will always learn" (p. 24), tenderness and compassion "for they do not embarrass the need to be firm and sure" (p. 25), and kindness "that patients find refreshment to continue their struggle with illness" (p. 25). Mathewson concluded with the rhetorical question: "Shall my road be one of service or just a job, a road that is professional but humble, a road to God, or just a road?" (p. 72).

It has been reported that with the opening of U.S nursing schools in the late 19th century and into the early 20th century, curricula were based on the model embraced by Florence Nightingale and advanced the profession of nursing through strict discipline, moral training and nursing education. In addition, character development was viewed as most important. Character qualities of "altruism, courage, fidelity, compassion and benevolence" were just a few of the characteristics desired in nurses of the time (Como, 2007, p. 37). These characteristics remain imprinted in the minds and hearts of today's senior nurses, whose education took place around the middle of the 20th century.

Later, in the 1970s and the 1980s, the newly introduced concepts of holistic health care and holistic nursing began to formally incorporate the spiritual dimension of caring into the profession. In holistic caring the ill person is envisioned as composed of body, mind, and spirit. Nurse authors began to focus on the incorporation of spirituality within holistic care in such books as *Holistic Nursing: A Handbook for Practice* (Dossey, Keegan, Guzzetta, & Kolkmeier, 1988) and journal articles such as "Spirituality: Cornerstone of Holistic Nursing Practice" (Nagai-Jacobson & Burkhart, 1989).

There are myriad descriptions of covenantal caring found in the biographical literature on nursing leaders of the previous century. Just a few examples include the caring and courageous trauma nursing of Edith Cavell (Judson, 1941), the advocacy and compassion for the sick urban poor of Lillian Wald (Dolan, 1978), the initiation of nursing care for poverty-stricken rural mothers through the founding of the Frontier Nursing Service by Mary Breckinridge (Raines & Wilson, 1996), and the heroic military nursing of Genevieve de Galard ("Nurse Heroes of the Century," 1999).

To conclude, covenant-oriented caring has been a central concept of care of the sick from the inception of informal nursing to the initiation of the formal training of professional nurses. Covenantal or covenant-oriented caring has been, and hopefully will always remain, a hallmark of the nursing service provided to all those seeking care.

▶ Spiritual Concepts in Nursing Theories of Caring

We are indebted to a number of pioneer and contemporary nurse theorists for the formalization of caring theory in professional nursing. Foremost among those early and later visionaries are Madeleine Leininger (Culture Care Theory), Jean Watson (Theory of Human Care/Theory of Transpersonal Caring), Simone Roach (Five Cs of Caring), Katie Eriksson (Caritative Theory), Marilyn Ray (Theory of Bureaucratic Caring), Kristen Swanson (Theory of Caring), Joanne Duffy (Quality Care Theory), and Anne Boykin and Savina Schoenhofer (Theory of Nursing as Caring). While this list is certainly not exhaustive, each of the nursing theorists mentioned contributed new insights and perceptions related to the concept of caring. Today's practitioners of nursing care stand on the shoulders of these distinguished theorists of caring.

Not all of the caring theorists have addressed the concept of the spirituality of caring directly. There is, nevertheless, an implicit spiritual undergirding in their writings. This is related to the nature of the concept of caring as an altruistic dimension of nursing practice.

Writing in 1981, Madeleine Leininger expressed the opinion that "Caring is the central and unifying domain for the body of knowledge and practices in nursing"

(p. 3). She added: "I believe caring helps to bridge human relatedness, concern and compassionate help to others" (p. 8). In a conceptual model describing "transcultural and ethnocaring constructs," Leininger included a number of spiritually related caring concepts such as "compassion," "empathy," "love," "presence," "succourance," and "trust" (p. 13). And, in 1984, Leininger asserted: "Caring is nursing and nursing is caring" (p. 83). Later, in articulating her Concept of Culture Care Diversity, Leininger taught that nursing care should be culture specific in the caregiver's sensitivity to values, beliefs, and practices of those for whom he or she cares (Leininger, 1991). Thus, the nurse's attention to patients' cultural beliefs and practices implicitly includes attention to religious and/or spiritually associated beliefs and practices.

Jean Watson described "caring science as sacred science" in 2005 and, under the heading "Divine Love," commented that "compassionate human service and authentic caring are ultimately motivated by love, both human and Cosmic . . . [and by] . . . connecting with our deep humanity, we find the foundation of love and caring" (p. 80). In defining "the core processes of caring," Watson identified "10 carative factors," several of which have distinctly spiritual orientations, such as, "the formation of humanistic-altruistic system of values"; "the instillation of faith-hope"; "the development of a helping-trusting relationship"; and "the provision for a supportive, protective and/or corrective mental, physical, sociocultural and spiritual environment" (pp. 2–3). Watson (2012), in discussing her concept of the Transpersonal Caring Relationship, explains that, "Caring, in this sense, is viewed as the moral ideal of nursing where there is the utmost concern for human dignity and preservation of humanity" (p. 75). Watson adds that, "Human caring begins when the nurse . . . is able to detect the other person's condition of being (spirit, soul)" (p. 75). Watson specifically addresses the spiritual dimension of the individual as "the world of the spirit and the soul," which, she notes, "becomes increasingly more important as a person grows and matures" (p. 68). Ultimately, Watson describes the inherent values in her theory as "associated with deep respect and openness for the wonders, mysteries and even miracles of life and the power of humans to change . . . to become . . . more in line with one's spiritual destiny, dignity and one's soul's code" (p. 88).

In her 1987 work, *The Human Act of Caring*, theorist Simone Roach addressed the theological nature of caring: "Examined in the theological perspective, caring is epitomized in the Old Testament in the God of the Covenant . . . God is revealed as the one who enters into a covenant with his people; as the one who restores the covenant and who fulfills the covenant" (p. 15). Ultimately, Roach asserts, "Caring is used to describe those rare, precious moments of unique encounter when the participants recognize their common base of humanity" (p. 19). "To be is to care," she concludes (p. 19). In relation to nursing theory, Simone Roach is generally referenced for her identification of the Five Cs of Caring, which are Compassion, Competence, Confidence, Conscience, and Commitment. These qualities, she notes, "evolved over time in response to the question, what is a nurse doing when she [or he] is caring?" (p. 58). Simone Roach later added a sixth "C" as an attribute of caring, that of Comportment. Roach described comportment as "meaning bearing, demeanor or to be in agreement or harmony with" another person (p. 67). "When we visit a special person," Roach asserted, "usually our mode of dress and choice of language are in keeping with the regard, esteem and respect with which the person is held" (p. 67). Writing on "comportment as a caring attribute" in 2010, Simone Roach and Colleen Maykut pointed out that comportment "has the potential to offer an opportunity to concurrently visually represent the intentionality of a nursing practice and demonstrate professionalism" (p. 22).

This latter "C" identified by Roach seems very much in keeping with the spiritual concept of respect for the sacredness of life and of the human person.

Katie Eriksson's (1994) Caritative Theory of Caring is based on the caritas motive, which she describes as "the core of caring": "Compassion is the force which motivates a person to care" (p. 13). This "caring, caritative love," Eriksson explains, "is based on the fact that we always try to save the 'distinction' by seeing 'the other,' and taking responsibility for another. In that sense, the love is total ethic. This presupposes deliberate spiritual reflection and awareness of the real value of the person and of that person's holiness" (p. 13). "True caring is based on compassion . . . the nurse's ability to feel compassion emerges from personal experiences of suffering and love" (p. 14). "Caritative caring," Eriksson (1992) observed, "means that we take 'caritas' into use when caring for the human being in health and suffering" (p. 204). Caritative caring, she adds, "has a caring effect through its very existence in a caring culture" (p. 204). And, "there is caritative caring in nursing practice which is derived from the original idea of human love and charity . . . faith, hope and love, the basic elements of caring, are conveyed through caring, playing and learning in both large and small everyday nursing tasks" (p. 204).

In the Theory of Bureaucratic Caring, Marilyn Ray also includes an overtly spiritual theme in considering the person as both a spiritual and a cultural being. She suggests that "persons are created by God, the mystery of being, and they engage co-creatively in human organizational and transcultural relationships to find meaning and value" (Coffman, 2010, p. 121). According to Ray, caring is "a complex, transcultural, relational process grounded in the ethical, spiritual context" (p. 118), and the practice of nursing is viewed as engaging in a "holistic, relational, spiritual and ethical" kind of caring that seeks to promote both the good of patients and organizations (p. 121). Ray includes a spiritual dimension in key elements of her theory.

Kristen Swanson's (1993) Theory of Caring includes attention to the physical, psychological, social, and spiritual needs of the individual. Swanson envisions persons as "unique beings who are in the midst of becoming and whose wholeness is made manifest in thoughts, feelings and behaviors" (p. 352). Swanson asserts that all individuals' attitudes and behaviors are affected by their "genetic heritage" and "spiritual "endowment": "spiritual endowment connects each being with an eternal and universal source of goodness, mystery, life, creativity and serenity. The spiritual endowment may be a soul, higher power/Holy Spirit, positive energy or simply grace" (p. 352). Swanson's understanding of caring in nursing relates to the caregiver's desire to achieve the highest good for the one being cared for.

Joanne Duffy's (2009) Quality Caring Model, developed in 2003, was "designed as a middle-range theory to support the understanding of the connections between quality health care and caring" (p. 35). The model is described as "integrating biomedical and psychosocioculturalspiritual factors associated with quality health care" (p. 35). Essentially, the Quality Caring Model was developed for the purpose of "improving patient outcomes and advancing professional nursing" (p. 40). A spiritual aspect of this model might be interpreted as relating to the "centrality of caring relationships" (p. 39), which are critical for persons seeking to participate in the needs and concerns of members, especially needy members, of the human family.

And, in their book, *Nursing as Caring: A Model for Transforming Practice,* Anne Boykin and Savina Schoenhofer (2001) define caring as "the intentional and authentic presence of the nurse with another who is recognized as a person living caring and growing in caring . . . each person grows in caring through interconnectedness with others" (p. 13). A basic assumption of the Nursing as Caring Theory is that "persons are caring by virtue of their humanness" (p. 1). This conceptualization of caring, with the nurse bringing his or her own human skill and talent to the process of caring, might be interpreted as a spirituality of caring in giving of oneself to the person in need of care. Citing the work of Cooper, Boykin and Schoenhofer observe that "as caring persons we see relationship (covenant) and honor the bond between self and other. The ultimate knowledge gained from this perspective is that we are related to one another (and to the universe) and that harmony (brotherhood and sisterhood) is present as we live out caring relationships" (p. 7).

A number of standardized instruments have been developed to measure and validate the process of caring in clinical nursing practice. As with the identified theories of caring, not all of the caring tools specifically address the spirituality of caring practice. Spirituality might, however, be considered implicit in caring tool items that measure concerns and needs "important" to the individual patient. Several caring instruments do include specific items related to the spiritual needs of those for whom the nurse is caring.

Some examples of measurement tools that evaluate the concept of caring include the Care-Q Instrument (Larson, 1984), the Caring Behaviors Inventory (Wolf, 1986), the Caring Behaviors Assessment (Cronin & Harrison, 1988), the Holistic Caring Inventory (Latham, 1988), and the Caring Attributes Scale (Nyberg, 1990). One example of a caring instrument item that directly measures patients' spiritual concerns is an item in the Caring Behaviors Assessment (Cronin & Harrison, 1988) that states "Consider my spiritual needs" (as cited in Watson, 2009, p. 95). Another example is in the Caring Attributes Scale (Nyberg, 1990): "Understand that spiritual forces contribute to human care" (as cited in Watson, 2009, p. 116).

▶ A Sacred Covenant Model of Caring for Nursing Practice

Although never fully conceptualized as a theory or model, the author's past nursing writing and research have included a number of references to a "sacred covenant." In research exploring the nurse's caring role in ministering to chronic renal failure patients, migrant workers, institutionalized and homebound elders, persons living with HIV/AIDS, and other acute and chronically ill patients, the sacred caring covenant of nursing emerged as a guiding principle. In a sense, the model was continually emerging, although it was never formalized.

Development of the Model

The formal Sacred Covenant Model of Caring for Nursing Practice has been developing for close to 30 years. While pursuing a graduate degree in theology, I became reacquainted with the concept of God's covenant with his people through one of my early courses in Old Testament Scripture. It immediately struck me that the commitment, the care, and the faithfulness of God's covenantal love provided a beautiful model for the nurse's caring for the sick.

An explanation of the nurse–patient relationship envisioned as a sacred covenant was first introduced in the original edition of *Spirituality in Nursing: Standing on Holy*

Ground (M. E. O'Brien, 1998, pp. 85–87). The idea of a nurse's caring being guided by the concept of a sacred covenant was explained briefly, presented as an introduction to a chapter discussing research on the spirituality of caring. The concept of caring as a sacred covenant was derived from data describing positive nurse–patient interactions as related by study participants. Some of the covenant-oriented themes identified from analysis of the qualitative data included a sacred calling, a sense of mission, touching the hand of God, a healing ministry, proddings of the Holy Spirit, praying a lot, and experiencing the divine.

The concept of nurses' caring as a sacred covenant relationship with the patient was next introduced in 2001, in the book *The Nurse's Calling: A Christian Spirituality of Caring for the Sick.* One example related to pediatric nursing:

> So tiny, so fragile, the small patient seems; almost lost amidst the wires and lines and monitoring devices which furnish her neonatal intensive care home. A miniature hand reaches out desperately seeking comfort in this strange new world into which the frail newborn has entered. Tenderly a NICU [neonatal intensive care unit] nurse allows the tiny fist to grasp her hand, to make a human connection, to make a spiritual connection. This is the nurse-patient covenant; this is a sacred covenant. (M. E. O'Brien, 2001, p. 11)

In 2003, the concept of nursing practice as a sacred covenant was presented in the chapter "Prayer and the Nurse–Patient Relationship" in the book *Prayer in Nursing: The Spirituality of Compassionate Caregiving* (M. E. O'Brien, 2003, pp. 57–58). The underlying rationale for linking prayer and the nurse's sacred covenant of caring was that in order to bring "the sacred covenant of God's love into nursing practice . . . we must establish our own personal relationship with the Lord" (p. 59).

Published in 2006, the book *The Nurse with an Alabaster Jar: A Biblical Approach to Nursing,* explored how the biblical concept of "God's sacred covenant" reflects "an underlying theme that guides interaction between nurses and their patients" (M. E. O'Brien, 2006, p. 95). The experiences of the author, as well as those of practicing nurses, were reported as confirming "the sacredness of the nurse–patient relationship."

In 2008, the book *A Sacred Covenant: The Spiritual Ministry of Nursing* included discussion of some of the specific elements of the sacred covenant of caring, including: "called with a holy calling," "called by name," "serve one another," "a sacred covenant," and "a nurse's prayer of covenant" (M. E. O'Brien, 2008, p. vii). In reflecting on the beautiful prayer of Saint Teresa of Avila, "Christ Has No Body Now but Yours," it was suggested that, "The choice and commitment, made by nurses, to be used by Jesus as His ministers to the sick may be envisioned as a 'sacred covenant,' as a lived experience of the spiritual ministry of nursing" (p. 2).

And, finally, recent research exploring nurses' caring, in relation to the concept of servant leadership, has continued to validate the existence of and appreciation for a covenantal or covenant-oriented model of caring in contemporary nursing practice. Elements of the Model of Servant Leadership in Nursing, published in *Servant Leadership in Nursing: Spirituality and Practice in Contemporary Health Care* (M. E. O'Brien, 2011), demonstrate the sacredness of nurses' perceptions of covenantal caring and their covenantal caring behaviors in clinical practice. Some of these include, under the label "Nursing Vocation Attitudinal Themes": "a blessed calling," "passionate caring," "ingrained in the spirit," "the extra mile," and "a privilege." "Nursing Servant Leader Behavioral Themes" included: "listening with the heart," "giving of yourself," "doing ministry," "assessing needs," "becoming an advocate," "discerning a decision," "making a difference," and "being there to serve" (p. 210).

Philosophy and Theology

The Sacred Covenant Model of Caring for Nursing Practice is grounded in the belief that caring is an essential concept included in the clinical practice of nursing the sick and, further, that professional nurses embrace the concept both theoretically and operationally. It is also believed that practicing nurses experience in their caring activities a "sacredness" related to their call to be of service to those in need. Associated with this "calling of service" are the closely related concepts of a blessed sense of trust and a commitment to reverence governing nurse–patient relationships. It is also understood that recipients of such covenant-oriented caring find solace and satisfaction in the caring interactions with nurses whose practice is guided by a covenantal model. Nurses find extraordinary meaning and personal satisfaction, as well, in practicing their profession guided by a philosophy of sacred covenant-oriented caring.

The theology supporting the Sacred Covenant Model of Caring for Nursing is derived from both Old and New Testament Scriptures. As noted earlier in the chapter, in discussing caring as a covenant, there are myriad examples of the concept of God's covenants with his people in the Old Testament: "I have made a covenant with my chosen one" (Psalm 89:3). Of major relevance is God's covenant with Moses and the people of Israel, and God's continuing faithfulness to his people. Even when the people turned away from God's laws and built for themselves an idol of a "Golden Calf," the Lord continued to care for the Israelites: "And the Lord changed his mind about the disaster that he planned to bring on his people" (Exodus 32:14). For a nurse, faithfulness to his or her vocation is central to the profession of caring. Even if a patient is decidedly noncompliant with a prescribed therapeutic regimen, the nurse must remain faithful to the commitment to caring to the best of his or her ability.

In exploring the theological perspective of caring, theorist Simone Roach (1987) agreed that "caring is epitomized in the Old Testament in the God of the Covenant" (p. 15). She noted: "In the Bible, God is revealed as the one who enters into a covenant with His people; as the one who restores the covenant and who fulfills the covenant. God is a faithful God; and his fidelity or faithfulness is frequently associated with his paternal goodness toward the people of the covenant" (p. 15). God's fulfilling of the covenant is generally understood as the sending of His Divine Son Jesus as the savior of mankind.

One of the salient New Testament passages in terms of the importance of covenantal caring is that of the "Good Samaritan," the man who saw an injured traveler and was "moved to pity": "He went to him and bandaged his wounds . . . then he put him on his own animal, brought him to an Inn and took care of him" (Luke 10:30, 33–34, 40). Also of relevance for the Sacred Covenant Model of Caring for Nursing is the message contained in Matthew 25:35–36: "For I was hungry and you gave me food, I was thirsty and you gave me something to drink, I was a stranger and you welcomed me," "I was naked and you gave me clothing," "I was sick and you took care of me," "I was in prison and you visited me . . . truly I tell you, just as you did it to one of the least of these who are members of my family, you did it to me."

In a meditation entitled "Compassionate Caregiving," a practicing nurse is described as asking the Lord how to better serve Him, and the Lord replies: "I am the hungry elder to whom you tenderly feed a cup of soup; I am the thirsty ICU patient whose parched tongue you solicitously moisten; I am the homeless stranger you compassionately welcome to your ER [emergency room]; I am the shivering post-op patient you caringly clothe; I am the homebound person you lovingly visit; and, It is my trembling arm round which you gently wrap your blood-pressure cuff" (M. E. O'Brien, 2003, p. 2).

Theory Synthesis and Focal Concepts

Lorraine Walker and Kay Avant (2011) explain that "the aim of theory synthesis is construction of a theory, an interrelated system of ideas, from evidence" (p. 140). Through theory or model synthesis "a theorist pulls together available information about a phenomenon. Concepts and statements are organized into a network or whole, a synthesized theory" (p. 140). Walker and Avant suggest three steps for theory synthesis: identification of "focal concepts" for the model, literature review on the key concepts and specification of the relationship among concepts, and organizing of concepts "into an integrated and efficient representation of the phenomena of interest" (p. 140).

For the present Sacred Covenant Model of Caring for Nursing Practice, the focal concepts include the "attributes of nursing," which have been identified as a calling of service, a blessed trust, and a commitment to reverence. These concepts, as well as the central concept of caring as a sacred covenant, have been defined both empirically and from the extant literature earlier in the chapter. Following are some empirical examples from the author's research with nurses engaged in current practice. A calling of service: "Most nurses I know see nursing as a calling of service . . . I think there is a quiet, deep inside knowing that this is what I am supposed to do. This feels right, and it is nourishing to me and others so this is the spiritual calling" (M. E. O'Brien, 2011, p. 103). A blessed trust: "All of nursing is a sacred trust, whether it be involved in direct patient care, administration, education or research . . . nursing is a blessing to be held in trust as a gift from God" (p. 159). A commitment to reverence: "Nursing is a sacred trust . . . holding something sacred demands an awareness of the sacredness of what it is, and also a commitment to reverence and real care" (p. 158). For a nurse who perceives the attributes of nursing to be a calling of service, a blessed trust, and a commitment to reverence, thus leading to the model of practice labeled caring as a sacred covenant, five covenantal nursing practice behavioral themes have been identified from both the literature and empirical data; these themes include: "respecting life," "being present," "comforting with compassion," "creating bonds," and "becoming an advocate."

Respecting Life

The idea of having respect or reverence for life is so integral to the practice of nursing that few articles on the topic exist in the professional literature. One exception is the commentary "The Ethics of Respect in Nursing." The author, nurse educator Dr. Constance Milton, reports that "the recipients of nursing services . . . voice concern over wanting to feel respected and call upon members of the healthcare team, including physicians and nurses, to offer respect for them and for one another" (2005, p. 22). Milton concludes with a powerful assertion in advising nurses that we "must listen to the society we serve . . . the value of our discipline and service to society should be manifested not only by the demonstrated abilities of our technological and mechanical skills, but with the transforming value of our services as we engage in the nurse-patient relationship" (p. 23). She adds a final hope: "May we be mindful of our responsibilities and engage in activities that are deemed honoring and respectful to those we serve and to one another" (p. 23). While admitting that "a culture of life must include an acceptance of death," Koppelman (2005) points out that "living with an awareness" of the transitory nature of all life can inspire people not to waste the gift of life, but to cherish it and to demonstrate a reverence for life by respecting all living things" (p. 351). In discussing the nursing of persons with intellectual disabilities, Herman Meininger (2005) notes that "understanding of the client and self-understanding of the caregiver . . . invites a respect for life in its openness toward the future and presupposes an openness toward other possible versions of the life narrative" (p. 106).

Numerous comments and anecdotes related by nurses in the author's past research studies reflect the importance placed on the concept of respecting and supporting the lives of those for whom they care. An ICU nurse spoke about needing to respect and reverence the very ill patients she cared for each day:

> You have these really sick patients who are fragile and afraid, and you have families who are "spacing out" over what's happening to their family member, and you have to give them 100%. Your head can't be someplace else when you're working in the unit; all of you, body, mind and soul, has to be there in this nursing . . . every day you have a mission; sometimes it seems like a mission impossible, but with God's help you can make it through the shift and leave feeling that you really have accomplished a mission of healing. (M. E. O'Brien, 2008, p. 48)

Another example of respect for life is embedded in the words of a community health nurse who worked with the poor and underserved:

> Most of my patients are underprivileged or underserved, and when I go talk to them or visit them at home, I see myself as being of service . . . I'm trying to find the right words, being as a servant . . . I see nursing as a blessed call to serve, especially those who are not as fortunate as I am. (M. E. O'Brien, 2011, p. 104)

Being Present

The words "presence and caring are ubiquitous terms within nursing" and often are used in a way as to be "substantively similar" (Finfgeld-Connett, 2008, p. 111). While admitting that presence is sometimes associated with caring in the literature, the author of a concept analysis of presence concluded that "presence is part of a holistic caring approach which involves integration of mind, body and spirit" (Gilje, 1992, p. 63). In a metasynthesis of presence, presence in nursing is defined as "an interpersonal process that is characterized by sensitivity, holism, intimacy, vulnerability and adaptation to unique circumstances" (Finfgeld-Connett, 2006, p. 708). Finfgeld-Connett adds that presence "consists of a process in which patients demonstrate a need for and openness to presence. In turn, nurses must be willing to enact presence and practice within an environment that is conducive to it" (p. 708).

In moving "toward a mid-range theory of presence," McMahon and Christopher (2011) present a nurse–client model that includes nurse characteristics, client characteristics, nurse–client dyad characteristics, and environmental factors (p. 74).

Zyblock (2010) attempted to clarify the concept of presence in nursing practice through a literature review that revealed, among other things, that "the act of being present should allow the patient to perceive a meaningful exchange between himself or herself and the nurse" (p. 121). Findings from a qualitative study of nurses' presence in an oncology unit also revealed the importance of nurse–patient trust in meaningful exchanges, as well as the potential for stressors that might intervene in the nurse's presence (Osterman, Schwartz-Barcott, & Asselin, 2010, p. 197). The research team concluded that: "Nurses can use presence as a way to provide emotional support to patients who are exposed to overwhelming threats to their mind, body and spiritual integrity" (p. 197). The value of the research of Osterman, Schwartz-Barcott, and Asselin is supported by the perception of ethicists Anne Bishop and John Scudder (1996), who point out the difficulty of attempting to define caring presence, noting that, "It's meaning, however, can be disclosed in concrete examples of nursing care" (p. 38).

A central component of therapeutic or caring presence is that of "listening," "listening with the ear of the heart," as described many centuries ago by the great monastic Saint Benedict. Benedict did not mean just listening with one's ears to the words being spoken, but truly listening in a heartfelt caring manner to the meaning of what the speaker wishes to convey. The nursing literature is replete with references to listening. It has been asserted that "listening is likely the most ancient of healthcare skills. It is a critical component of all aspects of nursing care and is necessary for meaningful interaction with patients" (Shipley, 2010, p. 125). Listening has also been described as the "oldest and conceivably most influential tool of healing" (Browning & Waite, 2010, p. 150). Listening is also linked to the concept of presence by Bunkers (2010), who observed that "true presence involves listening to what is important to the other and listening to what the meaning of a situation is in the moment for that person. It involves bearing witness to another's lived experience with love and compassion" (pp. 22–23).

Some examples of presence and listening contained in the comments of contemporary practicing nurses include:

> There is a way of having a caring presence with your patients. This is the time that you spend with the patients, listening with your heart to what they reflect in their attitude, their tone of voice, their facial concern . . . There is a feeling of trust, a feeling of presence in being there for them. (M. E. O'Brien, 2011, p. 134)
>
> I learned as a nurse that just listening to patients, really listening with the heart, was one of the greatest healers for many kinds of suffering. Listening with a caring heart can heal loneliness, fear, anger, grief and so many painful emotions that a patient may be suffering from. Listening is one of the key activities of nurses seeking to heal hurting patients. (M. E. O'Brien, 2011, p. 133)

Comforting with Compassion

In two papers exploring the implications of compassion for contemporary nursing, Collette Straughair (2012a, 2012b) addresses both the history of the concept from the Nightingale era and an understanding from current literature, which, she notes, "illustrates that compassion is a human emotion, borne out of an awareness of another's suffering and a desire to alleviate this" (p. 240). Similarly, compassion is described by Beth Perry (2009) as "sensing another person's suffering combined with a desire to alleviate or reduce such suffering" (p. 14). Dr. Maria Schantz (2007) pointed out that, "Compassion is a quality deemed *sine qua non* for nursing" (p. 48), and adds that "many a nurse will say that it was compassion for others that inspired her [sic] to become a nurse" (p. 54).

An expanded definition of compassion, which is particularly appropriate for nursing is that offered by theologian Michael Downey:

Compassion is the capacity to be attracted and moved by the fragility, weakness and suffering of another. It is the ability to be vulnerable enough to undergo risk and loss for the good of another. Compassion involves a movement to be of assistance to the other, but it ineluctably entails a movement of participation in the experience of the other in order to be present and available in solidarity and communion. Compassion requires sensitivity to what is weak and/or wounded, as well as the vulnerability to be affected by the other. It also demands action to alleviate pain and suffering. (Downey, 1993, pp. 192–193)

As two nurses explained it: "Seeing nursing as a calling, I think, makes me more compassionate as a nurse. I empathize with my patients. I can be more filled with compassionate care . . . these people are depending on me"; and "I was attracted to nursing out of a deep compassion for human beings and to be able to alleviate suffering in some way" (M. E. O'Brien, 2011, p. 146).

Creating Bonds

The concept of creating bonds as a behavioral outcome of nursing under the guidance of the Sacred Covenant Model of Caring relates to the sanctity of the nurse–patient relationship. The caring nurse–patient relationship has been described as "a helping relationship [that] provides nursing with an identity and differentiates it from other professions" (Gamez, 2009, p. 126). The nurse–patient relationship is considered to be "the core of nursing" (Halldorsdottir, 2008, p. 643). It is also asserted that "caring behaviors demonstrated by the nurse facilitate the nurse-patient relationship and may ultimately promote healing" (Spencer & Lunsford, 2010, p. 30).

As a nursing supervisor put it: "I feel that nursing in itself is a type of ministry to the sick. We have a special bond with patients that is unique . . . I feel that we are called to a higher calling as we are a spiritual profession in a way that we understand the whole person as he [or she] is" (M. E. O'Brien, 2011, p. 151). The concept of bonding with patients was echoed by a pediatric team leader: "You develop such solid relationships with patients; you connect with them. And I never realized how much a part of nursing that would be" (M. E. O'Brien, 2011, p. 154). A critical care nurse commented: "When you make a connection with people who are sick, as a nurse, it becomes personal. And you begin to realize that you have a real impact on their lives. You can't help but know that you are in a relationship that is something beyond the client and the person serving. You can say I helped [the patient]" (M. E. O'Brien, 2011, p. 152).

Becoming an Advocate

Nursing advocacy has been defined as integrating "aspects of individuality, professionalism and experiences of empowering . . . it is not a single event, but a process of analyzing, counseling, responding, shielding and whistleblowing activities in clinical nursing practice" (Vaartio, Leino-Kilpi, Salantera, & Suominen, 2006, p. 282). Advocacy is also described as "an essential component of the Registered Nurse professional role . . . Three core attributes of the concept of patient advocacy are identified [as]: (1) safeguarding patients' autonomy; (2) acting on behalf of patients; and (3) championing social justice in the provision of health care" (Bu & Jezewski, 2007, p. 101). In a phenomenological study of nursing advocacy among medical–surgical nurses, analysis of data revealed six emergent themes: "speaking out and speaking for patients; being compelled to act on unmet needs of patients; fulfillment and frustration; the patient is changed; primarily learned on the job; and confidence gained through practice" (Hanks, 2008, p. 468). Hanks's recommendation to continue study of the concept of advocacy is supported by nursing director Hannah MacDonald (2007), who noted that "advocacy is universally considered a moral obligation in nursing practice, and thus advancement of our knowledge about its nature in nursing is relevant to nursing across multiple contexts and cultures" (p. 119). Ultimately, Hanks (2010) asserted, "Although other health professionals advocate for their patients or clients, nursing has designated the advocate role as a central role of nursing practice (p. 107).

A medical–surgical nurse asserted: "You really have to become a patient advocate more than anything else. Nursing was a vocation 23 years ago when I started, and it is still a vocation now . . . I think the more you do it, the more you want to care for the patient because you know their needs, you know what needs to be done" (M. E. O'Brien, 2011, p. 170). A nurse educator added: "Nursing . . . is becoming a patient advocate. It is a profession that requires a lot of knowledge and related to that is responsibility and accountability in providing nursing care . . . being a patient advocate in nursing" (M. E. O'Brien, 2011, p. 170).

▶ The Sacred Covenant Model of Caring for Nursing Practice

As noted earlier the Sacred Covenant Model of Caring has evolved and continued to develop during the course of the author's research, with both patients and practicing nurses, over the past 30 years. The most recent study, from which a number of the previous comments are taken, was entitled "Called to Serve: The Lived Experience of a Nursing Vocation." Initially 75 nursing leaders were interviewed employing a hermeneutic phenomenological method; another 24 nurses were later interviewed in order to validate themes that emerged in the initial phase of the study. The study nurses were employed in a variety of positions including administration, management, education, research, and practice. Those nurses engaged in practice represented multiple settings such as hospital, clinic, long-term care and home care, and myriad nursing specialty areas including medical–surgical, critical care, pediatrics, psych–mental health, obstetrics and gynecology, community health, and others. The nurses' credentials included registered nurse (RN), associate degree nurse (ADN), baccalaureate degree nurse (BSN), master's degree nurse (MSN), doctorate in nursing science (DNSc), and doctor of philosophy in nursing (PhD, RN). The instrument employed for data collection was an investigator-developed "Nursing Vocation Interview Guide"; data were analyzed through a process of content analysis to identify key themes that emerged from the qualitative interviews.

The Sacred Covenant Model of Caring for Nursing Practice (see **FIGURE 17-1**) contains the key themes/focal concepts identified during multiple data analysis

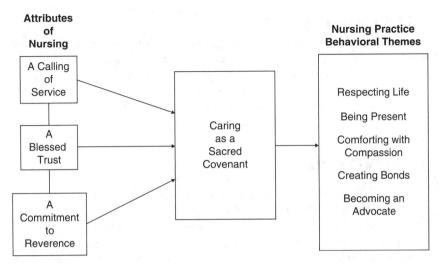

FIGURE 17-1   A Sacred Covenant Model of caring for nursing practice.
Note: "Attributes of Nursing" and "Nursing Practice Behavioral Themes" have been derived from study participants' comments made in research interviews with contemporary nurses practicing in a variety of clinical settings.

processes. As suggested earlier, significant attributes of nurses' caring reported by contemporary nurses are: a calling of service, a blessed trust, and a commitment to reverence, as identified on the left side of the model. Nurses who perceive and practice their profession possessed of these attributes are thus guided by the philosophy of caregiving that is labeled the Sacred Covenant of Caring Model. For nurses who practice under the guidance of this model, key nursing practice behavioral themes, as included on the right side of the figure, are respecting the sanctity of human life, being fully present and listening caringly to patients and family members, comforting suffering patients with compassion, creating bonds of caring within the nurse–patient relationship, and consistently advocating for the needs of patients and families. Empirical examples of these behaviors were cited earlier.

Hypotheses Derived from the Model

Several hypotheses may be derived from the Sacred Covenant Model of Caring for Nursing Practice. A broad hypothesis might be proposed that there will be a significant relationship between a nurse's practice being guided by the Sacred Covenant Model of Caring and the operationalization of behavioral concepts including respecting life, being present to patients, comforting with compassion, creating bonds, and becoming an advocate. Specifically, it can be hypothesized that a nurse who perceives and practices nursing as a "calling of service" will respect the life of his or her patients and be fully present to patients and families in need. It may also be hypothesized that a nurse who perceives and practices nursing as "a blessed trust" will create strong nurse–patient bonds and consistently advocate for his or her patients' needs. And, finally, it can be hypothesized that a nurse who perceives and practices nursing as "a commitment to reverence" will care and comfort with compassion those who are suffering.

Empirical Testing

Empirical testing of these hypotheses has begun with qualitative research to explore the concept of covenantal caring in contemporary nursing practice. Examples were presented earlier in the chapter. It is anticipated that the Sacred Covenant Model of Caring for Nursing Practice, including potential hypotheses, will continue to be tested in future research exploring the spirituality of caring in nursing.

▶ References

Baly, M. (Ed.). (1991). *As Miss Nightingale said . . . Florence Nightingale through her sayings: A Victorian perspective.* London, England: Scutari Press.

Barcott, J. (2006). The meaning of commitment. *The Washington Nurse, 36*(3), 11.

Barry, C. D. (1994). Nursing's values expressed in caring rituals. In D. A. Gaut & A. Boykin (Eds.), *Caring as healing: Renewal through hope* (pp. 66–82). New York, NY: National League for Nursing Press.

Baynham, B. (1993). Fidelity. In M. Downey (Ed.), *The new dictionary of Catholic spirituality* (p. 406). Collegeville, MN: The Liturgical Press.

Beck, M. B. (1945). *The nurse: Handmaid of the divine physician.* Philadelphia, PA: J. B. Lippincott.

Belcher, M. (2009). Graduate nurses' experiences of developing trust in the nurse-patient relationship. *Contemporary Nurse, 31*(2), 142–152.

Bell, L., & Duffy, A. (2009). A concept analysis of nurse-patient trust. *British Journal of Nursing, 18*(1), 46–51.

Biley, F. C., & Chiocchi, N. M. (2007). Nursing: A sacred healing dance. *Reflections on Nursing Leadership, 33*(3), 1–2.

Bishop, A., & Scudder, J. (1996). *Nursing ethics: Therapeutic caring presence.* Sudbury, MA: Jones & Bartlett Learning.

Boadt, L. (1984). *Reading the Old Testament: An introduction.* New York, NY: Paulist Press.

Boykin, A., & Schoenhofer, S. (2001). *Nursing as caring: A model for transforming practice.* Sudbury, MA: Jones & Bartlett Learning.

Bradshaw, A. (1997). The historical tradition of care. In G. Brykczynska (Ed.), *Caring: The compassion and wisdom of nursing* (pp. 10–31). London, England: Arnold.

Bradshaw, A. (1999). The virtue of nursing: The covenant of care. *Journal of Medical Ethics, 25*(1), 477–481.

Brilowski, G. A., & Wendler, M. C. (2005). An evolutionary concept analysis of caring. *Journal of Advanced Nursing, 50*(6), 641–650.

Browning, S., & Waite, R. (2010). The gift of listening; Just listening strategies. *Nursing Forum, 45*(3), 150–158.

Bruhn, J. G. (2005). The lost art of covenant: Trust as a commodity in health care. *The Health Care Manager, 24*(4), 311–319.

Bu, X., & Jezewski, M. A. (2007). Developing a mid-range theory of patient advocacy through concept analysis. *Journal of Advanced Nursing, 57*(1), 101–110.

Bunkers, S. (2010). The power and the possibility in listening. *Nursing Science Quarterly, 23*(1), 22–27.

Burnard, P. (1997). Why care? Ethical and spiritual issues in caring in nursing. In G. Brykczynska (Ed.), *Caring: The compassion and wisdom of nursing* (pp. 32–44). London, England: Arnold.

Carson, V. B. (1989). Spirituality and the nursing process. In V. B. Carson (Ed.), *Spiritual dimensions of nursing practice* (pp. 165–169). Philadelphia, PA: W.B. Saunders.

Chiang, Y.-C., Lee, H.-C., Chu, T.-L., Han, C.-Y., & Hsiao, Y.-C. (2016). The impact of nurses' spiritual health on their attitudes toward spiritual care, professional commitment and caring. *Nursing Outlook, 64*(3), 215–224.

Coffman, S. (2010). Maryilyn Ray: Theory of bureaucratic caring. In M. Alligood & A. Tomey (Eds.), *Nursing theorists and their work* (7th ed., pp. 113–136). Maryland Heights, MO: Mosby.

Como, J. M. (2007). Care and caring: A look at history, ethics and theory. *International Journal for Human Caring, 11*(4), 37–45.

Conn, J. (1990). Spirituality. In J. Komonchak, M. Collins, & D. Lane (Eds.), *The new dictionary of theology* (pp. 972–986). Collegeville, MN: The Liturgical Press.

Cooper, M. C. (1988). Covenantal relationships: Grounding for the nursing ethic. *Advances in Nursing Science, 10*(4), 48–59.

Cronin, S., & Harrison, B. (1988). Importance of nurse caring behaviors as perceived by patients after myocardial infarction. *Heart and Lung, 17*(4), 374–380.

DalPezzo, N. K. (2009). Nursing care: A concept analysis. *Nursing Forum, 44*(4), 256–264.

Davidson, J. (2009). The sacred place of nursing. *Creative Nursing, 15*(1), 14.

Desmond, M. E., Horn, S., Keith, K., Kelby, S., Ryan, L., & Smith, J. (2014). Incorporating caring theory into personal and professional nursing practice to improve perception of care. *International Journal for Human Caring, 18*(1), 35–44.

Dolan, J. (1978). *Nursing in society: A historical perspective* (2nd ed.). Philadelphia, PA: W. B. Saunders.

Dossey, B., Keegan, L., Guzzetta, C. E., & Kolkmeier, L. (Eds.). (1988). *Holistic nursing: A handbook for practice*. Rockville, MD: Aspen.

Downey, M. (1993). Compassion. In M. Downey (Ed.), *The new dictionary of Catholic spirituality* (pp. 192–193). Collegeville, MN: The Liturgical Press.

Duffy, J. (2009). *Quality caring in nursing: Applying theory to clinical practice, education and leadership.* New York, NY: Springer.

Dyess, S. M., Boykin, A., & Bulfin, M. J. (2013). Hearing the voice of nurses in caring theory-based practice. *Nursing Science Quarterly, 26*(2), 167–173.

Eley, D., Eley, R., Bertello, M., & Rogers-Clark, C. (2012). Why did I become a nurse? Personality traits and reasons for entering nursing. *Journal of Advanced Nursing, 68*(7), 1456–1555.

Emerson, C. T. (1914). The place of religion in the life of the nurse. *The American Journal of Nursing, 14*(10), 863–864.

Eriksson, K. (1992). Nursing: The caring practice "being there." In D. A. Gaut (Ed.), *The presence of caring in nursing* (pp. 201–210). New York, NY: National League for Nursing Press.

Eriksson, K. (1994). Theories of caring as health. In D. A. Gaut & A. Boykin (Eds.), *Caring as healing: Renewal through hope* (pp. 3–20). New York, NY: National League for Nursing Press.

Finfgeld-Connett, D. (2006). Meta-synthesis of presence in nursing. *Journal of Advanced Nursing, 55*(6), 708–714.

Finfgeld-Connett, D. (2008). Qualitative comparison and synthesis of nursing presence and caring. *International Journal of Nursing Terminologies and Classifications, 19*(3), 111–119.

Fry, S. (1991). A theory of caring: Pitfalls and promises. In D. A. Gaut & M. Leininger (Eds.), *Caring: The compassionate healer* (pp. 161–172). New York, NY: National League for Nursing Press.

Gamez, G. (2009). The nurse-patient relationship as a caring relationship. *Nursing Science Quarterly, 22*(2), 126–127.

Gardner, K. (1992). The historical conflict between caring and professionalization: A dilemma for nursing. In D. A. Gaut (Ed.), *The presence of caring in nursing* (pp. 241–255). New York, NY: National League for Nursing Press.

Garesche, E. F. (1929). *Ethics and the art of conduct for nurses.* Philadelphia, PA: W. B. Saunders.

Gerber, L. (2007). The sacred path. *Nursing 2007, 37*(5), 43.

Gilje, F. (1992). Being there: An analysis of the concept of presence. In D. A. Gaut (Ed.), *The presence of caring in nursing* (pp. 53–66). New York, NY: National League for Nursing Press.

Gregg, A. (2011). Message from the past president. *The Florida Nurse, 59*(4), 4–5.

Halldorsdottir, S. (2008). The dynamics of the nurse-patient relationship: Introduction of a synthesized theory from the patient's perspective. *Scandinavian Journal of Caring Science, 22*(1), 643–652.

Hanks, R. G. (2008). The lived experience of nursing advocacy. *Nursing Ethics, 15*(4), 468–477.

Hanks, R. G. (2010). The medical-surgical nurse perspective of the advocate role. *Nursing Forum, 45*(2), 97–107.

Harmer, B. (1922). *Textbook of the principles and practice of nursing.* New York, NY: Macmillan.

Hayes, E. J., Hayes, P. J. & Kelly, D. E. (1956). *Moral handbook of nursing.* New York, NY: Macmillan.

Hemsley, M., & Glass, N. (2006). Sacred journeys of nurse healers. *Journal of Holistic Nursing, 24*(4), 256–268.

Holland, P. D. (1990). Vocation. In J. Komonchak, M. Collins, & D. Lane (Eds.), *The new dictionary of theology* (pp. 1087–1092). Collegeville, MN: The Liturgical Press.

Huynh, T., Alderson, M., & Thompson, M. (2008). Emotional labour underlying caring: An evolutionary concept analysis. *Journal of Advanced Nursing, 64*(2), 195–208.

Judson, H. (1941). *Edith Cavell.* New York, NY: Macmillan.

Katz, A. (2011). Trust. *Nursing for Women's Health, 15*(2), 101–102.

Koppelman, K. (2005). The culture of life. *Illness, Crisis and Loss, 13*(4), 351–357.

Krebs, K. (2001). The spiritual aspect of caring: An integral part of health and healing. *Nursing Administration Quarterly, 25*(3), 55–60.

Larson, P. (1984). Important nurse caring behaviors perceived by patients with cancer. *Oncology Nursing Forum 11*(1), 46–50.

Lashley, M., Neal, M., Slunt, E., Berman, L., & Hultgren, F. (1994). *Being called to care.* Albany, NY: State University of New York Press.

Latham, C. (1988, March). *Measurement of caring in recipient-provider interactions.* Proceedings of Second Annual Measurement of Clinical and Educational Nursing Outcomes Conference, Sago, CA.

Leininger, M. (1981) *Caring: An essential human need.* Thorofare, NJ: Charles B. Slack.

Leininger, M. (1984). *Care: The essence of nursing and health.* Thorofare, NJ: Charles B. Slack.

Leininger, M. (1991). *Culture care diversity and universality: A theory of nursing.* New York, NY: National League for Nursing Press.

Lundmark, M. (2007). Vocation in theology-based nursing theories. *Nursing Ethics, 14*(6), 767–780.

MacDonald, H. (2007). Relational ethics and advocacy in nursing: Literature review. *Journal of Advanced Nursing, 57*(2), 119–126.

Mary's nurse. (1929). *The American Journal of Nursing, 29*(12), 1445–1446.

Mathewson, E. L. (1963). A creed for nurses. *The Catholic Nurse, XII*(1), 24–25; 72.

McDermott, M. S. (1926). Follow the gleam. *The Trained Nurse and Hospital Review, LXXVII*(5), 501–502.

McMahon, M. A., & Christopher, K. A. (2011). Toward a mid-range theory of nursing presence. *Nursing Forum, 46*(2), 71–82.

Meininger, H. P. (2005). Narrative ethics in nursing for persons with intellectual disabilities. *Nursing Philosophy, 6*(1), 106–118.

Miller, M. (1954). Modern Veronicas. *The Catholic Nurse, 2*(3), 20–22.

Milton, C. L. (2005). The ethics of respect in nursing. *Nursing Science Quarterly, 18*(1), 20–23.

Miriam, A. (1940). Vocational guidance and the nurse. *The Trained Nurse and Hospital Review, CIV*(5), 447–448.

A Mission Nurse. (1953). Nurses and vocations. *The Catholic Nurse, 2*(2), 15–17.

Montgomery, C. L. (1992). The spiritual connection: Nurses' perceptions of the experience of caring. In D. A. Gaut (Ed.), *The presence of caring in nursing* (pp. 39–52). New York, NY: National League for Nursing Press.

Montgomery, C. L. (1993). *Healing through communication: The practice of caring.* Newbury Park, NJ: Sage Publications.

Nagai-Jacobson, M. G., & Burkhart, M. A. (1989). Spirituality: Cornerstone of holistic nursing practice. *Holistic Nursing Practice, 3*(3), 18–26.

Nightingale, F. (1859). *Notes on nursing: What it is and what it is not.* London, England: Harrison, Bookseller to the Queen.

Nouwen, H. J. M. (2003). *Creative ministry.* New York, NY: Image Books.

Nowell, I. (1990). Covenant. In J. Komonchak, M. Collins, & D. Lane (Eds.), *The new dictionary of theology* (pp. 234–246). Collegeville, MN: The Liturgical Press.

Nurse heroes of the century. (1999). *Nursing Times, 95*(44), 34–35.

Nyberg, J. (1990). The effects of care and economics on nursing practice. *Journal of Nursing Administration, 20*(5), 13–18.

O'Brien, M. E. (1998). *Spirituality in nursing: Standing on holy ground.* Sudbury, MA: Jones & Bartlett Learning.

O'Brien, M. E. (2001). *The nurse's calling: A Christian spirituality of caring for the sick.* Mahwah, NJ: Paulist Press.

O'Brien, M. E. (2003). *Prayer in nursing: The spirituality of compassionate caregiving.* Sudbury, MA: Jones & Bartlett Learning.

O'Brien, M. E. (2006) *The nurse with an alabaster jar: A biblical approach to nursing.* Madison, WI: NCF Press.

O'Brien, M. E. (2008). *A sacred covenant: The spiritual ministry of nursing.* Sudbury, MA: Jones & Bartlett Learning.

O'Brien, M. E. (2011). *Servant leadership in nursing: Spirituality and practice in contemporary health care.* Sudbury, MA: Jones & Bartlett Learning.

O'Brien, T. C. (1979). Reverence. In P. Meagher, T. C. O'Brien, & C. Aherne (Eds.), *Encyclopedic dictionary of religion, vol. O–Z* (p. 3040). Washington, DC: Corpus Publications.

Okland, K. (2002). Remember reverence. *Nursing Management, 33*(6), 18.

Osterman, P., Schwartz-Barcott, D., & Asselin, M. E. (2010). An exploratory study of nurses' presence in daily care on an oncology unit. *Nursing Forum, 45*(3), 197–205.

Parse, R. R. (2009). Reverence. *Newsletter for the International Consortium of Parse Scholars, 18*(1), 1.

Perry, B. (2009). Conveying compassion through attention to the essential ordinary. *Nursing Older People, 21*(6), 14–20.

Pfeiffer, J. B., Gober, C., & Taylor, E. J. (2014). How Christian nurses converse with patients about spirituality. *Journal of Clinical Nursing, 23*(19/20), 2886–2095.

Piippo, J., & Aaltonen, J. (2008). Mental health care: Trust and mistrust in different caring contexts. *Journal of Clinical Nursing, 17*(1), 2867–2874.

Raatikainen, R. (1997). Nursing care as a calling. *Journal of Advanced Nursing, 25*(1), 1111–1115.

Raines, K. H., & Wilson, A. (1996). Frontier Nursing Service: A historical perspective on nurse-managed care. *Journal of Community Health Nursing, 13*(2), 123–127.

The Random House dictionary of the English language. (1966). New York, NY: Random House.

Ranheim, A., Karner, A., & Bertero, C. (2012). Caring theory and practice: Entering a simultaneous concept analysis. *Nursing Forum, 47*(2), 78–90.

Ranheim, A., Karner, A., & Bertero, C. (2011). Eliciting reflections on caring theory in elderly caring practice. *International Journal of Qualitative Studies in Health and Well-Being, 6*(2), 1–10.

Roach, S. (1987). *The human act of caring: A blueprint for the health professions.* Ottawa, Ontario: Canadian Hospital Association.

Roach, S., & Maykut, C. (2010). Comportment: A caring attribute in the formation of an intentional practice. *International Journal for Human Caring, 14*(4), 22–26.

Rykkje, L., Eriksson, K., & Raholm, M. (2011). A qualitative metasynthesis of spirituality from a caring science perspective. *International Journal for Human Caring, 15*(4), 40–53.

Sanctity and nursing. (1952). *The Catholic Nurse, 1*(1), 36–39.

Schantz, M. L. (2007). Compassion: A concept analysis. *Nursing Forum, 42*(2), 48–54.

Schmock, B., Breckenridge, D., & Benedict, K. (2009). Effect of sacred space environment on surgical patient outcomes: A pilot study. *International Journal for Human Caring, 13*(1), 49–59.

Schreiter, R. J. (1993). Trust. In M. Downey (Ed.), *The new dictionary of Catholic spirituality* (pp. 982–983). Collegeville, MN: The Liturgical Press.

Senior, D. (1993). Covenant. In M. Downey (Ed.), *The new dictionary of Catholic spirituality* (pp. 237–238). Collegeville, MN: The Liturgical Press.

Shipley, S. D. (2010). Listening: A concept analysis. *Nursing Forum, 45*(2), 125–134.

Snelson, C. (1992). Trust as a caring construct with the critically ill: A beginning exploration. In D. A. Gaut (Ed.), *The presence of caring in nursing* (pp. 157–166). New York, NY: National League for Nursing Press.

Sourial, S. (1997). An analysis of caring. *Journal of Advanced Nursing, 26*(6), 1189–1192.

Spence, D., & Smythe, E. (2008). Feeling like a nurse: Re-calling the spirit of nursing. *Journal of Holistic Nursing, 26*(4), 243–252.

Spencer, J., & Lunsford, V. (2010). Electronic documentation and the caring nurse-patient relationship. *International Journal of Human Caring, 14*(2), 30–35.

Stark, E. C. (1952). The spiritual care of the patient. *The Catholic Nurse, 1*(1), 48–49.

Stemler, M. M. (1955). The call to greatness. *The Catholic Nurse, 4*(1), 25–30.

Straughair, C. (2012a). Exploring compassion: Implications for contemporary nursing. Part 1. *British Journal of Nursing, 21*(3), 160–164.

Straughair, C. (2012b). Exploring compassion: Implications for contemporary nursing. Part 2. *British Journal of Nursing, 21*(4), 239–244.

Strumpf, N. E., & Asimos, K. (1996). Accountability: The covenant between patient and nurse practitioner. In J. V. Hickey, R. M. Ouimette, & S. L. Venegoni (Eds.), *Advance practice nursing: Changing roles and clinical applications* (pp. 176–186). Philadelphia, PA: Lippincott.

Sulzbach, J. (1954). Nursing: A privilege and a responsibility. *The Catholic Nurse, 2*(3), 57–58.

Sumner, J. (2006). Concept analysis: The moral construct of caring in nursing as communicative action. *International Journal for Human Caring, 10*(1), 8–16.

Swanson, K. M. (1993). Nursing as informed caring for the well-being of others. *Image: The Journal of Nursing Scholarship, 25*(4), 352–357.

Taylor, E. J., Park, C. G., & Pfeiffer, J. B. (2014). Nurse religiosity and spiritual care. *Journal of Advanced Nursing, 70*(11), 2612–2621.

Tschudin, V. (1997). The emotional cost of caring. In G. Brykczynska (Ed.), *Caring: The compassion and wisdom of nursing* (pp. 155–179). London, England: Arnold.

Vaartio, H., Leino-Kilpi, H., Salantera, S., & Suominen, T. (2006). Nursing advocacy: How it is defined by patients and nurses, what does it involve and how is it experienced? *Scandinavian Journal of Caring Science, 20*(1), 282–292.

Vaillot, M. C. (1962). *Commitment to nursing: A philosophic investigation.* Philadelphia, PA: Lippincott.

Walker, L. O., & Avant, K. C. (2011). *Strategies for theory construction in nursing.* Boston, MA: Prentice Hall.

Watson, J. (2005). *Caring science as sacred science.* Philadelphia, PA: F. A. Davis Company.

Watson, J. (2009). *Assessing and measuring caring in nursing and health science.* New York, NY: Springer.

Watson, J. (2012). *Human caring science: A theory of nursing* (2nd ed.). Burlington, MA: Jones & Bartlett Learning.

Webster's third new international dictionary. (2002). Springfield, MA: G. & C. Merriam.

White, F. S. (1923). At the gate of the temple. *The Public Health Nurse, XV*(6), 282–285.

Wolf, Z. R. (1986). The caring concept and nurse identified caring behaviors. *Topics in Clinical Nursing, 8*(2), 84–93.

Woods, R. (1993). Spirituality, Christian. In M. Downey (Ed.), *The new dictionary of Catholic spirituality* (pp. 938–946). Collegeville, MN: The Liturgical Press.

Wright, J. J. (1962). The nursing vocation. *The Catholic Nurse, 11*(2), 34–38.

Wright, S., & Neuberger, J. (2012). Why spirituality is essential for nurses. *Nursing Standard, 26*(40), 19–21.

Zyblock, D. M. (2010). Nursing presence in contemporary nursing. *Nursing Forum, 45*(2), 120–124.

CHAPTER 18

A Lived Experience of Caring in Nursing Practice: the Ministry of Catherine of Siena

"Your hands were made to serve your neighbors when you see them sick . . . your feet were given to you to serve by carrying your body to places that are holy and useful to you and your neighbors for the glory and praise of my Name."

Catherine of Siena, Dialogue, 144

> The most important part of our nursing vocation is the caring for those who are sick; using our hands to serve them with love. Caring is a spiritual thing. It is a blessing and a gift, not just for the patient but for the nurse as well.

Cecilia, Home Health-Care Nurse

In Chapter 17 a conceptual model reflecting dimensions of the spirituality of caring in nursing practice is presented. The framework is titled *"A Sacred Covenant of Caring for the Sick."* The attributes and behaviors identified and described in the theory were derived from the author's prior research with persons living with both acute and chronic illnesses. The model's concepts were also supported by the work of early and later theorists of caring in nursing.

The purpose of this chapter is to further explain and describe the "Sacred Covenant" model through exploring a "lived experience" of the spirituality of caring. This task has been approached from both a historical and a contemporary perspective. The historical figure, whose caring ministry was chosen as exemplar of the model is Catherine of Siena* described previously as the patroness of nursing. In order to understand the lived experience of Catherine's covenantal nursing ministry the method of hermeneutic phenomenology, as articulated by Max van Manen, was employed (van Manen, 1990).

The phenomenological method of study, van Manen (1990) described as a retrospective reflection on an individual's lived experience; it is "reflection on an experience that has already passed or been lived through" (p. 10). In order to initiate the exploration, an extensive literature review on Catherine of Siena's 14th-century care of the sick was carried out over the period of several years. Data reflecting Catherine's nursing ministry were collected through examining biographical/hagiographical, theological, spiritual, and historical works on her life. Primary data sources included: *Catherine of Siena: The Dialogue* (1980), *The Letters of Catherine of Siena, Volumes 1-4* (2000, 2001, 2007, 2008), *The Prayers of Catherine of Siena* (2001), *The Life of St. Catherine of Siena* by Blessed Raymond of Capua (2011), the *Leggenda Minore* (1868) and the *Supplimento Alla Vita di Santa Caterina da Siena* (2010) by Fra Tommaso D'Antonio Caffarini, and the anonymously authored *Miracoli of Catherine of Siena* (2005). Secondary sources included 28 biographies/hagiographies of Saint Catherine including the writings of such authors as: Augusta Theodosia Drane, Edmund Gardner, Johannes Jorgensen, Clare Mary Antony, Martin Gillet, Igino Giordani, Joseph Marie Perrin, Thomas Luongo, Giuliana Cavallini, Suzanne Noffke, Mary Ann Fatula, Arrigo Levasti, Alice Curtayne, Mary O'Driscoll, Sigred Undset, Catherine Meade, Thomas McDermott, and Giacinto D'Urso.

Data describing Catherine's nursing of the ill and infirm were also obtained through the review of 15 classic nursing history texts, including the works of James Walsh, Sr. Charles Marie Frank, Adelaide Nutting and Lavinia Dock, Josephine Dolan, Isabel Stewart and Anne Austin, Victor Robinson, Agnes Pavey, Minnie Goodnow, Lena Dietz and Aurelia Lehozky, M. Patricia Donahue, Josephine Dolan, H. Louise Fitzpatrick and Eleanor K. Herrman, Gladys Sellew and C. Joseph Nuesse, Lucy R. Seymer and Deborah Jensen, John Spaulding and Elwyn Cady, as well as through review of 31 journal articles, which touched on some dimension of Catherine's care of the sick.

▶ Catherine of Siena: Patroness of Nursing

Catherine of Siena, identified historically as the patroness of nursing, was born Caterina Benincasa in 1347, into a large loving family in Tuscan Italy. From her earliest years young Catherine had a desire to serve those in need; she frequently asked to give food and alms from the Benincasa household to those who were sick and poor. She would carry the items to needy families with her own hands. Catherine also developed a profound devotion to God and spent many hours in prayer during periods of childhood and adolescence. At the tender age of seven she is reported to have made a promise to commit her life to Christ and to the service of others. While this commitment was not initially well received by her parents, ultimately they came to accept their daughter's deep spirit of devotion and supported her in her chosen path. It was this path that led Catherine, at around the age of 18, to seek entrance into a Lay community called the Sisters of Penance of St. Dominic. The Sisters of Penance, or Mantellate, remained in their homes but devoted their lives to the service of the sick and the poor.

---

*A detailed exploration of Catherine of Siena's life and nursing ministry can be found in *Catherine of Siena: A Sacred Covenant of Caring for the Sick,* New Priory Press, 2015.

Catherine came of age as a young lay Dominican Sister shortly before a second wave of the *Black Death*, the bubonic plague, began ravaging much of Europe. As a "Mantellata," the informal title accorded Dominican women tertiaries of the era, her designated ministry was to care for the sick, especially the sick poor, in their homes and in the local hospitals. Saint Catherine carried out these nursing tasks with incredible tenderness and compassion, seeing in each poor sufferer the image of Christ, the beloved Spouse, to whom she had committed her life. Catherine's ministry to plague victims was described by one of her early companions: "Never did she appear more admirable than at this time. She was always with the plague stricken; she prepared them for death, she buried them with her own hands. I myself witnessed the joy with which she tended them" (Drane, 1880, pp. 221–222.)

The following discussion will identify and describe Catherine's spirituality of caring as reflected in the sacred covenant of her nursing ministry. The relevance of Catherine's example for contemporary caregivers is noted as well.

▶ Catherine's Covenantal Ministry

Three attributes of the spirituality of caring for the sick, "a calling of service," "a blessed trust," and a "commitment to reverence" direct the health-care minister to practice a covenantal model of caring. Five behavioral themes that flow from the caregiver's understanding of caring as a sacred covenant are "respecting life," "being present," "comforting with compassion," "creating bonds," and "becoming an advocate" (a further description of the attributes and behavioral themes of a covenantal ministry is included in the preceding chapter).

Those health-care ministers who view their profession as a vocation of service, given by God as a blessed trust, and containing within it a commitment to reverence, embrace a covenantal style of caring. For caregivers to the sick, whose practice is guided by this model, behavioral outcomes include: "respecting the sanctity of human life, being fully present and listening supportively to patients and family members, comforting suffering patients with understanding and compassion, creating bonds of caring within the nurse-patient relationship and consistently advocating for the needs of patients and families" (O'Brien, 2015, p. 162).

In this chapter Saint Catherine's covenantal care for the ill is described to provide inspiration for today's health-care ministers; specific nursing activities are identified within the context of the sacred covenant model of caring for the sick. A case example of Catherine's service to the ill and infirm is presented to illustrate each of the model's three attributes: a calling of service, a blessed trust, and a commitment to reverence, as well as the five behavioral themes: respecting life, being present, comforting with compassion, establishing bonds and becoming an advocate.

▶ Sacred Covenant Attributes

A Calling of Service

An example of Saint Catherine's response to "a calling of service" is that presented in an anecdote describing the gentle and selfless nursing care that she provided to a woman named Andrea suffering from the ravages of advanced breast cancer. One biographer affirmed:

> In addition to the poor . . . Catherine was attracted to the sick. She, who endured suffering so courageously, could not bear to see others suffer especially when their suffering separated them from God instead of drawing them nearer to Him. Catherine, the patroness of nurses and of all those who care for the sick, hovered lovingly around the beds of the sick and in certain instances carried her devotion to the point of heroism. For example, one cannot read the account of the care and conversion of Andrea without trembling before a spectacle which surpasses the expectations of human nature and disconcerts the most intrepid wills and the most generous hearts (Gillet, 1946, p. 172).

Catherine's first biographer and spiritual guide, Blessed Raymond of Capua, wrote that when Catherine learned of the illness and great suffering of Andrea, she immediately went to the woman's home and offered her services for as long as she was needed (at that time there were no known therapeutic remedies for breast cancer patients). Even though many of the nursing tasks were unpleasant Raymond asserted of Catherine: "She was with the sick woman continuously . . . unbandaging the sore, wiping it, washing it, dressing it, showing no signs of repulsion, seemingly unwearied by the length of time it took her, and doing everything with such grace and cheerfulness that the sick woman herself was amazed to see such constancy of soul, such warmth of affection and charity" (Raymond of Capua, 2011, p. 121). Another early biographer, August Theodosia Drane, also commented on Saint Catherine's care of Andrea: "Day after day, Catherine lavished on her patient the tenderest care; in spite of the repulsive nature of the services she had to perform, she never showed any sign of disgust or adopted any of those precautions which others had made use of in the tainted atmosphere of the sick room, lest by doing so she should give pain to Andrea's feelings" (Drane, 1880, p. 181).

Catherine's loving nursing ministry to Andrea reflected vividly the saint's perception that caring for the sick was indeed "a calling of service" given to her directly by God.

> Twenty-first century ministers to the sick, such as nurses, physicians, and chaplains, are also sometimes called to attend patients the sequellae of whose illnesses may make the caregiving challenging. While modern medicine provides for the alleviation of a number of the vicious symptom manifestations of illness and disease, in some cases unpleasant side effects remain. This is true for many chemotherapy patients, especially those with advanced disease. In her tender and committed ministry of nursing to the advanced cancer patient Andrea, Catherine of Siena teaches the true meaning of caring for the sick when envisioned as a sacred "calling of service." In serving Andrea, Catherine was also serving her Blessed Lord; she modeled for us how we also can serve Him in today's ministries to the ill and infirm (O'Brien, 2015, pp. 166–167).

A Blessed Trust

Catherine's many caregiving activities, carried out in the homes of the sick poor and the streets of Siena, as well as in the local hospitals, reflected the saint's perception that her ministry to the ill and infirm was a blessed mission entrusted to her by Christ

Himself; thus her nursing was embraced as a "blessed trust." A particular reflection of Catherine's perception of her ministry to the sick as "a blessed trust" was the fact that she seemed to possess an innate knowledge of how to approach persons with a certain disease or illness and what remedies to provide. We do not know, from any written sources, how the saint was educated in nursing the sick yet the following example demonstrates her understanding of both human physiology and human psychology" (O'Brien, 2015, p. 168).

A telling anecdote was described by a Dominican companion of Catherine of Siena, Fra Tommaso D'Antonio Caffarini:

> A woman of Siena named Gemma, a Sister of Penance of St. Dominic, attached to the Virgin so much that no leaf moved without her advice, complained to Catherine because she did nothing but sleep, especially when she wanted to pray and practice things pleasing to the Lord. The Virgin said: My sister, you are deceived; take strength and rest awake, and you will find the consolation of God.
>
> Then Gemma started to stay awake, but the following night she realized that she had hurt her left eye; it was red and swollen and she could barely see. She told the Virgin: "Well, as you see I listened to you and I got sick in one eye." The Virgin answered: "Just take a leaf of 'Sow Thistle' and put it on the eye."
>
> Hearing this, Gemma looked for and took up the leaf but having more faith in the Virgin than in the virtue of the plant, she sought a way to make Catherine touch it. Catherine, guessing the desire of her companion, took the leaf in her hand and then handed it back saying: "Put it on the eye." As soon as she (Gemma) had, her sight was regained (Caffarini, 2010, pp. 58–59).

An important revelation in this anecdote relates to the term *Cicerbita*, the Italian word used by Saint Catherine, which translates to "Sow Thistle" in English. Sow Thistle is, in fact, the name of an herbal plant possessed of a variety of healing properties including anti-inflammatory and anti-febrile characteristics. Currently one can find professional literature describing therapeutic uses for the plant. "One example is 'Validation of Medicinal Values of Traditionally Used *Sonchus Asper* (Prickly Sow Thistle) leaves for the treatment of skin ailments' (Upadhyay et al., 2013). Catherine recognized in her 14th century nursing care of a woman with a sore eye, the soothing and healing ability of a medicinal plant which remains valued in today's 21st century medicine" (O'Brien, 2015, p. 741.)

In this case example, Catherine of Siena's continuous follow up of her patient, who initially complained of fatigue, and then later of an irritated eye, demonstrated perception of her nursing care as "a sacred trust," which she held with both commitment and persistence in caring for one who was suffering. This is a blessed trust given as a gift to all of us who are contemporary ministers to the ill and infirm.

A Commitment to Reverence

An accompanying attribute to her covenantal caring perceptions of a sacred calling and a blessed trust, was Catherine's commitment to reverence for the holiness of all human life. In nursing activities in the homes of the ailing, in the Sienese hospitals of *Santa Maria della Scala, Casa della Misericordia,* and *San Lazzaro,* and when meeting plague victims in the streets, one finds Catherine demonstrating and practicing reverence for those who are suffering. The Virgin made "no distinctions; whether sinner or saint, she treated all with the reverence with which she would treat her Blessed Lord, whose image she saw in the sick poor under her care" (O'Brien, 2015, p. 170).

An example of this reverence lies in the account of Catherine's ministry to a woman named Palmarina who suddenly fell critically ill with an undiagnosed malady. Unfortunately, Palmarina, aware of Saint Catherine's holiness and commitment to care for the sick, was envious of her vocation. Thus, even though Catherine tried, as noted by Blessed Raymond (2011), to "placate her with acts of humility and kindness, the woman had nothing but contempt for them" (p. 115). Nevertheless, Catherine tried to support Palmarina by acts of concern and tender caring; she "frequently went to see her, appeared before her submissively, and with kind words and charming ways, did all she could to comfort her by endeavoring to serve her as much as she could in every possible way" (Raymond 2011, p. 115).

In the end Catherine's constancy in caring and her reverence finally won the heart of Palmarina and the ill woman recognized her fault and begged forgiveness. As soon as Catherine learned of this "she went with all speed to see Palmarina, who now manifested her pleasure and respect for her from whom she had formerly shrunk, and with what signs she could, and with words and gestures confessed her sin. And then, having received the sacraments, with great contrition of heart, she died" (Raymond 2011, p. 117).

Catherine so reverenced Palmarina's physical and spiritual well-being that she was determined to find the means to console her. "This commitment to reverence that Catherine modeled so profoundly is also demanded of present-day caregivers who minister in our complex and sometimes broken world. Today's ministers to the sick may at times also be called upon to serve 21st century 'Palmarinas'; may we be blessed with the loving reverence so willingly demonstrated by Saint Catherine of Siena" (O'Brien, 2015, pp. 171–172).

▶ Sacred Covenant Behaviors

Respecting Life

As well as exercising tender reverence for the sick, Saint Catherine respected the dignity of all human life, even the lives of those whom others considered sinners or practitioners of criminal behavior; she often described herself as a "sinner who was loved by the Lord." Catherine frequently visited prisoners in the Sienese jail and spent the night listening to their pain and praying with them. Blessed Raymond of Capua related an incident that demonstrates the saint's respect for the lives of two local townsmen condemned to be tortured and die as criminals" (O'Brien, 2015, pp. 172–173).

> By order of the chief justice two malefactors were arrested in Siena and for their heinous crimes condemned to a most cruel death; they were to be put in a cart, bound to a post, and tortured by the executioners in different parts of their bodies with hooks and red-hot pincers. Neither in prison nor on the point of being led out to die did they show any desire to repent of their misdeed nor would they confess to the priest. (Raymond of Capua, 2011, p. 181)

When Saint Catherine saw the criminals thus suffering, her heart was moved with pity and she begged the Lord to help them. It was reported that after Catherine's prayerful intercession, the men both repented of their sins and begged forgiveness of God and those they had harmed. The crowd who witnessed this were amazed at the criminals' sudden change of heart and even "the torturers themselves were moved by the sight of such devotion and did not dare to continue their cruelties" (Raymond, 2011, p. 183).

In this account of Catherine's concern for two condemned criminals we find a powerful example of her respect for life. Contemporary caregivers are also called to respect the dignity of human life. "Saint Catherine had no thought of condemning the criminals; she made no judgment. Instead the Virgin, who could not save the men's earthly lives, immediately took to prayer, begging the Lord to grant them the gift of repentance and thus the blessing of eternal salvation. While we may see only sinfulness in the criminal's behavior, Catherine saw only the potential for goodness; she respected the men's humanity and the Lord responded to her prayerful intercession" (O'Brien, 2015, p. 174).

Being Present

For all of us who care for the ill and infirm, in a variety of venues, the concept of presence or being available to listen, to support and to care is central to our vocation. For one who is experiencing suffering, whether physical, psychological, or spiritual, the presence of a loving caregiver is a gift rarely refused and generally deeply appreciated. Such supportive presence can greatly alleviate the feeling of "aloneness" often described by one who is ill.

One of the more dramatic acts of ministry described by numerous of Catherine's biographers was that of her "presence" to a Perugian nobleman named Niccolo di Toldo. The young man had been sentenced to execution by beheading for frivolously speaking critically of a city official. Dominican Friar Martin Gillet (1946) noted that the sentence was "quite common in that day, for political indiscretion" (p. 175). Niccolo was "condemned to death for a trifling thing, a few thoughtless words spoken out of bravado when under the influence of wine at a banquet" (p. 175).

After his sentencing, Niccolo became angry and despondent; he refused the visit of a priest and cursed God for his dreadful fate. While waiting for the sentence to be carried out, and in great anguish, the young man was told of Saint Catherine's holiness and care for all who were suffering, including prisoners; he finally begged her to visit him. An eyewitness to Catherine's visit, Fra Tommaso D'Antonio Caffarini, related:

> Indeed once I went to the communal prison with her (Catherine) to visit one condemned to death, a young nobleman from Perugia whose name was Niccolo di Toldo. He had been employed in some function by the then senator of Siena, and during some unrest had ill-famed the senator of something concerning the city-state. For this he found himself sentenced without remedy, and chose to throw himself into the abyss of desperation. The Virgin had heard of him and as she was entirely jealous for the health of souls, so it happened that he who had at first paced his cell like a ferocious and desperate lion, by means of the Virgin's presence was so restored that he went devout and willing, just like a gentle lamb born to the slaughter, to the place of beheading. And thus, he accepted death while still at a young

age, in the presence of the Virgin, and with her receiving his head into her hands, with such marvelous devotion that it was like the transitus of some devout martyr and not the death of one who was condemned for a human crime. And everyone watching, among whom I was one, was so moved internally and from the heart that I do not remember any previous burial accompanied by so much devotion as that one. (Caffarini, as cited in Luongo, 2006, pp. 91–92)

Saint Catherine herself, in a letter to her spiritual mentor Blessed Raymond, recounted the ministry of presence to young Niccolo:

I went to visit the one you know and he was so comforted and consoled that he confessed his sins and prepared himself very well. He made me promise for the love of God that when the time came for the execution I would be with him. This I promised and did. (Catherine of Siena, *The Letters of Catherine of Siena: Volume I*, 2000, p. 86)

Prior to the execution, Catherine took Niccolo to Mass and to reception of the Holy Eucharist and said to him:

Courage my dear brother, for soon we shall reach the wedding feast. You will go forth to it bathed in the sweet blood of God's Son, with the sweet name of Jesus, which I don't want to ever leave your memory. I shall wait for you at the place of execution . . . And, he said: "I shall go all joyful and strong, and when I think that you will be waiting for me there, it will seem a thousand years until I get there." (p. 87)

Catherine continued:

I waited for him at the place of execution. I waited there in continual prayer . . . I prayed and pleaded with Mary that I wanted this grace, that at his last moment she would give him light and peace of heart and afterwards see him return to his destination . . . Then he arrived like a meek lamb, and when he saw me he began to laugh and wanted me to make the sign of the Cross on him. When he had received the sign, I said "Down for the wedding, my dear brother, for soon you will be in everlasting life!" He knelt down very meekly; I placed his neck (on the block) and bent down and reminded him of the blood of the Lamb. His mouth said nothing but "Gesu" and "Caterina," and as he said this, I received his head into my hands, saying "I will!" with my eyes fixed on Divine Goodness. (p. 88)

Catherine concluded: "Now that he was hidden away where he belonged, my soul rested in peace and quiet" (p. 89).

In a contemporary article entitled "St. Catherine of Siena and the Spectacle of Public Execution," author Molly Morrison explained Catherine's presence and in-volvement at Niccolo di Toldo's decapitation as "an example of a successful comforting ritual." Morrison described such rituals as being "commonly carried out by members of medieval confraternities who aided criminals about to be publicly executed . . . the comforter's main function was to strengthen the condemned prisoner in the time remaining before his impending doom. Since the eternal salvation of the prisoner was paramount, the comforter was to prepare him to make his last confession and receive the Eucharist" (Morrison, 2013, p. 44).

Morrison concluded that Catherine's ministry of presence to Niccolo di Toldo "clearly shows her as a comforter" (p. 44), and added "Essentially the comforter's goal was to transform the gruesome event of public execution into a type of reenactment of the death of Christ or one of the martyrs. The comforter stayed with the condemned right up until the last, distracting him for the horror about to occur. Even the most dreaded moments were turned into a means of consolation" (p. 45).

Saint Catherine's presence to the young Niccolo, both during his incarceration and at the time of his execution, provides a powerful example of the importance a caregiver's presence can be to one who is suffering either physically, emotionally or spiritually.

> How often have we not heard ill persons share thoughts to the effect that they were not afraid of death, rather it was the "getting there" that worried them? Elders, in particular, often fear being alone when the end of life comes; will anyone be there to console and comfort them in their final moments? How blessed we are as caregivers to be able to provide that loving presence to a dying person; to, as is sometimes described by hospice nurses, "midwife" patients at their birth into eternal life. (O'Brien, 2015, pp. 178–179)

Comforting with Compassion

It was well known that Catherine was unfailingly merciful and compassionate to those who were ill. "She did not wish to see anyone suffer unnecessarily if she could provide care which might lead to either physical or spiritual healing" (O'Brien, 2015, p. 180). An example of Saint Catherine's compassionate caregiving was that extended to a woman named Bartolomea who was seriously injured in a fall on the balcony of her home. The balcony had collapsed while Bartolomea was standing on it and she received a multiplicity of cuts and bruises from the accident. Even though a physician attempted to treat her, the woman remained in great pain.

When Catherine heard about the injuries, she immediately went to Bartolomea to try and comfort her. "Seeing that she was suffering such agonies, Catherine touched the parts that were hurting her as though soothing them, and the victim allowed her to do so because she was sure that only good could come from contact with her" (Raymond of Capua, 2011, p. 203). Blessed Raymond explained that "as the Virgin's hand passed from one painful spot to another, the pain vanished" (p. 203). Bartolomea continued to beg Catherine to touch her injuries "until the moment came when she who a little while before had been unable to make the slightest bodily movement began to turn this way and that, obviously quite recovered" (p. 203).

Historical anecdotes describing Saint Catherine's care of the sick provide multiple examples of the saint's compassion: compassion for those with stigmatizing diseases such as leprosy or plague; compassion for those who were marginalized by poverty or lifestyle; compassion for prisoners. In those scenarios, as well as in the case of Bartolomea, "Catherine's example challenges today's caregivers not to fail in compassionate ministry to those who are sick. While present-day ministers to the ailing may not be possessed of Saint Catherine's miraculous gift of healing, we do have many tools in our therapeutic arsenals which may be used in compassionate care and comfort for a suffering patient" (O'Brien, 2015, p. 182).

Creating Bonds

The concept of nurses, and in fact all health-care ministers, bonding with patients, that is, creating bonds of caring and respect, is key to the sanctity of the caregiver–patient relationship. When real concern is evidenced on the part of a caregiver, "mutual bonds of caring, reflecting the covenantal nature of the partnership, may emerge" (O'Brien, 2015, p. 182).

Catherine had a unique ability to establish bonds with her companions as well as with those for whom she cared. One of the individuals with whom she had created a special bond was Matteo di Cenni dei Fazio, Rector of the Siena hospital *Casa della Miseracordia*, which Catherine often visited. During the height of the Black Death epidemic in Italy. The *Casa della Miseracordia* was considered one of the most important Sienese health-care facilities engaged in battling the plague.

For many weeks Rector Matteo and his nursing brothers had been working day and night to care for victims of the terrible disease. One day Matteo collapsed while nursing the sick and was carried to his room by the brothers. He was described, by some who observed him, as being "like one dead." A physician pronounced Matteo's condition grave and commented that he saw little hope of a cure. At this point Saint Catherine, known to be the rector's colleague and friend, was summoned to his bedside.

> As she (Catherine) was very fond of Matteo because of his virtues, she hastened to see him fired by charity and as though angry with the plague itself, and even before she reached him she started shouting from a distance: "Get up, Messer Matteo, get up; this is no time for lying in a soft bed." At the words of this command the fever and the swelling in the groin and all the pain immediately disappeared and Matteo felt as well as if he had never been ill at all. Nature had obeyed God through the mouth of the Virgin, and, at the sound of her voice, his body had been restored to health. (Raymond of Capua, 2011, p. 200)

In this anecdote we learn of the importance of patient–caregiver bonding. Catherine had gotten to know Rector Matteo well during her service at the *Casa dell Miseracordia* hospital. While some of his brothers and friends thought Matteo to be dying, Catherine trusted otherwise because of her knowledge of the patient. Thus, the saint who was reputedly gentle and kind to the ill, was confident in challenging Matteo with an urgent message that he must quickly recover in order to continue his service to others.

"Catherine teaches us that knowing our patients and bonding with them will help us understand how to approach and assist them in their illnesses; when to use gentle kindness and compassion and when a firm hand is in order. The ability to distinguish when to use either of these approaches is a blessed gift for the caregiver" (O'Brien, 2015, p. 184).

Becoming an Advocate

Patient advocacy may become a critically important component of the caregiving relationship for those who minister to the sick. If an ill person is unable to advocate for his or her own needs, it is frequently the nurse who must intervene to assure that a patient's needs are being met.

Catherine had a particular concern for and commitment to those who had received traumatic injuries associated with feud-related violence. She "believed in prevention and promotion of health and thus engaged in counseling and advocacy for those involved in local feuds whenever possible; her goal was to prevent injuries before they occurred. One of the Sienese citizens who came to Catherine's attention was a man well known for his involvement in feuding named Nanni di Ser Vanni" (O'Brien, 2015, p. 186).

Blessed Raymond (2011) described Nanni as suffering from "one of the city's worst characters; he was quite incapable of keeping the peace with anyone and was always starting private feuds; setting traps for people and then pretending to know nothing about it" (p. 188). Nanni di Ser Vanni was at the time involved in a particularly vicious feud in which one local citizen had been killed but he stubbornly refused to end the dispute.

When Saint Catherine learned of Nanni's latest feud she attempted to counsel him but initially to no avail even though she pointed out that his soul was in mortal peril. However, after a number of meetings and a great deal of prayer on Catherine's part, Nanni began to surrender to her advice and she became his advocate. Through the saint's prayers and counseling Nanni di Ser Vanni's heart was touched and he assented to her desire that he end his feuding. After doing so he admitted: "My God, how contented I now feel in my soul from having said I shall make peace" (p. 190). Ultimately, Raymond of Capua reported that Nanni's "devotion greatly increased, and he gave many gifts to the church because of the transformation of his life" (191–192).

In undertaking an advocacy role for one who is ill, a nurse may often need to employ significant creativity in the process of negotiating for a patient's needs. Catherine adopted such strategies in her counseling and prayerful support for Nanni di Ser Vanni. Nanni's life "was ultimately transformed by Saint Catherine's 14th century advocacy. Patient advocacy in the 21st century also has the potential to bring about a transformation in an ill person's life and illness trajectory" (O'Brien, 2015, pp. 187–188).

This chapter demonstrates, from a historical perspective, how a lived experience of the spirituality of caring was manifested in the ministry of a 14th-century nurse, Catherine of Siena. Catherine's vocation of service to the sick poor reflected a philosophy of covenantal caring, as identified in the previous chapter, including the attributes of: a calling of service, illustrated in the saint's tender nursing of Andrea suffering from advanced breast cancer; a blessed trust, which Catherine demonstrated in her consistent care for Gemma's physical complaints and a commitment to reverence, so powerfully evidenced in St. Catherine's ministry to Palmarina during her final illness. The saint's nursing practice also displayed each of the five sacred covenant behaviors: respecting life, in her concern for the eternal salvation of two condemned criminals; being present, in her ministry to young Niccolo di Toldo who was distraught over his forthcoming execution; comforting with compassion, in caring for Bartolomea who was suffering from severe pain; creating bonds, which enabled Catherine to guide Brother Matteo to recovery and becoming an advocate, reflected in her prayers for and counseling of Nanni di Ser Vanni.

Ultimately, Saint Catherine's medieval covenantal practice of nursing provides a powerful and inspiring model of the spirituality of caring for contemporary ministers to the ill and the infirm.

▶ References

Caffarini, T.di'A. (1868). *Leggenda minore di Santa Caterina da Siena e lettere dei suoi discepoli.* Bologna, Italy: Presso Gaetano Romagnoli.

Caffarini, T.di'A. (2010). *Supplemento all vita di S. Caterina da Siena. A cura di Angelo Belloni e Tito Centi.* Firenze, Italy: Edizioni Nerbini.

Catherine of Siena (1980). *The dialogue* (S. Noffke, Trans.). Mahwah, NJ: Paulist Press.

Catherine of Siena (2000, 2001, 2007, 2008). *The letters of Catherine of Siena: Volumes I–IV* (S. Noffke, Trans.). Tempe, AZ: ACMRS, Arizona Center for Medieval and Renaissance Studies.

Catherine of Siena (2001). *The prayers of Catherine of Siena.* (S. Noffke, Trans.). San Jose, CA: Author's Choice Press.

Drane, A. T. (1880). *The history of St. Catherine of Siena and her companions.* London, England: Burns and Oates.

Gillet, M. S. (1946). *The mission of St. Catherine.* (M. T. Lopez, Trans.). St. Louis, MO: B. Herder Book Company.

Lehmijoki-Gardner, M., & Bornstein, D. (Eds). (1374). The miracoli of Catherine of Siena. *Dominican penitent women.* Mahwah, NJ: Paulist Press.

Luongo, F. T. (2006). *The saintly politics of Catherine of Siena.* Ithaca, NY: Cornell University Press.

Morrison, M. (2013). St. Catherine of Siena and the spectacle of public execution. *Logos: A Journal of Catholic Thought and Culture, 16*(3), 43–55.

O'Brien, M. E. (2015). *Catherine of Siena: A sacred covenant of caring for the sick.* Chicago, IL: New Priory Press.

Raymond of Capua (2011). *The life of St. Catherine of Siena.* (G. Lamb, Trans.). Charlotte, NC: Tan.

Upadhyay, H., Kumar, A., Gupta, M. K., Sharma, A., & Rahal, A. (2013). Validation of medicinal values or traditionally used *sonchus asper* (prickly sow thistle) leaves for the treatment of skin ailments. *Advancement in Medicinal Plant Research, 1*(1): 29–35.

van Manen, M. (1990). *Researching lived experience. Human science for an action sensitive pedagogy.* New York, NY: The State University of New York Press.

Index

M